Recent Results in Cancer Research 183

Thomas Moehler • Hartmut Goldschmidt
(Editors)

Multiple Myeloma

Springer

Editors
Dr. Thomas Moehler
Department of Medicine V
University Hospital Heidelberg
Heidelberg
Germany

Present Address:
i3 research
Wiesbaden
Germany
thomas.moehler@i3global.com

Prof. Dr. Hartmut Goldschmidt
Department of Medicine V
University Hospital Heidelberg
and National Center for Tumor Disease
Heidelberg
Germany
hartmut_goldschmidt@med.uni-heidelberg.de

ISBN 978-3-540-85771-6 e-ISBN 978-3-540-85772-3
DOI 10.1007/978-3-540-85772-3
Springer Heidelberg Dordrecht London New York

Library of Congress Control Number: 2011925944

Cover design: estudioCalamar, Figueres/Berlin

Printed on acid-free paper

Springer is part of Springer Science + Business Media (www.springer.com)

Dedicated to the families of the authors for their patience and understanding.

Foreword

It is a great pleasure to introduce and preview this comprehensive new text on multiple myeloma.

In the last decade, therapy and diagnosis of multiple myeloma have seen more changes than ever before in the history of this life-threatening disease. Further, importantly, multiple myeloma has been recognized as a crucial indication for the proof of concept in oncology for novel compounds exemplified by the approval of lenalidomide and the approval of bortezomib for mantle cell lymphoma.

This book is a reference for all physicians who are involved in myeloma treatment with an emphasis on the description, and, most importantly, on the interpretation of new data available.

Clinical chapters are designed to concisely summarize new data as well as relevant data to current up-to-date recommendations regarding diagnostic procedures and treatment.

The important developments in therapy and diagnosis and introduction of new compounds would not be possible without the improved scientific knowledge and molecular information. Therefore three chapters in this book are devoted to the pathophysiology of multiple myeloma: molecular pathophysiology of multiple myeloma by B. Klein, A. Seckinger, T. Moehler, and D. Hose; angiogenesis and vasculogenesis by A. Vacca and D. Ribatti; immunology and immunotherapeutic approach in multiple myeloma by C. Schlude and P Beckhove.

The unique historical viewpoint is provided by R.A. Kyle and D.P. Steensma, which is accompanied by a thorough evaluation of the epidemiology of multiple myeloma by N. Becker.

The best approach to the patient, particularly regarding staging and imaging, is provided by J. Hillengass and S. Delorme and coauthors.

The emphasis of this book is on novel aspects of treatment, and renowned authors have contributed to summarize the state of the art but more importantly how to best integrate different therapeutic procedures into a patient-tailored treatment. The part on therapy starts with the chapter on novel drugs designed by K. Boyd, F.E. Davies, and G.J. Morgan, followed by chapters on the integration of current treatment options for first-line treatment by

M. Roussel, T. Facon, P. Moreau, J.-L. Harousseau, and M. Attal, and high-dose therapy and autologous treatment strategies by R. Haas, I. Bruns, G. Kobbe, and R. Fenk.

Approaches to treat patients in relapse are covered by the chapter by T. Moehler and H. Goldschmidt, which is followed by the chapter by G. Gahrton on the outcome possibilities that are provided by allogeneic transplantation.

Local therapies need to be integrated in the systemic treatment strategy and are delineated (radiotherapy by S. Krause, J. Debus, D. Neuhof and osteoplastic procedures by C. Kasperk and I. Grafe). Last but not least, H. Ludwig describes the important aspects of supportive therapy.

This book provides a guideline and rationale for patient care but also describes the pathway into the future. Congratulations to Prof. Goldschmidt and Dr. Moehler for producing such an excellent new text which will, I am sure, be an important addition for all interested in understanding the biology of myeloma and new approaches to treatment.

Los Angeles, CA, USA

B. Durie

Preface

Recent years have continued to deliver a fast growing body of preclinical and clinical data relevant for further improving the outcome of patients with multiple myeloma which is the ultimate goal of long-term remissions of this life-threatening disease.

We have attempted to provide an overview about the current state of the art in diagnosis and treatment of multiple myeloma with a particular emphasis on therapeutic strategies. This book is considered for practicing physicians and scientists who are working in this field. Moreover students, patients and caregivers can retrieve deeper information about this disease. In addition, clinical researchers in other indications can recapitulate the rationale and strategy for the development of novel agents as bortezomib and immunomodulatory drugs which could be providing important information for the development of these compounds in other indications.

We are very grateful to the panel of international experts that participated in this book project who revealed their interpretation of the vast array of data and translated into practical recommendations for diagnostic procedures and therapy.

Hartmut Goldschmidt
Thomas Moehler

Acknowledgements

We would like to express our thanks to all authors who contributed despite being involved in many other activities. Your expertise and dedication are the foundation for the scientific development of the field and for translation of scientific innovation into clinical improvements for our patients.

Several members of the Section Multiple Myeloma in Heidelberg actively contributed and supported organizational aspects. We thank you all and would in particular mention Dr. Christine Leist and Dr. Annemarie Angerer.

Furthermore we wish to thank all the patients for their faithful cooperation, especially in studies and clinical trials. Their confidence and sensible feedback forms an important basis for ongoing research and improvement of myeloma treatment.

Contents

Part I History and Epidemiology

Part III Clinical Features

Part IV Therapy

Contributors

Michel Attal, M.D.
Hématologie Clinique, CHU Purpan,
Toulouse, France

Andrea Baur-Melnyk, M.D.
Institute of Clinical Radiology,
Munich University Hospital Großhadern,
Munich, Germany

Nikolaus Becker, Ph.D.
Division of Cancer Epidemiology,
German Cancer Research Center,
Heidelberg, Germany

Philipp Beckhove, M.D.
Translational Immunology,
German Cancer Research Center, *and*
National Center of Tumor Disease,
Heidelberg, Germany

**Kevin Boyd, B.Sc., MB.BS.,
MRCP., FRCPath**
The Institute of Cancer Research
and The Royal Marsden Hospital,
Sutton, UK

Ingmar Bruns, M.D.
Department of Hematology,
Oncology and Clinical Immunology,
Heinrich-Heine-University,
Düsseldorf, Germany

Faith E. Davies, M.D., MRCP., FRCPath
The Institute of Cancer Research
and The Royal Marsden Hospital,
Sutton, UK

Jürgen Debus, M.D., Ph.D.
Department of Radiation Oncology,
University of Heidelberg,
Heidelberg, Germany

Stefan Delorme, M.D.
Department of Radiology,
German Cancer Research Center,
Heidelberg, Germany

Thierry Facon, M.D.
Maladies du Sang,
CHU C. Huriez,
Lille, France

Roland Fenk, M.D.
Department of Hematology,
Oncology and Clinical Immunology,
Heinrich-Heine-University, Düsseldorf,
Germany

Gösta Gahrton, M.D.
Department of Medicine,
Karolinska Institutet and Karolinska
University Hospital Huddinge,
Stockholm, Sweden

Hartmut Goldschmidt, M.D.
Department of Medicine V,
University Hospital Heidelberg and
National Center for Tumor Diseases,
Heidelberg, Germany

Ingo Grafe, M.D.
Department of Internal Medicine I
and Clinical Chemistry, Division of
Osteology, University of Heidelberg,
Heidelberg, Germany

Rainer Haas, M.D.
Department of Hematology,
Oncology and Clinical Immunology,
Heinrich-Heine-University,
Düsseldorf, Germany

Jean-Luc Harousseau, M.D.
CLCC René Gauducheau,
Nantes, France

Jens Hillengass, M.D.
Department of Medicine V,
University Hospital Heidelberg,
Heidelberg, Germany

Dirk Hose, dipl. phys., M.D.
Department of Medicine V,
University Hospital Heidelberg and
National Center for Tumor Diseases,
Heidelberg, Germany

Michael Hundemer, M.D.
Department of Medicine V,
University Hospital Heidelberg,
Heidelberg, Germany

Christian Kasperk, M.D., Ph.D., DDS
Department of Medicine I
and Clinical Chemistry,
University Hospital Heidelberg,
Heidelberg, Germany

Bernard Klein, Ph.D.
CHU Montpellier, Institute of
Research in Biotherapy,
Montpellier, France and
INSERM, U847, Montpellier,
France and
UFR Médecine, Université Montpellier 1,
Montpellier, France

Guido Kobbe, M.D.
Department of Hematology, Oncology
and Clinical Immunology,
Heinrich-Heine-University,
Düsseldorf, Germany

Sonja Krause, M.D.
Department of Radiation Oncology,
University of Heidelberg,
Heidelberg, Germany

Robert A. Kyle, M.D.
Department of Medicine, Division
of Hematology, Mayo Clinic,
Rochester, MN, USA

Heinz Ludwig, M.D.
Department of Medicine I,
Center of Oncology and Hematology,
Wilhelminenspital,
Vienna, Austria

Thomas Moehler, M.D.
Department of Medicine V,
University Hospital Heidelberg,
Heidelberg, Germany
Present Address:
i3 research, Wiesbaden,
Germany

Philippe Moreau, M.D.
Hématologie Clinique,
CHU Hôtel Dieu,
Nantes, France

Gareth J. Morgan, Ph.D., F.R.C.P., FRCPath
Section of Haemato-Oncology,
The Institute of Cancer Research,
UK

Dirk Neuhof, M.D.
Department of Radiation Oncology,
University of Heidelberg,
Heidelberg, Germany

Domenico Ribatti, M.D.
Department of Human Anatomy
and Histology, University of
Bari Medical School,
Bari, Italy

Murielle Roussel, M.D.
Hématologie Clinique, CHU Purpan,
Place du Docteur Baylac,
Toulouse, France

Christoph Schlude, dipl. biol.
Translational Immunology,
German Cancer Research Center, *and*
National Center of Tumor Disease,
Heidelberg, Germany

Anja Seckinger, M.D.
Deptartment of Medicine V,
University Hospital Heidelberg and
National Center for Tumor Diseases,
Heidelberg, Germany

David P. Steensma, M.D.
Department of Medical Oncology,
Dana-Farber Cancer Institute,
Boston, Massachusetts, USA

Angelo Vacca, M.D., Ph.D.
Department of Internal Medicine
and Clinical Oncology,
University of Bari Medical School,
Bari, Italy

Niklas Zojer, M.D.
Department of Medicine I,
Center of Oncology and Hematology,
Wilhelminenspital,
Vienna, Austria

Part I

History and Epidemiology

History of Multiple Myeloma

1

Robert A. Kyle and David P. Steensma

Contents

Abstract Multiple Myeloma has been recognized since Ancient Times. The first well-documented case was reported in 1844 by Samuel Solly. The most commonly recognized case is that of Thomas Alexander McBean, a highly respectable tradesman from London in 1850. Mr. McBean excreted a large amount of protein that was described by Henry Bence Jones in the middle of the 19th century. Jones was a well-known physician and made many contributions to medicine. One of the best known cases of multiple myeloma was that of Dr. Loos that was reported by Otto Kahler. The recognition of plasma cells and subsequently their product, a monoclonal protein has been described in detail. The authors have reviewed the treatment of multiple myeloma including the novel agents, thalidomide, bortezomib and lenalidomide.

R.A. Kyle (✉)
Department of Medicine, Division of Hematology, Mayo Clinic, 200 First Street SW, Stabile 6-28, Rochester, MN, USA
e-mail: kyle.robert@mayo.edu

T. Moehler and H. Goldschmidt (eds.), *Multiple Myeloma*,
Recent Results in Cancer Research 183, DOI: 10.1007/978-3-540-85772-3_1,

1.1 Ancient Origins

Although the first well-documented cases of multiple myeloma were described in the 1840s, the disease has undoubtedly existed for centuries and perhaps even for eons. Spheroid skeletal lesions that are "purely lytic," with sharply demarcated borders and without evidence of sclerosis or formation of new bone, are suggestive of multiple myeloma — especially when such lesions are multiple and occur in the axial skeleton and proximal long bones (Rothschild et al. 1998). Two human skeletons with this bony lesion pattern — both males, with estimated ages at death of between 40 and 60 years — were identified from among 905 individuals in necropoles excavated at Thebes-West and Abydos in Upper Egypt, dating from 3200 BC to 500 BC (Zink et al. 1999), while two similarly affected skeletons were found among 2,547 individuals entombed in a rural South German ossuary between AD 1400 and AD 1800 (Nerlich et al. 2006).

Additional possible multiple myeloma cases identified by paleopathologists include the skeleton of a middle-aged female from AD 1000 to AD 1400 recently discovered in Iceland (Gestsdottir and Eyjolfsson 2005), two calvaria from medieval Britain (Wells 1964), four American Indian skeletons from AD 200 to AD 1300 (Morse et al. 1974), and 14 pre-Columbian American skeletons dating back to 3300 BC (Steinbock 1976). Recently, the Wellcome Collection in London featured an exhibit on skeletons; the museum curators highlighted myeloma-like lesions in the bones of a 45-year-old Roman soldier. The remains of George Grenville (1712–1770), the Whig Prime Minister whose administration passed the notorious Stamp Act of 1765 that first alienated American colonists from Great Britain, reveal lytic lesions resembling those of multiple myeloma.

Multiple myeloma with Bence Jones proteinuria (see below) occurs spontaneously in contemporary animals (Hanna 2005), raising questions about whether myelomatous lesions might be reliably identified in prehistoric non-human fossils. Paleontologists have detected multiple lytic defects without evidence of bony remodeling in a few dinosaur skeletons from the Jurassic and Cretaceous periods, and these have been interpreted as evidence of an origin of multiple myeloma in the Mesozoic era or earlier, but caution is indicated in interpretation of such ancient specimens (Capasso 2005).

1.1.1 Early Well-Documented Cases

The first well-documented case of multiple myeloma was the second patient in a series of cases of "mollities ossium" (i.e., pathological bony softness and fragility) published in 1844 by Samuel Solly (1805–1871), a distinguished London surgeon (Solly 1844). The patient's name was Sarah Newbury, a 39-year-old housewife, who developed fatigue and severe back pain while stooping 4 years before her death. Two years later, pain in Mrs. Newbury's limbs increased, making movement difficult, and she was eventually confined to her room. On one occasion, she developed fractures of her femurs when her husband lifted her and carried her to the bed. This event was followed by fractures of the clavicles, right humerus, and right radius and ulna (Fig. 1.1).

On April 15, 1844, Mrs. Newbury was hospitalized at St. Thomas' Hospital in Southwark, London, where Dr. Solly was a lecturer on anatomy. Treatment consisted of an infusion of orange peel and a rhubarb pill, as well as opiates at night. She also received wine and arrowroot, a mutton chop, and a pint of porter daily. Arrowroot was an easily digestible starch from the roots of tubers imported from the West Indies to England in the eighteenth century (Stephens 1994). It was considered to be bland, and

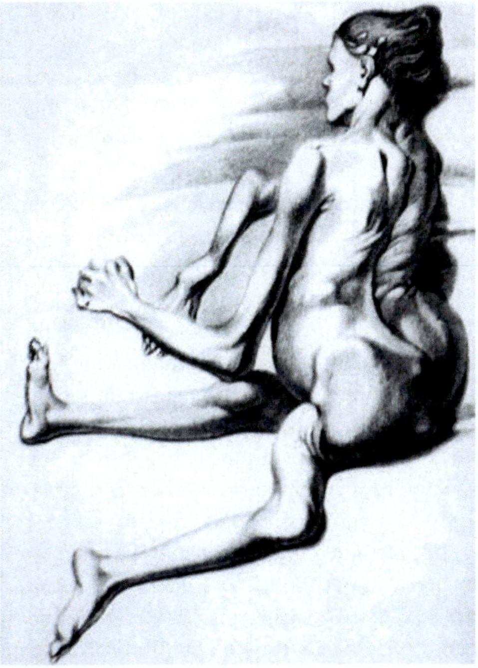

Fig. 1.1 Sarah Newbury. Fractures of femurs and right humerus

appropriate for persons who had difficulty with their digestion and were in poor condition (Felter and Lloyd 1898–1900). Porter, a dark, bitter ale made from black malted barley, was a popular drink among London working classes (especially porters and draymen) during the early eighteenth century, a time when clean, safe drinking water was difficult to obtain. Orange-based preparations, such as *infusum aurantii* made from oranges or orange peels, were often used to change the flavor of a medication. Rhubarb is a traditional gastrointestinal cathartic employed to treat dyspepsia and constipation, while opium compounds have been used since ancient times to produce pain relief.

Despite these ministrations, Mrs. Newbury died suddenly on April 20, 1844. At autopsy, Dr. Solly found that the cancellous portion of her sternum had been replaced by a peculiar red matter. The bone marrow cells were examined by Dr. Solly and a Mr. Burkett, who described the cells as "very clear, their edge being remarkably distinct and the clear oval outline enclosed one bright central nucleolus, rarely two, never more." Solly thought that the disease was an inflammatory process, and that it began with a "morbid action" of the blood vessels in which the "earthy matter of the bone is absorbed and thrown out by the kidneys in the urine" — remarkably prescient. Little did he know that, 150 years later, antiangiogenesis drugs such as thalidomide would be used for the treatment of multiple myeloma (Kyle 2000). Was Solly perhaps contemplating the role of angiogenesis in the pathophysiology of Mrs. Newbury's disease?

The best-known early case of multiple myeloma is that of Thomas Alexander McBean, "a highly respectable tradesman" in London, who was 45 years of age when he became ill. The patient developed fatigue and noted that his "body linen was stiffened by his urine." While on holiday in September 1844, he vaulted out of an underground cavern and suddenly "felt as if something had snapped or given way within the chest" and, for some minutes, he lay unable to move because of severe pain. A "strengthening plaster" was applied to the chest and the pain was temporarily relieved, but symptoms recurred 3 to 4 weeks later. Subsequently, "a pound of blood" (a pint — approximately one unit of red cells) was removed, and leeches were applied for "maintenance therapy."

Mr. McBean's bony pain eventually resolved, but he had considerable weakness for 2 to 3 months after this initial event. In the spring of 1845, his chest pain recurred; cupping and therapeutic phlebotomy were not helpful, and made him feel weaker. Dr. Thomas Watson, his physician, then prescribed steel and quinine, which was associated with rapid symptomatic improvement. Iron compounds had been used as tonics since the time of Paracelsus in the 1500s, while quinine was introduced to Europe in the late 1630s. Although quinine was given as a specific treatment for malaria in the early nineteenth century, many physicians recommended it for virtually every febrile illness, and the combination of quinine and iron was considered appropriate for severely debilitated patients (Day 1870).

The patient traveled to Scotland in the summer of 1845, where "he bounded over hills as nimbly as any of his companions" (Macintyre 1850). Unfortunately, after returning to London, he developed lumbar and sciatic pain. He was seen in consultation on October 30, 1845, by Dr. William Macintyre (*c.*1791–1857), a Harley Street consultant. Macintyre personally examined the urine because edema had been observed, and he found that it "abounded in animal matter." The following note and a sample of urine were sent to Henry Bence Jones, a chemist at St. George's Hospital:

> Saturday, Nov. 1st, 1845
>
> "Dear Dr. Jones,
>
> The tube contains urine of very high specific gravity. When boiled, it becomes slightly opaque. On the addition of nitric acid, it effervesces, assumes a reddish hue, and becomes quite clear; but as it cools, assumes the consistence and appearance which you see. Heat reliquifies it. What is it?"

Bence Jones confirmed the findings of Macintyre with respect to the urine, and calculated that the patient had excreted more than 60 g/day of protein. He concluded that the strange new protein was an oxide of albumin, specifically "hydrated deutoxide of albumen," and thought that chlorine caused this new protein to form from albumen (Bence Jones 1848). The connection between congealable protein in the urine, dropsy (edema), and kidney disease had been emphasized 20 years earlier by Richard Bright (1789–1858), a physician at Guy's Hospital in London, who published three classic papers on proteinuria and kidney disease beginning in 1827 (Steensma and Kyle 2007). Dr. Bright's practice was to use a spoon to detect protein in the urine, heating fresh urine over a candle and watching for the development of opacity.

Mr. McBean's pain persisted, despite a variety of attempted therapies, and he died on January 1, 1846 (Fig. 1.2). At autopsy, his bones were found to be soft, brittle, and readily fractured, and to contain "a gelatiniform substance of a blood-red colour and unctuous feel." Histologic examination of the bone marrow revealed round and oval-shaped cells that were one-half to twice as large as an average blood cell and contained one or two nuclei and a bright-colored nucleolus (Kyle 2000).

Because Macintyre, rather than Bence Jones, first identified the chemical properties of the

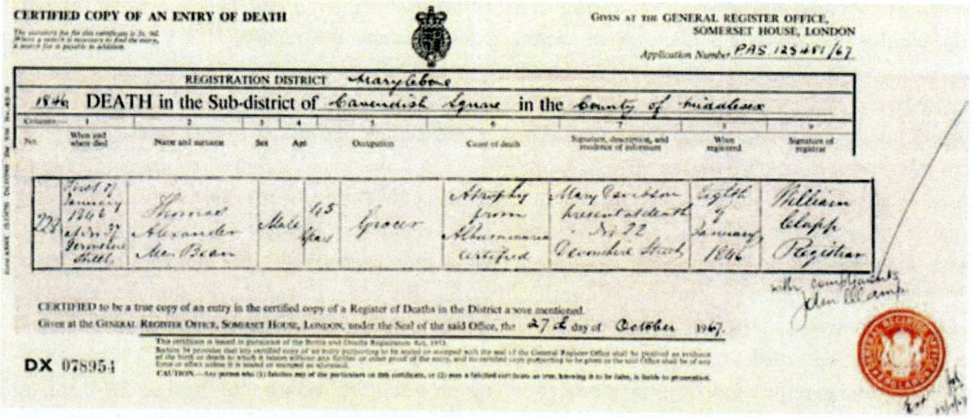

Fig. 1.2 Death certificate of Thomas Alexander McBean

unusual protein found in Mr. McBean's urine, some might suggest changing the common term "Bence Jones proteinuria" to "Macintyre proteinuria." However, although Macintyre described the heat properties of the urine, his case report describing Mr. McBean focused on the clinical course rather than the novel urinary findings (Macintyre 1850), and it was Bence Jones who emphasized the place of the new protein in the diagnosis of multiple myeloma generally: "I need hardly remark on the importance of seeking for this oxide of albumen in other cases of mollities ossium (softening of the bone)" (Bence Jones 1847).

1.2 Henry Bence Jones (1813–1873)

Henry Bence Jones was born on December 31, 1813, at Thorington Hall, in the parish of Thorington, just north of Yoxford in Suffolk, England (Kyle 2001). (The more famous Thorington Hall that is a National Trust property in Stoke-on-Nayland in the Stour River Valley is a different structure.) His childhood home had been loaned to his parents, Matilda Bence and Lieutenant Colonel William Jones (Dragoon guards), by Bence Jones' maternal grandfather, Reverend Mr. Bence Sparrow (d. 1824). Bence Jones' grandfather — the rector (parish priest) of Beccles, a village 10 miles north of Thorington — was sometimes known as Rev. Bence Bence, because he adopted the surname Bence in May 1804 upon inheriting Thorington Hall from his first cousin Anne Bence Golding.

Young Henry attended boarding school in Putney, a borough in south west London, in preparation for Harrow, one of the great English public schools. He said that he had learned little at Putney, but did enjoy walking in nearby Wimbledon Park. At Harrow, he was an accomplished cricketer and football and racquet player. He entered Trinity College, Cambridge, in 1831, where he rowed crew, and was a passable student, taking a second-class degree in January 1836. Although he attended Divinity lectures and attained a certificate for ordination, he decided not to pursue a career in the church.

Uncertain about his future, the young Bence Jones tried to find work with a relative in Liverpool, and also seriously considered immigrating to New Zealand (even proceeding with the necessary paperwork), but for unknown reasons, he did not leave England. His father suggested that he study medicine, and in 1836, he began working in the apothecary shop of John Hammerton where he prepared medicines under Hammerton's direction for 6 months. Years later, he said that this experience "was of the utmost use to me all my life" (Bence Jones 1929). He entered the Medical School at St. George's Hospital on October 1, 1838, where he began attending lectures in the dissecting room. Subsequently, he worked as a dresser in the surgeons' ward and then he turned to the physicians' ward. During medical school, he attended the lectures of the physicist Michael Faraday (1791–1867) on electricity at the Royal Institution, while Dr. James Hope, an assistant physician at St. George's, taught him use of the stethoscope. Bence Jones also noted that at the time he was a student, "the glorious discoveries of Dr. Bright [about renal disease] were not valued by any of our medical men" (Bence Jones 1929).

St. George's Hospital, where Bence Jones studied, had been established as a teaching facility and public infirmary in 1733 in what was then the open countryside outside the village of Knightsbridge — a site noted for its clean air, in stark contrast to the nearby overcrowded and filthy conditions prevalent in the city of London. Its faculty has included John Hunter, Edward Jenner, Thomas Young and Henry Gray (anatomist). After post–World War II reorganization as part of the National Health Service, St. George's Hospital moved to Tooting in South London in 1980; by then, the medical school had become a constituent institution of the University of London system. The Lanesborough Hotel is presently on the original hospital site at Hyde Park Corner. When the hospital was rebuilt and expanded in the 1820s into the Classical neo-Grecian structure that Bence Jones would have known, noted architect William Wilkins (1778–1839) was responsible for the design; Wilkins also designed the National Gallery in Trafalgar Square, and University College London.

Bence Jones's medical studies were interrupted when he developed rheumatic fever in the spring of 1839 and returned home for 6 weeks. Fortunately, he "recovered without complications of disease of the heart" (Bence Jones 1929) — at least none that were detectable at that time. Upon his return to London, he enrolled as a private pupil to Professor Thomas Graham (1805–1869), the "father of colloid chemistry" and discoverer of the principle of dialysis, at University College. Most of the teaching was done by Graham's assistant, George Fownes (1815–1849), a brilliant researcher who published his own chemistry textbook in 1844, and won the prestigious Royal Medal of the Royal Society in 1847 before ill health caused him to have to give up his research. Fownes, in turn, had studied with Justus von Liebig (1803–1873) in Giessen, Germany; von Liebig was a leading chemist of the age and a strident advocate of applying chemistry to the study of plant and animal physiology, against the opposition of others, including the vitalists, who advocated strict separation between inorganic and organic chemistry. The cost of a year's tuition for the course with Graham was £50. Bence Jones learned the principles of organic chemical analysis from Fownes and Graham, and analysis of the sulfur content in a cystine oxide calculus represented his first medical publication (Bence Jones 1842).

Bence Jones was admitted in the spring of 1841 as a licentiate of the College of Physicians, which allowed him to practice, but he had no University medical degree as of yet. On Easter Sunday in 1841, he left for Giessen, Germany, where he studied in von Liebig's laboratory for 6 months. There he learned some advanced analytical methods, and analyzed the proteins in the brain and egg yolk. Bence Jones remained in contact with von Liebig throughout his life, and shared von Liebig's passion for applying chemistry to medicine. Coincidentally, von Liebig and Bence Jones died 2 days apart in April 1873, and their obituaries appeared in the same issue of *Lancet*.

In May 1842, 28-year-old Bence Jones married a cousin, Lady Millicent Acheson (*c.*1812–1887), the youngest daughter of Mary Sparrow and Sir Archibald Acheson, the second Earl of Gosford, an Irish peer who had served as Governor General of British North America from 1835 to 1838. Together they would have seven children. The young couple settled at 30 Grosvenor Square, London, and Bence Jones began working at St. George's. He analyzed the calculi in the Museum of University College Hospital and published his second paper (Bence Jones 1845). He was asked to give a course of 100 lectures on chemistry at Middlesex Hospital, where he became known for insisting on the study of urine in diagnosis of disease. Three years later, he obtained an assistant physician position at St. George's Hospital, and became a full physician there the next year; he was affiliated with St. George's for the rest of his life. In 1846, he became a Fellow of the Royal Society and also received a doctoral degree in medicine from Cambridge. He became involved with the Royal Institution when he gave a series of lectures in 1851, and he served as secretary of that institution — dedicated to "diffusing science for the common purposes of life" — for more than 20 years.

Although his clinical practice grew quickly and was consuming, he vowed to "let no year pass without doing something original in natural science as applied to medicine" (Bence Jones 1929) (Fig. 1.3). Bence Jones was no classicist;

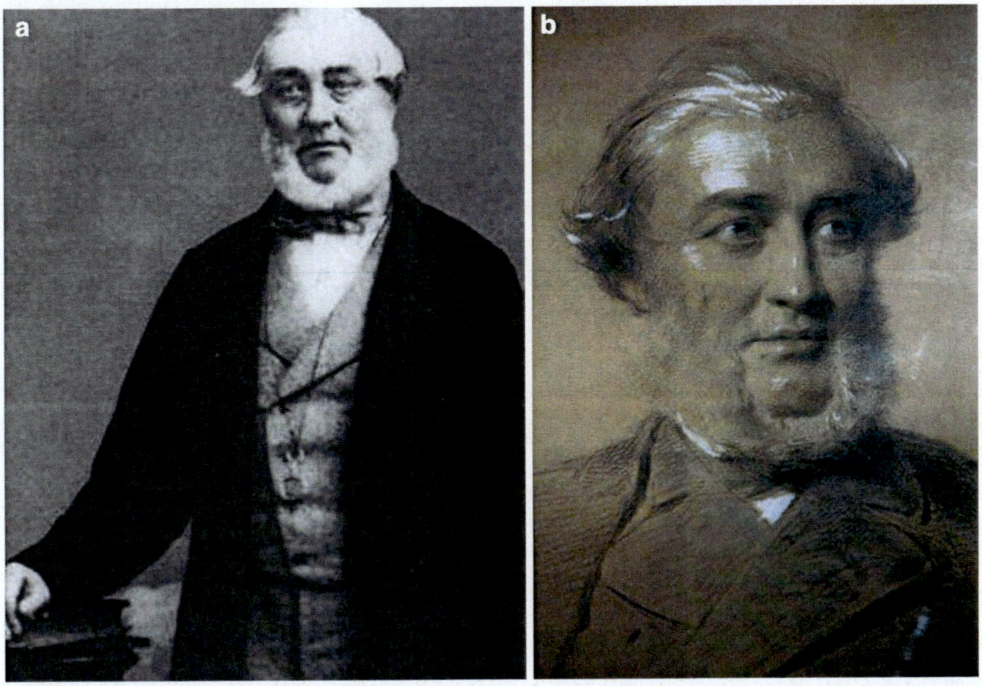

Fig. 1.3 (**a**, **b**) Portraits of Henry Bence Jones

he believed that medicine would be much better served if students spent more time acquiring knowledge of chemistry and physics, rather than memorizing Latin and Greek vocabulary and declensions. As a biochemist, he believed in nothing that he could not separate, test, and measure, scorning experience, tradition, and authority. His research resulted in a series of articles on the sediment, uric acid, calcium oxalate, and the alkaline and earthy phosphates of urine, but while his obituary in the *Medical Times and Gazette* listed 34 papers and six additional articles, no accurate, complete bibliography exists (obituary 1873). He believed that medication must diffuse throughout the tissues before they could produce any benefit and demonstrated that quinine reached its maximum level in tissues 3 h after ingestion.

Bence Jones' work habits were somewhat unusual. He began his laboratory work at 6 a.m. and then arrived at the hospital at approximately 1 p.m. for ward rounds. However, few students sought a clerkship with him because of his unpunctuality. He frequently chided students with the phrase, "Oh! Medical facts! Medical facts!" He taught students to "be as long as you like in forming your opinion on a case, but when you have thoroughly formed it, stick to it" (obituary 1873). His chief aim in the wards was to make therapeutics more scientific. He was unwilling to mix several medications together, a common practice of the day, and instead used simple, precise prescriptions. He was also skeptical of most of the therapeutic drugs of his day. Philosopher Herbert Spencer (1820–1903) wrote in his autobiography, "Speaking of drugs, Bence Jones said that there is scarcely one which may not, under different conditions, produce opposite effects…" (Rosenbloom 1919).

Bence Jones' medical practice grew rapidly and eventually became large and lucrative. In 1 year, his profits from practice were £7,400 — an enormous income for the time — and he bought a house at 84 Brook Street on one of the "grand avenues" of the posh Mayfair neighborhood in West London (obituary 1873). He was recognized widely as a "chemical" doctor, and thus, his practice drew the interest of other scientists. Charles Darwin (1809–1882), the great naturalist, was one of his patients. For Darwin, a noted hypochondriac, Bence Jones prescribed a "severe" diet for his indigestion, which "half-starved him to death" (Rosenbloom 1919). Other famous patients included Michael Faraday, about whom he wrote an affectionate biography in 1870 (Bence Jones 1870) and the biologist, Thomas Huxley ("Darwin's bulldog") (1825–1895). Nursing pioneer Florence Nightingale (1820–1910) once stated that Bence Jones was "the best chemical doctor in London" (Putnam 1993).

In the 1860s, Bence Jones' health began to fail. He noted frequent palpitations and diagnosed rheumatic heart disease in himself after hearing a mitral systolic murmur with his stethoscope in 1861. Reversing his earlier claim that he had suffered no ill effects from his bout of rheumatic fever in 1839, he realized that this illness and its sequelae had "done permanent damage to one of the valves" (Bence Jones 1929). In early 1866, congestive heart failure became more obvious; upon listening to his own lungs with a stethoscope, he stated, "I fancied that one side was half full of fluid" (Bence Jones 1929). His energy decreased, and by August 1870, in a letter to physicist John Tyndall (1820–1893), Bence Jones stated, "I am very lazy and feel unfit for any work and as neither eating, drinking, or sleeping come pleasantly to me, I am a useless mortal and had better be helping the worms and the grass to grow faster than they otherwise would do…" (Putnam 1993). Congestive hepatomegaly, ascites, and anasarca followed, and finally in 1873, Bence Jones was forced to both give up his clinical practice and resign as secretary of the Royal Institution. On April 20, 1873, he died at his home at 84 Brook Street in London of congestive heart failure, and was buried at Kensal Green Cemetery.

A Bence Jones ward exists at St. George's Hospital in Tooting, but it is devoted to gynecology patients rather than patients with multiple myeloma or kidney disease. Interestingly, Bence Jones' obituary in *Medical Times and Gazette* described his work on renal stones, diabetes mellitus, and malignant and tuberculous involvement of the kidney, as well as his emphasis on the clinical value of microscopic analysis of the urine, but there was no mention of the unique urinary protein that bears his name and would preserve that name for posterity (obituary 1873). Henry Bence Jones did not hyphenate his name, and a hyphen is not used in any of his papers or books published during his lifetime. The Royal College of Physicians and the *Dictionary of National Biography* enter him under "Jones." He signed his correspondence, "H. Bence Jones", and apparently did not like the name "Henry." His descendants added a hyphen more than a half-century after his death (Rosenfeld 1987).

1.3 Other Contributions to Bence Jones Proteinuria

In 1846, an Austrian clinical chemist, Johann Florian Heller (1813–1871), described a protein in the urine that precipitated when warmed above 50°C and then dissolved again on further heating (Heller 1846). Heller distinguished this protein from albumin and casein, and it is almost certain that this was Bence Jones protein, despite Heller's failure to recognize the reprecipitation of the protein when the urine cooled again. R. Fleischer, in 1880, is credited with the first publication to use the term "Bence Jones protein." (Fleischer 1880).

W. Kühne described a 40-year-old man with acute osteomalacia and an unusual urinary protein in 1883 (Kühne 1883). The patient's urine precipitated on warming to between 40°C and 50°C and cleared at 100°C. Kühne isolated the urinary protein, which he called "albumosurie," and found that the carbon, hydrogen, and nitrogen levels were similar to those described by Bence Jones, attributing minor differences in composition to the fact that his preparation was more pure than that of Henry Bence Jones.

Bence Jones recognized only a single type of protein, but in 1922, Stanhope Bayne-Jones (1888–1970) and D.W. Wilson at Johns Hopkins found that there are actually two distinct groups of Bence Jones proteins (Bayne-Jones and Wilson 1922). Leonhard Korngold and Rose Lipari, at Memorial Cancer Institute in New York, demonstrated a relationship between Bence Jones protein and the serum proteins of multiple myeloma in 1956 (Korngold and Lipari 1956). The two major classes of Bence Jones protein have been designated kappa and lambda in honor of Korngold and Lipari. Gerald Edelman (1929–) and Joseph A. Gally at the Rockefeller Institute in New York, 117 years after the description of the unique heat properties of Bence Jones protein, proved that the light chains prepared from an IgG myeloma protein and the Bence Jones protein from the same patient's urine had an identical amino acid sequence; similar spectrofluorometric behavior; identical appearance on chromatography with carboxymethylcellulose; and, on starch gel electrophoresis after reduction and alkylation, the same ultracentrifugal pattern, identical thermosolubility, and the same molecular weight (Edelman and Gally 1962). The light chains examined by Edelman and Galley precipitated when heated to between 40°C and 60°C, dissolved on boiling and reprecipitated when cooled to between 40°C and 60°C — identical to the physicochemical properties of Bence Jones protein.

1.4 Other Early Cases of Multiple Myeloma

In 1867, Hermann Weber reported a 40-year-old man with pain, tenderness, and deformity of the sternum. The patient also had severe pain in the lumbar area, and he died 3.5 months after the onset of pain. At postmortem examination, the patient's sternum was almost entirely replaced by a grayish-red substance that had the microscopic appearance of a sarcoma. There were several round defects in the skull, many of the ribs, several vertebrae and parts of the pelvis. Amyloid — described by Rudolf Virchow (1821–1902) in Berlin in 1854 — was found in the kidneys and spleen (Weber 1867).

Five years later, William Adams described a similar patient to Weber's with bone pain and fractures. At autopsy, it was observed that the cancellous portions of the bones had been replaced by a homogenous soft gelatinous substance consisting of small spherical and oval cells containing one oval nucleus (rarely two) with a bright nucleolus. "Lardaceous changes" (likely amyloidosis) were found in the liver and kidneys (Adams 1872).

J. Von Rustizky, a Russian pathologist working in the laboratory of Friedrich von Recklinghausen (1833–1910) in Strassburg in 1873, introduced the term "multiple myeloma." At autopsy, a 47-year-old patient examined had eight separate tumors of bone marrow, which Von Rustizky called "multiple myelomas," and he noted that the nucleus of the tumor cells was located in the periphery of the cell membrane — a morphology highly suggestive of plasma cells.

1.4.1 The Case of Dr. Loos

The term "Kahler's disease" was once used to describe myeloma; this eponym resulted from a case report of a physician named Dr. Loos by

Professor Otto Kahler of Prague. The patient, Dr. Loos, was a 46-year-old physician who developed severe thoracic pain in July 1879. During the next 2 years, intermittent pain aggravated by exercise occurred in Dr. Loos' ribs, spine, left shoulder, upper arm, and right clavicle. Albuminuria was found in September 1881, and pallor was seen 2 years later. Dr. Loos was first seen by Professor Kahler in 1885. Kahler found anemia, severe kyphosis, tenderness of many bones, and albumosuria. The urine of Dr. Loos was described in detail in 1889 by Karl Hugo Huppert (1832–1904), a German chemist and physician who was the Professor of Medicinal Chemistry in Prague. Kyphosis of the upper thoracic spine increased and the patient's chin pressed against the sternum producing a pressure ulcer. Dr. Loos died on August 26, 1887, 8 years after the onset of symptoms. At autopsy, soft gray-reddish masses were noted in the ribs and microscopic examination revealed large, round cells consistent with myeloma. The patient sustained a high fluid intake and took sodium bicarbonate on a regular basis, which may have helped prevent renal failure.

Otto Kahler, born in 1849, was the son of a well-known physician in Prague. After receiving his M.D. degree from the University of Prague in 1871, Kahler studied in Paris, where he met the French neurologists Jean Martin Charcot (1825–1893) and Guillaume-Benjamin-Amand Duchenne (1806–1875). Kahler became interested in neurology, particularly in neuroanatomy. He contributed to the understanding of the pathological anatomy of tabes dorsalis, localization of parietal central oculomotor paralysis, and the symptoms of gradual compression of the spinal cord. He then returned to Prague where he became head of the second medical clinic at the German University of Prague. In 1889, Kahler succeeded the Austrian internist Heinrich von Bamberger (1822–1888), as Professor at the University of Vienna (Fig. 1.4). Kahler finished his inaugural address in Vienna on May 13, 1889, with a statement, "Ars longa vita brevis" (the art [of medicine] is long, life is short) — words that proved prophetic in 1889, when he developed a malignant tumor of the tongue. Despite an attempted excision, carcinoma of the tongue recurred the following year, and Kahler died on January 24, 1893 (Nothnagel 1893). Kahler was known for being extremely kind to his patients and an excellent teacher. Incidentally, his obituaries and eulogies made no mention of his famous case report of Dr. Loos (Kahler 1889); the contributions of both Henry Bence Jones and Otto Kahler to multiple myeloma were not recognized during their lifetimes.

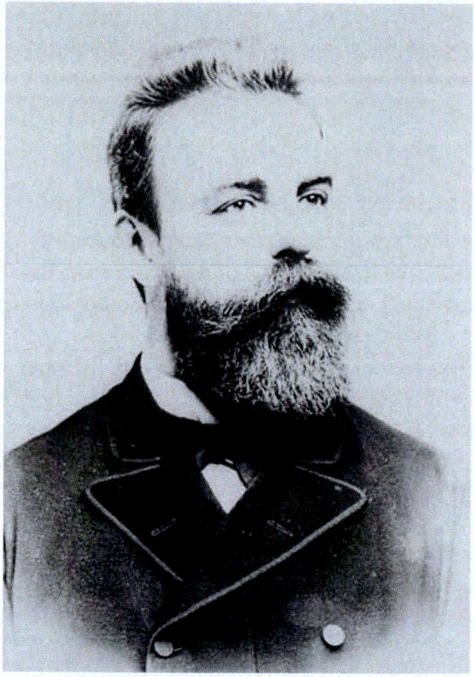

Fig. 1.4 Otto Kahler

1.4.2 The First Myeloma Case in America

Probably the first reported case of multiple myeloma in the United States was published by

James Herrick (1861–1954) and Ludvig Hektoen at Rush Medical College in Chicago in 1894 (Herrick and Hektoen 1894). A 40-year-old woman had lumbar pain for 16 months before painless nodules developed on the sternum, face, and chest. The right clavicle enlarged and then fractured without trauma. The hemoglobin level was less than half normal. The patient died 18 months after the onset of symptoms. Autopsy revealed tumors involving the sternum, ribs, spine, right clavicle, both humeri, and the skull, and microscopic examination revealed the round, lymphoid cells with large nuclei described in other reports.

1.4.3 Recognition of the Poor Prognosis Associated with Bence Jones Protein

Frederick Parkes Weber (1863–1962), an English physician who is the "Weber" in Klippel–Trenauney–Weber syndrome and Rendu–Osler–Weber disease, reported a case of multiple myeloma in 1898 and stated that in the future, the diagnosis might be "greatly facilitated by the employment of Röntgen's rays" (Weber 1898). Weber also claimed that bone marrow was the site of production of the Bence Jones protein and that its presence was of "fatal significance" and that it "nearly always, if not always, indicated that the patient was suffering from multiple myeloma" (Weber et al. 1903).

1.4.4 Case Series

In the first half of the twentieth century, case reports gave way to case series. In 1928, Charles F. Geschickter (1901–1987) and Murray M. Copeland (1902–1982) at Georgetown University in Washington, DC, presented an analysis of all 425 cases of multiple myeloma reported since 1848 (Geschickter and Copeland 1928). They emphasized six major features consisting of multiple involvement of the skeleton by tumors, pathologic fractures, Bence Jones proteinuria, back pain, anemia, and renal insufficiency. They did not recognize abnormalities of blood protein or elevation of the erythrocyte sedimentation rate. Bone marrow aspiration, described in 1929 by Mikahael Arinkin in Leningrad, greatly increased the antemortem recognition of multiple myeloma (Arinkin 1929). Rosenthal and Vogel reported that only three cases of multiple myeloma had been recognized in Mount Sinai Hospital in New York from 1916 to 1935, but that 13 cases were found in the succeeding 2.5 years (Rosenthal and Vogel 1938). Edwin Bayrd (1917–2007) and Frank Heck described 83 patients with histological proof of multiple myeloma who were seen at Mayo Clinic through 1945. Duration of survival ranged from 1 to 84 months (median 15 months) (Bayrd and Heck 1947).

1.4.5 Plasma Cells

The term "plasma cell" was first used in 1875 by Heinrich Wilhelm Gottfried von Waldeyer-Hartz (1836–1921), a German anatomist, but from the detailed description, it seems likely that he was observing tissue mast cells, rather than the antibody-producing cells that we currently call by that name (Waldeyer 1875). Plasma cells were described accurately by the great Spanish anatomist Santiago Ramón y Cajal (1852–1934) in 1890 during a study of syphilitic condylomas (Cajal 1896). Cajal believed that the unstained perinuclear area ("hof") contained the Golgi apparatus, and he felt that the plasma cells were likely normal constituents of connective tissue. T. von Marschalkó, a Hungarian pathologist, described the key characteristics of plasma cells in 1895, including blocked chromatin, eccentric position of the nucleus, a perinuclear pale area, and a spherical or irregular cytoplasm (Marschalko 1895). J.H. Wright thought that the tumor cells of myeloma consisted of plasma cells or their immediate descendants (Wright 1900).

1.4.6 Antibodies

In 1890, Emil Adolf von Behring (1854–1917), a German physiologist, and Japanese bacteriologist Shibasaburō Kisato (1853–1931) described a specific neutralizing substance in the blood of animals immunized with diphtheria and tetanus toxin — an observation that won them the first Nobel Prize in physiology or medicine in 1901. von Behring and Kisato and their successors noted that antitoxins — later called antibodies — could be found after the injection of most foreign proteins (von Behring and Kisato 1890). Although a Bence Jones protein had been detected in the serum by Jacobsen in 1917, it was not until 1928 that William A. Perlzweig (1891–1949) and his colleagues at Johns Hopkins recognized hyperproteinemia, when they described a patient with multiple myeloma who had 9 to 11 g of globulin in the serum (Perlzweig et al. 1928). The Johns Hopkins team also noted that it was almost impossible to obtain serum from clotted blood drawn from a hyperproteinemic patient, because the clot failed to retract even with prolonged centrifugation. Maxwell Wintrobe (1901–1986) and M.V. Buell, also at Johns Hopkins, recognized cryglobulinemia in 1933 (Wintrobe and Buell 1933), but the term "cryoglobulin" was introduced by medical student Aaron Lerner (1920–2007) and his research preceptor, C.J. Watson, at the University of Minnesota 14 years later (Lerner and Watson 1947). The patient described by Lerner and Watson had previously been reported as having allergic purpura with hypersensitivity to cold (Peters and Horton 1941).

1.4.7 Electrophoresis

Separation of serum proteins by electrophoresis was described by Swedish biochemist Arne Tiselius (1902–1971) in his doctoral dissertation in 1930; he published expanded observations using the moving boundary method of electrophoresis in 1937 (Tiselius 1937b). Interestingly, this article, which led to his 1948 Nobel Prize in chemistry and later to the Presidency of the Nobel Foundation, was rejected by the *Biochemical Journal* (Putnam 1993) — perhaps a note of encouragement for other frustrated authors. Later in 1937, Tiselius described the separation of serum globulins into three major protein components, which he termed alpha, beta, and gamma according to their electrophoretic mobility (Tiselius 1937a, b). Tiselius and an American postdoctoral fellow, Elvin A. Kabat (1914–2000), localized antibody activity to the gamma globulin region of the plasma proteins (Tiselius and Kabat 1939). However, they quickly recognized that some antibodies migrated in the fast gamma region and others in the slow gamma region, and that some sedimented in the ultracentrifuge as 7S and others as 19S molecules, suggesting further heterogeneity. The concept of a family of proteins with antibody activity was described by Belgian immunologist Joseph-Félix Heremans (d. 1975) in 1959 (Heremans 1959). Before 1960, the term "gamma globulin" was used for any protein that migrated in the gamma mobility region of the electrophoretic pattern; these gamma globulins are now referred to as immunoglobulins: IgG, IgA, IgM, IgD, and IgE.

In 1939, Lewis G. Longsworth and his colleagues at the Rockefeller Institute applied electrophoresis to the study of multiple myeloma, and demonstrated the tall, narrow-based "church spire peak" (Longsworth et al. 1939). The electrophoresis apparatus used by Longsworth and contemporaries was cumbersome and difficult to use; the original commercial models were 20-ft long and 5-ft high, and often occupied a separate laboratory room. A single electrophoretic run required a full day, and results could only be interpreted by an experienced operator (Putnam 1993). Subsequent technical refinements made electrophoresis simpler and more widely available. For instance, the use of filter paper as a support permitted the separation of proteins into discrete zones that could be stained with various dyes (Kunkel and Tiselius 1951), and cellulose acetate replaced filter paper. Currently, most laboratories now use agarose gel electrophoresis.

Immunoelectrophoresis was described by Grabar and Williams in 1953 (Grabar and Williams 1953). Eleven years later, Wilson reported immunofixation or "direct immunoelectrophoresis," in which he applied antisera on the surface of the agarose immediately after completion of electrophoresis. Rowe and Fahey isolated IgD monoclonal protein from a myeloma patient (Rowe and Fahey 1965). A year later, Ishizaka et al. described the final immunoglobulin isotype, IgE (Ishizaka et al. 1966).

1.4.8 Monoclonal Versus Polyclonal Gammopathies

A critical milestone was the concept of monoclonal versus polyclonal gammopathies, first presented in the Harvey Lecture Series by Swedish physician Jan Gosta Waldenstrom (1906–1996) in 1961 (Waldenstrom 1960–1961). He described patients with a narrow band of hypergammaglobulinemia on electrophoresis as having a monoclonal protein, and those with a broad band on electrophoresis and hypergammaglobulinemia as having a polyclonal increase in proteins. While polyclonal hypergammaglobulinemia was associated with nonmalignant disorders including inflammation or infection, patients with monoclonal proteins typically had multiple myeloma or macroglobulinemia. However, others with a monoclonal pattern had no evidence of malignancy, and Waldenstrom considered them to have "essential hypergammaglobulinemia" or a "benign monoclonal protein." Today the preferred term for this phenomenon is monoclonal gammopathy of undetermined significance (MGUS), because some such proteins will remain stable for many years and not cause clinical problems, but in other patients with MGUS, multiple myeloma, macroglobulinemia, light chain (AL) amyloidosis, or a related disorder may subsequently develop (Kyle 1978).

1.5 Alkylator and Corticosteroid-Based Therapy

Therapy of multiple myeloma has improved markedly since the days of Sarah Newbury's treatment with rhubarb pills and infusion of orange peel, or the phlebotomy, leeches, steel, quinine, and other ministrations that Thomas McBean had to endure. Despite the therapeutic advances of the last half-century, however, the cure of myeloma has proven elusive, and there is much work yet to be done.

1.5.1 Urethane

Nils Alwall (1904–1986), a Swedish hemodialysis pioneer, reported in 1947 that a patient with multiple myeloma who was treated with urethane (ethyl carbamate) had a reduction in serum globulin concentration from 5.9 g/dL to 2.2 g/dL, an increase in hemoglobin from 60% to 87%, disappearance of proteinuria, and a reduction in bone marrow plasma cells from 33% to 0% (Alwall 1947). Urethane became the standard of treatment for myeloma for more than 15 years, until a randomized trial showed that it was not effective. In 1966, chemotherapy pioneer James

F. Holland and colleagues randomized 83 patients with treated or untreated multiple myeloma to receive urethane or a placebo consisting of cherry- and cola-flavored syrup (Holland et al. 1966). No difference was seen in the objective response or in survival between the two treatment groups.

1.5.2 Melphalan

In 1958, Nikolai Nikolaevich Blokhin and colleagues in Moscow reported that three of six patients with multiple myeloma obtained benefit from sacrolysin (L-phenylalanine mustard, melphalan) (Blokhin et al. 1958). Four years later, Daniel E. Bergsagel, at MD Anderson, and his colleagues confirmed these findings, reporting significant improvement in 8 of 24 patients with multiple myeloma who were treated with melphalan; 6 other patients had more modest objective improvements (Bergsagel et al. 1962). In a later report, melphalan given as a loading dose for 1 week followed by maintenance therapy produced responses in 78% of 64 patients with newly diagnosed or previously treated multiple myeloma (Hoogstraten et al. 1967).

1.5.3 Prednisone

Prednisone also was found to be effective for multiple myeloma at about the same time that melphalan debuted. In a placebo-controlled double-blind trial published in 1962, prednisone as a single agent produced significant decreases in serum globulin levels and an increase in hematocrit, but no improvement in survival when compared with a placebo (Mass 1962). In another study, prednisone, in a single dose of 200 mg every other morning, produced benefit in eight of ten patients with poor-risk myeloma (Salmon et al. 1967). In an analysis of two Cancer and Leukemia Group B (CALGB) myeloma treatment protocols, prednisone as a single agent produced a 44% objective response (MacIntyre et al. 1985). The classic regimen of melphalan plus prednisone (MP) was established in a randomized trial of 183 myeloma patients published in 1969. This study, led by Raymond Alexanian and colleagues, found that survival was 6 months longer with MP compared with melphalan alone (Alexanian et al. 1969). Later, dexamethasone was found to offer some advantages over prednisone.

1.5.4 Alkylator Combinations

Harley et al. first reported a combination of alkylating agents — melphalan, cyclophosphamide, and carmustine (BCNU) in 1972 (Harley et al. 1972). A combination of carmustine, cyclophosphamide, melphalan, vincristine, and prednisone (M-2 protocol) produced excellent subjective and objective responses in 60% of 36 myeloma patients (Lee et al. 1974). Likewise, in a series of 73 patients with myeloma, the M-2 protocol produced an 87% response rate in 73 myeloma patients (Case et al. 1977).

However, when the CALGB cooperative group studied the combination of carmustine (BCNU), cyclophosphamide, melphalan, and prednisone (BCMP regimen) to MP in 252 patients by J.B. Harley and colleagues in 1979; there was no survival benefit from the BCMP regimen above MP (Harley et al. 1979). Other trials had similar negative results in terms of survival, even when objective response rates improved. The Myeloma Trialists Collaborative Group described a large meta-analysis of individual data of 4,930 persons from 20 randomized trials comparing MP with various combinations of therapeutic agents (Myeloma Trialists' Collaborative Group 1998). Although the response rates were higher with combination chemotherapy (60% vs MP 53%,

$P < 0.0001$), there was no significant difference in response duration or overall survival. MP thus remained the mainstay of myeloma treatment for decades.

1.6 Stem Cell Transplantation

E. Donnall Thomas and his colleagues in Cooperstown, New York, treated six patients (one had multiple myeloma) with total body irradiation or chemotherapy followed by an intravenous infusion of bone marrow cells in 1957 (Thomas et al. 1957), but technical obstacles prevented successful results. Thomas moved to Seattle in 1963 and continued to modify approaches to stem cell transplantation, which ultimately led to his Nobel Prize in 1990. The first successful syngeneic bone marrow transplantation for myeloma was reported in 1982; two physician brothers were the patients (Osserman et al. 1982). In 1986, Alexander Fefer and colleagues in Seattle described five myeloma patients who received a syngeneic bone marrow transplant (Fefer et al. 1986). The following year, Gösta Gahrton and colleagues in Sweden reported that 10 of 14 patients with multiple myeloma who received an allogeneic bone marrow transplant from an HLA-compatible sibling donor survived for a median of 12 months (Gahrton et al. 1987).

The first reported autologous bone marrow transplantation in a patient with plasma cell leukemia was reported in 1983 by Timothy McElwain (1937–1990) and Ray Powles at the Royal Marsen Hospital in Sutton, England (McElwain and Powles 1983). The patient was given melphalan 140 mg/m^2 followed by platelet support and antibiotics; he relapsed 16 months later and was again given 140 mg/m^2 of melphalan followed by an intravenous autograft obtained from his remission marrow. Two of four previously untreated myeloma patients treated similarly obtained a complete response, whereas one of four previously treated patients had a complete response (McElwain and Powles 1983). Eleven (27%) of forty-one patients with previously untreated multiple myeloma obtained a complete remission after a single intravenous dose of melphalan 140 mg/m^2. Unfortunately, most of the patients relapsed with a median duration of remission of 19 months. In 1987, Bart Barlogie and colleagues at MD Anderson in Houston reported use of melphalan 140 mg/m^2 and total body irradiation (150 cGy), followed by autologous or allogeneic bone marrow transplantation, in six patients with multiple myeloma refractory to chemotherapy (Barlogie et al. 1987). Barlogie subsequently developed intense treatment programs using autologous transplantation, which he called "total therapy" (a term and concept pioneered for childhood leukemia at St. Jude's Hospital in Memphis), which eventually played a major role in establishing high-dose therapy and stem cell rescue as standard therapy for myeloma.

1.6.1 Novel Agents

Beginning in the late 1990s, other active drug therapies emerged that finally supplanted MP as the standard of care for patients with multiple myeloma. These included thalidomide (Singhal et al. 1999), bortezomib (Richardson et al. 2003, 2005), and lenalidomide (Rajkumar et al. 2005; Richardson et al. 2006).

1.6.1.1 Thalidomide

Chemie Grünenthal, a German pharmaceutical company, introduced thalidomide (alpha-N-[phthalimidol] glutarimide) (as a sedative) on October 1, 1957. Three years later, it was sold in more than 40 countries, and became popular both as a sedative and as a treatment for morning sickness of pregnancy.

1

Widukind Lenz (1919–1995), a German pediatrician and geneticist, reported on November 18, 1961, that in utero thalidomide was associated with severe teratogenic malformations (Lenz 1962). Exposure to the drug during the first trimester of pregnancy produced the fetal malformations. Thalidomide was removed from the market in most countries by the end of 1961, but by then almost 10,000 infants had been affected. Dr. Francis Kelsey of the US Food and Drug Administration (FDA) was concerned about the lack of safety data and fortunately did not approve the drug for use in the USA. No significant activity was noted in two separate clinical trials for patients with advanced cancer (Grabstald and Golbey 1965; Olson et al. 1965). A few myeloma patients were admitted to these trials, but clinical activity was not apparent.

Despite removal from the market as a sedative, thalidomide continued to be used in the developing world for the treatment of leprosy and other ailments. Beginning in the 1980s, thalidomide was also found to be effective for Behçet disease, graft-versus-host disease, and HIV-associated oral ulcers and wasting. The FDA approved thalidomide for the treatment of erythema nodosum leprosum in 1998, with a prescribing and distribution safety system termed, "The System For Thalidomide Education and Prescribing Safety" program (STEPS).

The antiangiogenic properties of thalidomide in the rabbit cornea micropocket assay were described by Robert D'Amato and colleagues in Judah Folkman's laboratory in Boston (D'Amato et al. 1994). Based on the increasing awareness of angiogenesis and the pathogenesis of cancer, and the evidence of increased angiogenesis in myeloma, the spouse of an affected myeloma patient convinced Barlogie and colleagues at the University of Arkansas to initiate a compassionate-use trial of "antiangiogenic therapy." After a detailed telephone conversation with Folkman, Barlogie and colleagues designed a landmark trial that enrolled 84 myeloma patients for whom MP had failed (Singhal et al. 1999). Thirty-two percent of patients in this pilot study responded to thalidomide, making it the first new drug with single-agent activity for myeloma in more than three decades.

1.6.1.2 Bortezomib

The orderly degradation of eukaryocytic cellular proteins is mediated by the ubiquitin-proteasome pathway (Ciechanover 1994). The 26S proteasome consists of a core 20S catalytic complex and a 19S regulatory complex. Ubiquitin-tagged proteins are recognized by the 19S regulatory complex, where the ubiquitin tags are removed, and then the 20S proteasome cylinder hydrolyzes the formerly tagged proteins into small polypeptides. Inhibition of the proteasome leads to cellular apoptosis with malignant, transformed, and proliferating cells being particularly susceptible (Adams et al. 1999; Orlowski et al. 1998).

Several boronic acid–derived compounds, including bortezomib, were designed to inhibit the proteasome pathway in a specific manner (Adams et al. 1999; Orlowski et al. 1998). The initial clinical study with bortezomib in advanced hematologic malignancies was conducted by Robert Orlowski at the University of North Carolina (Orlowski et al. 2002). Leading up to the trial, Orlowski's laboratory was investigating the proteasome pathway — an area of research that his father, Marian Orlowski (1918–2006), had pioneered years earlier. Bortezomib demonstrated antimyeloma activity in the initial phase I study (Orlowski et al. 2002). It also showed activity against myeloma cells in several preclinical models in a series of experiments conducted in the laboratories of Kenneth Anderson at the Dana Farber Cancer Institute in Boston (Hideshima et al. 2001). Approximately one-third of the 202 patients with relapsed refractory myeloma responded to bortezomib (Richardson et al. 2003). These results led to the approval of bortezomib by the FDA in May 2003. In a subsequent randomized trial, time to disease progression was superior with bortezomib compared with dexamethasone alone in patients with relapsed, refractory myeloma (Richardson et al. 2005).

1.6.1.3 Lenalidomide

Several analogs of thalidomide were synthesized to try to minimize some of the adverse events (including, perhaps, teratogenicity) associated with thalidomide. Lenalidomide, a 4-aminosubstituted analog of thalidomide formerly called CC-5013, belongs to a class of thalidomide analogs termed "immunomodulatory drugs" by the manufacturer, Celgene Corporation.

Lenalidomide was tested in phase I trials in relapsed refractory myeloma at the Dana Farber Cancer Institute by Paul Richardson and colleagues, and the compound showed promise (Richardson et al. 2002). A multicenter randomized phase II trial of lenalidomide, also led by Richardson, enrolled 102 patients with relapsed/refractory myeloma, with an overall response rate of 17% (Richardson et al. 2006). In a phase II trial conducted at Mayo Clinic, 31 of 34 patients (91%) with newly diagnosed myeloma achieved an objective response with thalidomide plus dexamethasone (Rajkumar et al. 2005). Two large phase III trials have shown a significantly superior time to progression with lenalidomide plus dexamethasone compared with placebo plus dexamethasone in patients with relapsed myeloma (Dimopoulos et al. 2007; Weber et al. 2007). The combination of lenalidomide and dexamethasone was approved by the FDA in June 2006 for the treatment of myeloma in patients who have failed one prior regimen.

References

Adams W (1872) Mollities ossium. Trans Pathol Soc Lond 23:186–187

Adams J, Palombella VJ, Sausville EA, Johnson J, Destree A, Lazarus DD, Maas J, Pien CS, Prakash S, Elliott PJ (1999) Proteasome inhibitors: a novel class of potent and effective antitumor agents. Cancer Res 59:2615–2622

Alexanian R, Haut A, Khan AU, Lane M, McKelvey EM, Migliore PJ, Stuckey WJ Jr, Wilson HE (1969) Treatment for multiple myeloma. Combination chemotherapy with different melphalan dose regimens. JAMA 208:1680–1685

Alwall N (1947) Urethane and stilbamidine in multiple myeloma: report on two cases. Lancet 2:388–389

Arinkin MI (1929) Die intravitale Untersuchungsmethodik des Knochenmarks. Folia Haematologie 38:233–240

Barlogie B, Alexanian R, Dicke KA, Zagars G, Spitzer G, Jagannath S, Horwitz L (1987) High-dose chemoradiotherapy and autologous bone marrow transplantation for resistant multiple myeloma. Blood 70:869–872

Bayne-Jones S, Wilson DW (1922) Immunological reactions of Bence Jones proteins. II. Differences between Bence Jones proteins from various sources. Bull Johns Hopkins Hosp 33:119–125

Bayrd ED, Heck FJ (1947) Multiple myeloma: a review of eighty-three proved cases. JAMA 133:147–157

Bence Jones H (1842) On gravel, calculus and gout; chiefly an application of Professor Liebig's physiology to the prevention and cure of these diseases. Taylor & Walton, London

Bence Jones H (1845) On the state in which the uric acid exists in the urine. R. Kinder, London

Bence Jones H (1847) Chemical pathology. Lancet 2:88–92

Bence Jones H (1848) On the new substance occurring in the urine of a patient with mollities ossium. Philos Trans R Soc Lond 138:55–62

Bence Jones H (1870) The life and letters of Faraday. J. B. Lippincott, Philadelphia

Bence Jones H (1929) An autobiography (with elucidations at later dates by his son, A.B. Bence Jones). Crusha & Sons, London (privately printed)

Bergsagel DE, Sprague CC, Austin C, Griffith KM (1962) Evaluation of new chemotherapeutic

1

agents in the treatment of multiple myeloma. IV. L-Phenylalanine mustard (NSC-8806). Cancer Chemother Rep 21:87–99

Blokhin N, Larionov L, Perevodchikova N, Chebotareva L, Merkulova N (1958) Clinical experiences with sarcolysin in neoplastic diseases. Ann NY Acad Sci 68:1128–1132

Cajal SR (1896) Estudios histologicos sobre los tumores epiteliales. Rev Trimest Microgr 1:83–111

Capasso LL (2005) Antiquity of cancer. Int J Cancer 113:2–13

Case DC Jr, Lee DJ III, Clarkson BD (1977) Improved survival times in multiple myeloma treated with melphalan, prednisone, cyclophosphamide, vincristine and BCNU: M-2 protocol. Am J Med 63:897–903

Ciechanover A (1994) The ubiquitin-proteasome proteolytic pathway. Cell 79:13–21

D'Amato RJ, Loughnan MS, Flynn E, Folkman J (1994) Thalidomide is an inhibitor of angiogenesis. Proc Natl Acad Sci USA 91:4082–4085

Day WH (1870) On the hypophosphites of iron, quinine, and strychnia in cases of general debility and nervous exhaustion. Trans Clin Soc Lond 3:1–7

Dimopoulos M, Spencer A, Attal M, Prince HM, Harousseau JL, Dmoszynska A, San Miguel J, Hellmann A, Facon T, Foa R, Corso A, Masliak Z, Olesnyckyj M, Yu Z, Patin J, Zeldis JB, Knight RD (2007) Lenalidomide plus dexamethasone for relapsed or refractory multiple myeloma. N Engl J Med 357:2123–2132

Edelman GM, Gally JA (1962) The nature of Bence-Jones proteins. Chemical similarities to polypetide chains of myeloma globulins and normal gamma-globulins. J Exp Med 116:207–227

Fefer A, Cheever MA, Greenberg PD (1986) Identical-twin (syngeneic) marrow transplantation for hematologic cancers. J Natl Cancer Inst 76:1269–1273

Felter HW, Lloyd JU (1898–1900) King's American dispensatory. Ohio Valley Co, Cincinatti

Fleischer R (1880) Ueber das Vorkommen des sogenannten Bence Jones' schen Eiweisskorpers im normalen Knochenmark. Arch Pathol Anat Physiol Klin Med 80:842–849

Gahrton G, Tura S, Flesch M, Gratwohl A, Gravett P, Lucarelli G, Michallet M, Reiffers J, Ringden O, van Lint MT et al (1987) Bone marrow transplantation in multiple myeloma: report from the European Cooperative Group for Bone Marrow Transplantation. Blood 69:1262–1264

Geschickter CF, Copeland MM (1928) Multiple myeloma. Arch Surg 16:807–863

Gestsdottir H, Eyjolfsson GI (2005) Myeloma in an archaeological skeleton from Hofstadir in Myvatnssveit. Laeknabladid 91:505–509

Grabar P, Williams CA (1953) Method permitting the combined study of the electrophoretic and the immunochemical properties of protein mixtures; application to blood serum. Biochim Biophys Acta 10:193–194

Grabstald H, Golbey R (1965) Clinical experiences with thalidomide in patients with cancer. Clin Pharmacol Ther 6:298–302

Hanna F (2005) Multiple myelomas in cats. J Feline Med Surg 7:275–287

Harley JB, Ramanan SV, Kim I, Thiagarajan PV, Chen JH, Gomez R, Koppel D, Hyde F, Gustke S, Krall J (1972) The cyclic use of multiple alkylating agents in multiple myeloma. W V Med J 68:1–3

Harley JB, Pajak TF, McIntyre OR, Kochwa S, Cooper MR, Coleman M, Cuttner J (1979) Improved survival of increased-risk myeloma patients on combined triple-alkylating-agent therapy: a study of the CALGB. Blood 54:13–22

Heller JD (1846) Die mikroscopisch-chemisch-pathologische untersuchung. Braumuller & Seidel, Vienna

Heremans JF (1959) Immunochemical studies on protein pathology. The immunoglobulin concept. Clin Chim Acta 4:639–646

Herrick JB, Hektoen L (1894) Myeloma: report of a case. Med News, Philadelphia 65:239–242

Hideshima T, Richardson P, Chauhan D, Palombella VJ, Elliott PJ, Adams J, Anderson KC (2001) The proteasome inhibitor PS-341 inhibits growth, induces apoptosis, and overcomes drug resistance in human multiple myeloma cells. Cancer Res 61:3071–3076

Holland JR, Hosley H, Scharlau C, Carbone PP, Frei E III, Brindley CO, Hall TC, Shnider BI, Gold GL, Lasagna L, Owens AH Jr, Miller SP (1966) A controlled trial of urethane treatment in multiple myeloma. Blood 27:328–342

Hoogstraten B, Sheehe PR, Cuttner J, Cooper T, Kyle RA, Oberfield RA, Townsend SR, Harley JB, Hayes DM, Costa G, Holland JF (1967) Melphalan in multiple myeloma. Blood 30:74–83

Ishizaka K, Ishizaka T, Hornbrook MM (1966) Physicochemical properties of reaginic antibody. V. correlation of reaginic activity with gamma-E-globulin antibody. J Urol 97:840–853

Kahler O (1889) Zur symptomatologie des multiplen myeloms: Beobachtung von Albumosurie. Prager Med Wochenschr (Prague) 14:45
Korngold L, Lipari R (1956) Multiple myeloma proteins. III. The antigenic relationship of Bence Jones proteins to normal gammaglobulin and multiple myeloma serum proteins. Cancer 9: 262–272
Kühne (1883) Ueber Hemialbumose im Harn. Z Biol 19:209–227
Kunkel HG, Tiselius A (1951) Electrophoresis of proteins on filter paper. J Gen Physiol 35: 89–118
Kyle RA (1978) Monoclonal gammopathy of undetermined significance. Natural history in 241 cases. Am J Med 64:814–826
Kyle RA (2000) Multiple myeloma: an odyssey of discovery. Br J Haematol 111:1035–1044
Kyle RA (2001) Henry Bence Jones — physician, chemist, scientist and biographer: a man for all seasons. Br J Haematol 115:13–18
Lee BJ, Sahakian G, Clarkson BD, Krakoff IH (1974) Proceedings: combination chemotherapy of multiple myeloma with alkeran, cytoxan, vincristine, prednisone, and BCNU. Cancer 33: 533–538
Lenz W (1962) Thalidomide and congenital abnormalities. Lancet 1:45
Lerner AB, Watson CJ (1947) Studies of cryoglobulins; unusual purpura associated with the presence of a high concentration of cryoglobulin (cold precipitable serum globulin). Am J Med Sci 214:410–415
Longsworth AB, Shedlovsky T, MacInnes DA (1939) Electrophoretic patterns of normal and pathological human blood serum and plasma. J Exp Med 70:399–413
Macintyre W (1850) Case of mollities and fragilitas ossium, accompanied with urine strongly charged with animal matter. Med Chir Trans 33:211–232
Marschalko T (1895) Ueber die sogenannten plasmazellen, ein Beitrage zur Kenntniss der Herkunft der entzundlichen infiltrationszellen. Arch Dermatol Syph 30:241
Mass RE (1962) A comparison of the effect of prednisone and a placebo in the treatment of multiple myeloma. Cancer Chemother Rep 16:257–259
McIntyre OR, Pajak TF, Kyle RA, Cornwell GG, Leone L (1985) Response rate and survival in myeloma patients receiving prednisone alone. Med Pediatr Oncol 13(5):239–243
McElwain TJ, Powles RL (1983) High-dose intravenous melphalan for plasma-cell leukaemia and myeloma. Lancet 2:822–824
Morse D, Dailey RC, Bunn J (1974) Prehistoric multiple myeloma. Bull New York Acad Med 50:447–458
Myeloma Trialists' Collaborative Group (1998) Combination chemotherapy versus melphalan plus prednisone as treatment for multiple myeloma: an overview of 6,633 patients from 27 randomized trials. J Clin Oncol 16:3832–3842
Nerlich AG, Rohrbach H, Bachmeier B, Zink A (2006) Malignant tumors in two ancient populations: an approach to historical tumor epidemiology. Oncol Rep 16:197–202
Nothnagel H (1893) Hofrath Otto Kahler. Wien Klin Wochenschr (Wien) 6:79–80
Obituary (1873). Henry Bence Jones, M.D., F.R.C.P., F.R.S. Med Times Gaz 1:505
Olson KB, Hall TC, Horton J, Khung CL, Hosley HF (1965) Thalidomide (N-Phthaloylglutamimide) in the treatment of advanced cancer. Clin Pharmacol Ther 6:292–297
Orlowski RZ, Eswara JR, Lafond-Walker A, Grever MR, Orlowski M, Dang CV (1998) Tumor growth inhibition induced in a murine model of human Burkitt's lymphoma by a proteasome inhibitor. Cancer Res 58:4342–4348
Orlowski RZ, Stinchcombe TE, Mitchell BS, Shea TC, Baldwin AS, Stahl S, Adams J, Esseltine DL, Elliott PJ, Pien CS, Guerciolini R, Anderson JK, Depcik-Smith ND, Bhagat R, Lehman MJ, Novick SC, O'Connor OA, Soignet SL (2002) Phase I trial of the proteasome inhibitor PS-341 in patients with refractory hematologic malignancies. J Clin Oncol 20:4420–4427
Osserman EF, DiRe LB, DiRe J, Sherman WH, Hersman JA, Storb R (1982) Identical twin marrow transplantation in multiple myeloma. Acta Haematol 68:215–223
Perlzweig WA, Delrue G, Geschicter C (1928) Hyperproteinemia associated with multiple myelomas: report of an unusual case. JAMA 90:755–757
Peters GA, Horton BT (1941) Allergic purpura with special reference to hypersensitiveness to cold. Mayo Clin Proc 16:631–636
Putnam FW (1993) Henry Bence Jones: the best chemical doctor in London. Perspect Biol Med 36:565–579
Rajkumar SV, Hayman SR, Lacy MQ, Dispenzieri A, Geyer SM, Kabat B, Zeldenrust SR, Kumar S,

1

Greipp PR, Fonseca R, Lust JA, Russell SJ, Kyle RA, Witzig TE, Gertz MA (2005) Combination therapy with lenalidomide plus dexamethasone (Rev/Dex) for newly diagnosed myeloma. Blood 106:4050–4053

Richardson PG, Schlossman RL, Weller E, Hideshima T, Mitsiades C, Davies F, LeBlanc R, Catley LP, Doss D, Kelly K, McKenney M, Mechlowicz J, Freeman A, Deocampo R, Rich R, Ryoo JJ, Chauhan D, Balinski K, Zeldis J, Anderson KC (2002) Immunomodulatory drug CC-5013 overcomes drug resistance and is well tolerated in patients with relapsed multiple myeloma. Blood 100:3063–3067

Richardson PG, Barlogie B, Berenson J, Singhal S, Jagannath S, Irwin D, Rajkumar SV, Srkalovic G, Alsina M, Alexanian R, Siegel D, Orlowski RZ, Kuter D, Limentani SA, Lee S, Hideshima T, Esseltine DL, Kauffman M, Adams J, Schenkein DP, Anderson KC (2003) A phase 2 study of bortezomib in relapsed, refractory myeloma. N Engl J Med 348:2609–2617 [see comment]

Richardson PG, Sonneveld P, Schuster MW, Irwin D, Stadtmauer EA, Facon T, Harousseau JL, Ben-Yehuda D, Lonial S, Goldschmidt H, Reece D, San-Miguel JF, Blade J, Boccadoro M, Cavenagh J, Dalton WS, Boral AL, Esseltine DL, Porter JB, Schenkein D, Anderson KC (2005) Bortezomib or high-dose dexamethasone for relapsed multiple myeloma. N Engl J Med 352:2487–2498

Richardson PG, Blood E, Mitsiades CS, Jagannath S, Zeldenrust SR, Alsina M, Schlossman RL, Rajkumar SV, Desikan KR, Hideshima T, Munshi NC, Kelly-Colson K, Doss D, McKenney ML, Gorelik S, Warren D, Freeman A, Rich R, Wu A, Olesnyckyj M, Wride K, Dalton WS, Zeldis J, Knight R, Weller E, Anderson KC (2006) A randomized phase 2 study of lenalidomide therapy for patients with relapsed or relapsed and refractory multiple myeloma. Blood 108:3458–3464

Rosenbloom J (1919) An appreciation of Henry Bence Jones, M.D., F.R.S. (1814-1873). Ann Med Hist 2:262–264

Rosenfeld L (1987) Henry Bence Jones (1813–1873): the best "chemical doctor" in London. Clin Chem 33:1687–1692

Rosenthal N, Vogel P (1938) Value of the sternal puncture in the diagnosis of multiple myeloma. Mt Sinai J Med 4:1001–1019

Rothschild BM, Hershkovitz I, Dutour O (1998) Clues potentially distinguishing lytic lesions of multiple myeloma from those of metastatic carcinoma. Am J Phys Anthropol 105:241–250

Rowe DS, Fahey JL (1965) A new class of human immunoglobulins. I. A unique myeloma protein. J Exp Med 121:171–184

Salmon SE, Shadduck RK, Schilling A (1967) Intermittent high-dose prednisone (NSC-10023) therapy for multiple myeloma. Cancer Chemother Rep 51:179–187

Singhal S, Mehta J, Desikan R, Ayers D, Roberson P, Eddlemon P, Munshi N, Anaissie E, Wilson C, Dhodapkar M, Zeddis J, Barlogie B (1999) Antitumor activity of thalidomide in refractory multiple myeloma. N Engl J Med 341:1565–1571 [see comment] [erratum appears in N Engl J Med 3 Feb 2000; 342(5):364]

Solly S (1844) Remarks on the pathology of mollities ossium with cases. Med Chir Trans 27:435–461

Steensma DP, Kyle RA (2007) A history of the kidney in plasma cell disorders. Contrib Nephrol 153:5–24

Steinbock T (1976) Paleopathological diagnosis and interpretation. CC Thomas, Springfield

Stephens JL (1994) Arrowroot — *Maranta arundinacea L.* In: Fact Sheet HS-542. A series of the Horticultural Sciences Department, Florida Cooperative Extension Service, Institute of Food and Agricultural Services, University of Florida, Gainsville

Thomas ED, Lochte HL Jr, Lu WC, Ferrebee JW (1957) Intravenous infusion of bone marrow in patients receiving radiation and chemotherapy. N Engl J Med 257:491–496

Tiselius A (1937a) Electrophoresis of serum globulin. II. Electrophoretic analysis of normal and immune sera. Biochem J 31:1464–1477

Tiselius A (1937b) A new apparatus for electrophoretic analysis of colloidal mixtures. T Faraday Soc 33:524

Tiselius A, Kabat EA (1939) Electrophoretic study of immune sera and purified antibody preparation. J Exp Med 69:119–131

von Behring EA, Kisato S (1890) Ueber das Zustandekommen der Diphtherie-Immunitat und der Tetanus-Immunitat bei Theieren. Dtsch Med Wochenschr 49:1113–1114

Waldenstrom J (1960–1961) Studies on conditions associated with disturbed gamma globulin formation (gammopathies). Harvey Lect 56:211–231

Waldeyer W (1875) Ueber bindegewebszellen. Arch Microbiol Anat 11:176–194

Weber H (1867) Mollities ossium, doubtful whether carcinomatous or syphilitic. Trans Pathol Soc Lond 23:186–187

Weber FP (1898) General lymphadenomatosis of bones, one form of 'multiple myeloma'. J Pathol 5:59–64

Weber FP, Hutchinson R, Macleod JJR (1903) Multiple myeloma (myelomatosis), with Bence-Jones protein in the urine (myelopathic albumosuria of Bradshaw, Kahler's disease). Am J Med Sci 126:644–665

Weber DM, Chen C, Niesvizky R, Wang M, Belch A, Stadtmauer EA, Siegel D, Borrello I, Rajkumar SV, Chanan-Khan AA, Lonial S, Yu Z, Patin J, Olesnyckyj M, Zeldis JB, Knight RD (2007) Lenalidomide plus dexamethasone for relapsed multiple myeloma in North America. N Engl J Med 357:2133–2142

Wells C (1964) Two mediaeval cases of malignant disease. BMJ 1:1611–1612

Wintrobe MM, Buell MV (1933) Hyperproteinemia associated with multiple myeloma, with report of a case in which an extraordinary hyperproteinemia was associated with thrombosis of the retinal veins and symptoms suggesting Raynaud's disease. Bull Johns Hopkins Hosp 52:156–165

Wright JH (1900) A case of multiple myeloma. Trans Assoc Am Physician 15:137–147

Zink A, Rohrbach H, Szeimies U, Hagedorn HG, Haas CJ, Weyss C, Bachmeier B, Nerlich AG (1999) Malignant tumors in an ancient Egyptian population. Anticancer Res 19:4273–4277

Epidemiology of Multiple Myeloma

2

Nikolaus Becker

Contents

N. Becker
Division of Cancer Epidemiology,
German Cancer Research Center,
Im Neuenheimer Feld 581, D-69120
Heidelberg, Germany
e-mail: n.becker@dkfz.de

Abstract Multiple myelomas are a less frequent cancer site among both sexes. On a worldwide scale, it is estimated that about 86 000 incident cases occur annually, accounting for about 0.8% of all new cancer cases. About 63 000 subjects are reported to die from the disease each year, accounting for 0.9% of all cancer deaths. Geographically, the frequency is very unevenly distributed in the world with the highest incidence in the industrialised regions of Australia / New Zealand, Europe and North America. Incidence and mortality seem to be stable in Asian countries and to increase slowly over the decades among whites in the western countries. The etiology is poorly understood. This depends partly upon the fact that the risk factors which play a major role for malignant diseases in general, such as tobacco consumption and diet have not been found strongly involved into multiple myeloma etiology. Nevertheless, some consistency seems to be in the findings about a risk elevation with obesity and a slightly decreased risk with high fruit consumption. Despite some contradicting results, indications to a role of ionising radiation persist. Finally, infections with HIV and hepatitis C virus appear related to an elevated multiple myeloma risk. Currently, large efforts are undertaken to unravel the etiology of malignant lymphoma including those of multiple myeloma.

T. Moehler and H. Goldschmidt (eds.), *Multiple Myeloma*,
Recent Results in Cancer Research 183, DOI: 10.1007/978-3-540-85772-3_2,

2.1 Descriptive Epidemiology

Multiple myelomas are a less frequent cancer site among both sexes. On a worldwide scale, it is estimated that about 86,000 incident cases occur annually (47,000 males and 39,000 females), accounting for about 0.8% of all new cancer cases. About 63,000 subjects are reported to die from the disease each year (33,000 males and 30,000 females), accounting for 0.9% of all cancer deaths (Parkin et al. 2005). In terms of age-standardized rates, the annual incidence rates amount to 1.7 per 100,000 in males and 1.2 in females, and the mortality rates to 1.2 (males) and 0.9 (females). Among the hematological malignancies, the proportion of multiple myelomas ranges in a magnitude of 15–20% (Devesa et al. 1992; Becker et al. 2007).

Geographically, the frequency is very unevenly distributed in the world with the highest incidence in the industrialized regions of Australia/New Zealand, Europe, and North America (Fig. 2.1). The ethnic comparison within the population of the USA shows an almost doubled occurrence of multiple myeloma among the blacks compared to the whites, while people of Asian origin, especially Chinese and Japanese, experience a much lower incidence (Coleman et al. 2008; Parkin et al. 2005).

Incidence and mortality seem to be stable in Asian countries and to increase slowly over the decades among whites in the western countries and blacks in the USA (see Fig. 2.2). The rates and trends for the Asian immigrants into the USA resemble those of the respective countries of origin (Hirabayashi and Katanoda 2008).

The reasons for these differences and the increasing trend among the whites in the western countries are unknown.

The average 5-year survival is about 15–20% with a wide range of survival between some few years to 10 years or more.

2.2 Etiology

The etiology of multiple myeloma is poorly understood. This depends partly upon the low frequency of the disease which makes its investigation difficult; and it partly depends upon the fact that the risk factors which play a major role for malignant diseases in general, such as tobacco consumption and diet (see Wynder and Gori 1977, Doll and Peto 1981 or Harvard Report on Cancer Prevention 1996), have not been found obviously involved in multiple myeloma etiology. However, major efforts are currently undertaken to unravel the etiology of hematological malignancies in general and of multiple myeloma in particular (Boffetta et al. 2007).

2.2.1 Tobacco

In most of the studies which investigated a potential association to multiple myeloma, no risk increase has been found (Alexander et al. 2007). Nevertheless, in a more recent (Nieters et al. 2006a) and a few of the older studies cited in Alexander et al., an elevated risk was observed (RR=2.4 in males, RR=2.9 in females for current smoker, respectively) so that the matter appears to still be unresolved. The study of Nieters et al. indicated that the latency between tobacco consumption and occurrence of hematological malignancies might be particularly long, making the confirmation of an association difficult. On the other hand, the recent analysis of the large European Prospective Investigation

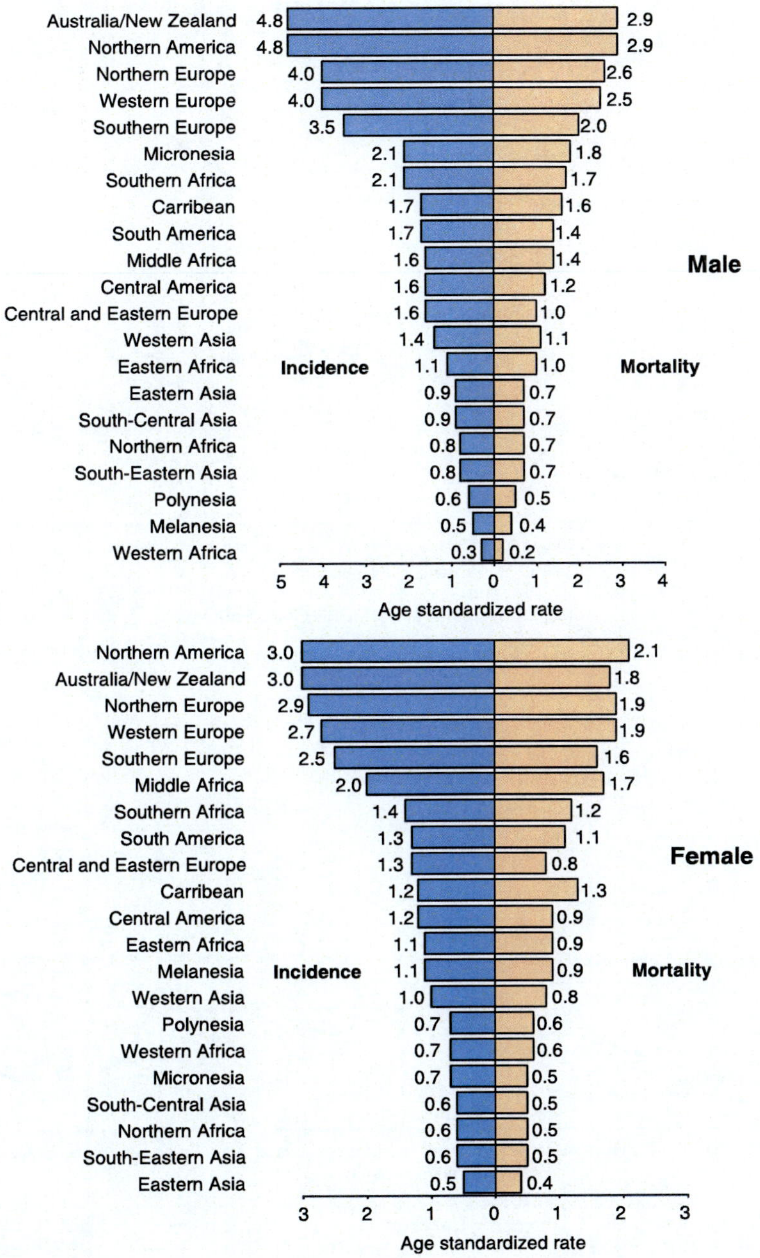

Fig. 2.1 Incidence and mortality rates for multiple myeloma. Rates are age-standardized with world standard as reference and given per 100,000 (Parkin et al. 2005)

2

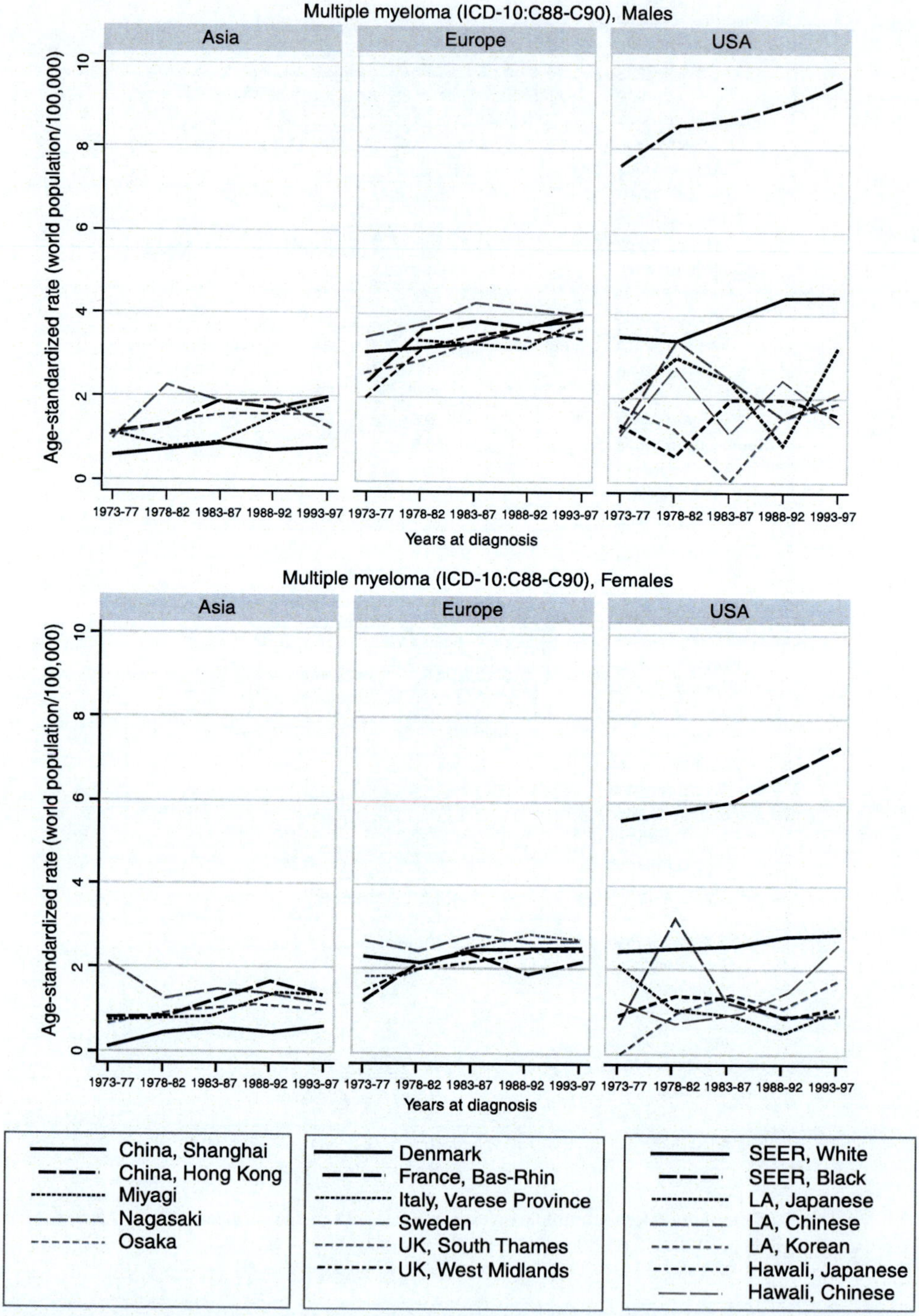

Fig. 2.2 Incidence of multiple myeloma in different parts of the world and different ethnic groups within the USA

into Cancer and Nutrition EPIC could not confirm this notion (Nieters et al. 2008). Thus, the currently available data strongly suggest that smoking is, if at all, at most a marginal risk factor for multiple myeloma.

2.2.2 Alcohol

Similarly, most investigations about the role of alcohol consumption reported a null result, only one an elevated risk in a particular combination of alcoholic beverages and two a decreased risk (Alexander et al. 2007). However, even those recent studies which reported a decreased relative risk with alcohol consumption for lymphoma in general could not observe this effect in multiple myeloma (Nieters et al. 2006a). Thus, also for alcohol consumption, the currently available data do not suggest a relevant contribution to multiple myeloma etiology.

2.2.3 Diet

A multitude of nutritional epidemiologic studies carried out over the past decades suggests divergent effects of different food groups on carcinogenesis. Thus, studies are usually focused on the respective food groups such as fruits and vegetable, meat, fish, etc. whose effects seem to range from potentially protective effects (e.g., high consumption of fruits and vegetable) for some cancer sites to risk elevations (high consumption of specified types of meat).

For multiple myeloma, several studies reported a decreased relative risk with a high consumption of fruits and vegetable (Tavani et al. 1997; Brown et al. 2001; Valjinac et al. 2003) which was confirmed by a recent evaluation of EPIC (Rohrmann et al. 2007). In this evaluation, an effect was seen for fruits, especially citrus fruits, but not for vegetable consumption. On the other hand, previous reports found inverse associations also for high vegetable consumption (see Alexander et al. 2007).

For meat consumption, a current, yet unpublished analysis of EPIC data provided overall a null result which is consistent with previous findings (see Alexander et al. 2007), but some indication to a potentially elevated relative risk for higher intake of chicken meat (S. Rohrmann 2009 personal communication).

Inconsistent results were reported from several studies on fish consumption from which several showed a decreased relative risk while a few also found risk increases (Alexander et al. 2007).

Thus, the current data on effects of diet on multiple myeloma are inconclusive, whereby the results on high intake of fruits and vegetable indicate the highest potential of a true, and potentially protective, effect.

2.2.4 Obesity

Elevated relative risks for obese subjects were reported from several epidemiologic studies, mainly case-control studies (Alexander et al. 2007; Bergström et al. 2001; Larsson and Wolk 2007). Though the recent evaluation of EPIC on body height and weight could not confirm an association to obesity or body fatness (Britton et al. 2008), with other prospective studies, an association could be confirmed (Birmann et al. 2001; Reeves et al. 2007). In the latter cohorts, the relative risk appeared to increase with increasing body weight. Thus, for obesity, the consistency of reports on a risk-increasing effect is relatively high though not yet finally conclusive. Supportive for a true association may be the fact that obese subjects seem to have elevated IL-6 levels and bioavailability of insulin growth factor which appears also related to development of multiple myeloma and survival from the disease (Ge and Rudikoff 2000; Xu et al. 1997), seems also to be affected by obesity (Bianchini et al. 2002; see also Birman et al. 2007).

2.2.5 Physical Activity

Physical activity is considered an established protective factor for several cancer sites (IARC 2002), but has not yet been investigated thoroughly for multiple myeloma. However, Birman et al. (2007) reported from three studies on obesity which also took physical activity into account. They did not observe any deviation of risk from unity (Blair et al. 2005; Oh et al. 2005; Pan et al. 2004). The results of Birman et al. (2007) were consistent to those null results.

2.2.6 Hormonal Factors

One reason for taking hormonal factors into account is that the risk for getting the disease is consistently higher in males than in females. Hormonal factors may affect this gender difference. Another reason is that lifestyle factors, such as obesity, may modulate the hormonal status of subjects (see above kaaks and Lukanova 2002).

Quite a number of studies referenced in Alexander et al. (2007) examined hormone replacement therapy (HRT), age at first birth, and number of pregnancies, the latter factors which have been found in several studies related to other lymphoma entities. None of them showed significant associations to multiple myeloma.

2.2.7 Environment and Occupation

Occupational settings are frequently used in epidemiology to investigate both occupational cancer risks as well as potential environmental hazards. Exposures which occur in the environment as well as in industry can in many instances better be investigated in the industrial environment since the exposures are frequently higher, can better be estimated or measured, and may have a longer and again better assessable duration during lifetime. Obtained results may be extrapolated by quantitative risk modeling to the exposure levels found in environmental settings.

A multitude of occupational-epidemiologic studies provided results for multiple myeloma and have been reviewed in Alexander et al. (2007). Particularly, exposures to pesticides, solvents, especially benzene, other chemicals, and hair dyes have been addressed. Though some studies reported increased relative risks and some other studies reported decreased relative risks, the overall balance appeared inconsistent and did not provide evidence for a major role of these agents on multiple myeloma etiology. The results for radiation will be presented separately below.

On the other hand, it must clearly be stated that many of the studies were based on small numbers which make – as already mentioned above – it difficult to detect moderate or late occurring hazards. Thus, further research will be needed and will move the inconclusive balance in the one or other direction. In this sense, a recent study of Costantini et al. (2008) reported an increased risk of multiple myeloma after benzene exposure and long latency.

2.2.8 Ionizing Radiation

Ionizing radiation was long considered an established risk factor for multiple myeloma based on the data of the atomic-bomb survivor studies (Alexander et al. 2007). However, later evaluations of these data taking a longer follow-up into account could not confirm the previous reports (Preston et al. 1994) so that the matter is open again. Preston et al. drew a parallel to CLL which are known to be unrelated to ionizing radiation and which have the origin from terminally differentiated B lymphocytes in common with multiple myeloma, suggesting biological plausibility that also multiple myeloma may be unrelated to ionizing radiation.

Other exposures to ionizing radiation may occur in medical applications in the context of diagnostic radiological imaging or radiotherapy for both patients as well as medical staff. None of these circumstances seemed to provide an excess risk for multiple myeloma.

A quite different setting may occur by occupational low-level radiation in nuclear industry since these exposures may be long-lasting in contrast to the shorter and high-dose atomic-bomb exposure. Though the overall balance about the existing studies appears also contradictorily, a recent carefully conducted large study provided indications to a statistically significant overall cancer risk and elevated excess risks for specified cancer sites including multiple myeloma. Nevertheless, the result for multiple myeloma was only marginally statistically significant and needs further confirmation (Cardis et al. 2007).

Finally, the effect of a chronic exposure to alpha-radiation could be investigated in the context of iatrogenically induced cancer death by administration of Thorotrast. Thorotrast was the brand name of a stabilized colloidal solution of thorium dioxide which was used as an X-ray contrast medium between 1930 and 1950. The administration of the medium led to a lifelong chronic α-particle irradiation by thorium decay products in the organs of deposition. Two of the overall four large cohort studies reported an increased myeloma risk among the exposed subjects (Visfeldt et al. 1995; Becker et al. 2008).

2.2.9 Inheritance

More consistent than for other candidate risk factors appear the data on a potential familial aggregation of multiple myeloma. Based on the Swedish family–cancer database, Hemminki et al. (2004) observed an elevated relative risk among offsprings of parents with a diagnosis of multiple myeloma. Several other studies reported more generally an increased risk in first-degree relatives of subjects with a diagnosis of multiple myeloma or hematopoietic malignancies in general (Alexander et al. 2007). The risk elevation was not found in second- or third-degree relatives and not for cancers other than of the hematopoietic system.

2.2.10 Medical History, Viruses, Immunological Conditions

Since lymphomas are malignancies of cells of the immune system, it is suggestive to look for associations with other immunological disorders. Thus, for B-cell lymphoma excluding multiple myeloma, previous studies reported relatively consistently an inverse association to atopic diseases. For multiple myeloma, however, the relationship is much more inconsistent. Alexander et al. (2007) summarized studies which observed an inverse association, but also studies with null results or even elevated relative risks in subjects with allergies. Thus, though more recent studies supported again the notion of an inverse association (Becker et al. 2004, 2007), the matter appears still unresolved.

Correspondingly, the results on associations with autoimmune diseases, childhood, or adult infections are inconclusive with two important exceptions: An elevated relative risk was shown in HIV-infected subjects (Goedert et al. 1998; Grulich et al. 1999) and among hepatitis C virus–infected subjects. The latter association was significant in a Swedish cohort (Duberg et al. 2005), and nonsignificant in a European case-control study (Nieters et al. 2006b).

2.3 Summary

In conclusion, most of the so far examined factors provided either null or inconsistent results (see Table 2.1). Some consistency seems to be in the findings about a risk elevation with obesity

2

Table 2.1 Summary of associations between established or suspected risk factors and multiple myeloma (Alexander et al. 2007)

Factor	Approximate range of observed associations	Comparison
Accepted risk factors		
Increasing age	12–16	<65 vs. ≥65
Male gender	1.5	Males vs. females
Black race	2–3	Black race vs. white race
Positive family history	1.5–5	Positive family history of MM or LHC in a first-degree relative with MM or LHC
MGUS	25+	MGUS positive vs. MGUS negative
Possible risk factors		
Obesity	1.2–2	Obese (BMI ≥ vs. normal range BMI) (BMI < 25)
Low fish consumption	1.2–1.7	Low vs. high fish consumption
Low green vegetable consumption	1.1–2.5	Low vs. high green vegetable consumption
AIDS	4–12	AIDS diagnosis vs. no AIDS diagnosis
Herpes zoster/shingles	1.2–2.6	History of infection vs. no history of infection
Epidemiologic data inconsistent		
Hair dye use		
Overall exposure	0.8–1.5	Any exposure vs. never exposed
Permanent hair dye	0,6–1.9	Permanent hair dye exposure vs. never exposed
Light hair dye coloring	0.9–1.3	Light hair dye vs. never exposed
Dark hair dye coloring	1.3–3	Dark hair dye exposure vs. never exposed
Farming occupation	1.1–1.2	Farmers vs. nonfarmers[a]
Wood dust or wood exposures	0.7–2.6	Wood dust or wood exposure vs. no exposure
Chronic immune stimulation conditions and/or vaccinations for such conditions[b]	0.7–2	History of chronic immune stimulation condition and/or vaccination vs. no exposure
Autoimmune disease (excluding AIDS		
General category	0.7–2	History of any autoimmune disease vs. no history of autoimmune disease
Rheumatoid arthritis	0.7–2.3	History of rheumatoid arthritis vs. no history of rheumatoid arthritis
Do not appear to be risk factors		
Smoking	0.8–1.3	Current smokers vs. never smokers
Alcohol	0.4–1.5	Alcohol consumption vs. no consumption
Pesticides[c]	0.8–1.4	Pesticide exposure vs. no
Organic solvents		
Overall exposure[d]	0.6–1.5	Any organic solvent exposure vs. no exposure
Benzene	0.7–1.4	Benzene exposure vs. no exposure

(continued)

Table 2.1 (continued)

Factor	Approximate range of observed associations	Comparison
Trichlorethylene	0.8–1.4	Trichlorethylene exposure vs. no exposure
Radiation		Radiation exposure vs. no exposure
Nuclear workers	0.7–1.1	Asbestos exposure vs. no exposure
Occupational therapeutic or diagnostic	0.7–1.4	History of allergic conditions vs. no allergic conditions
Asbestos	0.5–3	
Allergic conditions	0.6–2	

[a]Findings based on meta-analyses of 12–32 studies

[b]Chronic immune stimulation conditions include influenza, polio, smallpox, and tetanus immunizations and a history of tuberculosis, scarlet fever or rheumatic fever

[c]Findings based on general categories of exposure to pesticides or herbicides including applicators and sprayers.

[d]Findings based on studies of petroleum workers, painters, benzene, trichloroethylene, styrene, and general categories of organic solvents

and a decreased risk with high fruit consumption. Some indications to a role of ionizing radiation persist. Finally, infections with HIV and hepatitis C appear related to an elevated multiple myeloma risk. Current worldwide coordinated research activities promise to promote knowledge about the etiology of the disease.

References

Alexander D, Mink PJ, Adam HO, Cole P, Mandel JS, Oken MM, Trichopoulos D (2007) Multiple myeloma: a review of the epidemiologic literature. Int J Cancer 120:40–61

Becker N, Deeg E, Nieters A (2004) Population-based study of lymphomas in Germany: rationale, study design and first results. Leuk Res 28:713–724

Becker N, de Sanjosé S, Nieters A, Maynadié M, Foretova L, Cocco PL, Staines A, Alvaro T, Vornanen M, Brennan P, Boffetta P (2007) Birth order, allergies and lymphoma risk: results of the European collaborative research project Epilymph. Leuk Res 31:1365–1372

Becker N, Liebermann D, Wesch H, van Kaick G (2008) Mortality among Thorotrast-exposed patients and an unexposed comparison group in the German Thorotrast study. Eur J Cancer 44(9):1259–1268

Bergström A, Pisani P, Tenet V, Wolk A, Adami HO (2001) Overweight as an avoidable cause of cancer in Europe. Int J Cancer 91:421–430

Bianchini F, Kaaks R, Vainio H (2002) Weight control and physical activity in cancer prevention. Obes Rev 3:5–8

Birmann BM, Giovannucci E, Rosner B, Anderson KC, Colditz GA (2007) Body mass index, physical activity, and risk of multiple myeloma. Cancer Epidemiol Biomarkers Prev 16:1474–1478

Blair CK, Cerhan JR, Folsom AR, Ross JA (2005) Anthropometric characteristics and risk of multiple myeloma. Epidemiology 16:691–694

Boffetta P, Amstrong B, Linet M, Kasten C, Cozen W, Hartge P (2007) Consortia in cancer epidemiology: lessons from InterLymph. Cancer Epidemiol Biomarkers Prev 16(2):197–199

Britton JA, Khan AE, Rohrmann S, Becker N, Linseisen J, Nieters A, Kaaks R, TjØnneland A, Haljær J, Tang Serverinsen M, Overvad K, Rischon T, Boeing H, Trichopoulou A, Kalapothaki V, Trichopoulos D, Mattiello A,

2

Tagliabue G, Sacerdote C, Peeters PHM, Bueno-de-Mesquita B, Ardanaz E, Navarro C, Jakszyn P, Altzibar JM, Hallmans G, Malmer B, Berglund G, Manjer J, Allen N, Key T, Bingham S, Besson H, Ferrari P, Jenab M, Boffetta P, Vineis P, Riboli E (2008) Anthropometric characteristics and non-Hodgkin's lymphoma and multiple myeloma risk in the European Prospective Investigation into Cancer and Nutrition (EPIC). Haematologica 93(11):1666–1677

Brown LM, Gridley G, Pottern LM, Baris D, Swanso CA, Silvermann DT, Hayes RB, Greenberg RS, Swanson GM, Schoenberg JB, Schwartz AG, Fraumeni JF, Jr. (2001) Diet and nutrition as risk factors for multiple myeloma among blacks and whites in the United States. Cancer Causes Control 12:117–125

Cardis E, Vrijheid M, Blettner M, Gilbert E, Hakama M, Hill C, Howe G, Kaldor J, Muirhead CR, Schubauer-Berigan M, Yoshimura T, Bermann F, Cowper G, Fix J, Hacker C, Heinmiller B, Marshall M, Thierry-Chef I, Utterback D, Ahn Y-O, Amoros E, Ashmore P, Auvinen A, Bae J-M, Bernar J, Biau A, Cambalot E, Deboodt P, Diez Sacristan A, Eklöf M, Engels H, Engholm G, Gulis G, Habib RR, Holan K, Hyvonen H, Kerekes A, Kurtinaitis J, Malker H, Martuzzi M, Mastauskas A, Monnet A, Moser M, Pearce MS, Richardson DB, Rodriguez-Artalejo F, Rogel A, Tardy H, Telle-Lamberton M, Turai I, Usel M, Veress K (2007) Radiation Res 167:396–416

Coleman EA, Senner JW, Edwards BK (2008) Does multiple myeloma incidence vary by geographic area? J Ark Med Soc 105(4):89–91

Costantini AS, Benvenuti A, Vineis P, Kriebel D, Tumino R, Ramazzotti V, Rodella S, Stagnaro E, Crosignani P, Amadori D, Mirabelli D, Sommani L, Belletti I, Troschel L, Romea L, Miceli G, Tozzi GA, Mendico I, Maltoni SA, Miligi L (2008) Risk of leukemia and multiple myeloma associated with exposure to benzene and other organic solvents: Evidence from the Italian multicenter case-control study. Am J of Industrial Med 51: 803–811

Devesa SS, Fears T (1992) Non-Hodgkin´s Lymphoma time trends: United States and international data. Cancer Res (Suppl) 52:5432s–5440s

Doll R, Peto R (1981) The causes of cancer. J Natl Cancer Inst 66:1191–1308

Duberg AS, Nordstrom M, Torner A, Reichard O, Strauss R, Janzon R, Black E, Ekdahl K (2005) Non-Hodgkin´s lymphoma and other nonhepatic malignanies in Swedish patients with hepatitis C virus infection. Hepatology 41:652–659

Ge NL, Rudikoff S (2000) Insulin-like growth factor I is a dual effector of multiple myeloma cell growth. Blood 96:2856–2861

Goedert JJ, Cote TR, Virgo P, Scoppa SM, Kingma DW, Gail MH, Jaffe ES, Biggar RJ (1998) Spectrum of AIDS-assoicated malignant disorders. Lancet 351:1833–1839

Grulich AE, Wan X, Law MG, Coates M, Kaldo JM (1999) Risk of cancer in people with AIDS. AIDS 13:839–843

Harvard Report on Cancer Prevention (1996) Volume 1: Causes of human cancer. Cancer Causes Control 7(Suppl 1):S55–S58

Hemminki K, Li X, Czene K (2004) Familial risk of cance: data for clinical counseling and cancer genetics. Int J Cancer 108:109–114

IARC (2002) IARC Handbooks of cancer prevention. Volume 6. Weight control and physical activity. IARC Press, Lyon

Kaaks R, Lukanova A (2002) Effects of weight control and physical activity in cancer prevention: role of endogenous hormone metabolism. Ann NY Acad Sci 963:268–281

Larsson SC, Wolk A (2007) Body mass index and risk of multiple myeloma: a meta-analysis. Int J Cancer 121:2512–2516

Nieters A, Deeg E, Becker N (2006a) Tobacco and alcohol consumption and risk of lymphoma: results of a population-based case-control study in Germany. Int J Cancer 118:422–430

Nieters A, Kallinowski B, Brennan P, Ott M, Maynadié M, Benavente Y, Foretova L, Cocco PL, Staines A, Vornanen M, Whitby D, Boffetta P, Becker N, de Sanjosé S (2006b) Hepatitis C and risk of lymphoma: results of the European multicenter case-control study EPILYMPH. Gastroenterology 131:1879–1886

Nieters A, Rohrmann S, Becker N, Linseisen J, Ruediger T, Overvad K, TjØnneland A, Ohlsen A, Allen NE, Travis RC, Bingham S, Khaw KT, Ardanaz E, Redondo ML, Basterrechea M, Martinez C, Tormo MJ, Rosso S, Tagliabue G, Masala G, Mattiello A, Tumino R, Boeing H, Bergmann M, Kaaks R, Trichopoulou A, Trichopoulos D, Peeters PH, Bueno-de-Mesquita B, Boffetta P, Brennan P, Ferrari P, Neasham D, Lund E, Berglund G, Manjer J, Hallmans G, Johansson I, Vineis P, Riboli E (2008) Smoking and lymphoma risk in the European prospective investigation into cancer and nutrition. Am J Epidemiol 167:1081–1089

Oh SW, Yoon YS, Shin SA (2005) Effects of excess weight on cancer incidences dependng on cancer sites and histologic findings among men: Korea National Health Insurance Corporation Study. J Clin Oncol 23:4742–4754

Pan SY, Johnson KC, Ugnat AM, Wen SW, Mao Y (2004) Association of obesity and cancer risk in Canada. Am J Epidemiol 195:259–268

Parkin M, Bray F, Ferlay J, Pisani P (2005) Global cancer statistics, 2002. CA Cancer J Clin 55:74–108

Preston DL, Kusumi S, Tomonaga M, Izumi S, Ron E, Kuramoto A, Kamada N, Dohy H, Matsui T, Nonaka H, Thompson DE, Soda M, Mabuchi K (1994) Cancer incidence in atomic bomb survivors. Part III: Leukemia, lymphoma and multiple myeloma, 1950–1987. Radiat Res 137:S68–S97

Reeves GK, Pirie K, Beral V, Green J, Spencer E, Bull D, Million Women Study Collaboration (2007) Cancer incidence and mortality in relation to body mass index in the Million Women study: cohort study. BMJ 335(7630):1134, Epub 6 Nov 2007

Rohrmann S, Becker N, Linseisen J, Nieters A, Rüdiger T, Raaschou-Nielsen O, Tjonneland A, Johnsen HE, Overvad K, Kaaks R, Bergmann MM, Boeing H, Benetou V, Psaltopoulou T, Trichopoulou A, Masala G, Mattiello A, Krogh V, Tumino R, van Gils CH, Peeters PHM, Bas Bueno-de-Mesquita H, Ros MM, Lund E, Ardanaz E, Chirlaque M-D, Jakszyn P, Larranaga N, Losada A, Martinez-Garcia C, Agren A, Hallmans G, Berglund G, Manjer J, Allen NE, Key TJ, Bingham S, Khaw KT, Slimani N, Ferrari P, Boffetta P, Norat T, Vineis P, Riboli E (2007) Fruit and vegetable consumption and lymphoma risk in the European Prospective Investigation into Cancer and Nutrition (EPIC). Cancer Causes Control 18: 537–549

Tavani A, Pregnolato A, Negri E, Franceschi S, Serraino D, Carbone A, La Vecchia C (1997) Diet and risk of lymphoid neoplasms and soft tissue sarcomas. Nutr Cancer 27:256–260

Valjinac HD, Pekmezovic TH, Adanja BJ, Marinkovic JM, Kanazir MS, Suvajdizic ND, Colovic MD (2003) Case-control study of multiple myeloma with special reference to diet as risk factor. Neoplasma 50:79–83

Visfeldt J, Andersson M (1995) Pathoanatomical aspects of malignant haematological disorders among Danish patients exposed to thorium dioxide. APMIS 103:29–36

Wynder EL, Gori GB (1977) Contribution of the environment to cancer incidence: an epidemiologic exercise. JNCI 58:825–832

Xu F, Gardner A, Tu Y, Michl P, Prager D, Lichtenstein A (1997) Multiple myeloma cells are protected against dexamethasone-included apoptosis by insulin-like growth factors. Br J Haematol 97:429–440

Part II

Pathophysiology

Molecular Pathogenesis of Multiple Myeloma: Chromosomal Aberrations, Changes in Gene Expression, Cytokine Networks, and the Bone Marrow Microenvironment

3

Bernard Klein, Anja Seckinger, Thomas Moehler, and Dirk Hose

Contents

D. Hose (✉)
Department of Medicine V,
University of Heidelberg,
Im Neuenheimer Feld 410, 69120 Heidelberg,
Germany and
National Center for Tumor Diseases, Im
Neuenheimer Feld 460, 69120
Heidelberg, Germany
e-mail: dirk.hose@med.uni-heidelberg.de

T. Moehler and H. Goldschmidt (eds.), *Multiple Myeloma*,
Recent Results in Cancer Research 183, DOI: 10.1007/978-3-540-85772-3_3,

3

Abstract This chapter focuses on two aspects of myeloma pathogenesis: (1) chromosomal aberrations and resulting changes in gene and protein expression with a special focus on growth and survival factors of malignant (and normal) plasma cells and (2) the remodeling of the bone marrow microenvironment induced by accumulating myeloma cells. We begin this chapter with a discussion of normal plasma cell generation, their survival, and a novel class of inhibitory factors. This is crucial for the understanding of multiple myeloma, as several abilities attributed to malignant plasma cells are already present in their normal counterpart, especially the production of survival factors and interaction with the bone marrow microenvironment (niche). The chapter closes with a new model of pathogenesis of myeloma.

3.1 Survival, Growth, and Inhibitory Factors of Normal Plasma Cells

3.1.1 Survival and Growth Factors of Normal Plasma Cells and Their Generation

Plasma cells are mostly located in the bone marrow where they represent 0.25% of bone marrow mononuclear cells. Generated in the lymph node, due to their rarity, their generation and biology are poorly understood despite extensive studies during the last 10 years (Batista and Harwood 2009; Allen et al. 2007a, b). Naïve B cells entering into lymph node through high endothelial venules are selected by the antigen in the germinal center reaction, yielding selection of B cells with high affinity immunoglobulins and differentiation into memory B cells ($CD20^{+}CD19^{+}CD27^{+}CD38^{-}$) and early plasmablasts ($CD20^{-}CD19^{+}CD27^{++}CD38^{++}$).

The differentiation of B cells into plasma cells involves profound molecular changes yielding a cell able to produce large amounts of immunoglobulins for a long time. Two sets of transcription factors that repress each other are involved in this process (Cobaleda et al. 2007; Calame 2008); see Fig. 3.1). *Activation-dependent induction of Blimp-1*: The guardian of B cell phenotype is PAX5, which induces B cell genes and represses genes as *PRDM1* and *XBP1*, whose gene products – Blimp-1 and XBP1 – are critical for plasma cell generation and survival. BCL6 in association with MTA3 maintains the B cell phenotype and proliferation, down-regulating *PRDM1* expression. In the germinal center, activation of B cells through B cell receptor (BCR), CD40, and/or Toll like receptor (TLR) results in up-regulation of IRF4, down-regulation of BCL6 protein expression, and loss of *PRDM1* repression. This results in down-regulation of *PAX5* and then up-regulation of *XBP1*. In the centrocyte region, stimulation by IL-10, IL-21, or IL-6 results in STAT3 activation yielding *PRDM1* overexpression (Ettinger et al. 2007; Schmidlin et al. 2009).

This results in the full engagement of B cell differentiation into plasmablasts, in particular with the switch from surface to cytoplasmic immunoglobulins, and induction of the unfold protein response driven by XBP1. The detailed hierarchy of this molecular regulation is not fully understood and still a challenging issue.

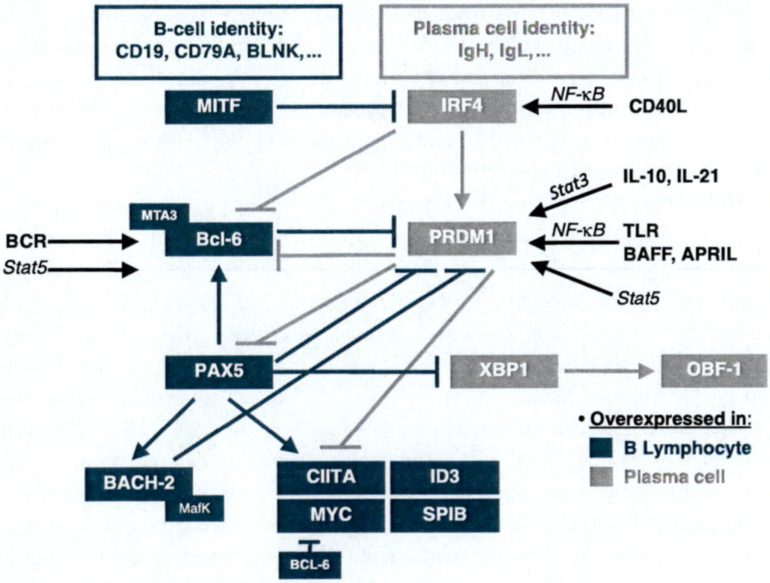

Fig. 3.1 *Plasma cell development.* Transcription factor network regulating B cell and plasma cell identity

Recent data suggest that PAX5 down-regulation and consecutive XBP1 up-regulation are the initial driving events in plasma cell generation independently of Blimp-1 expression (Kallies et al. 2007). Other data indicate a major role of IRF4 whose expression is triggered by NF-kB signaling (Saito et al. 2007).

Plasmablasts exit into peripheral blood and may survive for a short period only unless they are recruited into bone marrow, spleen, or mucosa-associated lymphoid tissues depending on their chemokine receptor expression (Arce et al. 2004; Gonzalez-Garcia et al. 2008; Mei et al. 2009). Expression of sphingosine 1 phosphate receptor 1 (S1P1) is important for the exit of lymph node plasmablasts into blood (Kabashima et al. 2006). In contact with their relevant niche, plasmablasts further differentiate into mature plasma cells that survive independently of antigen for several years yielding a long-term immunity. This explains why treatment with anti-CD20 antibody does not affect the level of circulating immunoglobulin that is insured by these long-term surviving plasma cells (DiLillo et al. 2008). The mechanisms of further differentiation of plasma cells and of homing are partly understood. Homing of plasmablasts into the bone marrow is driven in part by L selectin-induced rolling onto bone marrow endothelial cells, CXCR4 activation by CXCL12 produced by bone marrow stromal cells, as well as by VLA4 expression making adhesion to VCAM1^{+} bone marrow endothelial cells possible. Recruitment of plasmablasts into mucosa-associated lymphoma tissues is in part mediated by CCR10 expression, making recruitment through CCL28 produced in mucosa tissues possible (Kunkel and Butcher 2003).

These niches provide plasmablasts the factors to survive and further differentiate into long-living mature plasma cells (Tarlinton et al. 2008). CCR10 expressing IgA^{+} plasmablasts are mainly recruited to mucosa niche by the CCL28 chemokine (Kunkel and Butcher 2003). In the bone marrow, the plasma cell niche involves SDF-1 producing cells recruiting CXCR4^{+} plasmablasts and is shared by hematopoietic stem cells and pre-pro-B cells (Tokoyoda et al. 2004). The rarity of this niche explains the low amount of bone marrow plasma cells and is a matter of regulation of normal immunoglobulin production (Radbruch et al. 2006). "Young" plasma cells have to compete with the "old ones" to establish themselves in a niche (Odendahl et al. 2005). A hallmark of mature plasma cells is their large immunoglobulin secretion, a high expression of the syndecan-1 proteoglycan that is not expressed on B cells, and a lack of most B cell markers except CD19. These plasma cells also largely express CD38.

The intercellular communication signals that are critical to induce this B cell differentiation into plasmablastic cells and plasma cells are poorly known. Plasmablastic cells can be highly expanded in vivo in patients with acute or chronic inflammation. They comprise syndecan-1^{-} immature plasmablastic cells that can yield syndecan-1$^{\pm}$ plasmablastic cells (Jego et al. 1999).

We recently developed a three-step in vitro model of generation of polyclonal plasma cells starting from healthy donor's peripheral blood B cells (Jourdan et al. 2009; see Fig. 3.2). It involves a three-step and 10-day culture system comprising a 4-day step 1 to activate and amplify memory B cells using CD40 activation, TLR9 stimulation by CpG oligodeoxynucleotides (ODN) together with IL-2, IL-10, and IL-15. At day 4, the culture medium is removed and cells are cultured for 3 days with IL-2, IL-6, IL-10, and IL-15 to trigger plasmablastic differentiation (step 2), and in a final 3-day step 3 with IFN-α, IL-6, and IL-15 to trigger plasma cell differentiation. This model allows a better understanding of the mechanisms controlling survival of plasmablastic cells in the bone

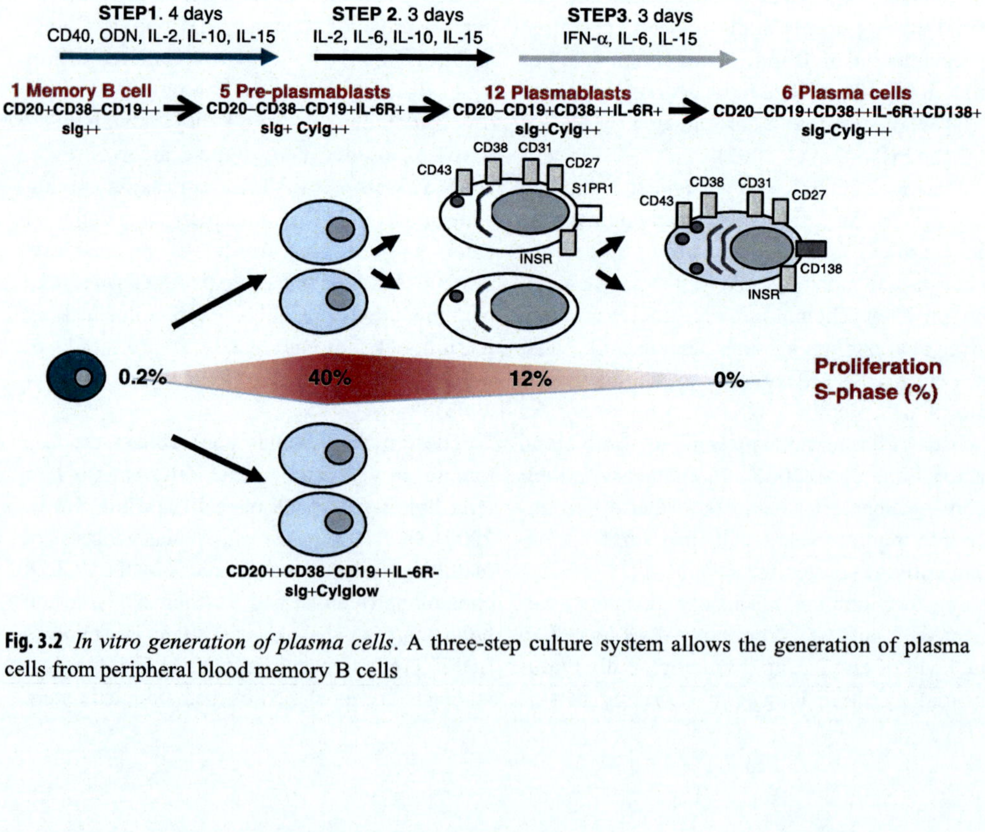

Fig. 3.2 *In vitro generation of plasma cells*. A three-step culture system allows the generation of plasma cells from peripheral blood memory B cells

marrow. A first requirement to induce plasma cell differentiation is the abrogation of CD40 stimulation. A second requirement is the activation of STAT3 through different cytokines as IL-10 and IL-6, yielding induction of *PRDM1*. A major role of IL-6 for the survival of plasmablasts from patients with reactive plasmacytosis was demonstrated by Jego et al. (1999). This property of IL-6 is not surprising since the IL-6 gene was initially cloned in 1988 as a B cell differentiation factor (Yamasaki et al. 1988). In addition, transgenic mice expressing an IL-6 gene driven by an Eμ promoter develop massive polyclonal plasmacytosis (Suematsu et al. 1989), whereas IL-6 knockout mice have a defect in the production of high affinity antibodies (Kopf et al. 1994). IL-21 is also a major cytokine driving plasma cell generation (Ozaki et al. 2002). For an overview of signal transduction pathways in normal and malignant plasma cells, see Fig. 3.3.

3.1.2 Inhibitory Factors Expressed by Normal Plasma Cells

Given the frequently long time from first diagnosis of early-stage plasma cell dyscrasias to overt myeloma and the mostly low proliferation rate of multiple myeloma cells (see below; Witzig et al. 1999), we hypothesize these to express a novel class of inhibitory factors of potential prognostic relevance. Due to their expression and ability to inhibit proliferation of myeloma and memory B cells (Ro et al. 2004; Kersten et al. 2005), bone morphogenic proteins (BMPs)

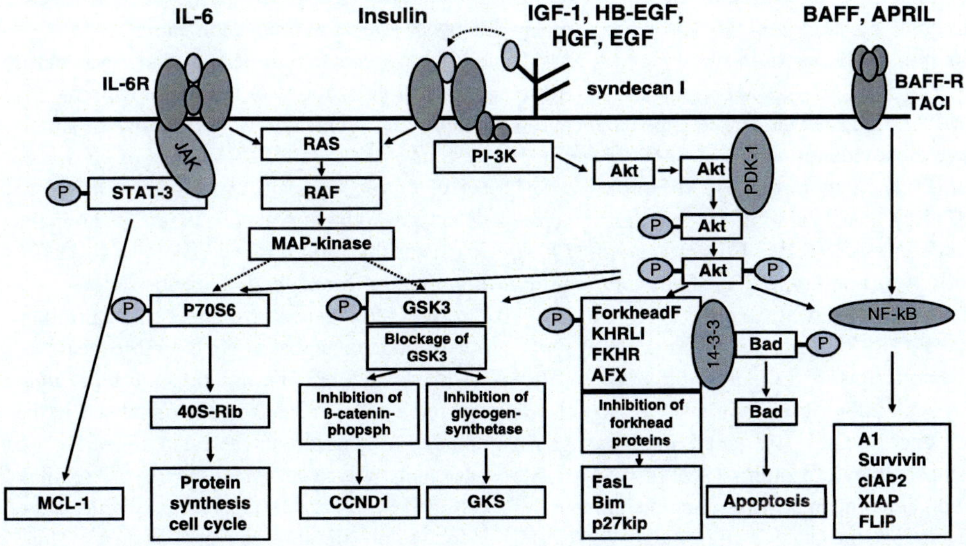

Fig. 3.3 *Signal transduction pathways in normal and malignant plasma cells*. The main signal transduction pathways in plasma cells comprise JAK/STAT signaling, MAPK-signaling, PI3K-signaling, and signaling via NF-kB. Syndecan-1 is a hallmark of normal and malignant plasma cells. It acts in concentration heparin-binding growth and survival factors (including IGF-1, HGF, BAFF, APRIL) at the cell surface and thus facilitates the interaction with the respective receptors. Insulin is a growth factor for normal plasma cells that acts via Insulin-R, and additionally an insulin/IGF1R hybrid receptor in malignant plasma cells. Inhibitory factors like BMP6 physiologically expressed by plasma cells act in terms of checks and balances on this network (not shown) (Modified from Klein et al. 2003)

represent possible candidates. Of these, BMP6 is the only BMP expressed by normal and malignant plasma cells (Seckinger et al. 2009; Zhan et al. 2002). Its expression is significantly lower in proliferating myeloma cells, myeloma cell lines, or plasmablasts. BMP6 significantly inhibits its proliferation of myeloma cell lines, survival of primary myeloma cells, and in vitro angiogenesis. High BMP6-expression in primary myeloma cell samples delineates significantly superior overall survival for patients undergoing high-dose chemotherapy independent of conventional prognostic factors (ISS-stage, beta-2-microglobulin; Seckinger et al. 2009). It likewise stimulates osteoblast differentiation (Ebisawa et al. 1999), osteoclast development (Wutzl et al. 2006), and bone formation (Cheng et al. 2003).

BMPs are members of the transforming growth factor-β superfamily, and act through binding to two different types of serine/threonine kinase receptors. Three type I receptors bind BMPs: activin-like kinase-2, (Alk-2, ACVR1), -3 (Alk-3, BMPR1A), and -6 (Alk-6, BMPR1B). Likewise, three type II receptors have been identified, i.e., BMP receptor II (BMPR2), activin type II receptor (ActRII, ACVR2), and activin type IIB receptor (ActRIIB, ACVR2B; Ebisawa et al. 1999). Both, type I and type II receptors are required for signaling (Kawabata et al. 1998). All BMPs use BMPR2, but utilize different BMP type I receptors. BMP6 preferably binds to ACVR1 (Ro et al. 2004). Intracellular BMP-signals are transduced mainly by small mothers against decapentaplegic proteins (SMADs). Alternate BMP-signaling pathways include prostanoid-generation via COX-2 (Ren et al. 2007) and MAPK-dependent activation of p38 or the Ras- and Erk-pathway (Nohe et al. 2004; Du et al. 2007). Both pathways have been reported to be present in myeloma cells (Trojan et al. 2006; Hoang et al. 2006).

BMP, and especially BMP6, are thus of high interest as a novel class of inhibitory and bone formation stimulating factors expressed already by normal plasma cells.

3.2 Chromosomal Aberrations

3.2.1 Background and Methods

A plethora of numerical and structural aberrations can be detected in myeloma cell samples of almost all patients, especially if CD138-purified plasma cells are used (Magrangeas et al. 2005; Kuehl and Bergsagel 2002; Chiecchio et al. 2006; Barlogie et al. 1985; Latreille et al. 1980; Tienhaara and Pelliniemi 1992; Drach et al. 1995; Flactif et al. 1995; Fig. 3.4; Table 3.1). Chromosomal aberrations lead to changes in gene and protein expression causing malignant properties of myeloma cells (Magrangeas et al. 2005), exemplified by aberrant expression of growth and survival factors (Sect. 3.6) but can likewise appear as epiphenomenon.

Three *methods* routinely used to assess chromosomal aberrations in multiple myeloma: (1) *metaphase cytogenetics* (mCG) allow the simultaneous assessment of aberrations of the whole set of chromosomes, but is largely unable to detect small changes or such in terminal regions (e.g., translocation t(4;14); Hallek et al. 1998). Importantly, for detection of aberrations, this method prerequisites myeloma cells to proliferate to obtain metaphases and therefore measures the frequency of aberrations in *proliferating* myeloma cells. mCG showed an increase in the number of aberrations detected in early- vs. late-stage patients and relapsed disease (Hallek et al. 1998). However, this basically reflects the increased proliferation rate in later stages (Hose et al. 2010). Using proliferation-independent methods, i.e., (2) interphase fluorescence in situ hybridization (iFISH; Drach et al. 1995 et seqq.) iFISH (Drach et al. 1995; Flactif et al. 1995; Nishida et al. 1997; Fonseca et al. 2001b; Avet-Loiseau et al. 1998) and (3)array-based comparative genomic hybridization (aCGH), an increasing frequency of aberrations from early-stage plasma cell dyscrasia to overt and

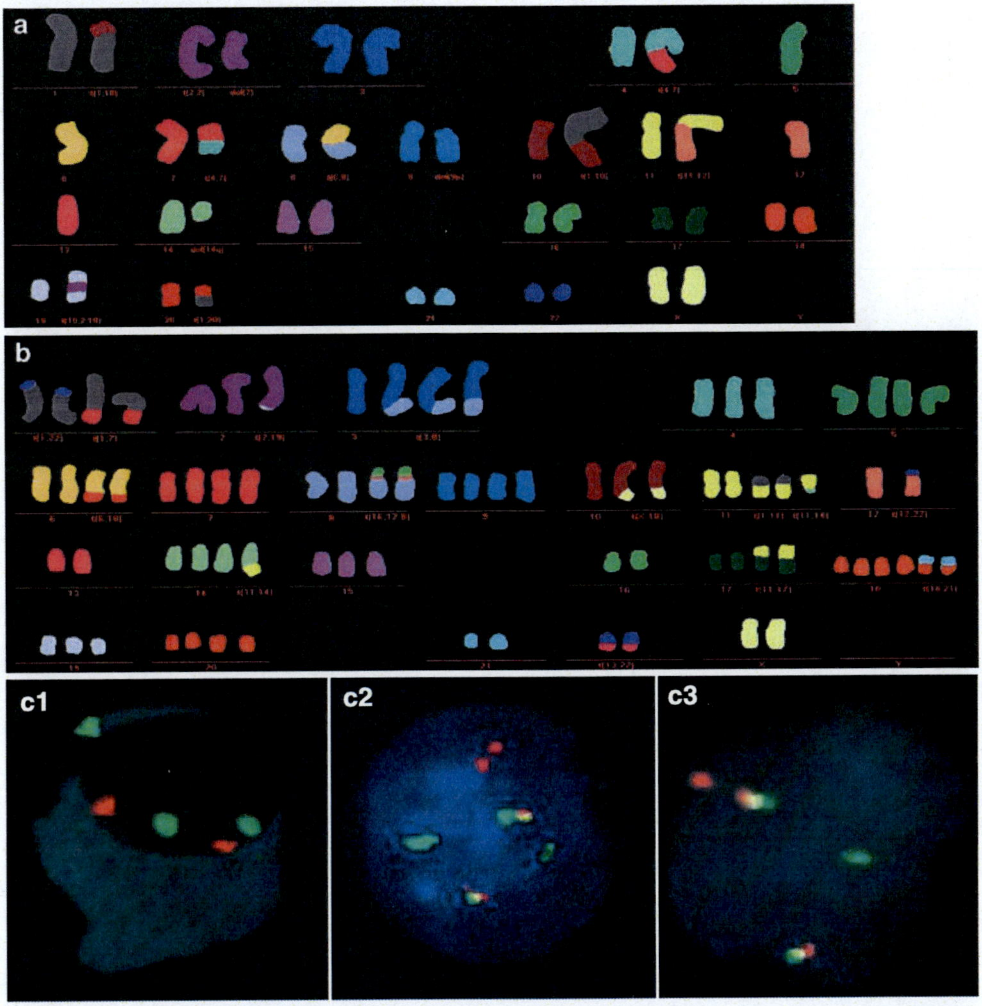

Fig. 3.4 *Metaphase multicolor-FISH.* (**a**) Non-hyperdiploid karyotype with several structural (translocations t(1;10), t(2;2), t(4;7), t(6;8), t(11;12), t(19;2;19), t(1;20)) and numerical (deletion of chromosomes or chromosomal regions 5, 13, and 14q, respectively). (**b**) Hyperdiploid karyotype with characteristic gain of odd numbered chromosomes, including 5, 9, 15, as well as several structural aberrations, including the recurrent translocation t(11;14), as well as nonrecurrent translocations, e.g., t(11;17) and t(1;11). (**c**) Frequent chromosomal aberrations as detected by iFISH. (**C1**) Gain of 11q13 (*green*), normal copy number of 9q34 (*red*). (**C2**) Translocation t(11:14). 11q13 (*green*), 14q32 (*red*). (**C3**) Translocation t(4;14). 4p16 (*green*), 14q32 (*red*)

relapsing myeloma has not been shown. iFISH in CD138-purified plasma cells is currently the workhorse of assessment of (prognostic) chromosomal aberrations and of clonal heterogeneity in terms of presence of subclones (Fig. 3.4, and see below). Before *iFISH* can be used, it is necessary to identify recurrent chromosomal aberrations to generate specific probes. *aCGH* does not have this prerequisite and allows assessment of copy number changes for hundreds of thousands of loci (Carrasco et al. 2006), but does not allow the detection of (prognostically

Table 3.1 Frequency of chromosomal aberrations in multiple myeloma (%)

	iFISH			mCG
	Neben et al. (2010) $n=312^a$	Avet-Loiseau et al. (2007) $n=1,000^a$	Chiecchio et al. (2006) $n=792^a$	Chiecchio et al. (2006) $n=213$
Hyperdiploidy	57	40	56	62
Non-hyperdiploidy	43	60	44	39
IgH-translocation (any)	n.a.	n.a.	45	52
t(4;14)	13	14	12	n.a.
t(11;14)	19	21	15	15
t(6;14)	n.a.	n.a.	n.a.	2
t(14;16)	2	n.a.	n.a.	3
t(14;20)	n.a.	n.a.	n.a.	4
Myc-translocations	n.a.	13	n.a.	n.a.
Deletion 17p13	10	11	9	n.a.
Deletion 13q14	46	45	48	48
1q21+	36	40	n.a.	n.a.

n.a. not assessed

[a]Different numbers of assessed patients; maximal number given (Neben et al. 2010; Avet-Loiseau et al. 2007; Chiecchio et al. 2006)

relevant) balanced translocations (e.g., translocation t(4;14)).

3.2.2 Types of Chromosomal Aberrations

Chromosomal aberrations in multiple myeloma can be grouped in (1) *structural* aberrations (mostly translocations, especially IgH-translocations), and (2) *numerical* aberrations of single chromosomes or chromosomal regions (e.g., deletion 13q14), or changes in *ploidy*, i.e., deviations from the diploid karyotype (aneuploidy). The latter are grouped according to the number of chromosomes: "hypodiploidy" (≤45; karyotypes with loss of Y-chromosome as single aberration are not considered abnormal), "pseudodiploidy" (46–47), "near tetraploidy" (≥75), and "hyperdiploidy" (HRD, 48–74; Chiecchio et al. 2006). Hypodiploid, near-tetraploid, and pseudodiploide karyotypes are summarized as non-hyperdiploid (non-HRD), in contrast to HRD. Both represent a broad category each comprising about 50% of abnormal karyotypes (Magrangeas et al. 2005): Hyperdiploid karyotypes show rather "global" changes in terms of *numerical* aberrations (gains), especially of the odd chromosomes 3, 5, 7, 9, 11, 15, 19, and 21. To the contrary, non-HRD karyotypes are mostly characterized by structural aberrations (Magrangeas et al. 2005). Frequently, these are IgH-translocations. In analogy to conventional karyotyping, iFISH can be applied to classify in HRD/non-HRD using a combination of frequently altered chromosomal regions as surrogate (Chiecchio et al. 2006; Wuilleme et al. 2005; Cremer et al. 2005). An example is to classify as HRD if at least two regions on chromosome 5, 9, and 15 are gained (Wuilleme et al. 2005). Alternatively, a value of (+1), (−1), and 0 is attributed for gain, loss, and lack of change for each if the regions 6q21, 8q21, 9q34, 11q23, 13q14, 15q22, 17p13, 19q13, and 22q11 are subsequently summed. For the resulting "copy-number score" (CS; Hose et al. 2004, 2005; Cremer et al. 2005), a value of CS ≥1 is defined as HRD, all others as non-HRD. The ploidy stage (HRD or non-HRD) usually does not change during disease progression (Chng et al. 2006).

Two further ways to classify chromosomal aberrations from a theoretical point of view are (1) whether they exclude each other ("*disjunct aberration*") or not ("*non-disjunct aberrations*"), and (2) whether they are involved in the initial pathogenesis ("*etiopathogenetic aberrations*"), the latter in most cases disjunct (e.g., t(11;14) and t(4;14)), or *additive aberrations* (non-disjunct, e.g., deletion of 17p).

3.2.3 Association of Chromosomal Aberrations

The appearance of several chromosomal aberrations is correlated: A t(4;14) or t(14;16) is in 85–90% of patients associated with a deletion of chromosome 13q14 (Kuppers and Dalla-Favera 2001; Keats et al. 2003; Fonseca et al. 2001a). A deletion 13 can be found in 85% of non-HRD malignant plasma cells, but in 30–35% of HRD malignant plasma cells (Smadja et al. 2001; Santra et al. 2003). Myeloma cells carrying a t(11;14), t(14;16), or t(4;14) are mostly non-HRD (Fonseca et al. 2003b; Magrangeas et al. 2005), those with nonrecurrent 14q32 translocations more frequently HRD. Avet-Loiseau et al. found an association between del(13) and t(4;14), del(17p) and del(13), but not between del(17p) and t(4;14) (Avet-Loiseau et al. 2007). Respective associations are not described for gains of 1q21 or losses of 17p13, see below.

3.2.4 Clonal, Subclonal, and Progression-Related Aberrations and Chromosomal Instability

Chromosomal aberrations can appear in different percentages within the malignant plasma cell population of a given patient. Whereas IgH-translocations as t(4;14) or ploidy state usually appear in the majority of myeloma cells, the frequency of malignant plasma cells in which a deletion 13q14 can be detected varies between 20% and 100% (Magrangeas et al. 2005); the same holds true for deletion of 17p13 or gains of 1q21 (Cremer et al. 2005). If one chromosomal aberration appears in ≥70% of myeloma cells whereas another only in a smaller percentage of this population (20–60%), a so-called subclonal aberration is present. Their appearance can be seen as a sign for an evolution of the malignant plasma cell clone (Cremer et al. 2005), in which the subclonal aberration appeared after the clonal aberration (Fig. 3.5). Neither the absolute number of chromosomal aberrations nor presence of subclonal aberrations tested by iFISH were significantly different between myeloma cells

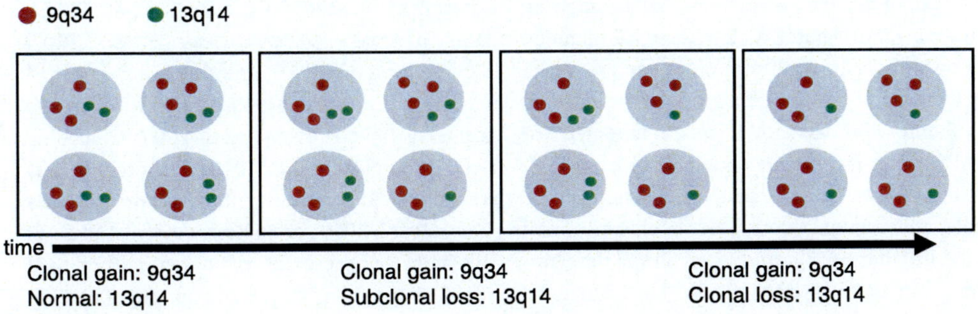

Fig. 3.5 *Subclonal aberrations and chromosomal instability*. Initially (*left*) a clonal gain of 9q34 (*red*) and a normal copy number regarding 13q14 (*green*) are present in all four depicted nuclei (*grey*). With time, a loss of 13q14 appears in a subfraction of myeloma cells (*middle-left*, 25%). This fraction increases (*middle-right*, 50%) until it has become a clonal aberration (100%, *right*). The detection of a subclonal aberration can be seen as an indicator for a present or past clonal instability

showing a gene expression–based proliferation index above vs. below the median (Hose et al. 2011). The appearance of some chromosomal aberrations seems to be associated with an evolution of the malignant plasma cell clone: Gains of 1q21, e.g., are found in none of 14 individuals with MGUS, 43% (206/479) of newly diagnosed and 71% (32/45) of relapsing myeloma patients, as well as in 91% (21/23) of investigated human myeloma cell lines (Hanamura et al. 2006). The percentage of myeloma cells carrying a $1q21^{+}$ as well as the number of copies of 1q21 within myeloma cells of a given patient increase with disease progression. 1q21-aberrations are frequent in terminal malignant diseases, e.g., in non-Hodgkin lymphoma (Le et al. 2001; Itoyama et al. 2002), Wilms-tumor (Lu et al. 2002), Ewing-sarcoma (Hattinger et al. 2002), ovarian cancer (Cheng et al. 2004), and breast cancer (Cheng et al. 2004; Zudaire et al. 2002). Malignant plasma cells of patients harboring a disease progression–associated gain of 1q21 or deletion of 13q14.3 show a significantly higher gene expression-based proliferation index, whereas patients with gain of chromosome 9, 15, or 19 (hyperdiploid samples) show a significantly lower one, see below (Hose et al. 2011).

It seemed logical that the multitude of chromosomal aberrations, the increase of their percentage in mCG from MGUS to relapsing myeloma, and the presence of subclonal aberrations could be taken as evidence of an ongoing chromosomal instability. However, as detailed above, only in the proliferation-dependent mCG an increase of the frequency of aberrations can be found. This has not been documented for proliferation-independent methods like iFISH. It thus seems that at least on a macroscopic scale, there might have been a chromosomal instability during a period of myeloma development, but there is currently no hard evidence that this process is continuously ongoing. This picture might, however, change, when high-resolution techniques like deep sequencing become available.

3.2.5 Prognostic Relevance of Chromosomal Aberrations

Several chromosomal aberrations show prognostic relevance (see Table 3.2). Already presence of an abnormal karyotype in mCG and detection of abnormal metaphases are associated with shorter survival in multiple myeloma (Chiecchio et al. 2006).

iFISH allows a risk stratification with presence of a translocation t(4;14) and/or deletion of 17p13 being the best-documented adverse prognostic factors (Avet-Loiseau et al. 2007; Chiecchio et al. 2006; Keats et al. 2003; Fonseca et al. 2003a; Moreau et al. 2002; Chang et al. 2004). Of etiology-associated aberrations (e.g., IgH-translocations), the translocation t(4;14) present in about 15% of patients represents a specific disease entity and is an independent risk factor despite conventional or high-dose treatment (Avet-Loiseau et al. 2007; Chiecchio et al. 2006; Keats et al. 2003; Fonseca et al. 2003a; Moreau et al. 2002; Chang et al. 2004). Treatment with bortezomib or lenalidomide containing regimen seems to reduce the negative prognostic impact of this aberration (Barlogie et al. 2008; San Miguel et al. 2008; Avet-Loiseau et al. 2009; Knop et al. 2009; Reece et al. 2009).

Regarding aberrations associated with disease progression, deletion of 17p13 (Avet-Loiseau et al. 2007; Chiecchio et al. 2006), gains of 1q21 (Avet-Loiseau et al. 2007; Hanamura et al. 2006), and deletions of 13q14 in univariate analyses are associated with adverse prognosis (Avet-Loiseau et al. 2007; Chiecchio et al. 2006; Neben et al. 2010). Different results are published regarding multivariate analyses (Neben et al. 2010; Avet-Loiseau et al. 2007). If adjusted for presence of deletion 17p and t(4;14), deletion of 13q14.3 is no longer considered to define adverse risk (Neben et al. 2010; Avet-Loiseau et al. 2007). Deletion of 17p13 remains an adverse prognostic factor in multivariate analyses. It likewise remains an adverse

Table 3.2 Prognostic relevance of chromosomal aberrations as detected by mCG and iFISH: Patients treated with high-dose therapy and autologous stem cell transplantation (Neben et al. 2010; Avet-Loiseau et al. 2007) and patients with conventional as well as high-dose therapy and autologous stem cell transplantation (Chiecchio et al. 2006), respectively.

Aberration	Neben et al. (2010)		Avet-Loiseau et al. (2007)		Chiecchio et al. (2006)					
	iFISH 36 months survival		iFISH 41 months survival		mCG Median survival		iFISH & mCG[b] Median survival		iFISH (all) Median survival	
	(%)	P	Months	P	Months	P	Months	P	Months	P
Abnormal karyotype	n.a.	n.a.	n.a.	n.a	24 vs. 45	0.001	–	–	–	–
Abnormal metaphases	n.a.	n.a.	n.a.	n.a	12 vs. 45	<0.001	–	–	–	–
Del 13q	72 vs. 82	0.037	68 vs. 83	<0.001	15 vs. 50	<0.001	24 vs. n.r.	<0.001	29 vs. 47	<0.001
Any IgH-TL	n.a.	n.a.	n.a.	n.a	24 vs. 41	0.038	–	–	–	–
t(4;14)	49 vs. 82	0.005	41.3[a] vs. 79	<0.001	9 vs. 41	<0.001	19 vs. n.r.	0.004	19 vs. 44	0.002
t(11;14)	79 vs. 77	0.855	80 vs. 74	0.28	n.e. vs. 33	0.787	n.r. vs. 33	0.540	n.r. vs. 36	0.229
t(14;16)	n.a.	n.a.	n.a.	n.a.	16 vs. 40	0.354	–	–	–	–
t(14;20)	n.a.	n.a.	n.a.	n.a.	7 vs. 40	0.109	–	–	–	–
Deletion 17p	50 vs. 81	<0.001	22[a] vs. 75	<0.001	15 vs. 41	0.048	21 vs. 40	0.069	19 vs. 43	<0.001
Hypodiploid	n.a.	n.a.	n.a.	n.a.	21 vs. 40	0.064	–	–	–	–
Non-hyperdiploid	51 vs. 77	0.041	70 vs. 82	0.006	21 vs. 41	0.003	26 vs. n.r.	0.036	33 vs. 47	0.041

Prognostic role of presence of the respective aberration vs. all patients without presence of the respective aberration

TL translocation

[a]Months survival (instead of %)

[b]Simultaneous

prognostic factor for bortezomib- and lenalidomide-based protocols (Knop et al. 2009; Reece et al. 2009).

Many investigations have shown the prognostic relevance of chromosomal aberrations to be independent of clinical parameters, in particular beta-2-microglobulin. Combining these parameters results in powerful prognostic models, in particular those of Facon et al. (beta-2-microglobulin and deletion 13; Facon et al. 2001), Avet-Loiseau et al. (model including t(4;14), del (17p), and serum beta-2-microglobulin >4 mg/dL Avet-Loiseau et al. 2007), or Neben et al. (model including t(4;14), del (17p), and ISS-stage; Neben et al. 2010).

3.3 Changes in Gene Expression in Multiple Myeloma

Multiple myeloma cells harbor a high median number of chromosomal aberrations (Cremer et al. 2005; Fonseca et al. 2004) as discussed above, and multiple changes in gene expression compared to normal bone marrow plasma cells (Andersen et al. 2009, 2010; Zhan et al. 2002, 2006). This molecular heterogeneity is thought to transmit into the very different survival times ranging from a few months to 15 or more years (Barlogie et al. 2006), with a median survival after conventional treatments of 3–4 and 5–9 years after high-dose melphalan treatment followed by autologous stem cell transplantation (Harousseau and Moreau 2009; Barlogie et al. 2008). On a molecular level, it seems that many and multiple myelomas exist (Fonseca 2003).

Gene expression profiling performed on $CD138^+$ purified myeloma cells allows assessing expression of (almost) all genes simultaneously without the need of a preselection of interesting genes or regions. Profiling of gene expression can be used (1) to classify patients due to molecular entities (mostly based on unsupervised clustering algorithms grouping patients according to the similarity of their expression profile), (2) to assess progression of pathophysiologically relevant target genes (e.g., aurora-kinase), (3) in expression and (to a certain extent) molecular entity–based risk assessment.

3.3.1 Gene Expression–Based Classifications in Myeloma

Three gene expression–based classifications delineate molecular groups in myeloma: the "molecular classification" based on differential gene expression in which three of seven groups ("proliferation," MAF-expression, and MMSET-overexpression) show different survival (Zhan et al. 2006), the TC-classification based on translocations and D-type cyclin (CCND) without prognostic relevance (Bergsagel and Kuehl 2005; Bergsagel et al. 2005), and the EC-classification based on chromosomal aberrations and resulting changes in gene expression with only one of four groups (t(4;14) and FGFR3-expression) showing adverse prognosis (Hose et al. 2004, 2005). Biological classifications likely remain relatively stable in contrast to prognostic factors prone to change with different treatment schedules (see below).

The molecular classification of Shaughnessy et al. (Zhan et al. 2006; groups denoted MS, MF, PR, Hy, D1, D2, LB) is based on unsupervised clustering and prediction of clustered groups, whereas the TC-classification by Bergsagel et al. (Bergsagel et al. 2005; groups denoted TC1-7) is centered on the hypothesis that CCND-expression is an early unifying event in multiple myeloma. The EC-classification delineates groups based on expression of CCND and underlying chromosomal aberrations. In EC1.1 and EC1.2, aberrant expression of CCND1, mediated by a gain of 11q13 (the CCND1-locus; Hoechtlen-Vollmar et al. 2000) in EC1.1, or a translocation involving this locus in EC1.2 (Specht et al. 2004;

Wlodarska et al. 2004) is present. Patients in EC1.1 and EC2.1 are almost all hyperdiploid, patients in EC1.2 (mostly) and EC2.2 (all) non-hyperdiploid. In groups EC2.1 and EC2.2, myeloma cells overexpress of the "physio logic" CCND2 involved in the proliferation of plasma cell precursors (i.e., polyclonal plasma cells), and expressed at a low level in normal bone marrow plasma cells. EC2.1 comprises patients with a hyperdiploid karyotype and few patients with rare translocations indicated by the respective expression pattern (e.g., t(14;16), MAF, (4/128), t(14;20), MAFB, (1/128), and FGFR2 (1/128)), and patients with t(4;14) without FGFR3 overexpression (3/128). EC2.2 is characterized by the presence of the translocation t(4;14) and FGFR3 overexpression. CCND2-overexpression seems to be correlated with hyperdiploidy, or triggered by aberrations in physiological plasma cell proliferation pathways like MAF (Hurt et al. 2004) or APRIL/TACI (via MAF; Moreaux et al. 2005). CCND3 expression does not show significant differences between normal bone marrow plasma cells, polyclonal plasma cells, or any of the groups. As an aberrant expression of CCND does not seem sufficient for oncogenic transformation, it is intriguing that in EC2.1 myeloma cells carry a higher number of aberrantly expressed growth factors compared to low (EC1.1) or high (EC1.2) intrinsic CCND1 expression. Therefore, intrinsic expression of CCND might mimic the effect of growth factor stimulation, thereby reducing the dependence of myeloma cells on external stimuli for proliferation and survival.

Despite methodological differences, in all classifications (1) a group with translocation t(4;14) (MS, TC7, EC2.2) and *MMSET* (with or without *FGFR3* expression) is identified and (2) a group with translocation t(11;14)/t(11;v) with high *CCND1* overexpression (EC1.2, TC2, subdivided in D1, D2 (*CCND1* or *CCND3* overexpression)). EC1.1 corresponds with TC3 (low *CCND1*, hyperdiploid), but correlates low *CCND1* overexpression with gain of 11q13 detected by iFISH. EC1.1 together with EC2.1 corresponds with Hy (hyperdiploid). EC2.1 also comprises patients with rare translocations like the MAF-translocations (the latter form separate groups, i.e., MF, TC8) or t(4;14) without *FGFR3* overexpression. We also observed simultaneous *CCND1* and *CCND2* expression as defining TC4, but interpret this either as an evolving aberration 11q13^{+} (on the background of physiological *CCND2* expression, which is down-regulated simultaneously with *CCND1* up-regulation), or the presence of two (sub) clones. No correspondence with our groups could be found for TC6 (no *CCND*), as all patients expressed at least one of the CCND, LB (low bone disease), as it was not significantly different distributed between the groups, and PR (proliferation), which seems to be a characteristic acquirable in all groups.

Taken together, gene expression profiling can be used to delineate different groups in myeloma. Some of these represent different entities, but it remains to be shown which are exclusive (disjunct), and which features can appear independent of delineated groups, e.g., emerging of a proliferative geno- and phenotype.

3.3.2 Gene Expression and Risk Stratification

Risk stratification by gene expression profiling is applied using four different strategies: (1) grouping multiple myeloma into "molecular groups" (entities, Sect. 3.4.1) subsequently investigating differences in survival between these groups, (2) assessing expression of a gene representing a potential therapeutic target and investigate its prognostic relevance, (3) assessing surrogates of biological variables and their respective prognostic relevance, and (4) assessing (high) risk based on association of gene expression with survival. The second possibility is exemplified by expression of Aurora-A

(Hose et al. 2009b) delineating significantly inferior survival in two independent cohorts of patients undergoing high-dose chemotherapy, independent from conventional prognostic factors. Gene expression profiling could here allow selecting (only) patients with aurora-kinase expression, which in turn have an adverse prognosis, for treatment with aurora-kinase inhibitors. The third possibility is exemplified by a gene expression–based proliferation index (see Sect. 3.5). Proliferation of malignant plasma cells, as determined by several methods, has been shown to be a strong adverse prognostic factor (Boccadoro et al. 1984; Greipp et al. 1988, 1993; San Miguel et al. 1995; Gastinne et al. 2007), independent of clinical prognostic factors, e.g., beta-2-microglobulin (Greipp et al. 1993), and can likewise be assessed by gene expression–based proliferation indices (Zhan et al. 2002, 2006; Bergsagel and Kuehl 2005; Bergsagel et al. 2005; Hose et al. 2011); see below). The fourth strategy comprises the high risk-scores of the University of Arkansas for Medical Sciences (UAMS; 17/70 genes; Shaughnessy et al. 2007) and the Intergroup Francophone du Myélome (IFM; 15 genes; Decaux et al. 2008) by building a score over a set of genes associated with survival. Both scores allow delineating a small group of patients (13% and 25%, respectively) with very adverse prognosis in the IFM and total therapy 2 (TT2-) dataset (both not including bortezomib), whereas in the TT3-cohort only the UAMS-score remains significant in univariate analysis. Thus, the UAMS-score remains its prognostic relevance if bortezomib is added to the treatment regimen (TT2 vs. TT3; Shaughnessy et al. 2007; Decaux et al. 2008). In relapsed patients treated with bortezomib within the APEX, SUMMIT, and CREST trials ($n=188$), both scores significantly delineate different outcome, whereas in patients treated with dexamethasone within these trials ($n=76$), only the UAMS-score significantly delineates a high risk group. No data are currently published in terms of independence of these scores of lenalidomide treatment.

3.4 Proliferation and Cell Cycle Regulation

3.4.1 "Potential to Proliferate" of Normal Plasma Cells

Cell cycle progression is regulated by several classes of cyclin-dependent kinases and their inhibitors (Sherr and Roberts 1999). Following Murry (2004), three basic levels of cell cycle regulation can be delineated: (1) The "cell cycle machinery" mediating the continuing fluctuations of cyclin-levels and activity of associated Cdk, (2) the subsequent targets of this machinery (DNA-replication, mitosis), and (3) signal transduction pathways regulating this machinery in response to external stimuli (Murray 2004). Signal transduction pathways of several growth and survival factors converge on CCND, crucial for G_0/G_1-S progression.

Bone marrow plasma cells have the "potential to proliferate." In contrast to their precursors (see Sect. 3.2.1), normal bone marrow plasma cells do not proliferate (Witzig et al. 1999; Drewinko et al. 1981; Hose et al. 2011) but have the "potential to proliferate": They express necessary parts of the cell cycle machinery, e.g., CDK4/6, but likewise cell cycle breaks, e.g., Kip/Cip (p21, p27) and INK4-family members (p18). Molecular integration of pro-proliferative (e.g., CCND2-expression due to growth factor stimulation, e.g., via TACI/c-maf) and thus CCND2/CDK4/6 promotion of G_0/G_1-transgression and anti-proliferative signals including a cell cycle arrest as part of the terminal B cell differentiation (Klein et al. 2003), i.e., *BCL6*-expression necessary for proliferation being suppressed by *PAX5*-expression necessary for terminal differentiation (see Sect.

3.2.1), result in a domination of the latter (as no proliferation is found).

On the background of this balanced "potential to proliferate" of normal plasma cells, it is not surprising that aberrations in signaling or components of the cell cycle machinery can lead to (in the beginning slow) accumulation of plasma cells.

3.4.2 D-Type Cyclin Expression in Myeloma

Changes in signal transduction chains can lead to an increased (e.g., c-myc – CCND2) or aberrant CCND-expression, as can be mediated directly due to chromosomal aberrations at the cyclin-loci (e.g., translocation t(11;14) – aberrant expression of CCND1). An over or aberrant expression of CCND, frequent in malignant diseases (Sherr 1996; Sherr and Roberts 2004), is a hallmark of multiple myeloma (Bergsagel and Kuehl 2003). Compared to normal bone marrow plasma cells, almost all myeloma cells show a higher expression of at least one of the CCND. About half of the myeloma patients show an overexpression of CCND2 (expressed in bone marrow plasma cells) the other half an aberrant expression of CCND1 (not expressed in bone marrow plasma cells or cells of the B cell lineage). Aberrant expression of CCND3 is rare (<5% of myeloma patients). Aberrant expression can be caused by direct mechanisms: translocations involving the 11q13-locus and the heavy chain (IgH)-locus, 14q32, i.e., a t(11;14) leading to high CCND1-expression, rarely of light chain genes (t(2;11), t(11;22)). Linked to hyperdiploidy, gains of 11q13 lead to an aberrant CCND1-expression (lower compared to the one by t(11;14)). CCND3-expression (at least high) is mediated by a t(6;14) translocation involving the CCND3-locus at 6p21. In contrast, CCND2-overexpression is mostly indirectly mediated, i.e., by alterations in the signal transduction chain (e.g., t(4;14); aberrant FGFR3-expression).

CCND exemplify the general concept that different molecular alterations converge onto the same oncogenic pathways.

3.4.3 Proliferation of Malignant Plasma Cells

Despite a general CCND (over)expression (Bergsagel and Kuehl 2003; Hose et al. 2004, 2005) malignant plasma mostly show only a low proliferation rate (Drewinko et al. 1981; see Fig. 3.6). This rate increases from MGUS-patients over newly diagnosed and relapsed patients (Witzig et al. 1999; Bergsagel et al. 2005; Hose et al. 2011). Proliferation of malignant plasma cells is measured by various methods including 3H-thymidine uptake (Latreille et al. 1982; Boccadoro et al. 1984), Bromodeoxyuridine uptake (Schambeck et al. 1995; Lokhorst et al. 1986; Greipp et al. 1987), cell cycle analysis using propidium iodide, percentage of Ki67-expressing myeloma cells (Alexandrakis et al. 2004), and gene expression–based proliferation indices based on selected genes (Rosenwald et al. 2003; Bergsagel et al. 2005; Zhan et al. 2006). An example of the latter is the index by Shaughnessy et al. using the normalized expression-values of 11 genes associated with proliferation (*TOP2A*, *BIRC5*, *CCNB2*, *NEK2*, *ANAPC7*, *STK6*, *BUB1*, *CDC2*, *C10orf3*, *ASPM*, and *CDCA1*) scaled to the maximum within 22 normal bone marrow plasma cell samples (proliferation index of bone marrow plasma cells defined as 1; Zhan et al. 2006). Bergsagel et al. used the median of 12 genes associated with proliferation (*TYMS*, *TK1*, *CCNB1*, *MKI67*, *KIAA101*, *KIAA0186*, *CKS1B*, *TOP2A*, *UBE2C*, *ZWINT*, *TRIP13*, and *KIF11*) scaled to the maximum values over all samples (Bergsagel et al. 2005). Our group

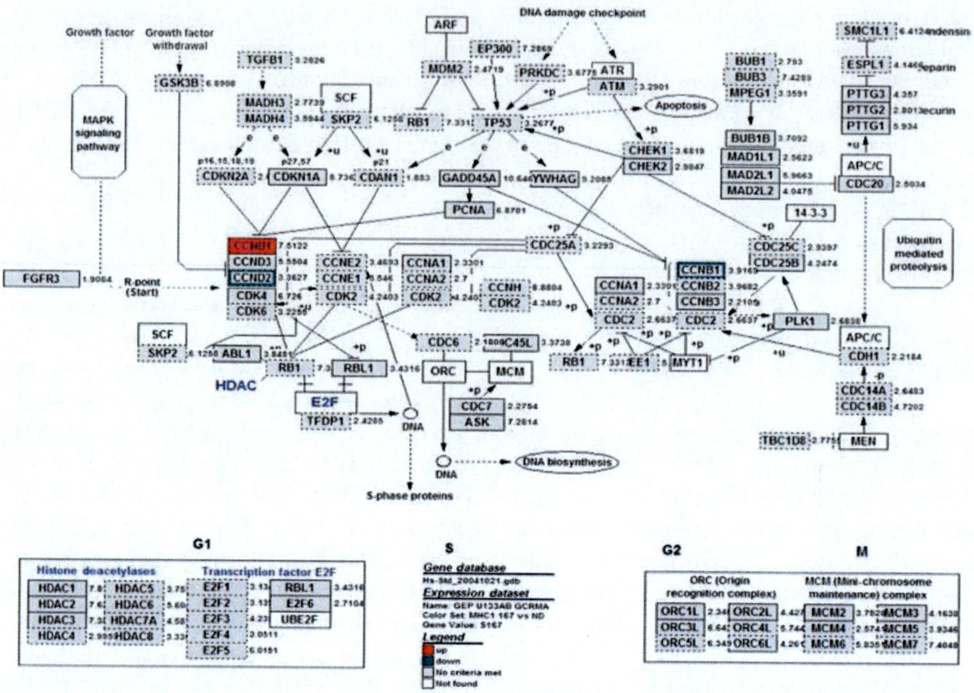

Fig. 3.6 *Cell cycle analysis*. Depicted is the core cell cycle machine for a particular patient (S167/02) relative to the median expression of the respective gene in seven bone marrow plasma cell (BMPC) samples. The patient harbors a hyperdiploid karyotype, gain of 11q13 without the presence of a translocation t(11;14), and an aberrant CCND1 expression (i.e., overexpression compared to BMPCs in which CCND1 is not expressed). In terms of molecular classification, the patient is attributed to EC1.1, TC4p16, and Hy (hyperdiploid) in the molecular classification (see Sect. 3.4.1). Overexpressed genes are depicted in *red* (e.g., CCND1), under-expressed in *green*. A *green border* depicts down-regulation if a gene is represented by more than one probeset (here CCND2 is down-regulated for one probeset compared to BMPCs). *Grey* implies no differential expression. Structures not encoded by a single gene (e.g., APC) are depicted in *white*. Note that this myeloma cell sample shows a relatively unaltered cell cycle

proposed a gene expression–based proliferation index consisting of 50 genes (Hose et al. 2011). Proliferation of malignant plasma cells as assessed by different methods appears as strong prognostic factors in several analyses (Boccadoro et al. 1984; Greipp et al. 1988; San Miguel et al. 1995; Greipp et al. 1993; Gastinne et al. 2007; Zhan et al. 2006; Shaughnessy et al. 2007), independent of conventional prognostic factors, e.g., beta-2-microglobulin (Greipp et al. 1993), ISS, or presence of translocation t(4;14) (Hose et al. 2011).

3.5 Myeloma Cell Survival and Proliferation Factors

Numerous studies have been devoted to the identification of myeloma cell growth factors and to the signaling pathways leading to survival and/or proliferation of myeloma cells. A first category of factors activates the PI-3 kinase/AKT and MAP kinase pathways (IGF-1, insulin,

EGF family, HGF). A second category activates the JAK/STAT and MAP kinase pathways (IL-6, IFNα, IL-10, IL-21) and a third category the NF-kappa B pathways (BAFF/APRIL, TNF). See Fig. 3.3.

3.5.1 Interferon Alpha/Interleukin-6 Family and Activation of the JAK/STAT and MAP Kinase Pathways

IL-6 binds to a specific receptor (IL-6R) and the complex IL-6/IL-6R binds and induces the homodimerization of the gp130 IL-6 transducer (Heinrich et al. 2003). A remarkable feature of IL-6R is that its soluble form (sIL-6R) is an agonist molecule. It binds IL-6 with the same affinity as membrane IL-6R and the complex IL-6/sIL-6R binds and activates gp130 (Heinrich et al. 2003). The evidences of a major role of IL-6 in the survival and proliferation of malignant plasma cells are accumulated since the initial reports by others and us 14 years ago (Klein et al. 1989; Kawano et al. 1988). These evidences are the following:

1. Antibodies to IL-6 block myeloma cell proliferation and reduce the number of myeloma cells in cultures of patients' bone marrow cells in vitro by 50% (Klein et al. 1989; Zhang et al. 1992).
2. Injection of anti-IL-6 mAb inhibited myeloma cell proliferation in patients with terminal disease (Klein et al. 1991; Bataille et al. 1995) if the antibody was injected at a sufficient concentration to block the large IL-6 production in vivo (Lu et al. 1995a).
3. Serum levels of IL-6 and soluble IL-6R are increased in patients with multiple myeloma in association with a poor prognosis (Bataille et al. 1989; Gaillard et al. 1993).
4. IL-6 is overproduced by the bone marrow environment of patients with multiple myeloma, mainly by monocytes, myeloid cells, and stromal cells (Klein et al. 1989; Portier et al. 1991; Mahtouk et al. 2010). This production of IL-6 by the tumor environment is mostly mediated by IL-1 that is produced by monocytes and myeloma cells (Klein et al. 1989; Mahtouk et al. 2010; Costes et al. 1998). IL-1 induces PGE2 synthesis that further triggers IL-6 production (Costes et al. 1998). Thus inhibitors of IL-1 as the IL-1 receptor antagonists or of PGE2 synthesis might be interesting to block IL-6 production in patients with multiple myeloma. A similar mechanism was shown in the model of murine plasmacytoma in BALB/C mice. The generation of plasmacytomas was blocked by chronic administration of indomethacin that inhibited PGE2 synthesis and the large IL-6 production by the inflammatory environment (Hinson et al. 1996). Myeloma cells can also directly trigger IL-6 production by direct contact with bone marrow stromal cells by unidentified mechanisms (Uchiyama et al. 1993).
5. Cell lines whose survival is dependent on addition of exogenous IL-6 can be obtained from patients with extramedullary proliferation (Zhang et al. 1994a).
6. Mice transgenic with an IL-6 gene driven by the Eμ promoter develops massive polyclonal plasmacytosis (Suematsu et al. 1989). When crossed with murine BALB/c mice that spontaneously develop plasmacytomas, these crossed mice develop malignant plasma cells (Suematsu et al. 1992). In addition, knockout of IL-6 gene abrogated the generation of malignant plasmacytomas in BALB/C mice primed with mineral oil (Lattanzio et al. 1997).

Other cytokines of the IL-6 family are also myeloma cell growth factors due to the expression of specific receptors: OSM, CNTF, IL-11, LIF (Zhang et al. 1994b). But these factors are likely not involved in the emergence of the disease in vivo as they are weakly produced by the tumor or its environment (Mahtouk et al. 2010). In our hands, we found that interferon-alpha (IFNα) is also a myeloma cell survival factor that is independent of IL-6 (Jourdan et al. 1991; Ferlin-Bezombes et al. 1998). IFNα activated the JAK/STAT and MAP kinase pathways as IL-6, in particular STAT3 phosphorylation (Lu et al. 1995a). Other groups found that IFNα could block myeloma cell proliferation. This discrepancy might be explained by the ability of IFNα to induce P19 inhibitor in some cell lines yielding to apoptosis (Arora and Jelinek 1998). Finally, IL-10 and IL-21 are also myeloma cell growth factors (Lu et al. 1995b; Menoret et al. 2008). IL-10 works through induction of autocrine loops of cytokines of the IL-6 family (Gu et al. 1996).

The myeloma cell survival activity of these cytokines is partly mediated by the phosphorylation of STAT3 by JAK kinases activated by the gp130 IL-6 transducer or IFN receptor. Blockade of JAK/STAT pathway by AG490 inhibits STAT3 phosphorylation and induces myeloma cell apoptosis (De Vos et al. 2000). STAT3 binding elements are found in the promoters of several anti-apoptotic proteins: MCL-1, bcl-2, bcl-xL. Among ten anti-apoptotic and pro-apoptotic proteins, we found that only MCL-1 was regulated by IL-6 or IFNα (Jourdan et al. 2000). Other groups suggested that bcl-xL was the main anti-apoptotic protein controlled by IL-6 in myeloma cells (Catlett-Falcone et al. 1999; Puthier et al. 1999), but a study emphasized that only a blockade of MCL-1, unlike bcl-2 or bcl-xL, could inhibit myeloma cell survival (Derenne et al. 2002). In addition, we found that induction of the constitutive production of MCL-1 by retroviral vector is sufficient to promote myeloma cell proliferation independently of IL-6 (Jourdan et al. 2003). IL-6 was reported to activate AKT kinase in myeloma cells that is able to trigger various signaling pathways (Tu et al. 2000). AKT activation can be mediated by STAT3 that can trigger PI-3 kinase activation (Pfeffer et al. 1997). In our experience, we found a weak AKT phosphorylation in only some IL-6-dependent cell lines. Actually, the IL-6-induced AKT phosphorylation in myeloma cells is weak and transient as compared to that induced by IL-6 (Mitsiades et al. 2002). PI-3 kinase-mediated AKT phosphorylation appears critical in promoting proliferation of myeloma cell lines since PI-3 kinase inhibitors abrogate it unlike MAP kinase inhibitors (Qiang et al. 2002; Pene et al. 2002).

3.5.2 Factors Activating the PI-3 and MAP Kinase Pathways: Insulin-Like Growth Factor 1, Heparin-Binding Growth Factors

3.5.2.1 Insulin-Like Growth Factor 1 (IGF-1)

IGF-1 plays likely a major role in myeloma in vivo. It is a survival and proliferation factor for most myeloma cell lines and primary myeloma cells (Georgii-Hemming et al. 1996; Jelinek et al. 1997). The reason is that IGF-1 receptor (IGF-1R) is aberrantly expressed by myeloma cells in association with poor prognosis (Sprynski et al. 2009). Indeed, IGF-1R is not expressed by normal plasma cells generated in vitro or in vivo. The reason for aberrant IGF-1R expression on myeloma cells is not known.

Large amount of IGF-1 are present in the bone marrow from patients (Hose et al. 2009a). First, IGF-1 gene is induced in the process of B to plasma cell differentiation and is also highly expressed by malignant plasma cells (Mahtouk et al. 2010). IGF-1 is also produced by osteoclasts (Mahtouk et al. 2010). Large amount of IGF-1 circulate in the blood in the form of a trimeric complex with IGF-BP3 and acid labile subunit in healthy individuals. IGF-1 plasma levels are not increased in patients with multiple myeloma but are predictive of a poor survival (Standal et al. 2002). The biology of IGF-1 is complex since several IGF-binding proteins, mostly IGF-BP3, circulate at high concentrations and neutralize IGF-1 (Duan 2002). Cells may also express IGF-binding proteins that contribute to the biological activity of IGF-1 and disrupt the circulating IGF/IGF-BP complexes (Mahtouk et al. 2010). Myeloma cells also highly express the proteoglycan syndecan-1 (CD138) and can thus bind these trimeric complexes through IGF-BP3 (Beattie et al. 2005). This results in a weakening of the acid labile subunit binding and release of IGF-1 at the cell membrane of myeloma cells. Thus, IGF-1R is aberrantly expressed by myeloma cells, which produced IGF-1 and are bathed in vivo in large concentrations of IGF-1.

Regarding the transduction pathways, IGF-1 activates mainly PI-3 kinase pathway and in particular the phosphorylation of AKT protein (Sprynski et al. 2009; Ge and Rudikoff 2000) and its effect is independent of an activation of the JAK/STAT pathway (Jelinek et al. 1997; Ferlin et al. 2000). IGF-1 also induces MAP kinase phosphorylation (Sprynski et al. 2009; Ge and Rudikoff 2000). An inhibitor of PI-3 kinase pathway unlike a MAP kinase inhibitor (Qiang et al. 2002; Sprynski et al. 2009) blocks the myeloma growth factor activity of IGF-1. One mechanism of action of AKT is the phosphorylation of the pro-apoptotic protein Bad that induces its sequestration by the 14-13-3 protein and prevents its migration to mitochondrial membrane (Ge and Rudikoff 2000). The PI-3 kinase/AKT pathway in myeloma cells phosphorylates other proteins: the P70S6-kinase, forkhead proteins, and the glycogen synthase kinase-3 beta (GSK3b; Qiang et al. 2002; Pene et al. 2002; Hideshima et al. 2001). Phosphorylation of these proteins contributes to blockade of apoptosis and activation of cell cycle in various models. In particular, IGF-1 induces CCND1 and Skp2 expression and down-regulation of P27kip1 in myeloma cells (Pene et al. 2002). In addition, it was shown in one myeloma cell line that the PI-3 kinase/AKT pathway may activate the NF-kappa B pathway and expression of several targets of NF-kappa B involved in cell survival: A1/Bfl1, cIAP2, XIAP, survivin, FLIP (Mitsiades et al. 2002).

Transfection of myeloma cells with an activated AKT enhances tumor growth and protects from dexamethasone-induced apoptosis and expression of AKT dominant negative results in inhibition of IL-6-induced proliferation of myeloma cells (Hsu et al. 2002). The importance of the PI-3 kinase/AKT pathways for the survival and proliferation of myeloma cells is emphasized by deletion/mutation of the PTEN gene in some myeloma cells (Ge and Rudikoff 2000). PTEN is a phosphatase inhibiting the PI-3 kinase/AKT pathway and its deletion results in a high activation of PI-3 K/AKT pathway.

3.5.2.2 Insulin

Insulin and IGF-1 as well as their receptors are closely related molecules but both factors bind to the receptor of the other one with a weak affinity. Large levels of insulin are available in the blood plasma, produced by pancreatic beta cells in response to glucose level. The role of insulin in multiple myeloma was poorly studied. We have shown that insulin receptor (INSR) is increased throughout normal plasma cell differentiation (Sprynski et al. 2009). The *INSR* gene is also expressed by myeloma cells of newly diagnosed patients. Insulin is a myeloma cell growth factor as potent as IGF-1 at physiological concentrations and requires the presence of insulin/IGF-1 hybrid receptors, stimulating $INSR^{+}IGF\text{-}1R^{+}$ myeloma cells, unlike $INSR^{+}IGF\text{-}1R^{-}$ or $INSR^{-}IGF\text{-}1R^{-}$ myeloma cells (Sprynski et al. 2009). Immunoprecipitation experiments indicated that INSR is linked with IGF-1R in myeloma cells and that insulin induced both IGF-1R and INSR phosphorylation and vice versa. Further therapeutic strategies targeting the IGF-IGF-1R pathway have to take into account neutralizing the IGF-1R-mediated insulin myeloma cell growth factor activity.

3.5.3 Heparin-Binding Factors

A hallmark of plasma cell differentiation is the expression of the proteoglycan syndecan-1 (CD138; Wijdenes et al. 1996; Costes et al. 1999). This heparan-sulfate protein has many biological activities and in particular is able to bind heparin-binding growth factors and present them to their specific receptors (Sanderson and Yang 2008). Thus, it is not surprising that several myeloma cell growth factors are heparin-binding molecules. Antibodies against CD138 are used for myeloma cell purification in clinical routine.

3.5.3.1 Heparin-Binding Epidermal Growth Factors

Using Atlas microarrays, we initially found that myeloma cell lines overexpress HB-EGF gene compared to EBV-transformed B cell lines or normal plasmablastic cells and that inhibitors of HB-EGF can block the IL-6-dependent survival of these myeloma cell lines (De Vos et al. 2001). Actually, we found that myeloma cells can bind large levels of EGF family molecules through heparan-sulfate chain of syndecan-1 molecules (Mahtouk et al. 2006). Myeloma cells express the four receptors of EGF family, ErbB1 through ErbB4. ErbB1 and ErbB2 are also expressed by normal plasma cells while ErbB3 and ErbB4 are aberrantly expressed by myeloma cells (Mahtouk et al. 2005). EGF members trigger the PI-3 kinase/AKT and MAPK pathways in myeloma cells, unlike STAT3 phosphorylation (Mahtouk et al. 2004). An inhibitor of the tyrosine kinase activity of these receptors can kill myeloma cells as well as primary myeloma cells (Mahtouk et al. 2004). We have also found that the EGF family members cooperate with IL-6 to trigger an optimal survival of myeloma cells, likely through an interaction between the transducer chains, gp130, and EGF receptors (Wang et al. 2002). These data indicate that ErbB inhibitors can potentiate dexamethasone-induced apoptosis of myeloma cell lines and of primary myeloma cells of most patients and suggest that they might improve treatment of patients with multiple myeloma.

3.5.3.2 Hepatocyte Growth Factor (HGF)

A study has shown that HGF is also a growth factor for myeloma cell lines (Derksen et al. 2002). HGF activity is blocked by removal of heparan-sulfate chains of syndecan-1 with heparitinase. This result indicates that syndecan-1 is critical to capture heparin-binding HGF and to present it to its receptor, cMet. Whether HGF cooperates with IL-6 to trigger myeloma cell survival was not investigated. Noteworthy, the XG-1 cell line used in this study was initially obtained in our laboratory and produces a low amount of autocrine IL-6 (Jourdan et al. 2005) that is sufficient to induce the HB-EGF activity. HGF is likely involved in the biology of myeloma. Indeed, HGF is expressed by 75% of myeloma cell samples, its serum level is increased and it is a prognostic factor in patients with multiple myeloma (Seidel et al. 1998). As HGF increases bone resorption, it may also be involved in the abnormal osteoclast resorption in patients with multiple myeloma (Hjertner et al. 1999).

3.5.3.3
Fibroblast Growth Factor (FGF)

A role of FGF in myeloma is suggested by the finding of a t(4;14) translocation affecting the FGF receptor type 3 in 15% of patients with multiple myeloma (Avet-Loiseau et al. 1998) (see Sect. 3.3.5). FGFs likely play an important role in myeloma biology because they bind syndecan-1 as HB-EGF or HGF and activation of FGFR3 induces the PI-3 kinase/AKT pathway that is critical for myeloma cell survival and proliferation.

3.5.4
Factors Activating NF-Kappa B: BAFF Family

BAFF and APRIL belong to the TNF family and activate at least three receptors of the TNF receptor family: BAFF-R, BCMA, and TACI. BAFF proteins are critical for the survival of B cells and may be involved in systematic lupus erythematosus. Activation of BAFF receptor family results in triggering the NF-kappa B pathway and likely other unidentified pathways (Mackay and Schneider 2009). Using DNA microarray or flow cytometric analysis, we and others found myeloma cells to express the two BAFF receptors, BCMA and TACI (Moreaux et al. 2004, 2009; Novak et al. 2004). BAFF-R is rarely expressed by myeloma cells (Moreaux et al. 2009). This observation prompted us to look for a role of the BAFF/APRIL in the survival/proliferation of myeloma cells. We found that two BAFF family proteins, BAFF or APRIL, are potent survival and proliferation factors of myeloma cells, depending on their expression of BAFF-R or TACI. In addition, BAFF or APRIL can protect myeloma cells from dexamethasone-induced apoptosis (Moreaux et al. 2004). Only a part of human myeloma cell lines do express TACI (Moreaux et al. 2007). As for primary myeloma cells, the $TACI^+$ myeloma cells have a mature plasma cell gene expression profiling (Moreaux et al. 2005). The results prompted us to perform a phase I trial with a BAFF/APRIL inhibitor, a TACI receptor fused with Fc fragment of human immunoglobulin (Rossi et al. 2009). TACI-Fc is a dimer. We observed a lack of toxicity of the treatment, a decrease in the concentration of polyclonal immunoglobulins in some patients indicating an inhibition of the survival of normal plasma cells. A stabilization of the disease was found for some of these patients with refractory disease (Rossi et al. 2009).

3.5.5
Hierarchy of Myeloma Cell Growth Factors and Potential Clinical Applications

In the end, a minimum amount of growth factors need to be present in conjunction with chromosomal aberrations (see Sect. 3.3) to overcome the cell cycle break present in normal plasma cells (see Sect. 3.5). Some of the different components seem to be interchangeable, to a certain degree. High intrinsic CCND-expression (e.g., CCND1 as present in t(11;14)) might reduce the dependence on extrinsic growth factor stimulation. As reviewed above, several growth factors of myeloma cells have been documented, in particular because they are also critical for the generation of normal plasma cells: IL-6, IL-10, IL-21, IFNα, BAFF, and APRIL.

An exception is IGF-1 whose receptor is aberrantly expressed by about 50% of primary myeloma cells of newly diagnosed patients in association with a poor prognosis and 90% of myeloma cell lines (Sprynski et al. 2009). This aberrant IGF-1R expression confers a major myeloma cell growth activity to IGF-1 but also to insulin, both molecules being abundant in vivo.

In agreement with this pathophysiological observation, we and others have found IGF-1 being the major growth factor for myeloma cells, the effect of other growth factors being dependent in part on the activation of IGF-1R by IGF-1. This is the case for IL-6, IL-21, EGF family members, and HGF (Menoret et al. 2008; Sprynski et al. 2009). The effect of IGF-1 is dependent on the expression of CD45 by myeloma cells. Indeed, the phosphatase CD45 can dephosphorylate and inactivate IGF-1R, conferring an important role for IL-6 to trigger the growth of $CD45^+$ myeloma cells (Descamps et al. 2006).

Another major point is the role played by syndecan-1 in myeloma biology. Syndecan-1 with three heparan-sulfate chains and two chondroitin-sulfate ones is mandatory for human myeloma cell growth in animal models. Targeting syndecan-1 or the heparan-sulfate chain synthesis blocks myeloma cell growth in vivo (Reijmers et al. 2010). Syndecan-1 may bind large amounts of growth factors (Mahtouk et al. 2006) and mobilize them close to growth factor receptors. This is likely the case for IGF-1, which circulates at a large concentration in the form of an inactive complex that can be disrupted by binding to syndecan-1.

Clinical implications of these findings are that targeting IGF-1R should be of major interest. One has to be aware of using inhibitors blocking both IGF-1 activation of IGF-1R homodimeric receptors and also insulin activation of IGF-1R/INSR hybrid receptors. IL-6 inhibitors should be also of major interest. These growth factor inhibitors have not to be used alone, since at the stop of the treatment, resumption of tumor growth will occur. This was observed in patients treated with anti-IL-6 antibodies. Inhibitors of myeloma cell growth factors have to be used in combination with cytotoxic agents as melphalan, dexamethasone, or bortezomib. Indeed, these growth factors can increase the resistance of myeloma cells to these drugs in vivo. In particular, we have documented the rise of large amounts of IL-6 9 days after high-dose melphalan in vivo (Condomines et al. 2010). This huge concentration of IL-6 will facilitate melphalan-resistant myeloma cells to repair their lesions in vivo. We have performed a phase II trial with anti-IL-6 antibody in association with high-dose melphalan (Rossi et al. 2005). This trial has shown the lack of toxicity of blocking IL-6 throughout high-dose melphalan and stem cell transplantation. It has also shown that patients treated with high-dose melphalan, stem transplantation, and anti-IL-6 had a survival advantage when mixed with a large series of matched patients treated with melphalan and stem cell transplantation alone (Rossi et al. 2005). In addition, drugs targeting efficiently the heparan-sulfate chains of syndecan-1, highly expressed by myeloma cells, will inhibit the biological effect of the majority of myeloma cell growth factors.

3.6 Multiple Myeloma Cells and the Microenvironment

Multiple myeloma is characterized by a progressive accumulation of myeloma cells within the bone marrow and a concomitant transformation of the bone marrow microenvironment. Hallmarks of the transformation process in the bone marrow are development of bone disease, impaired cellular immunity, and (increased) bone marrow angiogenesis (Chap. 4). We discuss in the following in depth the reciprocal interaction of myeloma cells and bone turnover as an example.

3.6.1
Pathogenesis of Myeloma-Induced Bone Disease

As normal plasma cells, myeloma cells are in tight *bidirectional* interaction with other cellular populations of the microenvironment as well as the extracellular matrix (Nagasawa 2006; Yaccoby et al. 2004; Abe et al. 2004). On the one hand, the bone marrow microenvironment forms a niche influencing plasma and myeloma cells being essential for their survival: Growth and survival factors like APRIL or IGF-1 are produced by osteoclasts (Moreaux et al. 2004; Sprynski et al. 2009), or, like IGF-1, liberated when bone-matrix is degraded during bone turnover. Additionally, a direct, e.g., integrin-mediated, interaction with fibronectin within the bone-matrix takes place (Shain et al. 2009; Tai et al. 2003). Furthermore, osteoclasts stimulate myeloma cell survival and proliferation via direct interaction (Yaccoby et al. 2004; Abe et al. 2004), especially involving $\alpha_4\beta_1$-integrin (Mori et al. 2004). On the other hand, myeloma cells influence the bone marrow microenvironment by increasing the number and activity of osteoclasts while reducing number and activity of osteoblasts, and destroying the three-dimensional structure of the bone remodeling compartment (BRC; see Fig. 3.7).

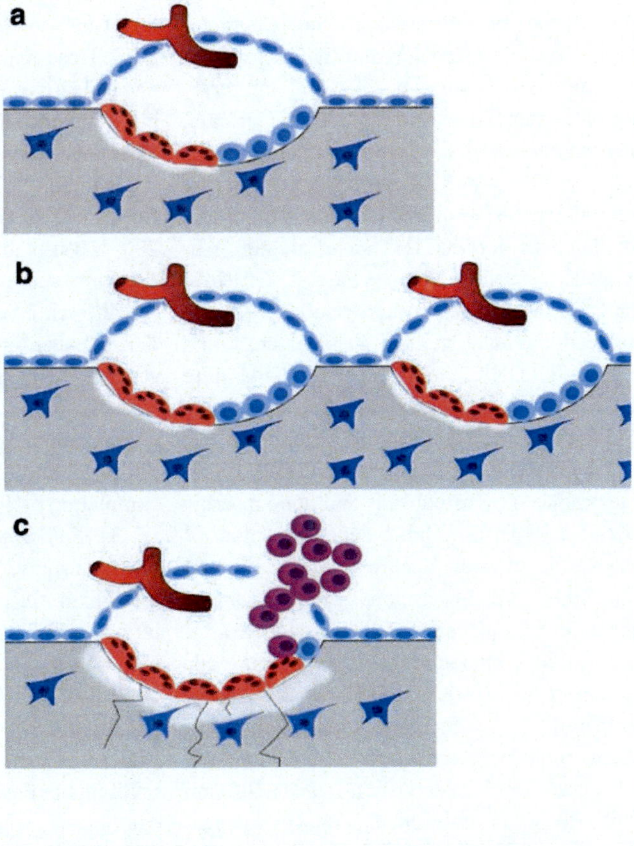

Fig. 3.7 *Myeloma-induced bone defects*. (**a**) Physiological situation. Bone formation by osteoblasts (*light blue*) and bone resorption by osteoclasts (*red*) are coupled. (**b**) In multiple myeloma, initially a higher bone resorption is found while bone formation keeps the pace (intact "bone remodeling compartments", BRCs). (**c**) If BRCs are disrupted due to interaction with myeloma cells (*violet*), bone resorption is increased and bone formation almost completely abrogated

3

(1) *Increase in osteoclast number and activity*: Normal and malignant plasma cells produce osteoclast-activating or osteoclast-generating mediators like vascular endothelial growth factor A (VEGFA; (Hose et al. 2009a). In a co-culture model of osteoclasts and myeloma cells, a simultaneous inhibition of VEGF and osteopontin inhibits angiogenesis and bone resorption almost completely (Tanaka et al. 2007). In vitro, VEGF can substitute the stimulating effect of macrophage-colony stimulating factor (M-CSF) on differentiation of osteoclasts (Niida et al. 1999). Further factors are macrophage inflammatory proteins (MIP)-1α and MIP-1β (Terpos et al. 2003a), which directly increase production rate and resorption activity of osteoclasts by binding to the receptors CCR1 and CCR5 (Oba et al. 2005). At the same time, they increase expression of receptor activator nuclear factor kappa B ligand (RANKL)- and IL-6 expression by bone marrow stromal cells and indirectly stimulate osteoclasts (Abe et al. 2002; Oba et al. 2005; see below). Furthermore, myeloma cells shift the OPG:RANKL-ratio on osteoblasts by aberrant expression of Wnt-signaling inhibitors like dickkopf 1 (DKK1; Tian et al. 2003) or secreted frizzled related protein-2 (sFRP-2; Oshima et al. 2005). Physiologically, DKK1 is produced by bone marrow stromal cells and osteoblasts. DKK1 inhibits Wnt3A-signaling via LRP5/6 leading to a consecutive shift in the OPG:RANKL-expression on osteoblasts in favor of RANKL. Osteoprotegerin (OPG) likewise produced by osteoblasts and bone marrow stromal cells is, as soluble decoy-receptor for RANKL, its physiological antagonist (Simonet et al. 1997). OPG-secretion by bone marrow stromal cells and osteoblasts is reduced after direct cellular interaction with myeloma cells (Pearse et al. 2001; Giuliani et al. 2001). Compared to healthy individuals, myeloma patients show increased RANKL- and decreased OPG-serum levels (Pearse et al. 2001; Giuliani et al. 2001; Politou et al. 2004). Increasing serum-RANKL:OPG-ratios correlate with extent of disease and survival (Terpos et al. 2003b). Whether RANKL is also expressed by primary myeloma cells or myeloma cell lines is discussed controversially (Sezer et al. 2002; Giuliani et al. 2001, 2002; Yaccoby et al. 2007; Haaber et al. 2008). Increased RANKL-expression by osteoblasts and bone marrow stromal cells (Pearse et al. 2001) is a central feature. Interaction with receptor activator of nuclear factor-κB (RANK) on osteoclast-precursors and osteoclasts stimulates production and resorption activity of osteoclasts (Lacey et al. 1998).

(2) *Reducing the number of osteoblasts*: Myeloma cells express functional inhibitors of the differentiation from mesenchymal stromal (stem) cells to osteoblasts. An example is HGF. HGF is expressed by malignant plasma cells of about 60% of myeloma patients (Standal et al. 2007; Hose et al. 2009a). High serum-HGF-level correlate here negatively with the serum level of bone-specific alkaline phosphatase (as marker of osteoblast activity; Standal et al. 2007). In vitro, HGF inhibits BMP-induced osteoblastogenesis from mesenchymal stromal cells (Standal et al. 2007). It lifts the BMP-induced arrest of proliferation of mesenchymal stromal cells necessary for differentiation. A direct cell-to-cell interaction between myeloma cells and bone marrow stromal cells leads to increased IL-6 and RANKL-production whereas OPG-production is concomitantly reduced (Giuliani et al. 2001; Shipman and Croucher 2003), in turn again stimulating osteoclastogenesis.

(3) *(Self-)limiting interaction*: We and others have shown recently that normal as well as malignant plasma cells produce factors stimulating osteoblast differentiation and activity, e.g., BMP6 (Seckinger et al. 2009) or adrenomedullin (Cornish et al. 1997; see Sect. 3.2.2). This could be eventually interpreted as self-limitation of the impact of plasma and myeloma cells on bone turnover, in analogy to osteoblasts, which likewise produce RANKL *and* OPG.

Taken together, myeloma cells have the ability to induce a reduced number of osteoblasts with a RANKL:OPG-ratio shifted to RANKL (osteoclastogenesis), and an increased number and activity of osteoclasts (see Fig. 3.7). To understand the in vivo situation, however, the microanatomical structure of bone remodeling and interaction with myeloma cells needs to be understood.

(4) *Role of intact "bone remodeling compartments"*: Histomorphometric investigations report myeloma patients to show an increase in number and activity of osteoclasts (Valentin-Opran et al. 1982; Taube et al. 1992; Bataille et al. 1991). The number of osteoblasts in early stages of myeloma is likewise increased, but decreases over time together with osteoblast activity in patients with bone lesions (see Fig. 3.7; Bataille et al. 1990, 1991; Giuliani et al. 2005; Standal et al. 2007). Andersen et al. published recently a very insightful analysis of the role of the BRCs and an intact canopy of osteoblast like cells on the magnitude of bone resorption/formation activities (Andersen et al. 2009, 2010). They compared the extent of erosion and osteoid surfaces (1) in control bone, (2) in myeloma biopsies showing more than 75% of the total erosion under intact BRC canopies (MM-I), and (3) in those with at least 75% erosion under disrupted BRC canopies (MM-D). MM-I biopsies show increased erosion surface, osteoclast surface, and osteoid surface compared to controls. MM-D biopsies show even more increased erosion surface and osteoclast surface compared to MM-I biopsies, but in contrast, their osteoid surface falls below control levels, thereby indicating lack of bone formation despite increased bone resorption. In control and MM-I biopsies, increased osteoid surface parallels increased erosion surface, indicating coupling between bone formation and resorption. In contrast, in MM-D biopsies, erosion surface increases strongly without corresponding increase in osteoid surface, indicating absence of coupling between bone formation and resorption. Thus, bone formation responds commensurately to bone resorption only when the BRC canopy is continuous. The same conclusion holds true if the analysis is based on osteoclast surface and if the myeloma biopsies are grouped according to the proportion of osteoclast surface in intact BRCs. Bone formation occurs very preferentially in intact BRCs as also seen when analyzing the proportion of osteoid in intact BRCs; this proportion averages 75% in all three groups of biopsies, despite their differences in overall extent of osteoid surface. This is in marked contrast with erosion, which proceeds whether BRCs are intact or not and becomes even higher in the latter case. The authors deduced a close link between the integrity of BRC canopies and the magnitude of osteoclast and osteoblast activities. In summary, if BRCs are disrupted, bone resorption tends to increase and bone formation to be prevented (Andersen et al. 2009, 2010), whereas in intact BRCs present in controls, MM-I, and patients with hyperparathyroidism, bone formation increases with bone resorption (Andersen et al. 2009; Hauge et al. 2001).

3.6.2 Patterns and Healing of Bone Defects

Nothing is currently known about causes of different *patterns of bone defects* in multiple myeloma, e.g., diffuse and focal patterns. Healing of bone defects, if present, appears also in patients with complete remission at orders of magnitude slower as compared to the healing of fractures (Epstein and Walker 2006), comparable with the delayed healing of osteoporotic fractures; likewise, the reason remains unclear. Possible scenarios are the presence of remaining residual myeloma cells, which maintain a continuous stimulation of bone resorption vs. bone formation (Esteve and Roodman 2007), a loss of the stimulus to repair bone defects, and a "scorched earth" left over by destroyed BRCs and pathological remodeling in bone defects. At the same time, the bone marrow microenvironment might remember former presence of myeloma cells over years. Evidence is given by in vitro differentiated osteoblasts from myeloma patients, which show a different expression pattern compared to those differentiated from normal donors (Corre et al. 2007).

3.6.3 Therapeutic Strategies for Treatment and Prevention of Myeloma Bone Disease

Amino-bisphosphonates like zoledronate induce apoptosis in osteoclasts (Kellinsalmi et al. 2005) and significantly reduce skeletal events in patients with malignant bone destruction (Rosen et al. 2004). Amino-bisphosphonates show – albeit limited – activity against myeloma cells (Aviles et al. 2007). RANKL-antibodies like denosumab show direct inhibition of osteoclastogenesis (Lewiecki 2006). Novel agents used in myeloma treatment like proteasome inhibitors (bortezomib) or IMiDs (lenalidomide) exhibit at systemic application besides their activity against malignant plasma cells an impact on osteoblast and osteoclast function. Lenalidomide inhibits resorption by osteoclasts, but seems not to influence osteoblast function (Breitkreutz et al. 2008; De et al. 2009). Bortezomib induces apoptosis in myeloma cells (Richardson et al. 2005), inhibits bone resorption by osteoclasts (von Metzler et al. 2007), and stimulates osteoblast activity (Heider et al. 2006). The latter is of special interest; as with parathyroid hormone, only one bone-anabolic compound is approved for systemic application. For local use, BMP2 and BMP7 are approved (Gautschi et al. 2007; Tsuji et al. 2006).

An appropriate functionalization of biomaterials using pathophysiological knowledge for local treatment of bone defects in multiple myeloma especially with bone formation promoting agents seems thus to be a promising approach.

3.7 Pathogenetic Model of Multiple Myeloma

We will conclude this chapter with some more general reflections on factors influencing myeloma cell accumulation and a proposal for a new pathogenetic model of multiple myeloma (Fig. 3.8).

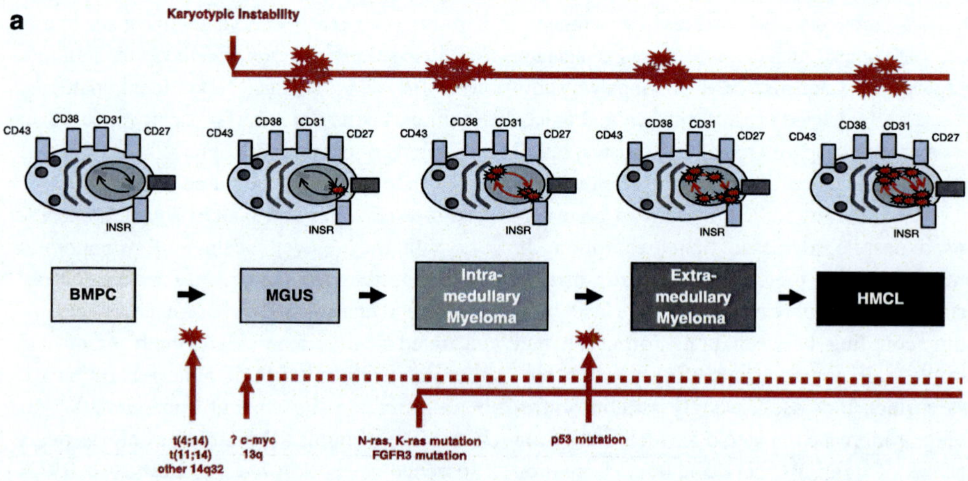

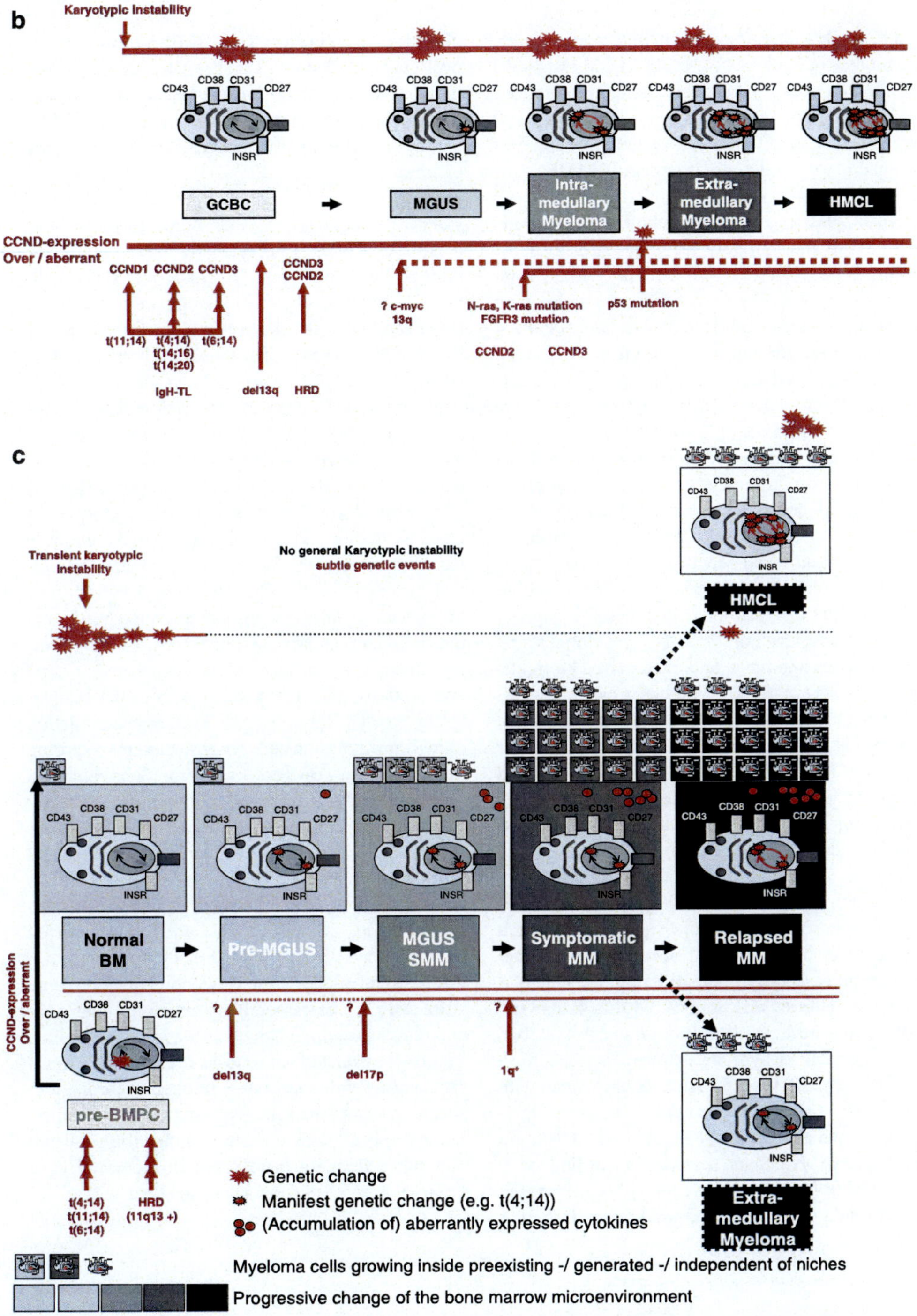
b
Karyotypic instability
CD43
CD38
CD31
CD27
INSR
GCBC
MGUS
Intra-medullary Myeloma
Extra-medullary Myeloma
HMCL
CCND-expression
Over / aberrant
CCND1 CCND2 CCND3
CCND3
CCND2
t(11;14)
t(4;14)
t(14;16)
t(14;20)
t(6;14)
IgH-TL
del13q
HRD
? c-myc
13q
N-ras, K-ras mutation
FGFR3 mutation
p53 mutation
CCND2
CCND3
c
Transient karyotypic instability
No general Karyotypic instability
subtle genetic events
HMCL
Normal BM
Pre-MGUS
MGUS SMM
Symptomatic MM
Relapsed MM
CCND-expression
Over / aberrant
pre-BMPC
?
?
?
del13q
del17p
1q+
t(4;14)
t(11;14)
t(6;14)
HRD
(11q13 +)
Extra-medullary Myeloma
Genetic change
Manifest genetic change (e.g. t(4;14))
(Accumulation of) aberrantly expressed cytokines
Myeloma cells growing inside preexisting -/ generated -/ independent of niches
Progressive change of the bone marrow microenvironment

Fig. 3.8 *Models of pathogenesis of multiple myeloma.* The models of Hallek et al. 1998(A) and Bergsagel et al. 2005(B) focus on a sequel of genetic aberrations driving changes of gene expression on (malignant) plasma cells that in turn lead to a transformation of the bone marrow microenvironment (BMME). Our model (C) proposes the accumulation of hijacked "normal" plasma cells accumulating in the bone marrow and thus initially driving changes in the bone marrow microenvironment. **(a)** Model from Hallek et al. 1998. The model proposes an ongoing karyotypic instability (indicated by *red stars*) starting at MGUS-stage and leads to multiple accumulating genetic lesion (*red stars* with *black border*). Bone marrow plasma cells (BMPCs) or precursors are targeted by recurrent IgH-translocations. Plasma cells progress from a premalignant MGUS-stage in a sequel from intramedullary to extramedullary myeloma with human myeloma cell lines (HMCLs) being the end stage. Each step of this sequel is driven by an additional genetic event. Dysregulation of c-myc is thought to appear early, ras-mutation and eventually mutations of FGFR3 appear beginning with the intramedullary myeloma-stage. p53 mutations appear as late event. **(b)** The model from Bergsagel et al. (2005) focuses on the earliest oncogenic changes that are thought to involve three overlapping pathways and occur in germinal center B cells (GCBC). They are present in MGUS thought to be premalignant tumors. Two partially overlapping pathways, indicated by IgH-translocations and multiple trisomies, generate non-hyperdiploid and hyperdiploid tumors, respectively. A third pathway (del13q) leading to monosomy of chromosome 13 or deletion of 13q14 can be present in both types of tumors, but occurs with a higher prevalence in non-hyperdiploid tumors, where it occurs in almost all tumors with t(4;14) and t(14;16), but infrequently in tumors with t(11;14). The essentially invariant dysregulation of a CCND (aberrant/overexpression) is associated with these early oncogenic changes. Recurrent IgH-translocations and the dysregulation of CCND are used to group MGUS and myeloma according to the TC-classification (see Sect. 3.4.1). **(c)** Proposed new model. Two principal pathways targeting plasma cell precursors (pre-BMPCs), most likely post-germinal-center B cells, i.e., translocations most often involving the IgH-locus, and a hyperdiploid pathway. Both lead to increased CCND-expression, overexpression (CCND2) or aberrant expression (CCND1, CCND3). Karyotypic instability is in place only at this time (indicated by *red stars*). Targeted pre-BMPCs home to the normal plasma cell niche (indicated by a *grey box*). The BMME (*light-grey box*) is unaltered. These cells already have a slightly dysregulated cell cycle (hijacked "normal" plasma cells) and the tendency to accumulate (see text for details). In pre-MGUS-stage, the transformation process of the BMME begins slowly. Initially, pre-MGUS cells share the niche with BMPCs. A further accumulation leads to MGUS/smoldering MM (SMM) stage without the necessity of further genetic events. The BMME is slowly transformed by normal BMPC-factors (indicated by the increasingly *dark grey*) and aberrantly expressed factors (*red dots*). Aberrant expression is driven mainly by the changing microenvironment, not accumulating genetic alterations. Malignant plasma cells populate existing BMPC-niches (*light-grey boxes*), recruit new niches (*dark grey boxes*) and partially gain independence from the BMME (plasma cell without a box). Further accumulation of malignant plasma cells leads to therapy-requiring myeloma. The BMME transformation continues (*darkening grey*, increased number of aberrantly expressed factors) in a positive feedback loop. A further selection pressure to recruit new niches and grow independently of niches is in place. HMCLs can be derived from therapy-requiring or relapsed myeloma, i.e., cells that already gained partial independence of the BMME. They do represent a further step of myeloma development. The same holds true for extramedullary myeloma that does not regularly appear, even in end-stage patients. Progression-related aberrations (del17p, 1q21 gain) can appear with increasing frequency throughout accumulation of malignant plasma cells; these aberrations appear with a certain probability and are thus more frequent in relapsed myeloma; at least $1q21^{+}$. For detailed discussion, see Sect. 3.8

3.7.1 Disease Activity, Tumor Load, and Molecular Characteristics of Myeloma Cells

3.7.1.1 Describing Disease Activity

Main determinants of *disease activity* at a *given time* are the *tumor-load* (total number of plasma cells) and *molecular characteristics* of myeloma cells. Tumor-load and molecular characteristics are to a certain degree independent at a given time (e.g., an aggressive lesion can be present together with high and low tumor mass), but interdependent, if the time course is taken into account (an aggressive lesion will lead faster to a higher tumor mass and might have, e.g., a higher bone turnover stimulating capacity).

Molecular characteristics at a given time represent a flash image of (1) myelomagenesis (etiology), (2) entity (e.g., HRD/non-HRD, t(4;14)-myeloma, GEP-based group), and (3) accumulated evolutionary (progression-related) aberrations (e.g., gain of 1q21, loss of p53-expression). Whereas as a matter of definition etiologic aberrations cannot change over time, for the disease entity this depends on the definition of the latter. iFISH-based entities (e.g., t(4;14), HRD myeloma) seem to be constant throughout the course of myeloma. This likewise holds true for GEP-based groups with the exception of the proliferation group within the molecular classification (Zhan et al. 2006) to which patient-attributed other groups can progress, e.g., patients from MS (t(4;14)) at diagnosis to PRL in relapse.

Molecular characteristics comprise a further important feature of myeloma cells: their "biological activity", e.g., potential to generate bone lesions, induce angiogenesis, or immunosuppression (e.g., expression of cancer testis antigens; Condomines et al. 2007, 2009 or CD200; Barclay et al. 2002; Moreaux et al. 2006). This biological activity is not necessarily connected to disease etiology or entity as exemplified by the promotion of bone disease by DKK1-expression.

The *total number of plasma cells* is mediated by five main variables: (1) The proliferation rate, i.e., speed of cell division; (2) the survival (or death-) rate, comprising of (a) apoptosis rate ("suicide") and (b) (T-)cell mediated elimination-rate ("killing," a host factor), the first two taken together as growth rate, (3) the dissemination rate, i.e., the ability of myeloma cells to spread to different bone marrow parts and niches therein, (4) the rate of transforming the bone marrow microenvironment and thus the creation of additional niches, and (5) the rate of gaining independence of niches. Regarding the latter factors, whereas normal bone marrow plasma cells depend on *extrinsic* survival signals provided within a special niche, myeloma cells can gain a certain independence of these by autocrine production (e.g., IL-6), induction of the production in the bone marrow microenvironment, e.g., IL-6 via amphiregulin produced by myeloma cells, and recruitment of factors abundant in serum (e.g., IGF-1) by expression of respective receptors (Sprynski et al. 2009; see Fig. 3.8). An additional, less understood, mechanism is an *intrinsic* loss of dependence on these factors, e.g., by aberrant CCND1-expression due to presence of a t(11;14) mimicking a respective growth factor stimulation converging on the G_0/G_1-transition. Human myeloma cell lines, carrying a plethora of chromosomal aberrations and being only dependent on serum factors in their culture medium, are a special example. These variables are partially interdependent, e.g., transformation of the bone marrow microenvironment and recruitment of additional survival factors can influence apoptosis rate. Over time, the proliferation *(growth) rate* becomes a very important feature, also transmitting to prognostic significance (see Sect. 3.5).

A further important characteristic of myeloma cells within one patient is their potential intrapatient-*heterogeneity*. Evidence is given by the presence of subclonal-, and the emergence of "progression-related" aberrations like gains of 1q21 (see Sect. 3.3). It is therefore an interesting question whether the two possibilities of myeloma cell accumulation – generation of niches and obtaining the ability to grow independently of these – take part in the generation of intra-patient clonal heterogeneity. This heterogeneity might likewise be present in terms of a part of the myeloma cell population being "myeloma stem cells," a controversial discussion outside the scope of this chapter.

3.7.1.2 Interpatient Heterogeneity: Many and Multiple Myelomas

Discernable chromosomal aberrations (e.g., IgH-translocations vs. hyperdiploidy) and a plethora of changes in gene expression are present in different multiple myeloma patients, i.e., a huge molecular interpatient heterogeneity. Clinically, multiple myeloma is on the one hand a rather homogeneous disease, with plasma cell accumulation in the bone marrow, and almost all patients developing increased bone marrow angiogenesis and bone lesions. On the other hand, multiple myeloma is very heterogeneous in terms of survival (see Sects. 3.3.5 and 3.4.2). As discussed above, on a molecular level, almost all patients show the presence of either an IgH-translocation or a hyperdiploidy driven pathway, and almost all show a CCND dysregulation. This notion has lead to the idea of "many and multiple myelomas" (Fonseca 2003).

Thus, the same clinical phenotype (e.g., accumulation of plasma cells, induction of bone disease and angiogenesis) can be reached by different molecular phenotypes, i.e., different alterations of DNA and gene expression. For example, there has been up to now no single unifying aberration or change in gene expression found explaining bone disease or angiogenesis in myeloma (Hose et al. 2009a).

From a theoretical point of view, there are two possible explanations: (1) Targets of aberrations converge on a limited number of intermediary molecules of signal transduction ("*molecular hubs*"). If a certain intermediary is needed to be activated for myeloma cell survival/proliferation or a specific feature of myeloma cells like induction of bone disease, selection pressure could lead on different ways to this necessary alteration. If, e.g., increased ras-signaling would be critical, this could be due to, e.g., (a) autocrine IL-6 production, (b) increased IL-6 production in the bone marrow microenvironment by AREG-expression of myeloma cells, and (c) IGF-1 expression via ras/MAPK signal transduction, or constitutive ras-activation in myeloma (Klein et al. 2003; Neri et al. 1989; Liu et al. 1996). Another example is given by *D-type cyclin* expression – the hallmark of multiple myeloma – which can be due to several molecular causes (see Sect. 3.5). Here, CCND could exemplify a final integrator of signal transduction by external (growth factor stimulation) and internal (aberrant CCND-expression) signals. (2) Myeloma cells are "just hijacked" normal plasma cells in terms of an initially (subtle) takeover of cell cycle control leading to a slow induction of accumulation of plasma cells but otherwise use of (physiological) plasma cell features explaining clinical features of myeloma. This could easily explain why different aberrations targeting cell cycle and especially CCND lead to the same clinical phenotype of multiple myeloma (see also the following). According to this model, a low number of aberrations targeting the cell cycle takes place very early in the development of myeloma, i.e., in post-germinal center B cells. The accumulation of plasma cell-like myeloma cells, i.e., hijacked "normal" plasma cells, then changes the bone marrow microenvironment. Not investigated up to now, expression changes in myeloma cells could be attributed to epigenetic changes driven by the changing bone marrow microenvironment, not primary genetic events.

3.7.2 Multistep Transformation of Myeloma Cell Model

This model initially described by Hallek et al. (Hallek et al. 1998; Fig. 3.8a) is based on a proposed *sequel of progressive genetic* events that profoundly change the pathophysiological features of myeloma cells at each step and then lead to the ordered progression from a normal plasma cell to MGUS, where the cells are immortalized, but not transformed, and do not progressively accumulate or cause bone destruction; to intramedullary myeloma, where the cells are confined to the bone marrow microenvironment, accumulate and cause bone destruction; to extramedullary myeloma, where the cells proliferate more rapidly and grow in the blood (plasma cell leukemia) or other extramedullary sites; and to a myeloma cell line, where the cells may be propagated in vitro. Critical oncogenic events in myeloma cells are thought either to occur after or do not interfere with most of the normal differentiation process involved in generating a long-lived plasma cell. The model evokes a karyotypic instability thought to appear in MGUS and continues throughout all stages of tumor progression, giving rise to the different molecular events in relation to clinical progression. 14q32-translocations are seen as a potential early event, concordant with isotype switch recombination, so that it precedes MGUS. Some translocations (e.g., t(11;14)) were thought to lead more rapidly to fulminant disease, eventually bypassing an MGUS-stage. For other aberrations, the timing was not clear but nonetheless thought to be in some kind of 7der, including monosomy 13 or dysregulation of c-myc. In patients with aberrant FGFR3 expression caused by t(4;14), a mutation of FGFR3 could lead to ligand independence and clinical progression (Sibley et al. 2002). Mutations of N- and K-ras are not present in MGUS, but are present in intramedullary myeloma, with an increasing incidence as the disease progresses. Mutations of p53 are a late event associated with aggressive extramedullary myeloma.

Current additions are the presence of a presumed second pathway (i.e., hyperdiploid myeloma) independent of IgH-translocations (Fig. 3.6; Bergsagel and Kuehl 2005; Bergsagel et al. 2005; Fig. 3.8b).

This model basically focuses (1) on the genetic changes within myeloma cells (i.e., genetic alterations causing aberrant expression) as driving force for myeloma cell progression and *concomitantly* for changes within the bone marrow microenvironment; the changes within the bone marrow microenvironment are thus driven by the "malignant features" of malignant plasma cells; and (2) on an underlying broad chromosomal instability as a driving force.

As of now, parts of this concept need to be reevaluated: First, there is currently only evidence for rather subtle changes, and an ongoing genetic instability has never been proven with nonproliferation-dependant methods (see Sect. 3.3 and below). Second, several features attributed to myeloma cells are already such of normal plasma cells, including the ability to induce angiogenesis (see Sect. 3.8.3.1). As mentioned before, part of the change within the bone marrow microenvironment could be driven by accumulation of "semi-normal" plasma cell–like myeloma cells. "Semi-normal" here refers to this change being due to normal plasma cell features in cells "hijacked" to limited proliferation. Third, the proposed sequel from normal plasma cells, MGUS, intramedullary multiple myeloma, extramedullary and cell line–like myeloma seems to be rather an exception than the rule. Extramedullary myeloma is a special feature in a subpopulation of patients, and eventually, even in these, a subpopulation of myeloma cells. Myeloma cell lines are only obtainable in less than 10% of patients and almost never in hyperdiploid multiple myeloma (Fig. 3.6).

3.7.3 Transformation of Bone Marrow Microenvironment Model

3.7.3.1 Features of Normal Plasma Cells as Explanation for Those of Myeloma Cells

Capabilities of malignant plasma cells are partly explainable by physiological functions of their normal counterpart, bone marrow plasma cells. The primary feature of the latter is being antibody-production facilities. Evidence is given that they re-structure their surroundings (bone marrow microenvironment) according to their needs: (1) by securing their own supply by a basal angiogenic stimulus, e.g., the production of VEGFA (Hose et al. 2009a); (2) bone marrow plasma cells can interact with the microenvironment and bone remodeling by production of factors like BMP6 (see Sect. 3.2.2; Seckinger et al. 2009); (3) connected to this or via an independent process, bone marrow plasma cells are able to *create to a certain extent their survival niche*. The niche is critical to allow normal plasma cells surviving for several years (see Sect. 3.2.1). The number of survival niches is thought to be limited and thus help in maintaining a fairly constant number of plasma cells over life, evidenced by a constant level of polyclonal immunoglobulin, despite the ability of the immune system to adapt to novel antigen challenges, and thus the creation of novel plasma cells that have to compete for a survival niche; thus, "niching" per se is a dynamic process. Furthermore, bone marrow plasma cells can create niches under certain conditions, as exemplified in cases of reactive plasmacytosis, in which their number can increase for a prolonged amount of time. Much less is known about the ability of bone marrow plasma cells to interact with the hematopoietic and the immune system. Taken together, molecular alterations in the pre-bone marrow plasma cell are according to our concept a crucial factor for molecular pathogenesis of myeloma, as the proliferation arrest is removed and the "potential to proliferate" liberated, leading to accumulation of hijacked "normal" plasma cells, which by itself generates changes in the bone marrow microenvironment without the a priori need for enforced selection of myeloma cell variants with additional aberrations.

3.7.3.2 Pre-MGUS-Stage

At this stage, founder cells (myeloma cells) are present, but the "disease" activity is far below the (detection) limit defining "MGUS," even by molecular techniques. Initial *etiological chromosomal aberrations* (probably related to a hyperdiploid and a non-hyperdiploid pathway, see Sect. 3.3.2) lead to subtle cell cycle alteration (direct or indirect CCND over or aberrant expression). Cell cycle breaks are initially unaltered leading to a very low proliferation rate with doubling times of months or even years. T cell–mediated elimination of aberrant cells is intact. The apoptosis rate is comparable to the one of normal plasma cells. These cells presumably populate the same survival niche as normal bone marrow plasma cells allowing their longevity. Pre-MGUS myeloma cells are basically hijacked "normal" plasma cells.

3.7.3.3 MGUS-Stage/Smoldering Myeloma

Continuing accumulation of myeloma cells in the bone marrow leads to a detectable but asymptomatic "disease" – MGUS. It is now clear that MGUS consistently precedes myeloma (Landgren et al. 2009). The accumulation slowly transforms the bone marrow microenvironment, initially mainly by factors already produced by normal bone marrow plasma cells (e.g., VEGFA). The total production of these factors is increased due to the increasing number of hijacked "normal" plasma cells/myeloma cells. At the same time, a selection pressure for myeloma cells is in place due to the limited number of niches – either to create new niches comparable to those of normal bone marrow plasma cells, or gain a certain independence by recruiting new sources of growth and survival factors, i.e., by aberrantly producing such factors (e.g., HGF, amphiregulin, IL-6) or by inducing their production within the bone marrow microenvironment (e.g., IL-6) to increase the availability of growth factors present in serum (e.g., IGF-1 by better blood vessel supply (angiogenesis)), access to growth factors for which myeloma cells carry receptors, but the bone marrow microenvironment does not express ligands (e.g., FGF:FGFR3). A further tappable source of growth and survival factors is the alteration of bone turnover. Initially, BRCs are relatively intact (see Sect. 3.7) and the surrounding bone marrow unaltered. Some leaking out of these complexes (e.g., of IGF-1 liberated from bone-matrix) is likely. An increased bone turnover would lead to an increase of total leaking despite BRCs being intact. At a later stage, largely increased liberation will appear as a consequence of disrupted BRCs, leading in turn to lytic bone lesions (see Sect. 3.7). Interaction of myeloma cells with the BRCs (osteoblasts and osteoclasts) is presumably initially mostly driven by factors already expressed by normal plasma cells, e.g., BMP6. Nevertheless, myeloma cells aberrantly express such factors as exemplified by the Wnt-antagonist DKK1 (Li et al. 2006). We hypothesize these factors to be already expressed at the earliest stage, in agreement with complete lack of evidence of an appearance only in disease progression.

3.7.3.4 Symptomatic Myeloma

Further accumulation of myeloma cells leads to an increasing concentration of plasma cell and aberrantly expressed myeloma cell growth factors. As mentioned above, this aberrant expression is not necessarily the consequence of genetic alteration but could also be driven by the changing bone marrow microenvironment, in turn leading to expression changes within hijacked "normal" plasma cells driving these to an increasingly abnormal expression pattern. This could explain the plethora of expression changes (see also Sect. 3.4) without the prerequisite of an ongoing genetic instability. The factors act together in terms of a positive feedback mechanism: better growth conditions lead to an increased speed of accumulation of myeloma cells and in turn a better adaption of the bone marrow microenvironment according to the need of myeloma cells. The increasing transforms of the bone marrow microenvironment become clinically visible in terms of (1) increased angiogenesis, (2) bone destruction (breakup of BRCs and subsequent generation of osteolysis and generalized osteopenia), (3) reduced tumor surveillance, and (4) increased plasma cell infiltration based on generation additional survival niches for myeloma cells. As mentioned above, we hypothesize that accumulation of plasma cell-like myeloma cells could already explain a basic appearance of these features without the a priori necessity of directed extensive molecular changes within the myeloma cells (see above). This could also elegantly explain the lack of one myeloma typical aberration. Several aberrations ultimately converge on hubs and at least in part on CCND (see Sect. 3.8.1). A positive feedback loop would be a good explanation for a scenario of relatively long slow growth by creating additional niches with a subsequent "outbreak" of therapy-requiring myeloma once an additional source is tapped (as a BRC).

The possible explanation that pathogenetic features of myeloma are driven by cell cycle targeted "hijacking" of normal plasma cell functions is of fundamental interest, as it takes away the necessity of the requirement of accumulation of further chromosomal aberrations for progression within the sequel from MGUS to overt myeloma and plasma cell leukemia as proposed in the model of Hallek et al. (see Sect. 3.8.2; Hallek et al. 1998). The proposed principal role of plasma cell accumulation notwithstanding, a likely subtle selection pressure may be present in terms of factors promoting (faster) plasma cell accumulation (Sect. 3.8.1.1). To this end, growth factor stimulation substantially present due to the changing bone marrow microenvironment might lead to an increased tendency to proliferate and "overrule" cell cycle checkpoints inhibiting growth of cells, in particular with chromosomal aberrations, again in a positive feedback mechanism. Secondary chromosomal aberrations (e.g., del17p, loss of p53) and mutations (e.g., ras) would further increase independence of cell cycle checkpoints. It has to be emphasized that this seems to be a rather subtle process, not the presence of an *ongoing* and widespread chromosomal instability. This nonewithstanding, there seems to have been at a certain (early) time during myelomagenesis for a set period such an instability, explaining the plethora of chromosomal aberrations, but again, it could not be taken as proven explanation for the disease progression from early MGUS to smoldering and therapy-requiring myeloma. As depicted in Sect. 3.3.1, only metaphase (proliferation dependent) cytogenetics show a prominent increase in the number of chromosomal aberrations with disease progression (Jonveaux and Berger 1992) and are therefore not representative for the presence of chromosomal aberrations. This increase has indeed up to now not been verified by (proliferation independent) iFISH data on large cohorts of patients. Further investigations including next generation sequencing will show whether this relative stableness is also present if a genome-wide screen for mutations is performed. If it holds true that the main features of myeloma cells might be already in place during pre-MGUS-stage as a consequence of "hijacked" normal plasma cells, another consequence would be that our perception of "monoclonal gammopathy of unknown significance" might change, and, speculatively, the last two words eventually will be dropped (see Fig. 3.8c).

We would like to finish this chapter with an urban myth – the attributed blessing, or curse, of a Chinese philosopher for a newborn – to live in interesting times. Whatever the true origin, this has surely become true for myeloma research – in a positive sense.

Acknowledgments This work was supported by grants from the Ligue Nationale Contre le Cancer (équipe labellisée 2009), France, from INCA (PL06_070), the Hopp-Foundation, Germany, and the Deutsche Forschungsgemeinschaft (DFG) Transregio TRR79, Germany.

References

Abe M, Hiura K, Wilde J, Moriyama K, Hashimoto T, Ozaki S, Wakatsuki S, Kosaka M, Kido S, Inoue D, Matsumoto T (2002) Role for macrophage inflammatory protein (MIP)-1alpha and MIP-1beta in the development of osteolytic lesions in multiple myeloma. Blood 100(6): 2195–2202

Abe M, Hiura K, Wilde J, Shioyasono A, Moriyama K, Hashimoto T, Kido S, Oshima T, Shibata H, Ozaki S, Inoue D, Matsumoto T (2004) Osteoclasts enhance myeloma cell growth and survival via cell-cell contact: a vicious cycle between bone destruction and myeloma expansion. Blood 104(8):2484–2491

Alexandrakis MG, Passam FH, Kyriakou DS, Dambaki K, Niniraki M, Stathopoulos E (2004)

Ki-67 proliferation index: correlation with prognostic parameters and outcome in multiple myeloma. Am J Clin Oncol 27(1):8–13

Allen CD, Okada T, Cyster JG (2007a) Germinal-center organization and cellular dynamics. Immunity 27(2):190–202

Allen SJ, Crown SE, Handel TM (2007b) Chemokine: receptor structure, interactions, and antagonism. Annu Rev Immunol 25:787–820

Andersen TL, Soe K, Sondergaard TE, Plesner T, Delaisse JM (2010) Myeloma cell-induced disruption of bone remodelling compartments leads to osteolytic lesions and generation of osteoclast-myeloma hybrid cells. Br J Haematol 148(4): 551–561

Andersen TL, Sondergaard TE, Skorzynska KE, Dagnaes-Hansen F, Plesner TL, Hauge EM, Plesner T, Delaisse JM (2009) A physical mechanism for coupling bone resorption and formation in adult human bone. Am J Pathol 174(1):239–247

Arce S, Luger E, Muehlinghaus G, Cassese G, Hauser A, Horst A, Lehnert K, Odendahl M, Honemann D, Heller KD, Kleinschmidt H, Berek C, Dorner T, Krenn V, Hiepe F, Bargou R, Radbruch A, Manz RA (2004) CD38 low IgG-secreting cells are precursors of various CD38 high-expressing plasma cell populations. J Leukoc Biol 75(6):1022–1028

Arora T, Jelinek DF (1998) Differential myeloma cell responsiveness to interferon-alpha correlates with differential induction of p19(INK4d) and cyclin D2 expression. J Biol Chem 273(19):11799–11805

Avet-Loiseau H, Li JY, Facon T, Brigaudeau C, Morineau N, Maloisel F, Rapp MJ, Talmant P, Trimoreau F, Jaccard A, Harousseau JL, Bataille R (1998) High incidence of translocations t(11;14)(q13;q32) and t(4;14)(p16;q32) in patients with plasma cell malignancies. Cancer Res 58(24):5640–5645

Avet-Loiseau H, Attal M, Moreau P, Charbonnel C, Garban F, Hulin C, Leyvraz S, Michallet M, Yakoub-Agha I, Garderet L, Marit G, Michaux L, Voillat L, Renaud M, Grosbois B, Guillerm G, Benboubker L, Monconduit M, Thieblemont C, Casassus P, Caillot D, Stoppa AM, Sotto JJ, Wetterwald M, Dumontet C, Fuzibet JG, Azais I, Dorvaux V, Zandecki M, Bataille R, Minvielle S, Harousseau JL, Facon T, Mathiot C (2007) Genetic abnormalities and survival in multiple myeloma: the experience of the Intergroupe Francophone du Myelome. Blood 109(8):3489–3495

Avet-Loiseau H, Moreau P, Mathiot C, Charbonnel C, Caillot D, Facon T, Attal M, Benboubker L, Hulin C, Marit G, Minvielle S, Harousseau JL (2009) Induction with velcade®/dexamethasone partially overcomes the poor prognosis of t(4;14), but not that of del(17p), in young patients with multiple myeloma. ASH Annu Meeting Abstr 114(22):957

Aviles A, Nambo MJ, Neri N, Castaneda C, Cleto S, Huerta-Guzman J (2007) Antitumor effect of zoledronic acid in previously untreated patients with multiple myeloma. Med Oncol 24(2): 227–230

Barclay AN, Wright GJ, Brooke G, Brown MH (2002) CD200 and membrane protein interactions in the control of myeloid cells. Trends Immunol 23(6):285–290

Barlogie B, Alexanian R, Dixon D, Smith L, Smallwood L, Delasalle K (1985) Prognostic implications of tumor cell DNA and RNA content in multiple myeloma. Blood 66(2):338–341

Barlogie B, Tricot GJ, van Rhee F, Angtuaco E, Walker R, Epstein J, Shaughnessy JD, Jagannath S, Bolejack V, Gurley J, Hoering A, Vesole D, Desikan R, Siegel D, Mehta J, Singhal S, Munshi NC, Dhodapkar M, Jenkins B, Attal M, Harousseau JL, Crowley J (2006) Long-term outcome results of the first tandem autotransplant trial for multiple myeloma. Br J Haematol 135(2):158–164

Barlogie B, Anaissie EJ, van Rhee F, Shaughnessy JD Jr, Haessler J, Pineda-Roman M, Hollmig K, Epstein J, Crowley JJ (2008) Total therapy (TT) for myeloma (MM)–10% cure rate with TT1 suggested by >10 year continuous complete remission (CCR): bortezomib in TT3 overcomes poor-risk associated with T(4;14) and DelTP53 in TT2. J Clin Oncol (Meeting Abstracts) 26(15):8516

Bataille R, Jourdan M, Zhang XG, Klein B (1989) Serum levels of interleukin 6, a potent myeloma cell growth factor, as a reflect of disease severity in plasma cell dyscrasias. J Clin Invest 84(6):2008–2011

Bataille R, Chappard D, Marcelli C, Rossi JF, Dessauw P, Baldet P, Sany J, Alexandre C (1990) Osteoblast stimulation in multiple myeloma lacking lytic bone lesions. Br J Haematol 76(4):484–487

3

Bataille R, Chappard D, Marcelli C, Dessauw P, Baldet P, Sany J, Alexandre C (1991) Recruitment of new osteoblasts and osteoclasts is the earliest critical event in the pathogenesis of human multiple myeloma. J Clin Invest 88(1):62–66

Bataille R, Barlogie B, Lu ZY, Rossi JF, Lavabre-Bertrand T, Beck T, Wijdenes J, Brochier J, Klein B (1995) Biologic effects of anti-interleukin-6 murine monoclonal antibody in advanced multiple myeloma. Blood 86(2):685–691

Batista FD, Harwood NE (2009) The who, how and where of antigen presentation to B cells. Nat Rev Immunol 9(1):15–27

Beattie J, Phillips K, Shand JH, Szymanowska M, Flint DJ, Allan GJ (2005) Molecular recognition characteristics in the insulin-like growth factor (IGF)-insulin-like growth factor binding protein-3/5 (IGFBP-3/5) heparin axis. J Mol Endocrinol 34(1):163–175

Bergsagel PL, Kuehl WM (2003) Critical roles for immunoglobulin translocations and cyclin D dysregulation in multiple myeloma. Immunol Rev 194:96–104

Bergsagel PL, Kuehl WM (2005) Molecular pathogenesis and a consequent classification of multiple myeloma. J Clin Oncol 23(26):6333–6338

Bergsagel PL, Kuehl WM, Zhan F, Sawyer J, Barlogie B, Shaughnessy J Jr (2005) Cyclin D dysregulation: an early and unifying pathogenic event in multiple myeloma. Blood 106(1): 296–303

Boccadoro M, Gavarotti P, Fossati G, Pileri A, Marmont F, Neretto G, Gallamini A, Volta C, Tribalto M, Testa MG (1984) Low plasma cell 3(H) thymidine incorporation in monoclonal gammopathy of undetermined significance (MGUS), smouldering myeloma and remission phase myeloma: a reliable indicator of patients not requiring therapy. Br J Haematol 58(4):689–696

Breitkreutz I, Raab MS, Vallet S, Hideshima T, Raje N, Mitsiades C, Chauhan D, Okawa Y, Munshi NC, Richardson PG, Anderson KC (2008) Lenalidomide inhibits osteoclastogenesis, survival factors and bone-remodeling markers in multiple myeloma. Leukemia 22(10): 1925–1932

Calame K (2008) Activation-dependent induction of Blimp-1. Curr Opin Immunol 20(3):259–264

Carrasco DR, Tonon G, Huang Y, Zhang Y, Sinha R, Feng B, Stewart JP, Zhan F, Khatry D, Protopopova M, Protopopov A, Sukhdeo K, Hanamura I, Stephens O, Barlogie B, Anderson KC, Chin L, Shaughnessy JD Jr, Brennan C, Depinho RA (2006) High-resolution genomic profiles define distinct clinico-pathogenetic subgroups of multiple myeloma patients. Cancer Cell 9(4):313–325

Catlett-Falcone R, Landowski TH, Oshiro MM, Turkson J, Levitzki A, Savino R, Ciliberto G, Moscinski L, Fernandez-Luna JL, Nunez G, Dalton WS, Jove R (1999) Constitutive activation of Stat3 signaling confers resistance to apoptosis in human U266 myeloma cells. Immunity 10(1):105–115

Chang H, Sloan S, Li D, Zhuang L, Yi QL, Chen CI, Reece D, Chun K, Keith SA (2004) The t(4;14) is associated with poor prognosis in myeloma patients undergoing autologous stem cell transplant. Br J Haematol 125(1):64–68

Cheng H, Jiang W, Phillips FM, Haydon RC, Peng Y, Zhou L, Luu HH, An N, Breyer B, Vanichakarn P, Szatkowski JP, Park JY, He TC (2003) Osteogenic activity of the fourteen types of human bone morphogenetic proteins (BMPs). J Bone Joint Surg Am 85-A(8):1544–1552

Cheng KW, Lahad JP, Kuo WL, Lapuk A, Yamada K, Auersperg N, Liu J, Smith-McCune K, Lu KH, Fishman D, Gray JW, Mills GB (2004) The RAB25 small GTPase determines aggressiveness of ovarian and breast cancers. Nat Med 10(11):1251–1256

Chiecchio L, Protheroe RK, Ibrahim AH, Cheung KL, Rudduck C, Dagrada GP, Cabanas ED, Parker T, Nightingale M, Wechalekar A, Orchard KH, Harrison CJ, Cross NC, Morgan GJ, Ross FM (2006) Deletion of chromosome 13 detected by conventional cytogenetics is a critical prognostic factor in myeloma. Leukemia 20(9):1610–1617

Chng WJ, Winkler JM, Greipp PR, Jalal SM, Bergsagel PL, Chesi M, Trendle MC, Ahmann GJ, Henderson K, Blood E, Oken MM, Hulbert A, Wier SA, Santana-Davila R, Kyle RA, Gertz MA, Lacy MQ, Dispenzieri A, Fonseca R (2006) Ploidy status rarely changes in myeloma patients at disease progression. Leuk Res 30(3):266–271

Cobaleda C, Schebesta A, Delogu A, Busslinger M (2007) Pax5: the guardian of B cell identity and function. Nat Immunol 8(5):463–470

Condomines M, Hose D, Raynaud P, Hundemer M, De Vos J, Baudard M, Moehler T, Pantesco V, Moos M, Schved JF, Rossi JF, Reme T, Goldschmidt H, Klein B (2007) Cancer/testis genes in multiple myeloma: expression patterns and prognosis value determined by microarray analysis. J Immunol 178(5):3307–3315

Condomines M, Hose D, Reme T, Requirand G, Hundemer M, Schoenhals M, Goldschmidt H, Klein B (2009) Gene expression profiling and real-time PCR analyses identify novel potential cancer-testis antigens in multiple myeloma. J Immunol 183(2):832–840

Condomines M, Veyrune JL, Larroque M, Quittet P, Latry P, Lugagne C, Hertogh C, Kanouni T, Rossi JF, Klein B (2010) Increased plasma-immune cytokines throughout the high-dose melphalan-induced lymphodepletion in patients with multiple myeloma: a window for adoptive immunotherapy. J Immunol 184(2):1079–1084

Cornish J, Callon KE, Coy DH, Jiang NY, Xiao L, Cooper GJ, Reid IR (1997) Adrenomedullin is a potent stimulator of osteoblastic activity in vitro and in vivo. Am J Physiol 273(6 Pt 1): E1113–E1120

Corre J, Mahtouk K, Attal M, Gadelorge M, Huynh A, Fleury-Cappellesso S, Danho C, Laharrague P, Klein B, Reme T, Bourin P (2007) Bone marrow mesenchymal stem cells are abnormal in multiple myeloma. Leukemia 21(5):1079–1088

Costes V, Portier M, Lu ZY, Rossi JF, Bataille R, Klein B (1998) Interleukin-1 in multiple myeloma: producer cells and their role in the control of IL-6 production. Br J Haematol 103(4):1152–1160

Costes V, Magen V, Legouffe E, Durand L, Baldet P, Rossi JF, Klein B, Brochier J (1999) The Mi15 monoclonal antibody (anti-syndecan-1) is a reliable marker for quantifying plasma cells in paraffin-embedded bone marrow biopsy specimens. Hum Pathol 30(12):1405–1411

Cremer FW, Bila J, Buck I, Kartal M, Hose D, Ittrich C, Benner A, Raab MS, Theil AC, Moos M, Goldschmidt H, Bartram CR, Jauch A (2005) Delineation of distinct subgroups of multiple myeloma and a model for clonal evolution based on interphase cytogenetics. Genes Chromosomes Cancer 44(2):194–203

De Vos J, Jourdan M, Tarte K, Jasmin C, Klein B (2000) JAK2 tyrosine kinase inhibitor tyrphostin AG490 downregulates the mitogen-activated protein kinase (MAPK) and signal transducer and activator of transcription (STAT) pathways and induces apoptosis in myeloma cells. Br J Haematol 109(4):823–828

De Vos J, Couderc G, Tarte K, Jourdan M, Requirand G, Delteil MC, Rossi JF, Mechti N, Klein B (2001) Identifying intercellular signaling genes expressed in malignant plasma cells by using complementary DNA arrays. Blood 98(3): 771–780

De Matteo M, Brunetti AE, Maiorano E, Cafforio P, Dammacco F, Silvestris F (2009) Constitutive down-regulation of Osterix in osteoblasts from myeloma patients: in vitro effect of Bortezomib and Lenalidomide. Leuk Res 34(2):243–249

Decaux O, Lode L, Magrangeas F, Charbonnel C, Gouraud W, Jezequel P, Attal M, Harousseau JL, Moreau P, Bataille R, Campion L, Avet-Loiseau H, Minvielle S (2008) Prediction of survival in multiple myeloma based on gene expression profiles reveals cell cycle and chromosomal instability signatures in high-risk patients and hyperdiploid signatures in low-risk patients: a study of the Intergroupe Francophone du Myelome. J Clin Oncol 26(29):4798–4805

Derenne S, Monia B, Dean NM, Taylor JK, Rapp MJ, Harousseau JL, Bataille R, Amiot M (2002) Antisense strategy shows that Mcl-1 rather than Bcl-2 or Bcl-x(L) is an essential survival protein of human myeloma cells. Blood 100(1): 194–199

Derksen PW, Keehnen RM, Evers LM, van Oers MH, Spaargaren M, Pals ST (2002) Cell surface proteoglycan syndecan-1 mediates hepatocyte growth factor binding and promotes Met signaling in multiple myeloma. Blood 99(4): 1405–1410

Descamps G, Wuilleme-Toumi S, Trichet V, Venot C, Debussche L, Hercend T, Collette M, Robillard N, Bataille R, Amiot M (2006) CD45neg but not CD45pos human myeloma cells are sensitive to the inhibition of IGF-1 signaling by a murine anti-IGF-1R monoclonal antibody, mAVE1642. J Immunol 177(6): 4218–4223

DiLillo DJ, Hamaguchi Y, Ueda Y, Yang K, Uchida J, Haas KM, Kelsoe G, Tedder TF (2008) Maintenance of long-lived plasma cells and serological memory despite mature and memory B cell depletion during CD20 immunotherapy in mice. J Immunol 180(1):361–371

Drach J, Schuster J, Nowotny H, Angerler J, Rosenthal F, Fiegl M, Rothermundt C, Gsur A, Jager U, Heinz R (1995) Multiple myeloma: high incidence of chromosomal aneuploidy as detected by interphase fluorescence in situ hybridization. Cancer Res 55(17):3854–3859

Drewinko B, Alexanian R, Boyer H, Barlogie B, Rubinow SI (1981) The growth fraction of human myeloma cells. Blood 57(2):333–338

Du J, Yang S, Wang Z, Zhai C, Yuan W, Lei R, Zhang J, Zhu T (2008) Bone morphogenetic protein 6 inhibit stress-induced breast cancer cells apoptosis via both smad and P38 pathways. J Cell Biochem 103(5):1584–1597

Duan C (2002) Specifying the cellular responses to IGF signals: roles of IGF-binding proteins. J Endocrinol 175(1):41–54

Ebisawa T, Tada K, Kitajima I, Tojo K, Sampath TK, Kawabata M, Miyazono K, Imamura T (1999) Characterization of bone morphogenetic protein-6 signaling pathways in osteoblast differentiation. J Cell Sci 112(Pt 20):3519–3527

Epstein J, Walker R (2006) Myeloma and bone disease: "the dangerous tango". Clin Adv Hematol Oncol 4(4):300–306

Esteve FR, Roodman GD (2007) Pathophysiology of myeloma bone disease. Best Pract Res Clin Haematol 20(4):613–624

Ettinger R, Sims GP, Robbins R, Withers D, Fischer RT, Grammer AC, Kuchen S, Lipsky PE (2007) IL-21 and BAFF/BLyS synergize in stimulating plasma cell differentiation from a unique population of human splenic memory B cells. J Immunol 178(5):2872–2882

Facon T, Avet-Loiseau H, Guillerm G, Moreau P, Genevieve F, Zandecki M, Lai JL, Leleu X, Jouet JP, Bauters F, Harousseau JL, Bataille R, Mary JY (2001) Chromosome 13 abnormalities identified by FISH analysis and serum {beta}2-microglobulin produce a powerful myeloma staging system for patients receiving high-dose therapy. Blood 97(6):1566–1571

Ferlin M, Noraz N, Hertogh C, Brochier J, Taylor N, Klein B (2000) Insulin-like growth factor induces the survival and proliferation of myeloma cells through an interleukin-6-independent transduction pathway. Br J Haematol 111(2):626–634

Ferlin-Bezombes M, Jourdan M, Liautard J, Brochier J, Rossi JF, Klein B (1998) IFN-alpha is a survival factor for human myeloma cells and reduces dexamethasone-induced apoptosis. J Immunol 161(6):2692–2699

Flactif M, Zandecki M, Lai JL, Bernardi F, Obein V, Bauters F, Facon T (1995) Interphase fluorescence in situ hybridization (FISH) as a powerful tool for the detection of aneuploidy in multiple myeloma. Leukemia 9(12):2109–2114

Fonseca R (2003) Many and multiple myeloma(s). Leukemia 17(10):1943–1944

Fonseca R, Oken MM, Greipp PR (2001a) The t(4;14)(p16.3;q32) is strongly associated with chromosome 13 abnormalities in both multiple myeloma and monoclonal gammopathy of undetermined significance. Blood 98(4):1271–1272

Fonseca R, Oken MM, Harrington D, Bailey RJ, Van Wier SA, Henderson KJ, Kay NE, Van NB, Greipp PR, Dewald GW (2001b) Deletions of chromosome 13 in multiple myeloma identified by interphase FISH usually denote large deletions of the q arm or monosomy. Leukemia 15(6):981–986

Fonseca R, Blood E, Rue M, Harrington D, Oken MM, Kyle RA, Dewald GW, Van Ness B, Van Wier SA, Henderson KJ, Bailey RJ, Greipp PR (2003a) Clinical and biologic implications of recurrent genomic aberrations in myeloma. Blood 101(11):4569–4575

Fonseca R, Debes-Marun CS, Picken EB, Dewald GW, Bryant SC, Winkler JM, Blood E, Oken MM, Santana-Davila R, Gonzalez-Paz N, Kyle RA, Gertz MA, Dispenzieri A, Lacy MQ, Greipp PR (2003b) The recurrent IgH translocations are highly associated with nonhyperdiploid variant multiple myeloma. Blood 102(7):2562–2567

Fonseca R, Barlogie B, Bataille R, Bastard C, Bergsagel PL, Chesi M, Davies FE, Drach J, Greipp PR, Kirsch IR, Kuehl WM, Hernandez JM, Minvielle S, Pilarski LM, Shaughnessy JD Jr, Stewart AK, Avet-Loiseau H (2004) Genetics and cytogenetics of multiple myeloma: a workshop report. Cancer Res 64(4):1546–1558

Gaillard JP, Bataille R, Brailly H, Zuber C, Yasukawa K, Attal M, Maruo N, Taga T, Kishimoto T, Klein B (1993) Increased and highly stable levels of functional soluble interleukin-6 receptor in sera of patients with monoclonal gammopathy. Eur J Immunol 23(4):820–824

Gastinne T, Leleu X, Duhamel A, Moreau AS, Franck G, Andrieux J, Lai JL, Coiteux V, Yakoub-Agha I, Bauters F, Harousseau JL, Zandecki M, Facon T (2007) Plasma cell growth fraction using Ki-67 antigen expression identifies a subgroup of multiple myeloma patients displaying short survival within the ISS stage I. Eur J Haematol 79(4):297–304

Gautschi OP, Frey SP, Zellweger R (2007) Bone morphogenetic proteins in clinical applications. ANZ J Surg 77(8):626–631

Ge NL, Rudikoff S (2000) Insulin-like growth factor I is a dual effector of multiple myeloma cell growth. Blood 96(8):2856–2861

Georgii-Hemming P, Wiklund HJ, Ljunggren O, Nilsson K (1996) Insulin-like growth factor I is a growth and survival factor in human multiple myeloma cell lines. Blood 88(6):2250–2258

Giuliani N, Bataille R, Mancini C, Lazzaretti M, Barille S (2001) Myeloma cells induce imbalance in the osteoprotegerin/osteoprotegerin ligand system in the human bone marrow environment. Blood 98(13):3527–3533

Giuliani N, Colla S, Sala R, Moroni M, Lazzaretti M, La MS, Bonomini S, Hojden M, Sammarelli G, Barille S, Bataille R, Rizzoli V (2002) Human myeloma cells stimulate the receptor activator of nuclear factor-kappa B ligand (RANKL) in T lymphocytes: a potential role in multiple myeloma bone disease. Blood 100(13):4615–4621

Giuliani N, Colla S, Morandi F, Lazzaretti M, Sala R, Bonomini S, Grano M, Colucci S, Svaldi M, Rizzoli V (2005) Myeloma cells block RUNX2/CBFA1 activity in human bone marrow osteoblast progenitors and inhibit osteoblast formation and differentiation. Blood 106(7):2472–2483

Gonzalez-Garcia I, Rodriguez-Bayona B, Mora-Lopez F, Campos-Caro A, Brieva JA (2008) Increased survival is a selective feature of human circulating antigen-induced plasma cells synthesizing high-affinity antibodies. Blood 111(2):741–749

Greipp PR, Witzig TE, Gonchoroff NJ, Habermann TM, Katzmann JA, O'Fallon WM, Kyle RA (1987) Immunofluorescence labeling indices in myeloma and related monoclonal gammopathies. Mayo Clin Proc 62(11):969–977

Greipp PR, Katzmann JA, O'Fallon WM, Kyle RA (1988) Value of beta 2-microglobulin level and plasma cell labeling indices as prognostic factors in patients with newly diagnosed myeloma. Blood 72(1):219–223

Greipp PR, Lust JA, O'Fallon WM, Katzmann JA, Witzig TE, Kyle RA (1993) Plasma cell labeling index and beta 2-microglobulin predict survival independent of thymidine kinase and C-reactive protein in multiple myeloma. Blood 81(12):3382–3387

Gu ZJ, Costes V, Lu ZY, Zhang XG, Pitard V, Moreau JF, Bataille R, Wijdenes J, Rossi JF, Klein B (1996) Interleukin-10 is a growth factor for human myeloma cells by induction of an oncostatin M autocrine loop. Blood 88(10):3972–3986

Haaber J, Abildgaard N, Knudsen LM, Dahl IM, Lodahl M, Thomassen M, Kerndrup GB, Rasmussen T (2008) Myeloma cell expression of 10 candidate genes for osteolytic bone disease. Only overexpression of DKK1 correlates with clinical bone involvement at diagnosis. Br J Haematol 140(1):25–35

Hallek M, Bergsagel PL, Anderson KC (1998) Multiple myeloma: increasing evidence for a multistep transformation process. Blood 91(1):3–21

Hanamura I, Stewart JP, Huang Y, Zhan F, Santra M, Sawyer JR, Hollmig K, Zangarri M, Pineda-Roman M, van Rhee F, Cavallo F, Burington B, Crowley J, Tricot G, Barlogie B, Shaughnessy JD Jr (2006) Frequent gain of chromosome band 1q21 in plasma-cell dyscrasias detected by fluorescence in situ hybridization: incidence increases from MGUS to relapsed myeloma and is related to prognosis and disease progression following tandem stem-cell transplantation. Blood 108(5):1724–1732

Harousseau JL, Moreau P (2009) Autologous hematopoietic stem-cell transplantation for multiple myeloma. N Engl J Med 360(25):2645–2654

Hattinger CM, Potschger U, Tarkkanen M, Squire J, Zielenska M, Kiuru-Kuhlefelt S, Kager L, Thorner P, Knuutila S, Niggli FK, Ambros PF, Gadner H, Betts DR (2002) Prognostic impact of chromosomal aberrations in Ewing tumours. Br J Cancer 86(11):1763–1769

Hauge EM, Qvesel D, Eriksen EF, Mosekilde L, Melsen F (2001) Cancellous bone remodeling occurs in specialized compartments lined by cells expressing osteoblastic markers. J Bone Miner Res 16(9):1575–1582

Heider U, Kaiser M, Muller C, Jakob C, Zavrski I, Schulz CO, Fleissner C, Hecht M, Sezer O (2006) Bortezomib increases osteoblast activity in myeloma patients irrespective of response to treatment. Eur J Haematol 77(3):233–238

Heinrich PC, Behrmann I, Haan S, Hermanns HM, Muller-Newen G, Schaper F (2003) Principles of interleukin (IL)-6-type cytokine signalling and its regulation. Biochem J 374(Pt 1):1–20

3

Hideshima T, Chauhan D, Podar K, Schlossman RL, Richardson P, Anderson KC (2001) Novel therapies targeting the myeloma cell and its bone marrow microenvironment. Semin Oncol 28(6): 607–612

Hinson RM, Williams JA, Shacter E (1996) Elevated interleukin 6 is induced by prostaglandin E2 in a murine model of inflammation: possible role of cyclooxygenase-2. Proc Natl Acad Sci USA 93(10):4885–4890

Hjertner O, Torgersen ML, Seidel C, Hjorth-Hansen H, Waage A, Borset M, Sundan A (1999) Hepatocyte growth factor (HGF) induces interleukin-11 secretion from osteoblasts: a possible role for HGF in myeloma-associated osteolytic bone disease. Blood 94(11):3883–3888

Hoang B, Zhu L, Shi Y, Frost P, Yan H, Sharma S, Sharma S, Goodglick L, Dubinett S, Lichtenstein A (2006) Oncogenic RAS mutations in myeloma cells selectively induce cox-2 expression, which participates in enhanced adhesion to fibronectin and chemoresistance. Blood 107(11):4484–4490

Hoechtlen-Vollmar W, Menzel G, Bartl R, Lamerz R, Wick M, Seidel D (2000) Amplification of cyclin D1 gene in multiple myeloma: clinical and prognostic relevance. Br J Haematol 109(1):30–38

Hose D, Rossi JF, Ittrich C, DeVos J, Benner A, Reme T, Bila J, Grau V, Raab M, Kaukel P, Jourdan E, Moos M, Theil AC, Jauch A, Goldschmidt H, Klein B, Cremer FW (2004) A new molecular classification of multiple myeloma using gene expression profiling and fluorescence in situ hybridisation as predictor for event free survival. ASH Ann Meeting Abstr 104(11):73

Hose D, Rossi J-F, Ittrich C, DeVos J, Rème T, Benner A, Mahtouk K, del Val C, Moreaux J, Hotz-Wagenblatt A, Jonnakut S, Raab M, Kaukel P, Moos M, Grau V, Jauch A, Jourdan E, Cremere FW, Klein B, Goldschmidt H (2005) Molecular classification of multiple myeloma (MM) based on gene expression profiling (GEP) and fluorescence in situ hybridisation (FISH) is an independent predictor for event free survival (EFS). Blood 106(111):150a

Hose D, Moreaux J, Meissner T, Seckinger A, Goldschmidt H, Benner A, Mahtouk K, Hillengass J, Reme T, De VJ, Hundemer M, Condomines M, Bertsch U, Rossi JF, Jauch A, Klein B, Mohler T (2009a) Induction of angiogenesis by normal and malignant plasma cells. Blood 114(1):128–143

Hose D, Reme T, Meissner T, Moreaux J, Seckinger A, Lewis J, Benes V, Benner A, Hundemer M, Hielscher T, Shaughnessy JD Jr, Barlogie B, Neben K, Kramer A, Hillengass J, Bertsch U, Jauch A, De VJ, Rossi JF, Mohler T, Blake J, Zimmermann J, Klein B, Goldschmidt H (2009b) Inhibition of aurora kinases for tailored risk-adapted treatment of multiple myeloma. Blood 113(18):4331–4340

Hose D, Reme T, Hielscher T, Moreaux J, Meissner T, Seckinger A, Benner A, Shaughnessy JD, Barlogie B, Zhou Y, Hillengass J, Bertsch U, Neben K, Mohler T, Rossi JF, Jauch A, Klein B, Goldschmidt H. (2011) Proliferation is a central independent prognostic factor and target for personalized and risk adapted treatment in multiple myeloma. Haematologica 96(1):87–95

Hsu JH, Shi Y, Hu L, Fisher M, Franke TF, Lichtenstein A (2002) Role of the AKT kinase in expansion of multiple myeloma clones: effects on cytokine-dependent proliferative and survival responses. Oncogene 21(9):1391–1400

Hurt EM, Wiestner A, Rosenwald A, Shaffer AL, Campo E, Grogan T, Bergsagel PL, Kuehl WM, Staudt LM (2004) Overexpression of c-maf is a frequent oncogenic event in multiple myeloma that promotes proliferation and pathological interactions with bone marrow stroma. Cancer Cell 5(2):191–199

Itoyama T, Nanjungud G, Chen W, Dyomin VG, Teruya-Feldstein J, Jhanwar SC, Zelenetz AD, Chaganti RS (2002) Molecular cytogenetic analysis of genomic instability at the 1q12-22 chromosomal site in B-cell non-Hodgkin lymphoma. Genes Chromosomes Cancer 35(4):318–328

Jego G, Robillard N, Puthier D, Amiot M, Accard F, Pineau D, Harousseau JL, Bataille R, Pellat-Deceunynck C (1999) Reactive plasmacytoses are expansions of plasmablasts retaining the capacity to differentiate into plasma cells. Blood 94(2):701–712

Jelinek DF, Witzig TE, Arendt BK (1997) A role for insulin-like growth factor in the regulation of IL-6-responsive human myeloma cell line growth. J Immunol 159(1):487–496

Jonveaux P, Berger R (1992) Chromosome studies in plasma cell leukemia and multiple myeloma in transformation. Genes Chromosomes Cancer 4(4):321–325

Jourdan M, Zhang XG, Portier M, Boiron JM, Bataille R, Klein B (1991) IFN-alpha induces autocrine production of IL-6 in myeloma cell lines. J Immunol 147(12):4402–4407

Jourdan M, De Vos J, Mechti N, Klein B (2000) Regulation of Bcl-2-family proteins in myeloma cells by three myeloma survival factors: interleukin-6, interferon-alpha and insulin-like growth factor 1. Cell Death Differ 7(12):1244–1252

Jourdan M, Veyrune JL, De VJ, Redal N, Couderc G, Klein B (2003) A major role for Mcl-1 antiapoptotic protein in the IL-6-induced survival of human myeloma cells. Oncogene 22(19):2950–2959

Jourdan M, Mahtouk K, Veyrune JL, Couderc G, Fiol G, Redal N, Duperray C, De VJ, Klein B (2005) Delineation of the roles of paracrine and autocrine interleukin-6 (IL-6) in myeloma cell lines in survival versus cell cycle. A possible model for the cooperation of myeloma cell growth factors. Eur Cytokine Netw 16(1):57–64

Jourdan M, Caraux A, De VJ, Fiol G, Larroque M, Cognot C, Bret C, Duperray C, Hose D, Klein B (2009) An in vitro model of differentiation of memory B cells into plasmablasts and plasma cells including detailed phenotypic and molecular characterization. Blood 114(25): 5173–5181

Kabashima K, Haynes NM, Xu Y, Nutt SL, Allende ML, Proia RL, Cyster JG (2006) Plasma cell S1P1 expression determines secondary lymphoid organ retention versus bone marrow tropism. J Exp Med 203(12):2683–2690

Kallies A, Hasbold J, Fairfax K, Pridans C, Emslie D, McKenzie BS, Lew AM, Corcoran LM, Hodgkin PD, Tarlinton DM, Nutt SL (2007) Initiation of plasma-cell differentiation is independent of the transcription factor Blimp-1. Immunity 26(5):555–566

Kawabata M, Imamura T, Miyazono K (1998) Signal transduction by bone morphogenetic proteins. Cytokine Growth Factor Rev 9(1):49–61

Kawano M, Hirano T, Matsuda T, Taga T, Horii Y, Iwato K, Asaoku H, Tang B, Tanabe O, Tanaka H (1988) Autocrine generation and requirement of BSF-2/IL-6 for human multiple myelomas. Nature 332(6159):83–85

Keats JJ, Reiman T, Maxwell CA, Taylor BJ, Larratt LM, Mant MJ, Belch AR, Pilarski LM (2003) In multiple myeloma, t(4;14)(p16;q32) is an adverse prognostic factor irrespective of FGFR3 expression. Blood 101(4):1520–1529

Kellinsalmi M, Monkkonen H, Monkkonen J, Leskela HV, Parikka V, Hamalainen M, Lehenkari P (2005) In vitro comparison of clodronate, pamidronate and zoledronic acid effects on rat osteoclasts and human stem cell-derived osteoblasts. Basic Clin Pharmacol Toxicol 97(6): 382–391

Kersten C, Sivertsen EA, Hystad ME, Forfang L, Smeland EB, Myklebust JH (2005) BMP-6 inhibits growth of mature human B cells; induction of Smad phosphorylation and upregulation of Id1. BMC Immunol 6(1):9

Klein B, Zhang XG, Jourdan M, Content J, Houssiau F, Aarden L, Piechaczyk M, Bataille R (1989) Paracrine rather than autocrine regulation of myeloma-cell growth and differentiation by interleukin-6. Blood 73(2):517–526

Klein B, Wijdenes J, Zhang XG, Jourdan M, Boiron JM, Brochier J, Liautard J, Merlin M, Clement C, Morel-Fournier B (1991) Murine anti-interleukin-6 monoclonal antibody therapy for a patient with plasma cell leukemia. Blood 78(5): 1198–1204

Klein B, Tarte K, Jourdan M, Mathouk K, Moreaux J, Jourdan E, Legouffe E, De Vos J, Rossi JF (2003) Survival and proliferation factors of normal and malignant plasma cells. Int J Hematol 78(2):106–113

Knop S, Gerecke C, Liebisch P, Topp MS, Platzbecker U, Sezer O, Vollmuth C, Falk K, Glasmacher A, Maeder U, Einsele H, Bargou RC (2009) Lenalidomide, adriamycin, and dexamethasone (RAD) in patients with relapsed and refractory multiple myeloma: a report from the German Myeloma Study Group DSMM (Deutsche Studiengruppe Multiples Myelom). Blood 113(18):4137–4143

Kopf M, Baumann H, Freer G, Freudenberg M, Lamers M, Kishimoto T, Zinkernagel R, Bluethmann H, Kohler G (1994) Impaired immune and acute-phase responses in interleukin-6-deficient mice. Nature 368(6469): 339–342

Kuehl WM, Bergsagel PL (2002) Multiple myeloma: evolving genetic events and host interactions. Nat Rev Cancer 2(3):175–187

Kunkel EJ, Butcher EC (2003) Plasma-cell homing. Nat Rev Immunol 3(10):822–829

Kuppers R, Dalla-Favera R (2001) Mechanisms of chromosomal translocations in B cell lymphomas. Oncogene 20(40):5580–5594

Lacey DL, Timms E, Tan HL, Kelley MJ, Dunstan CR, Burgess T, Elliott R, Colombero A, Elliott G,

3

Scully S, Hsu H, Sullivan J, Hawkins N, Davy E, Capparelli C, Eli A, Qian YX, Kaufman S, Sarosi I, Shalhoub V, Senaldi G, Guo J, Delaney J, Boyle WJ (1998) Osteoprotegerin ligand is a cytokine that regulates osteoclast differentiation and activation. Cell 93(2):165–176

Landgren O, Kyle RA, Pfeiffer RM, Katzmann JA, Caporaso NE, Hayes RB, Dispenzieri A, Kumar S, Clark RJ, Baris D, Hoover R, Rajkumar SV (2009) Monoclonal gammopathy of undetermined significance (MGUS) consistently precedes multiple myeloma: a prospective study. Blood 113(22):5412–5417

Latreille J, Barlogie B, Dosik G, Johnston DA, Drewinko B, Alexanian R (1980) Cellular DNA content as a marker of human multiple myeloma. Blood 55(3):403–408

Latreille J, Barlogie B, Johnston D, Drewinko B, Alexanian R (1982) Ploidy and proliferative characteristics in monoclonal gammopathies. Blood 59(1):43–51

Lattanzio G, Libert C, Aquilina M, Cappelletti M, Ciliberto G, Musiani P, Poli V (1997) Defective development of pristane-oil-induced plasmacytomas in interleukin-6-deficient BALB/c mice. Am J Pathol 151(3):689–696

Le BP, Leroux D, Dascalescu C, Duley S, Marais D, Esmenjaud E, Sotto JJ, Callanan M (2001) Novel evidence of a role for chromosome 1 pericentric heterochromatin in the pathogenesis of B-cell lymphoma and multiple myeloma. Genes Chromosomes Cancer 32(3):250–264

Lewiecki EM (2006) RANK ligand inhibition with denosumab for the management of osteoporosis. Expert Opin Biol Ther 6(10):1041–1050

Li J, Sarosi I, Cattley RC, Pretorius J, Asuncion F, Grisanti M, Morony S, Adamu S, Geng Z, Qiu W, Kostenuik P, Lacey DL, Simonet WS, Bolon B, Qian X, Shalhoub V, Ominsky MS, Zhu KH, Li X, Richards WG (2006) Dkk1-mediated inhibition of Wnt signaling in bone results in osteopenia. Bone 39(4):754–766

Liu P, Leong T, Quam L, Billadeau D, Kay NE, Greipp P, Kyle RA, Oken MM, Van NB (1996) Activating mutations of N- and K-ras in multiple myeloma show different clinical associations: analysis of the Eastern Cooperative Oncology Group Phase III Trial. Blood 88(7):2699–2706

Lokhorst HM, Boom SE, Bast BJ, Ballieux RE (1986) Determination of the plasma cell labelling index with bromodeoxyuridine in a double fluorescence technique. Br J Haematol 64(2): 271–275

Lu ZY, Brailly H, Wijdenes J, Bataille R, Rossi JF, Klein B (1995a) Measurement of whole body interleukin-6 (IL-6) production: prediction of the efficacy of anti-IL-6 treatments. Blood 86(8):3123–3131

Lu ZY, Gu ZJ, Zhang XG, Wijdenes J, Neddermann P, Rossi JF, Klein B (1995b) Interleukin-10 induces interleukin-11 responsiveness in human myeloma cell lines. FEBS Lett 377(3):515–518

Lu YJ, Hing S, Williams R, Pinkerton R, Shipley J, Pritchard-Jones K (2002) Chromosome 1q expression profiling and relapse in Wilms' tumour. Lancet 360(9330):385–386

Mackay F, Schneider P (2009) Cracking the BAFF code. Nat Rev Immunol 9(7):491–502

Magrangeas F, Lode L, Wuilleme S, Minvielle S, Avet-Loiseau H (2005) Genetic heterogeneity in multiple myeloma. Leukemia 19(2):191–194

Mahtouk K, Jourdan M, De Vos J, Hertogh C, Fiol G, Jourdan E, Rossi JF, Klein B (2004) An inhibitor of the EGF receptor family blocks myeloma cell growth factor activity of HB-EGF and potentiates dexamethasone or anti-IL-6 antibody-induced apoptosis. Blood 103(5): 1829–1837

Mahtouk K, Hose D, Reme T, De Vos J, Jourdan M, Moreaux J, Fiol G, Raab M, Jourdan E, Grau V, Moos M, Goldschmidt H, Baudard M, Rossi JF, Cremer FW, Klein B (2005) Expression of EGF-family receptors and amphiregulin in multiple myeloma. Amphiregulin is a growth factor for myeloma cells. Oncogene 24(21):3512–3524

Mahtouk K, Cremer FW, Reme T, Jourdan M, Baudard M, Moreaux J, Requirand G, Fiol G, De VJ, Moos M, Quittet P, Goldschmidt H, Rossi JF, Hose D, Klein B (2006) Heparan sulphate proteoglycans are essential for the myeloma cell growth activity of EGF-family ligands in multiple myeloma. Oncogene 25(54):7180–7191

Mahtouk K, Moreaux J, Hose D, Reme T, Meissner T, Jourdan M, Rossi JF, Pals ST, Goldschmidt H, Klein B (2010) Growth factors in multiple myeloma: a comprehensive analysis of their expression in tumor cells and bone marrow environment using Affymetrix microarrays. BMC Cancer 10:198

Mei HE, Yoshida T, Sime W, Hiepe F, Thiele K, Manz RA, Radbruch A, Dorner T (2009) Blood-borne human plasma cells in steady state are derived from mucosal immune responses. Blood 113(11):2461–2469

Menoret E, Maiga S, Descamps G, Pellat-Deceunynck C, Fraslon C, Cappellano M, Moreau P, Bataille R, Amiot M (2008) IL-21 stimulates human myeloma cell growth through an autocrine IGF-1 loop. J Immunol 181(10):6837–6842

Mitsiades CS, Mitsiades N, Poulaki V, Schlossman R, Akiyama M, Chauhan D, Hideshima T, Treon SP, Munshi NC, Richardson PG, Anderson KC (2002) Activation of NF-kappaB and upregulation of intracellular anti-apoptotic proteins via the IGF-1/Akt signaling in human multiple myeloma cells: therapeutic implications. Oncogene 21(37):5673–5683

Moreau P, Facon T, Leleu X, Morineau N, Huyghe P, Harousseau JL, Bataille R, Avet-Loiseau H (2002) Recurrent 14q32 translocations determine the prognosis of multiple myeloma, especially in patients receiving intensive chemotherapy. Blood 100(5):1579–1583

Moreaux J, Legouffe E, Jourdan E, Quittet P, Reme T, Lugagne C, Moine P, Rossi JF, Klein B, Tarte K (2004) BAFF and APRIL protect myeloma cells from apoptosis induced by interleukin 6 deprivation and dexamethasone. Blood 103(8):3148–3157

Moreaux J, Cremer FW, Reme T, Raab M, Mahtouk K, Kaukel P, Pantesco V, De Vos J, Jourdan E, Jauch A, Legouffe E, Moos M, Fiol G, Goldschmidt H, Rossi JF, Hose D, Klein B (2005) The level of TACI gene expression in myeloma cells is associated with a signature of microenvironment dependence versus a plasmablastic signature. Blood 106(3):1021–1030

Moreaux J, Hose D, Reme T, Jourdan E, Hundemer M, Legouffe E, Moine P, Bourin P, Moos M, Corre J, Mohler T, De VJ, Rossi JF, Goldschmidt H, Klein B (2006) CD200 is a new prognostic factor in multiple myeloma. Blood 108(13):4194–4197

Moreaux J, Hose D, Jourdan M, Reme T, Hundemer M, Moos M, Robert N, Moine P, De VJ, Goldschmidt H, Klein B (2007) TACI expression is associated with a mature bone marrow plasma cell signature and C-MAF overexpression in human myeloma cell lines. Haematologica 92(6):803–811

Moreaux J, Sprynski AC, Dillon SR, Mahtouk K, Jourdan M, Ythier A, Moine P, Robert N, Jourdan E, Rossi JF, Klein B (2009) APRIL and TACI interact with syndecan-1 on the surface of multiple myeloma cells to form an essential survival loop. Eur J Haematol 83(2):119–129

Mori Y, Shimizu N, Dallas M, Niewolna M, Story B, Williams PJ, Mundy GR, Yoneda T (2004) Anti-alpha4 integrin antibody suppresses the development of multiple myeloma and associated osteoclastic osteolysis. Blood 104(7): 2149–2154

Murray AW (2004) Recycling the cell cycle: cyclins revisited. Cell 116(2):221–234

Nagasawa T (2006) Microenvironmental niches in the bone marrow required for B-cell development. Nat Rev Immunol 6(2):107–116

Neben K, Jauch A, Bertsch U, Heiss C, Hielscher T, Seckinger A, Mors T, Muller NZ, Hillengass J, Raab MS, Ho AD, Hose D, Goldschmidt H (2010) Combining information regarding chromosomal aberrations t(4;14) and del(17p13) with the International Staging System classification allows stratification of myeloma patients undergoing autologous stem cell transplantation. Haematologica 95(7):1150–1157

Neri A, Murphy JP, Cro L, Ferrero D, Tarella C, Baldini L, Dalla-Favera R (1989) Ras oncogene mutation in multiple myeloma. J Exp Med 170(5):1715–1725

Niida S, Kaku M, Amano H, Yoshida H, Kataoka H, Nishikawa S, Tanne K, Maeda N, Nishikawa S, Kodama H (1999) Vascular endothelial growth factor can substitute for macrophage colony-stimulating factor in the support of osteoclastic bone resorption. J Exp Med 190(2):293–298

Nishida K, Tamura A, Nakazawa N, Ueda Y, Abe T, Matsuda F, Kashima K, Taniwaki M (1997) The Ig heavy chain gene is frequently involved in chromosomal translocations in multiple myeloma and plasma cell leukemia as detected by in situ hybridization. Blood 90(2):526–534

Nohe A, Keating E, Knaus P, Petersen NO (2004) Signal transduction of bone morphogenetic protein receptors. Cell Signal 16(3):291–299

Novak AJ, Darce JR, Arendt BK, Harder B, Henderson K, Kindsvogel W, Gross JA, Greipp PR, Jelinek DF (2004) Expression of BCMA, TACI, and BAFF-R in multiple myeloma: a mechanism for growth and survival. Blood 103(2):689–694

Oba Y, Lee JW, Ehrlich LA, Chung HY, Jelinek DF, Callander NS, Horuk R, Choi SJ, Roodman GD (2005) MIP-1alpha utilizes both CCR1 and CCR5 to induce osteoclast formation and

3

increase adhesion of myeloma cells to marrow stromal cells. Exp Hematol 33(3):272–278

Odendahl M, Mei H, Hoyer BF, Jacobi AM, Hansen A, Muehlinghaus G, Berek C, Hiepe F, Manz R, Radbruch A, Dorner T (2005) Generation of migratory antigen-specific plasma blasts and mobilization of resident plasma cells in a secondary immune response. Blood 105(4):1614–1621

Oshima T, Abe M, Asano J, Hara T, Kitazoe K, Sekimoto E, Tanaka Y, Shibata H, Hashimoto T, Ozaki S, Kido S, Inoue D, Matsumoto T (2005) Myeloma cells suppress bone formation by secreting a soluble Wnt inhibitor, sFRP-2. Blood 106(9):3160–3165

Ozaki K, Spolski R, Feng CG, Qi CF, Cheng J, Sher A, Morse HC III, Liu C, Schwartzberg PL, Leonard WJ (2002) A critical role for IL-21 in regulating immunoglobulin production. Science 298(5598):1630–1634

Pearse RN, Sordillo EM, Yaccoby S, Wong BR, Liau DF, Colman N, Michaeli J, Epstein J, Choi Y (2001) Multiple myeloma disrupts the TRANCE/osteoprotegerin cytokine axis to trigger bone destruction and promote tumor progression. Proc Natl Acad Sci USA 98(20): 11581–11586

Pene F, Claessens YE, Muller O, Viguie F, Mayeux P, Dreyfus F, Lacombe C, Bouscary D (2002) Role of the phosphatidylinositol 3-kinase/Akt and mTOR/P70S6-kinase pathways in the proliferation and apoptosis in multiple myeloma. Oncogene 21(43):6587–6597

Pfeffer LM, Mullersman JE, Pfeffer SR, Murti A, Shi W, Yang CH (1997) STAT3 as an adapter to couple phosphatidylinositol 3-kinase to the IFNAR1 chain of the type I interferon receptor. Science 276(5317):1418–1420

Politou M, Terpos E, Anagnostopoulos A, Szydlo R, Laffan M, Layton M, Apperley JF, Dimopoulos MA, Rahemtulla A (2004) Role of receptor activator of nuclear factor-kappa B ligand (RANKL), osteoprotegerin and macrophage protein 1-alpha (MIP-1a) in monoclonal gammopathy of undetermined significance (MGUS). Br J Haematol 126(5):686–689

Portier M, Rajzbaum G, Zhang XG, Attal M, Rusalen C, Wijdenes J, Mannoni P, Maraninchi D, Piechaczyk M, Bataille R (1991) In vivo interleukin 6 gene expression in the tumoral environment in multiple myeloma. Eur J Immunol 21(7):1759–1762

Puthier D, Derenne S, Barille S, Moreau P, Harousseau JL, Bataille R, Amiot M (1999) Mcl-1 and Bcl-xL are co-regulated by IL-6 in human myeloma cells. Br J Haematol 107(2): 392–395

Qiang YW, Kopantzev E, Rudikoff S (2002) Insulinlike growth factor-I signaling in multiple myeloma: downstream elements, functional correlates, and pathway cross-talk. Blood 99(11):4138–4146

Radbruch A, Muehlinghaus G, Luger EO, Inamine A, Smith KG, Dorner T, Hiepe F (2006) Competence and competition: the challenge of becoming a long-lived plasma cell. Nat Rev Immunol 6(10):741–750

Reece D, Song KW, Fu T, Roland B, Chang H, Horsman DE, Mansoor A, Chen C, Masih-Khan E, Trieu Y, Bruyere H, Stewart DA, Bahlis NJ (2009) Influence of cytogenetics in patients with relapsed or refractory multiple myeloma treated with lenalidomide plus dexamethasone: adverse effect of deletion 17p13. Blood 114(3):522–525

Reijmers RM, Groen RW, Rozemuller H, Kuil A, de Haan-Kramer A, Csikos T, Martens AC, Spaargaren M, Pals ST (2010) Targeting EXT1 reveals a crucial role for heparan sulfate in the growth of multiple myeloma. Blood 115(3): 601–604

Ren R, Charles PC, Zhang C, Wu Y, Wang H, Patterson C (2007) Gene expression profiles identify a role for cyclooxygenase 2-dependent prostanoid generation in BMP6-induced angiogenic responses. Blood 109(7):2847–2853

Richardson PG, Sonneveld P, Schuster MW, Irwin D, Stadtmauer EA, Facon T, Harousseau JL, Ben-Yehuda D, Lonial S, Goldschmidt H, Reece D, San-Miguel JF, Blade J, Boccadoro M, Cavenagh J, Dalton WS, Boral AL, Esseltine DL, Porter JB, Schenkein D, Anderson KC (2005) Bortezomib or high-dose dexamethasone for relapsed multiple myeloma. N Engl J Med 352(24):2487–2498

Ro TB, Holt RU, Brenne AT, Hjorth-Hansen H, Waage A, Hjertner O, Sundan A, Borset M (2004) Bone morphogenetic protein-5, -6 and -7 inhibit growth and induce apoptosis in human myeloma cells. Oncogene 23(17):3024–3032

Rosen LS, Gordon DH, Dugan W Jr, Major P, Eisenberg PD, Provencher L, Kaminski M, Simeone J, Seaman J, Chen BL, Coleman RE (2004) Zoledronic acid is superior to pamidronate for the treatment of bone metastases in breast carcinoma patients with at least one osteolytic lesion. Cancer 100(1):36–43

Rosenwald A, Wright G, Wiestner A, Chan WC, Connors JM, Campo E, Gascoyne RD, Grogan TM, Muller-Hermelink HK, Smeland EB, Chiorazzi M, Giltnane JM, Hurt EM, Zhao H, Averett L, Henrickson S, Yang L, Powell J, Wilson WH, Jaffe ES, Simon R, Klausner RD, Montserrat E, Bosch F, Greiner TC, Weisenburger DD, Sanger WG, Dave BJ, Lynch JC, Vose J, Armitage JO, Fisher RI, Miller TP, LeBlanc M, Ott G, Kvaloy S, Holte H, Delabie J, Staudt LM (2003) The proliferation gene expression signature is a quantitative integrator of oncogenic events that predicts survival in mantle cell lymphoma. Cancer Cell 3(2):185–197

Rossi JF, Fegueux N, Lu ZY, Legouffe E, Exbrayat C, Bozonnat MC, Navarro R, Lopez E, Quittet P, Daures JP, Rouille V, Kanouni T, Widjenes J, Klein B (2005) Optimizing the use of anti-interleukin-6 monoclonal antibody with dexamethasone and 140 mg/m2 of melphalan in multiple myeloma: results of a pilot study including biological aspects. Bone Marrow Transplant 36(9):771–779

Rossi JF, Moreaux J, Hose D, Requirand G, Rose M, Rouille V, Nestorov I, Mordenti G, Goldschmidt H, Ythier A, Klein B (2009) Atacicept in relapsed/refractory multiple myeloma or active Waldenstrom's macroglobulinemia: a phase I study. Br J Cancer 101(7):1051–1058

Saito M, Gao J, Basso K, Kitagawa Y, Smith PM, Bhagat G, Pernis A, Pasqualucci L, Della-Favera R (2007) A signaling pathway mediating down-regulation of BCL6 in germinal center B cells is blocked by BCL6 gene alterations in B cell lymphoma. Cancer Cell 12(3):280–292

San Miguel JF, Garcia-Sanz R, Gonzalez M, Moro MJ, Hernandez JM, Ortega F, Borrego D, Carnero M, Casanova F, Jimenez R (1995) A new staging system for multiple myeloma based on the number of S-phase plasma cells. Blood 85(2):448–455

San Miguel JF, Schlag R, Khuageva NK, Dimopoulos MA, Shpilberg O, Kropff M, Spicka I, Petrucci MT, Palumbo A, Samoilova OS, Dmoszynska A, Abdulkadyrov KM, Schots R, Jiang B, Mateos MV, Anderson KC, Esseltine DL, Liu K, Cakana A, van de Velde H, Richardson PG (2008) Bortezomib plus melphalan and prednisone for initial treatment of multiple myeloma. N Engl J Med 359(9):906–917

Sanderson RD, Yang Y (2008) Syndecan-1: a dynamic regulator of the myeloma microenvironment. Clin Exp Metastasis 25(2):149–159

Santra M, Zhan F, Tian E, Barlogie B, Shaughnessy J Jr (2003) A subset of multiple myeloma harboring the t(4;14)(p16;q32) translocation lacks FGFR3 expression but maintains an IGH/MMSET fusion transcript. Blood 101(6):2374–2376

Schambeck CM, Wick M, Bartl R, Lamerz R, Fateh-Moghadam A (1995) Plasma cell proliferation in monoclonal gammopathies: measurement using BU-1 antibody in flow cytometry and microscopy: comparison with serum thymidine kinase. J Clin Pathol 48(5):477–481

Schmidlin H, Diehl SA, Blom B (2009) New insights into the regulation of human B-cell differentiation. Trends Immunol 30(6):277–285

Seckinger A, Meissner T, Moreaux J, Goldschmidt H, Fuhler GM, Benner A, Hundemer M, Reme T, Shaughnessy JD Jr, Barlogie B, Bertsch U, Hillengass J, Ho AD, Pantesco V, Jauch A, De VJ, Rossi JF, Mohler T, Klein B, Hose D (2009) Bone morphogenic protein 6: a member of a novel class of prognostic factors expressed by normal and malignant plasma cells inhibiting proliferation and angiogenesis. Oncogene 28(44):3866–3879

Seidel C, Borset M, Turesson I, Abildgaard N, Sundan A, Waage A (1998) Elevated serum concentrations of hepatocyte growth factor in patients with multiple myeloma. The Nordic Myeloma Study Group. Blood 91(3):806–812

Sezer O, Heider U, Jakob C, Eucker J, Possinger K (2002) Human bone marrow myeloma cells express RANKL. J Clin Oncol 20(1):353–354

Shain KH, Yarde DN, Meads MB, Huang M, Jove R, Hazlehurst LA, Dalton WS (2009) Beta1 integrin adhesion enhances IL-6-mediated STAT3 signaling in myeloma cells: implications for microenvironment influence on tumor survival and proliferation. Cancer Res 69(3):1009–1015

Shaughnessy JD Jr, Zhan F, Burington BE, Huang Y, Colla S, Hanamura I, Stewart JP, Kordsmeier B, Randolph C, Williams DR, Xiao Y, Xu H, Epstein J, Anaissie E, Krishna SG, Cottler-Fox M, Hollmig K, Mohiuddin A, Pineda-Roman M, Tricot G, van Rhee F, Sawyer J, Alsayed Y, Walker R, Zangari M, Crowley J, Barlogie B (2007) A validated gene expression model of

3

high-risk multiple myeloma is defined by deregulated expression of genes mapping to chromosome 1. Blood 109(6):2276–2284
Sherr CJ (1996) Cancer cell cycles. Science 274(5293):1672–1677
Sherr CJ, Roberts JM (1999) CDK inhibitors: positive and negative regulators of G1-phase progression. Genes Dev 13(12):1501–1512
Sherr CJ, Roberts JM (2004) Living with or without cyclins and cyclin-dependent kinases. Genes Dev 18(22):2699–2711
Shipman CM, Croucher PI (2003) Osteoprotegerin is a soluble decoy receptor for tumor necrosis factor-related apoptosis-inducing ligand/Apo2 ligand and can function as a paracrine survival factor for human myeloma cells. Cancer Res 63(5):912–916
Sibley K, Fenton JA, Dring AM, Ashcroft AJ, Rawstron AC, Morgan GJ (2002) A molecular study of the t(4;14) in multiple myeloma. Br J Haematol 118(2):514–520
Simonet WS, Lacey DL, Dunstan CR, Kelley M, Chang MS, Luthy R, Nguyen HQ, Wooden S, Bennett L, Boone T, Shimamoto G, DeRose M, Elliott R, Colombero A, Tan HL, Trail G, Sullivan J, Davy E, Bucay N, Renshaw-Gegg L, Hughes TM, Hill D, Pattison W, Campbell P, Sander S, Van G, Tarpley J, Derby P, Lee R, Boyle WJ (1997) Osteoprotegerin: a novel secreted protein involved in the regulation of bone density. Cell 89(2):309–319
Smadja NV, Bastard C, Brigaudeau C, Leroux D, Fruchart C (2001) Hypodiploidy is a major prognostic factor in multiple myeloma. Blood 98(7):2229–2238
Specht K, Haralambieva E, Bink K, Kremer M, Mandl-Weber S, Koch I, Tomer R, Hofler H, Schuuring E, Kluin PM, Fend F, Quintanilla-Martinez L (2004) Different mechanisms of cyclin D1 overexpression in multiple myeloma revealed by fluorescence in situ hybridization and quantitative analysis of mRNA levels. Blood 104(4):1120–1126
Sprynski AC, Hose D, Caillot L, Reme T, Shaughnessy JD Jr, Barlogie B, Seckinger A, Moreaux J, Hundemer M, Jourdan M, Meissner T, Jauch A, Mahtouk K, Kassambara A, Bertsch U, Rossi JF, Goldschmidt H, Klein B (2009) The role of IGF-1 as a major growth factor for myeloma cell lines and the prognostic relevance of the expression of its receptor. Blood 113(19):4614–4626
Standal T, Borset M, Lenhoff S, Wisloff F, Stordal B, Sundan A, Waage A, Seidel C (2002) Serum insulin like growth factor is not elevated in patients with multiple myeloma but is still a prognostic factor. Blood 100(12):3925–3929
Standal T, Abildgaard N, Fagerli UM, Stordal B, Hjertner O, Borset M, Sundan A (2007) HGF inhibits BMP-induced osteoblastogenesis: possible implications for the bone disease of multiple myeloma. Blood 109(7):3024–3030
Suematsu S, Matsuda T, Aozasa K, Akira S, Nakano N, Ohno S, Miyazaki J, Yamamura K, Hirano T, Kishimoto T (1989) IgG1 plasmacytosis in interleukin 6 transgenic mice. Proc Natl Acad Sci USA 86(19):7547–7551
Suematsu S, Matsusaka T, Matsuda T, Ohno S, Miyazaki J, Yamamura K, Hirano T, Kishimoto T (1992) Generation of plasmacytomas with the chromosomal translocation t(12;15) in interleukin 6 transgenic mice. Proc Natl Acad Sci USA 89(1):232–235
Tai YT, Podar K, Catley L, Tseng YH, Akiyama M, Shringarpure R, Burger R, Hideshima T, Chauhan D, Mitsiades N, Richardson P, Munshi NC, Kahn CR, Mitsiades C, Anderson KC (2003) Insulin-like growth factor-1 induces adhesion and migration in human multiple myeloma cells via activation of beta1-integrin and phosphatidylinositol 3′-kinase/AKT signaling. Cancer Res 63(18):5850–5858
Tanaka Y, Abe M, Hiasa M, Oda A, Amou H, Nakano A, Takeuchi K, Kitazoe K, Kido S, Inoue D, Moriyama K, Hashimoto T, Ozaki S, Matsumoto T (2007) Myeloma cell-osteoclast interaction enhances angiogenesis together with bone resorption: a role for vascular endothelial cell growth factor and osteopontin. Clin Cancer Res 13(3):816–823
Tarlinton D, Radbruch A, Hiepe F, Dorner T (2008) Plasma cell differentiation and survival. Curr Opin Immunol 20(2):162–169
Taube T, Beneton MN, McCloskey EV, Rogers S, Greaves M, Kanis JA (1992) Abnormal bone remodelling in patients with myelomatosis and normal biochemical indices of bone resorption. Eur J Haematol 49(4):192–198
Terpos E, Politou M, Szydlo R, Goldman JM, Apperley JF, Rahemtulla A (2003a) Serum levels of macrophage inflammatory protein-1 alpha (MIP-1alpha) correlate with the extent of bone disease and survival in patients with

multiple myeloma. Br J Haematol 123(1): 106–109

Terpos E, Szydlo R, Apperley JF, Hatjiharissi E, Politou M, Meletis J, Viniou N, Yataganas X, Goldman JM, Rahemtulla A (2003b) Soluble receptor activator of nuclear factor kappaB ligand-osteoprotegerin ratio predicts survival in multiple myeloma: proposal for a novel prognostic index. Blood 102(3):1064–1069

Tian E, Zhan F, Walker R, Rasmussen E, Ma Y, Barlogie B, Shaughnessy JD Jr (2003) The role of the Wnt-signaling antagonist DKK1 in the development of osteolytic lesions in multiple myeloma. N Engl J Med 349(26):2483–2494

Tienhaara A, Pelliniemi TT (1992) Flow cytometric DNA analysis and clinical correlations in multiple myeloma. Am J Clin Pathol 97(3): 322–330

Tokoyoda K, Egawa T, Sugiyama T, Choi BI, Nagasawa T (2004) Cellular niches controlling B lymphocyte behavior within bone marrow during development. Immunity 20(6):707–718

Trojan A, Tinguely M, Vallet S, Seifert B, Jenni B, Zippelius A, Witzens-Harig M, Mechtersheimer G, Ho A, Goldschmidt H, Jager D, Boccadoro M, Ladetto M (2006) Clinical significance of cyclooxygenase-2 (COX-2) in multiple myeloma. Swiss Med Wkly 136(25–26):400–403

Tsuji K, Bandyopadhyay A, Harfe BD, Cox K, Kakar S, Gerstenfeld L, Einhorn T, Tabin CJ, Rosen V (2006) BMP2 activity, although dispensable for bone formation, is required for the initiation of fracture healing. Nat Genet 38(12):1424–1429

Tu Y, Gardner A, Lichtenstein A (2000) The phosphatidylinositol 3-kinase/AKT kinase pathway in multiple myeloma plasma cells: roles in cytokine-dependent survival and proliferative responses. Cancer Res 60(23):6763–6770

Uchiyama H, Barut BA, Mohrbacher AF, Chauhan D, Anderson KC (1993) Adhesion of human myeloma-derived cell lines to bone marrow stromal cells stimulates interleukin-6 secretion. Blood 82(12):3712–3720

Valentin-Opran A, Charhon SA, Meunier PJ, Edouard CM, Arlot ME (1982) Quantitative histology of myeloma-induced bone changes. Br J Haematol 52(4):601–610

von Metzler I, Krebbel H, Hecht M, Manz RA, Fleissner C, Mieth M, Kaiser M, Jakob C, Sterz J, Kleeberg L, Heider U, Sezer O (2007) Bortezomib inhibits human osteoclastogenesis. Leukemia 21(9):2025–2034

Wang YD, De Vos J, Jourdan M, Couderc G, Lu ZY, Rossi JF, Klein B (2002) Cooperation between heparin-binding EGF-like growth factor and interleukin-6 in promoting the growth of human myeloma cells. Oncogene 21(16): 2584–2592

Wijdenes J, Vooijs WC, Clement C, Post J, Morard F, Vita N, Laurent P, Sun RX, Klein B, Dore JM (1996) A plasmocyte selective monoclonal antibody (B-B4) recognizes syndecan-1. Br J Haematol 94(2):318–323

Witzig TE, Timm M, Larson D, Therneau T, Greipp PR (1999) Measurement of apoptosis and proliferation of bone marrow plasma cells in patients with plasma cell proliferative disorders. Br J Haematol 104(1):131–137

Wlodarska I, Meeus P, Stul M, Thienpont L, Wouters E, Marcelis L, Demuynck H, Rummens JL, Madoe V, Hagemeijer A (2004) Variant t(2;11)(p11;q13) associated with the IgK-CCND1 rearrangement is a recurrent translocation in leukemic small-cell B-non-Hodgkin lymphoma. Leukemia 18(10):1705–1710

Wuilleme S, Robillard N, Lode L, Magrangeas F, Beris H, Harousseau JL, Proffitt J, Minvielle S, Avet-Loiseau H (2005) Ploidy, as detected by fluorescence in situ hybridization, defines different subgroups in multiple myeloma. Leukemia 19(2):275–278

Wutzl A, Brozek W, Lernbass I, Rauner M, Hofbauer G, Schopper C, Watzinger F, Peterlik M, Pietschmann P (2006) Bone morphogenetic proteins 5 and 6 stimulate osteoclast generation. J Biomed Mater Res A 77(1):75–83

Yaccoby S, Wezeman MJ, Henderson A, Cottler-Fox M, Yi Q, Barlogie B, Epstein J (2004) Cancer and the microenvironment: myeloma-osteoclast interactions as a model. Cancer Res 64(6):2016–2023

Yaccoby S, Ling W, Zhan F, Walker R, Barlogie B, Shaughnessy JD Jr (2007) Antibody-based inhibition of DKK1 suppresses tumor-induced bone resorption and multiple myeloma growth in vivo. Blood 109(5):2106–2111

Yamasaki K, Taga T, Hirata Y, Yawata H, Kawanishi Y, Seed B, Taniguchi T, Hirano T, Kishimoto T (1988) Cloning and expression of the human interleukin-6 (BSF-2/IFN beta 2) receptor. Science 241(4867):825–828

3

Zhan F, Hardin J, Kordsmeier B, Bumm K, Zheng M, Tian E, Sanderson R, Yang Y, Wilson C, Zangari M, Anaissie E, Morris C, Muwalla F, van Rhee F, Fassas A, Crowley J, Tricot G, Barlogie B, Shaughnessy J Jr (2002) Global gene expression profiling of multiple myeloma, monoclonal gammopathy of undetermined significance, and normal bone marrow plasma cells. Blood 99(5):1745–1757

Zhan F, Huang Y, Colla S, Stewart JP, Hanamura I, Gupta S, Epstein J, Yaccoby S, Sawyer J, Burington B, Hollmig K, Pineda-Roman M, Tricot G, van Rhee F, Walker R, Zangari M, Crowley J, Barlogie B, Shaughnessy JD Jr (2006) The molecular classification of multiple myeloma. Blood 108(6):2020–2028

Zhang XG, Bataille R, Widjenes J, Klein B (1992) Interleukin-6 dependence of advanced malignant plasma cell dyscrasias. Cancer 69(6):1373–1376

Zhang XG, Gaillard JP, Robillard N, Lu ZY, Gu ZJ, Jourdan M, Boiron JM, Bataille R, Klein B (1994a) Reproducible obtaining of human myeloma cell lines as a model for tumor stem cell study in human multiple myeloma. Blood 83(12):3654–3663

Zhang XG, Gu JJ, Lu ZY, Yasukawa K, Yancopoulos GD, Turner K, Shoyab M, Taga T, Kishimoto T, Bataille R et al (1994b) Ciliary neurotropic factor, interleukin 11, leukemia inhibitory factor, and oncostatin M are growth factors for human myeloma cell lines using the interleukin 6 signal transducer gp130. J Exp Med 179(4):1337–1342

Zudaire I, Odero MD, Caballero C, Valenti C, Martinez-Penuela JM, Isola J, Calasanz MJ (2002) Genomic imbalances detected by comparative genomic hybridization are prognostic markers in invasive ductal breast carcinomas. Histopathology 40(6):547–555

Angiogenesis and Vasculogenesis in Multiple Myeloma: Role of Inflammatory Cells

4

Angelo Vacca and Domenico Ribatti

Contents

A. Vacca (✉)
Department of Internal Medicine and Clinical Oncology, University of Bari Medical School, Policlinico – Piazza Giulio Cesare, 11, I-70124 Bari, Italy
e-mail: a.vacca@dimo.uniba.it

Abstract Angiogenesis plays a central role in the progression of both solid and hematologic tumors. We have focused our attention on multiple myeloma (MM) and on bone marrow stromal cells. These, in fact, both support tumor cell survival and participate in angiogenesis by releasing a broad number of angiogenic cytokines. Macrophages and mast cells may participate in this process through other mechanisms, such as vasculogenic mimicry. Lastly, it has been shown that hematopoietic stem and progenitor cells (HSPCs) are involved in vasculogenesis in MM.

4.1 Introduction

New blood vessels form through two steps: vasculogenesis and angiogenesis. In the first step (vasculogenesis), mesoderm-derived angioblasts proliferate and organize into a primitive vascular plexus (Risau and Lemmon 1995). In contrast, angiogenesis, i.e., the formation of new blood vessels from existing blood vessels, takes place in several conditions, both physiological (e.g., corpus luteum formation) and pathological, such as chronic inflammation and tumors (Risau 1997). In addition, extensive data have illustrated the

T. Moehler and H. Goldschmidt (eds.), *Multiple Myeloma*,
Recent Results in Cancer Research 183, DOI: 10.1007/978-3-540-85772-3_4,

existence of endothelial progenitor cells and their contribution to the formation of new blood vessels in adults (Ribatti et al. 2005). Their discovery has led to the new concept that vasculogenesis and angiogenesis may occur simultaneously in postnatal life because endothelial progenitor cells differentiate through a mechanism that recapitulates embryo vasculogenesis. Lastly, other vascularization mechanisms occur in tumors, e.g., vascular co-option of existing vessels and vascular mimicry (Ribatti et al. 2003).

Under physiological conditions, angiogenesis depends on the balance of positive and negative angiogenic modulators within the vascular microenvironment (Hanahan and Folkman 1996). It requires the functional activities of a number of molecules, including angiogenic factors, extracellular matrix proteins, adhesion receptors, and proteolytic enzymes. Tumor angiogenesis is linked to a switch in this balance, and mainly depends on the release by neoplastic cells of growth factors specific for endothelial cells and able to stimulate the growth of the host's blood vessels (Ribatti et al. 2007).

Solid tumor growth comprises an avascular and a subsequent vascular phase (Ribatti et al. 1999). If this second phase is dependent on angiogenesis and the release of angiogenic factors, acquisition of angiogenic capability can be seen as an expression of the progression from neoplastic transformation to tumor growth and metastasis. The role of angiogenesis in the growth and survival of leukemias and other hematological malignancies has become evident since 1994; in a series of demonstrations, it was clearly shown that the progression of several forms is related to their degree of angiogenesis (Ribatti and Vacca 2008).

4.2 Angiogenesis and Antiangiogenesis in Multiple Myeloma

In 1994, we demonstrated for the first time that in multiple myeloma (MM) bone marrow, angiogenesis measured as microvascular density increases with progression from monoclonal gammopathy of undetermined significance (MGUS) to nonactive MM and active MM, and is related with the plasma cell labeling index (Vacca et al. 1994). Assuming that microvascular density depends on angiogenesis, these results are consistent with the notion that angiogenesis favors expansion of the MM mass by promoting plasma cell proliferation. Subsequent studies have confirmed the observation of increased angiogenesis in active MM compared to healthy individuals or patients with MGUS (Vacca and Ribatti 2006).

Myeloma plasma cells induce angiogenesis directly via the secretion of angiogenic cytokines, such as vascular endothelial growth factor (VEGF) and fibroblast growth factor-2 (FGF-2), and indirectly by induction of host inflammatory cell infiltration, and degrade the extracellular matrix with their matrix-degrading enzymes, such as matrix metalloproteinase-2 and -9 (MMP-2 and MMP-9) and urokinase-type plasminogen activator (Vacca and Ribatti 2006). Although it is well established that MM cells drive angiogenesis by the secretion of angiogenic factors, there is also evidence of loss of antiangiogenic activity on the part of bone marrow plasma cells with disease progression (Kumar et al. 2004; Mangieri et al. 2008). Moreover, bone marrow MM endothelial cells secrete growth factors, including VEGF and interleukin-6 (IL-6), which promote MM cell growth in the bone marrow milieu (Vacca et al. 2003). Bone marrow angiogenesis can be targeted by new agents. For example, thalidomide inhibits bone marrow endothelial cell proliferation, capillarogenesis and secretion of VEGF, FGF-2 and hepatocyte growth factor (HGF) in patients with MM (Vacca et al. 2005).

Reciprocal positive and negative interactions between plasma cells and bone marrow stromal cells (BMSCs), namely hematopoietic stem and progenitor cells (HSPCs), fibroblasts, osteoblasts, osteoclasts, chondroclasts, endothelial cells, endothelial progenitor cells, T cells, macrophages and mast cells, are mediated by an array of cytokines, receptors, and adhesion molecules, and modulate the angiogenic response in

MM (Ribatti et al. 2006). Interactions between these components determine the proliferation, migration, and survival of plasma cells, as well as their acquisition of drug resistance and the development of disease (Ribatti et al. 2006).

BMSCs increase the concentration of angiogenic factors and matrix-degrading enzymes in the BM microenvironment by direct secretion or by stimulation of MM cells or endothelial cells through paracrine interactions (Ribatti et al. 2006). BMSCs, osteoclasts, osteoblasts, and endothelial cells secrete several factors, including VEGF, FGF-2, tumor necrosis factor-alpha (TNF-α), IL-6, B-cell activating factor, stromal cell–derived factor 1α (SDF1α, also known as CXCL12), and various Notch family members, which are further upregulated by tumor cell adhesion to extracellular matrix proteins and/or BMSCs (Hideshima et al. 2007).

BMSCs and other accessory cells supporting MM cell survival in the bone microenvironment constitute potential therapeutic targets. In this context, BM endothelial cells are the targets of diverse classes of antiangiogenic molecules (Hideshima et al. 2007).

4.3 The Role of Inflammatory Cells in Tumor Angiogenesis

Inflammatory cells regulate endothelial cell functions related to physiological angiogenesis as well as inflammatory and tumor-associated angiogenesis. It was Rudolf Virchow in 1863, who critically recognized the presence of inflammatory cells infiltrating neoplastic tissues and first established a causative connection between the "lymphoreticular infilitrate" at sites of chronic inflammation and cancer.

In neoplastic tissues, inflammatory cells act in concert with tumor cells, stromal cells, and endothelial cells to create a microenvironment that is critical for the survival, development, and diffusion of the neoplastic mass. These synergies may represent important mechanisms for tumor development and metastasis by providing an efficient vascular supply and an easy escape pathway. Indeed, the most aggressive human cancers, such as malignant melanoma, breast carcinoma, and colorectal adenocarcinoma, are associated with a dramatic host response composed of various inflammatory cells, especially macrophages and mast cells.

Cells belonging to the monocyte-macrophage lineage are a major component of the leukocyte infiltration in tumors, and there is growing evidence that they are part of inflammatory circuits that promote tumor progression, and favor invasion and metastasis (Mantovani et al. 1992; Balkwill and Mantovani 2001). The stimulating effect exerted by tumor-associated macrophages on the growth of the tumor mass is partly related to the angiogenic potential of these cells. Tumor-associated macrophages are a rich source of potent proangiogenic cytokines and growth factors, such as VEGF, TNF-α, IL-8, and FGF-2. They also express a broad array of angiogenesis-modulating enzymes, including MMP-2, MMP-7, MMP-9, MMP-12, and cycloxygenase-2 (COX-2) (Sunderkotter et al. 1991; Lewis et al. 1995; Klimp et al. 2001; Ribatti et al. 2006). The many proangiogenic factors they secrete may promote tumor spread and help to explain the correlation between increased tumor-associated macrophage density and the augmented tumor vasculature recognized during experimental and human carcinogenesis.

Moreover, macrophages take part in neovascularization by "drilling" tunnels for new vasculature, producing tubular destruction of the matrix, distributing to form columns and capillary-like structures containing erythrocytes (Moldovan et al. 2000), localizing in microvessels embedded in bundles of fibrillar collagen (Anghelina et al. 2006), and adhering to injured vessel walls, thus accelerating re-endothelization of the vascular barrier (Fujiyama et al. 2003).

In healthy subjects, cells of the monocyte lineage generate endothelial progenitor cells (Rehman et al. 2003), or act as pluripotent stem cells (Zhao et al. 2003). They develop an endothelial cell phenotype when stimulated by VEGF and/or FGF-2 (Fernandez Pujol et al. 2000; Zhao et al. 2003), and produce a functional capillary-like mesh (Schmeisser et al. 2001) permeable by blood cells (Anghelina et al. 2004). By contrast with these reports of the vascular ability of monocytes, mature macrophages form capillary-like lumina and branching patterns in vitro. This confirms their propensity to participate in new microvessel formation (Anghelina et al. 2004).

Experimental evidence points to mast cells as key host cells in the tumor infiltrate with important consequences for the fate of tumor cells. On the one hand, they are detrimental to tumor growth by producing molecules that kill tumor cells and by inducing an inflammatory reaction. On the other hand, they favor a tumor's progression by promoting expansion of its vascular supply, degradation of the tumor extracellular matrix, and immunosuppression (Theoharides and Conti 2004).

Mast cells are a rich source of preformed and newly synthesized angiogenic cytokines and growth factors, such as VEGF, FGF-2, TNF-α, IL-8, as well as of angiogenic proteases, such as tryptase and chymase, which are all contained in their secretory granules, that favor new vessel formation either directly or via local recruitment of activated inflammatory cells (Ribatti et al. 2004). In addition, mast cell–derived MMPs degrade the interstitial tumor stroma and hence release matrix-bound angiogenic factors. Several studies in human and experimental tumors have demonstrated that mast cells play a critical role in the support of tumor angiogenesis (Ribatti et al. 2004; Crivellato et al. 2008).

4.4 The Involvement of Macrophages in Vascular Mimicry in MM

We have recently shown that when bone marrow macrophages from MM patients are exposed to VEGF and FGF-2, which are major angiogenic cytokines secreted by plasma cells (Bellamy et al. 1999; Vacca et al. 1999), and present in the bone marrow microenvironment at 4–5-fold higher levels than in peripheral blood (Di Raimondo et al. 2000), they transform into cells functionally and phenotypically similar to paired MM endothelial cells, and generate capillary-like networks mimicking those of MM endothelial cells (Scavelli et al. 2008). By contrast, macrophages from nonactive MM, MGUS, and benign anemia patients display similar, albeit weaker features. Endothelial cell-like macrophages and apparently typical macrophages contribute sizably to the formation of the neovessel wall in patients with active MM, whereas their vascular supply is minimal in nonactive MM, and absent in MGUS patients and control patients (Scavelli et al. 2008). In patients with active MM, FACS analyses on freshly isolated BM mononuclear cells revealed higher percentages of CD14/CD68 double-positive cells than in those with nonactive disease and MGUS. Furthermore, in active MM patients, BM biopsies displayed macrophages with both endothelial cell-like (i.e., CD68/FVIII-RA double positive) and apparently typical (i.e., CD68 positive/FVIII-RA negative) features located in the microvessel wall and collaborating with MM endothelial cells to line the vessel lumen. Figures of this type were rare in nonactive MM patients and absent in MGUS. Thus, macrophage involvement in the vasculogenic pathway proceeds in step with MM activity, and with progression of plasma cell tumors as well (Scavelli et al. 2008).

Overall, these data suggest that in active MM, macrophages contribute to neovascularization through a vasculogenic pathway, and that in nonactive MM and MGUS, they are prone to behave accordingly, marching in step with progression, hence with the vascular switch (Kumar et al. 2004) (Fig. 4.1).

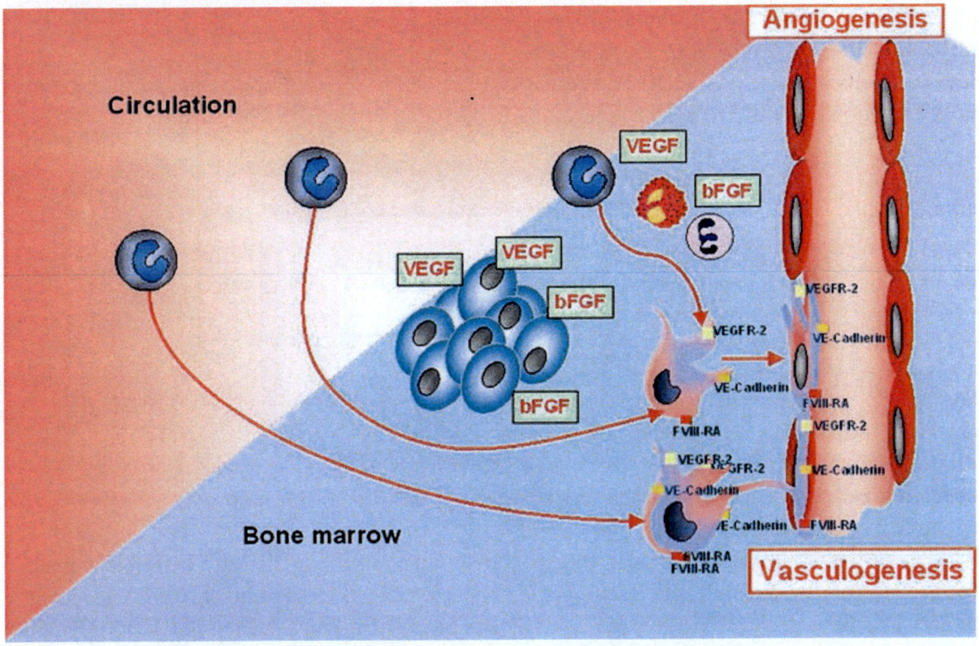

Fig. 4.1 Possible recruitment of macrophages for neovessel assembly by vasculogenesis in multiple myeloma. Circulating monocytes and macrophages from the resident BM pool are recruited by VEGF and FGF-2 (or bFGF) secreted by plasma cells and induced to differentiate into endothelial-like cells

4.5 The Involvement of Mast Cells in Vascular Mimicry in MM

We have previously demonstrated that bone marrow angiogenesis, evaluated as microvessel area, and mast cell density counts are highly correlated in patients with nonactive and active MM and in those with MGUS, and that both parameters increase simultaneously in active MM (Ribatti et al. 1999). Angiopoietin-1 (Ang-1) is a crucial promoter of MM cell growth by stimulating angiogenesis. Experimental evidence indicates that Ang-1 secreted by primary murine mast cells promote marked neovascularization in an in vivo transplantation assay (Nakayama et al. 2004). These authors demonstrated that primary mast cells accelerate tumor growth by established plasmocytoma cell lines, while Ang-1-neutralizing antibodies significantly reduced the growth of plasmocytomas containing mast cells.

We have recently demonstrated that at the ultrastructural level, vessels from MM biopsies are lined by mast cells whose cytoplasms are filled with numerous and irregularly shaped electron-dense granules (Nico et al. 2008). Moreover, thick endothelial cells, containing endocytotic vesicles, but lacking granules, are connected by a junctional system with the mast cells lining the vessel wall, whereas the vessels from MGUS biopsies are lined with thin endothelial cells, often surrounded by mast cells (Nico et al. 2008).

These ultrastructural findings have been confirmed by confocal laser microscopy using double anti-tryptase (to mark mast cells) and

4

anti-FVIII-RA (to mark endothelial cells) antibodies. Vessels from MM biopsies displayed regions stained by FVIII-RA alternating with regions stained by both tryptase and FVIII-RA. In the MGUS biopsies, the vessels were uniformly stained by the anti-FVIII-RA antibody only, while tryptase-positive mast cells were only recognizable perivascularly (Nico et al. 2008).

Overall, these data suggest that in MM patients, mast cells contribute to neovascularization. The BM of MM patients, in fact, displays typical tryptase-positive mast cells in the vessel wall that collaborate with endothelial cell to line the lumina. Since mast cells keep their lineage marker, they can be regarded as cells that do not transdifferentiate into endothelial cells. This behavior of mast cells can thus be regarded as another example of vasculogenic mimicry (Maniotis et al. 1999).

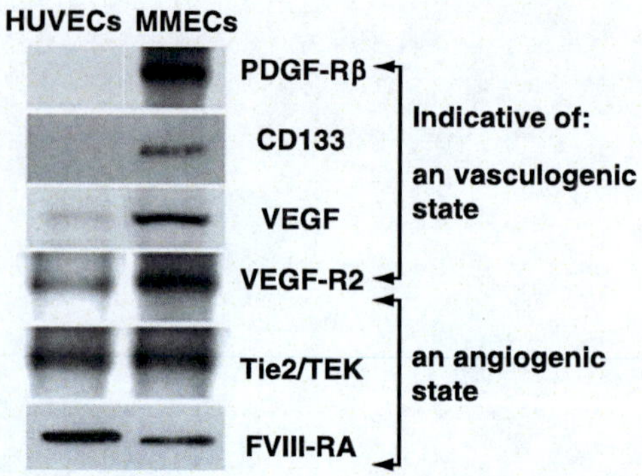

Fig. 4.2 MM endothelial cells (MMECs) express markers indicative of both an angiogenic and a vasculogenic state.

4.6 Vasculogenesis by Hematopoietic Stem and Progenitor Cells

At variance from normal human unbilical vein endothelial cells (HUVECs), we found that MM endothelial cells express some markers indicative of vasculogenesis, i.e., formation of new vessels from immature hematopoietic stem and progenitor cells (HSPCs). As shown in Fig. 4.2, these vasculogenic markers are CD133 and PDGF receptor beta (PDGF-Rβ) (Ria et al. 2008; Coluccia et al. 2008). PDGF-Rβ is shared with plasma cells and other stromal cells, and is a target for anti-plasma cell and anti-endothelial cell therapy with dasatinib (Coluccia et al. 2008). Thus, we tested the hypothesis that HSPCs from MM patients could be a source of endothelial cells via a vasculogenic pathway (Ria et al. 2008). HSPCs from MM patients at diagnosis were harvested from peripheral blood before conditioning therapy, using apheresis and an anti-CD133 antibody. Cells seeded on fibronectin and exposed to VEGF, bFGF, and insulin-like growth factor (IGF) were able to differentiate into cells with an MM endothelial cell phenotype after a 3-week culture. HSPCs gradually lost CD133 and acquired VEGF receptor-2 (VEGFR2/KDR), factor-VIII-related antigen (FVIII-RA) and VE-cadherin, indicative of a mature MM endothelial cell phenotype. In addition, cells adhered to fibronectin, spread, and acquired a typical endothelial cell shape. On day 21, differentiated cells formed a closely knit capillary network on the Matrigel surface. At variance from nonactive MM, MGUS, and benign anemia (control) patients, BM biopsies of the active MM showed cells co-expressing FVIII-RA and CD133, VEGFR2, or VE-cadherin involved in the formation of the microvessel wall. We hypothesize that VEGF, FGF-2, and IGF released by MM plasma cells and inflammatory cells during the active disease possibly induce the differentiation of CD133+ HSPCs into MM endothelial cells that contribute to the development of the MM vasculature through vasculogenesis (Fig. 4.3).

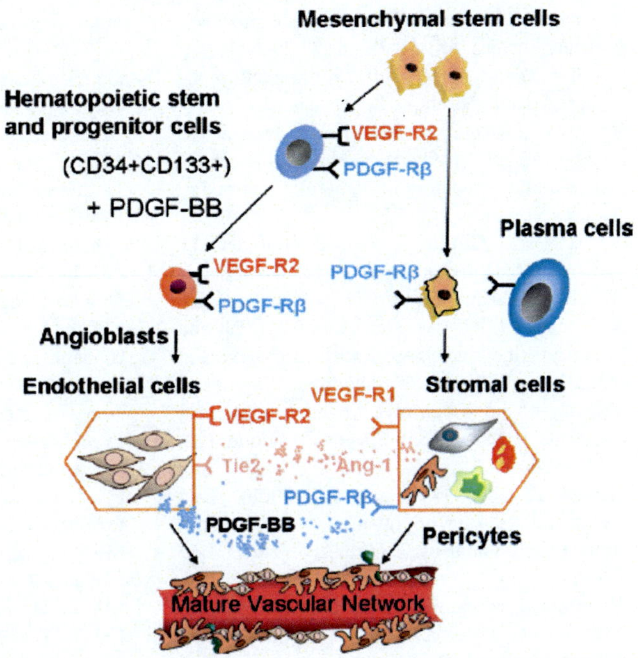

Fig. 4.3 Hypothetical differentiation of hematopoietic stem and progenitor cells into endothelial cells in multiple myeloma. This differentiation pathway is marked by expression of PDGF-Rβ and VEGFR-2 at high levels

4.7 Concluding Remarks

The pathogenesis of most cancers includes complex and mutual interactions that affect the number and phenotype of the tumor cells and host stromal cells. In this context, angiogenesis in MM is the result of a complex balance between pro- and antiangiogenic stimuli generated in the tissue milieu. The evidence summarized in this chapter highlights the importance of the stromal microenvironment during angiogenesis in MM and provides a novel perspective for the complex interplay between several stromal and vascular components in the BM microenvironment in MM. In this context, it seems of primary importance to further understand the contribution of inflammatory cells to angiogenesis in MM.

Acknowledgments This work was supported in part by grants from Associazione Italiana per la Ricerca sul Cancro (AIRC), Milan; the Ministry of Education, University and Research (MIUR, PRIN Projects 2007), Rome; the Ministry of Health, Progetto Oncologia 2006, Rome; Humanitas Mirasole S.p.A., Rome; Fondazione Cassa di Risparmio di Puglia, Bari, Italy.

References

Anghelina M, Krishnan P, Moldovan L, Moldovan NI (2004) Monocytes and macrophages form branched cell columns in matrigel: implications for their role in neovascularization. Stem Cells Dev 13:665–676

Anghelina M, Krishnan P, Moldovan L, Moldovan NI (2006) Monocytes/macrophages cooperate with progenitor cells during neovascularization and tissue repair: conversion of cell columns into fibrovascular bundles. Am J Pathol 168:529–541

Balkwill F, Mantovani A (2001) Inflammation and cancer: back to Virchow. Lancet 357:539–545

Bellamy WT, Richter L, Frutiger Y, Grogan TM (1999) Expression of vascular endothelial growth factor and its receptors in hematological malignancies. Blood 59:728–733

Coluccia AML, Cirulli T, Neri P, Mangieri D, Colanardi MC, Gnoni A, Di Renzo N, Tassone P, Ribatti D, Dammacco F, Gambacorti-Passerini C, Vacca A (2008) Validation of PDGFRβ and c-Src tyrosine kinases as tumor/vessel targets in patients with multiple myeloma: preclinical efficacy of the novel, orally available inhibitor dasatinib (BMS-354825/Sprycel®). Blood 112: 1346–1356

Crivellato E, Nico B, Ribatti D (2008) Mast cells and tumour angiogenesis: new insight from experimental carcinogenesis. Cancer Lett 269:1–6

Di Raimondo F, Azzaro MP, Palombo G, Bagnato S, Giustolisi G, Floridia P, Sortino G, Giustolisi R (2000) Angiogenic factors in multiple myeloma: higher levels in bone marrow than in peripheral blood. Haematologica 85:800–805

Fernandez Pujol B, Lucibello FC, Gehling UM, Lindemann K, Weidner N, Zuzarte ML, Adamkiewicz J, Elsasser HP, Muller R, Havemann K (2000) Endothelial-like cells derived from human CD14 positive monocytes. Differentiation 65:287–300

Fujiyama S, Amano K, Uehira K, Yoshida M, Nishiwaki Y, Nozawa Y, Jin D, Takai S, Miyazaki M, Egashira K, Imada T, Iwasaka T, Matsubara H (2003) Bone marrow monocyte lineage cells adhere on injured endothelium in a monocyte chemoattractant protein-1-dependent manner and accelerate re-endothelization as endothelial progenitor cells. Circ Res 93:980–989

Hanahan D, Folkman J (1996) Patterns and emerging mechanisms of the angiogenic switch during tumorigenesis. Cell 86:353–364

Hideshima T, Mitsiades C, Tonon G, Richardson PG, Anderson KC (2007) Understanding multiple myeloma pathogenesis in the bone marrow to identify new therapeutic targets. Nat Rev Cancer 7:585–598

Klimp AH, Hollema H, Kempinga C, van der Zee AG, De Vries EG, Daemen T (2001) Expression of cyclooxygenase-2 and inducible nitric oxide synthase in human ovarian tumors and tumor-associated macrophages. Cancer Res 61:7305–7309

Kumar S, Witzig TE, Timm M, Huang J, Wellik L, Kimlinger TK, Griepp PR, Rajkumar SV (2004) Bone marrow angiogenic ability and expression of angiogenic cytokines in myeloma: evidence favouring loss of marrow angiogenesis inhibitory activity with disease progression. Blood 104:1159–1165

Lewis CE, Leek R, Harris A, Mc Gee JO (1995) Cytokine regulation of angiogenesis in breast cancer: the role of tumor-associated macrophages. J Leukoc Biol 57:747–751

Mangieri D, Nico B, Benagiano V, De Giorgis M, Vacca A, Ribatti D (2008) Angiogenic activity of multiple myeloma endothelial cells in vivo in the chick embryo chorioallantoic membrane assay is associated to a down-regulation in the expression of endogenous endostatin. J Cell Mol Med 12:1023–1028

Maniotis AJ, Folberg R, Hess A, Seftor EA, Gardner LM, Pe'er J, Trent JM, Meltzer PS, Hendrix MJ (1999) Vascular channel formation by human melanoma cells in vivo and in vitro: vasculogenic mimicry. Am J Pathol 155:739–752

Mantovani A, Bottazzi B, Colotta F, Sozzani S, Ruco L (1992) The origin and function of tumor-associated macrophages. Immunol Today 13:265–270

Moldovan NI, Goldschmidt-Clermont PJ, Parker-Thornburg J, Shapiro SD, Kolattukudy E (2000) Contribution of moncytes/macrophages to compensatory neovascularization: the drilling of metalloelastase-positive tunnels in ischemic myocardium. Circ Res 87:378–384

Nakayama T, Yao L, Tosato G (2004) Mast cell-derived angiopoietin-1 plays a role in the growth of plasma cell tumors. J Clin Invest 114:1317–1325

Nico B, Mangieri D, Crivellato E, Vacca A, Ribatti D (2008) Mast cells contribute to vasculogenic mimicry in multiple myeloma. Stem Cells Dev 17:19–22

Rehman J, Li J, Orschell CM, March KL (2003) Peripheral blood "endothelial progenitor cells" are derived from monocyte/macrophages and secrete angiogenic growth factors. Circulation 107:1164–1169

Ria R, Piccoli C, Cirulli T, Falzetti F, Mangialardi G, Guidolin D, Tabilio A, Di Renzo N, Guarini A, Ribatti D, Dammacco F, Vacca A (2008) Endothelial differentiation of hematopoietic stem and progenitor cells from patients with multiple myeloma. Clin Cancer Res 14:1678–1685

Ribatti D (2007) The discovery of endothelial progenitor cells. An historical review. Leuk Res 31:439–444

Ribatti D, Vacca A (2008) Angiogenesis and anti-angiogenesis in haematological diseases. MEMO 1:31–33

Ribatti D, Vacca A, Nico B, Quondamatteo F, Ria R, Minischetti M, Marzullo A, Herken R, Roncali L, Dammacco F (1999) Bone marrow angiogenesis and mast cell density increase simultaneously with progression of human multiple myeloma. Br J Cancer 79:451–455

Ribatti D, Vacca A, Dammacco F (2003) New non-angiogenesis dependent pathways for tumor growth. Eur J Cancer 39:1835–1841

Ribatti D, Crivellato E, Roccaro AM, Ria R, Vacca A (2004) Mast cell contribution to angiogenesis related to tumor progression. Clin Exp Allergy 34:1660–1664

Ribatti D, Nico B, Crivellato E, Vacca A (2005) Endothelial progenitor cells in health and disease. Histol Histopathol 20:1351–1358

Ribatti D, Nico B, Vacca A (2006) Importance of the bone marrow microenvironment in inducing the angiogenic response in multiple myeloma. Oncogene 25:4257–4266

Ribatti D, Nico B, Crivellato E, Roccaro AM, Vacca A (2007) The history of the angiogenic switch concept. Leukemia 21:44–52

Risau W (1997) Mechanisms of angiogenesis. Nature 386:671–674

Risau W, Lemmon D (1995) Vasculogenesis. Annu Rev Cell Dev Biol 11:73–91

Scavelli C, Nico B, Cirulli T, Ria R, Di Pietro G, Mangieri D, Bacigalupo A, Mangialardi G, Coluccia AML, Caravita T, Molica S, Ribatti D, Dammacco F, Vacca A (2008) Vasculogenic mimicry by bone marrow macrophages in patient with multiple myeloma. Oncogene 27:663–674

Schmeisser A, Garlichs CD, Zhang H, Eskafi S, Graffy C, Ludwig J, Strasser RH, Daniel WG (2001) Monocytes coexpress endothelial and macrophagocytic lineage markers and form cord-like structures in Matrigel® under angiogenic conditions. Cardiovasc Res 49:671–680

Sunderkotter C, Goebeler M, Schiltze-Osthoff K, Bhardway R, Sorg C (1991) Macrophages-derived angiogenesis factors. Pharmacol Ther 51:195–216

Theoharides TC, Conti P (2004) Mast cells: the Jeckyll and Hyde of tumor growth. Trends Immunol 25:235–241

Vacca A, Ribatti D (2006) Bone marrow angiogenesis in multiple myeloma. Leukemia 20: 193–199

Vacca A, Ribatti D, Roncali L, Ranieri G, Serio G, Silvestris F, Dammacco F (1994) Bone marrow angiogenesis and progression in multiple myeloma. Br J Haematol 87:503–508

Vacca A, Ribatti D, Presta M, Minischetti M, Iurlaro M, Ria R, Albini A, Bussolino F, Dammacco F (1999) Bone marrow neovascularization, plasma cell angiogenic potential and matrix metalloproteinase-2 secretion parallel progression of human multiple myeloma. Blood 93:3064–3073

Vacca A, Ria R, Semeraro F, Merchionne F, Coluccia M, Boccarelli A, Scavelli C, Nico B, Gernone A, Bottelli F, Tabilio A, Guidolin D, Petrucci MT, Ribatti D, Dammacco F (2003) Endothelial cells in the bone marrow of patients with multiple myeloma. Blood 102:3340–3348

Vacca A, Scavelli C, Montefusco V, Di Pietro G, Neri A, Mattioli M, Bicciato S, Nico B, Ribatti D, Dammacco F, Corradini P (2005) Thalidomide downregulates angiogenic genes in bone marrow endothelial cells of patients with active multiple myeloma. J Clin Oncol 23:5334–5346

Zhao Y, Glesne D, Huberman E (2003) A human peripheral blood monocyte-derived subset acts as pluripotent stem cells. Proc Natl Acad Sci USA 100:2426–2431

Immunology and Immunotherapeutic Approaches in Multiple Myeloma

5

Christoph Schlude and Philipp Beckhove

Contents

Abstract Immunotherapy for patients suffering from multiple myeloma is a lively and emerging field in cancer research. Immunotherapeutic approaches offer unique treatment opportunities for this, to date, mostly incurable disease. Respective basic findings and recent clinical approaches are introduced and discussed. Although several obstacles still need to be overcome, it appears that clinically efficient immunotherapies will become available for multiple myeloma patients in the future.

5.1 Introduction

While the understanding of the mechanisms underlying the development, maintenance, and expansion of malignant plasma cells has strongly increased during the past decade, multiple myeloma remains, with few exceptions, an incurable disease. One of the major challenges lies in a long-lasting control of minimal residual disease and the immune system might represent a powerful tool to achieve such control or to even eradicate disseminated tumor cells (Hsu et al. 1997; Stevenson et al. 2004).

The capacity of the immune system, particularly of T cells, to eradicate malignant hematological tumors became apparent in the late 1980s.

P. Beckhove (✉)
Translational Immunology,
German Cancer Research Center,
NCT Building, Im Neuenheimer Feld 460,
69120 Heidelberg, Germany
e-mail: p.beckhove@dkfz-heidelberg.de

T. Moehler and H. Goldschmidt (eds.), *Multiple Myeloma*,
Recent Results in Cancer Research 183, DOI: 10.1007/978-3-540-85772-3_5,

At this time, autologous stem cell transplantation was developed and clinically applied. Interestingly, relapse rates turned out to be significantly lower in those patients who received allogeneic transplants containing donor T lymphocytes compared to patients treated with autologous or T cell depleted allogeneic transplants. Improved survival was based on the capacity of cytolytic T cell clones to specifically recognize tumor cell-associated antigens expressed by the malignant clone – resulting in tumor cell eradication (graft versus leukemia effect) (Gale et al. 1989; Hughes et al. 1989). In an allogeneic setting, donor T cells regularly respond against a broad repertoire of non-self minor histocompatibility (minor H) antigens exclusively expressed by host cells. Since expression of minor H antigens is not restricted to malignant cells, a graft versus leukemia effect is often associated with donor T cell activity against normal host cells, resulting in variable, but often fatal, degree of graft versus host disease.

Since the late 1980s, it has therefore been a major goal of tumor immunotherapy to target T cell responses selectively against antigens that are differentially expressed by malignant cells. These attempts have led to the discovery of a large panel of antigens expressed by tumors, including multiple myeloma (MM), which can now be used for eliciting specific T cell responses.

5.2 Myeloma-Associated Antigens

A variety of tumor-associated antigens have been identified in multiple myeloma cell lines or freshly isolated MM cells. Among them are a number of cancer testis antigens. Antigens from this class are expressed only at immune privileged sites of the testes. In healthy individuals, they are not accessible for specific T cells but can be recognized and attacked when expressed on malignant tumors elsewhere in the body. Still, cancer testis antigens are presented in the thymus, where central tolerance is induced. Therefore, T cells recognize these antigens generally with only intermediate affinity. SPAN-XB (Frank et al. 2008), MAGE-A1, MAGE-A3, SSX or CT7 (Lendvai et al. 2010), or NY-ESO-1 (van Rhee et al. 2005) are expressed on myeloma cells and therefore may represent suitable target antigens for T cell-based immunotherapy. In addition to cancer testis antigens, further antigens are overexpressed on myeloma cells such as Wilms' tumor antigen (WT1) (Azuma et al. 2004), MUC1 (Choi et al. 2005), the Lewis-y (Le(y)) antigen (Peinert et al. 2010), Dickkopf 1 (DKK1) (Qian et al. 2007), the receptor for hyaluronic acid-mediated motility (RHAMM) (Schmitt et al. 2008) or HM1.24. The latter has been identified as a surface molecule preferentially expressed on terminally differentiated B cells, and its overexpression is observed in multiple myeloma and also other malignancies (Hundemer et al. 2006). Besides common tumor antigens, the idiotype protein secreted by the malignant plasma cell clone represents a unique, though individual, MM antigen. Experimental and some clinical data show that the anti-Id immune response is able to kill MM tumor cells in vitro and in vivo (Li et al. 2000; Wen et al. 2001).

Due to the virtually unavoidable risk of graft versus host disease during allogeneic T cell transplantation, many researchers have focused on the induction of tumor-specific T cells in an autologous setting, for example, by vaccination. However, induced autologous T cell responses against tumor-associated self-antigens, due to central tolerance mechanisms in the thymus, are only of limited TCR affinity. This raised the concern that related therapeutic approaches may be less likely to efficiently control tumor progression. Therefore, researchers addressed the question of spontaneous immunogenicity of multiple myeloma and the prognostic impact of spontaneous immune responses. Meanwhile, multiple studies described spontaneous T cell and B cell responses against virtually all described multiple myeloma antigens, involving idiotype protein (Yi et al. 1995), MUC1 (Choi et al. 2005), NY-ESO-1 (van Rhee et al. 2005) or MAGE-A3, CT7 and SSX (Lendvai et al. 2010). Moreover, it was clearly shown that spontaneous T cell responses against myeloma antigens correlated with prolonged survival (Raitakari et al. 2003; Brown et al. 1997).

These findings provide a rationale for boosting preexisting and for inducing de novo myeloma-specific T cell responses in an autologous setting and are currently pursued in the context of various clinical vaccination trials.

5.3 Vaccination

Various clinical studies in MM have shown the capacity of vaccination to elicit myeloma-specific immune responses. These studies exploited a variety of different strategies. These are based on the application of whole tumor cells or tumor cell lysates, tumor peptides, peptide-loaded tumor cell-derived heat shock proteins, or antigen-encoding DNA and are often complemented by adjuvants and cytokines or presented through professional antigen presenting cells.

A critical issue of tumor vaccination is the choice of the antigen. Most immunotherapies are directed against MM target antigens expressed by mature myeloma cells. However, the small population of self-renewing, largely treatment-resistant "tumor initiating cells" (Matsui et al. 2004) may resemble a much more relevant target and the repertoire of antigens expressed by this population needs to be characterized for selective immunotherapeutic targeting in future trials.

A major drawback of tumor vaccines lies in the clonal selection of antigen loss variants, resulting in immune escape and tumor progression despite persistent immune response. To date, it appears therefore questionable if vaccination with a single antigen can effectively eradicate or control MM. The combination of multiple defined antigens, the use of tumor lysate or tumor cell-derived heat shock proteins provides the theoretical advantage of avoiding the selection of immune escape variants.

Ideal target antigens should play an essential role for maintenance of the malignant phenotype of the cell, exclusively but broadly expressed by tumor cells and not be subject to induction of central T cell tolerance in the thymus. Up to date, such antigen has not been identified in MM. However, with regard to tumor selectivity, the antibody idiotype expressed by the malignant clone represents a unique antigen not expressed in any other cell type, including the thymus. A major caveat, however, lies in the fact that idiotype-specific vaccination requires a patient-tailored treatment which is extremely costly, laborious, and has to overcome major regulatory hurdles. Nevertheless, many clinical approaches focused on this antigen, and recently a clinical benefit of such an approach was demonstrated by a phase III trial in patients with advanced B cell lymphoma (Schuster et al. 2009).

Intradermal vaccination with purified autologous M protein in conjunction with GM-CSF and IL-12 elicited Id-specific immune responses that were associated with prolonged time to progression in several patients (Hansson et al. 2007). More sophisticated approaches of anti-idiotype vaccination are based on purified Id protein or light and heavy chain variable regions linked to adjuvant molecules, such as keyhole limpet hemocyanin or immunostimulatory cytokines such as IL-2, IL-12, or GM-CSF (King et al. 1998; Osterborg et al. 1998), (Rasmussen et al. 2003; Stritzke et al. 2003). Moreover, a DNA vaccine has been constructed that encodes the gene for a single chain of the rearranged idiotype protein and can be fused with adjuvants such as the sequence of the tetanus toxoid as an enhancer of concomitant T cell help. This approach revealed high immunogenicity and is under evaluation in clinical trials (Stevenson et al. 2004).

5

In contrast to idiotype protein defined antigens commonly overexpressed on a majority of myeloma cells are generally applicable to all patients. Some antigens, involving HM1.24, MAGE-A3, SPAN-XB, DKK1, WT1-specific CTL and NY-ESO-1 are in early phases of clinical development (Chiriva-Internati et al. 2003; Rew et al. 2009), while a recent Phase 1 clinical trial of RHAMM-R3 peptide vaccination already showed a reduction of free light chains in the serum of two out of four MM patients (Schmitt et al. 2008).

In order to avoid the problem of antigen escape variants, several approaches focus on the application of multiple myeloma antigens. One such strategy is based on vaccination with purified heat shock proteins. Heat shock proteins are chaperones that are capable of binding peptide fragments of multiple proteins within the tumor cell, involving tumor-associated antigens. It was shown recently, that pooled heat shock proteins isolated from various myeloma cell lines induce immune responses against a broad spectrum of myeloma-associated antigens and may provide a therapeutic option for immunotherapy of multiple myeloma (Qian et al. 2009).

A personalized strategy of multiepitope vaccination has been developed by Cell Genesys with the Gvax® myeloma vaccine. The i.d. vaccine consists of irradiated, autologous myeloma cells that are administered with K562 bystander cells, genetically engineered to produce GM-CSF as an adjuvant to recruit professional antigen presenting cells to the vaccination site. Seventeen patients were vaccinated in the frame of a phase I/II trial following chemotherapy and autologous stem cell transplantation with promising clinical results (Borrello et al. 2004).

Direct vaccination with naked proteins, peptides, or DNA requires a complex course of events. This includes the recruitment and local activation of professional antigen-presenting cells, namely, dendritic cells (DC) followed by antigen uptake and -processing, the migration of antigen-presenting cells into draining lymph nodes, and finally the upregulation of costimulatory molecules and presentation of antigen fragments to naïve and memory T cells. DC in patients with myeloma often lack the capacity to express the costimulatory molecules CD80 and CD86, which are indispensable for the induction of protective T cell responses. Therefore, vaccination in myeloma patients might favor from approaches to generate antigen-pulsed activated DC from autologous precursor cells ex vivo under appropriate conditions for i.d. application (Reichardt et al. 1999).

Several studies have investigated the use of idiotype protein or peptide-pulsed DC after high-dose therapy and autologous peripheral blood stem cell transplantation (Reichardt et al. 1999; Lim and Bailey-Wood 1999; Liso et al. 2000; Yi et al. 2003) as well as after conventional therapy (Reichardt et al. 1999; Tarte et al. 1997; Dabadghao et al. 1998; Titzer et al. 2000; Ridgway 2003; Zeis et al. 1998). DC-based idiotype vaccination of myeloma patients is feasible and safe and can induce specific immune responses. A specific question of interest is the requirement of adjuvants for the recruitment and activation of bystander immune cells and for the stimulation of strong helper T cell responses. In many approaches, DC were not only pulsed with the idiotype antigen but also with KLH, which strongly stimulates T helper cells and thereby promoted strong anti-idiotype cytotoxic T cell responses (Reichardt et al. 1999; Liso et al. 2000) and also promising clinical results (Curti et al. 2007). This strategy was further developed by the addition of GM-CSF (Reichardt et al. 2003; Rice and Hart 2002) or IL-2 (Yi et al. 2003).

In conclusion, these early clinical trials clearly demonstrate that myeloma-specific T cell responses can be elicited through vaccination and also point to the possibility that such strategy may improve the prognosis of MM patients. However, clinical effects were observed only in proportions of patients and it remains questionable whether these will be long lasting. Thus, clinical efficacy still appears low and needs to be demonstrated by randomized prospective trials. A major challenge in the future will be to understand why vaccines remain inefficient in some patients and to develop methods to overcome these limitations. A strategy to circumvent this problem is the development of biomarkers for selection of only those patients that will benefit from a vaccine.

5.4 Immune Evasion

Immunotherapy of multiple myeloma is particularly challenging, since MM is associated with a variety of immune defects. These may influence the efficiency of immunotherapies and need to be addressed by future immunotherapeutic strategies (Cook and Campbell 1999). It is known for a long time that myeloma patients are prone to infections due to a general state of immune suppression (Zinneman and Hall 1954; Glenchur et al. 1959; Perri et al. 1981).

MM tumor cells secrete a variety of immune modulatory factors such as IL-6, IL-10, VEGF, and TGFβ (Brown et al. 2004; Cook et al. 1999; Campbell et al. 2001; Oyama et al. 1998). Through these factors, the malignant clone generates a microenvironment in the bone marrow that on the one hand supports growth, differentiation, and survival of the tumor cells and on the other hand impairs the host immune response and tumor rejection. One target cell population of myeloma-associated immune suppression are dendritic cells. MM patient–derived DCs exert phenotypic and functional defects that are characterized by a reduced expression of molecules required for antigen presentation and T-cell stimulation, such as CD40, CD80, and HLA-DR and by a reduced capacity to activate virus or myeloma-specific T cells. Interestingly, blockade of myeloma-derived IL-6 could partially restore DC function (Wang et al. 2006). However, even in the case that functional myeloma-reactive T cells have been generated spontaneously or in the course of immunotherapy, antitumor efficacy of such T cells appears to be reduced. Verdonck et al. demonstrated that MM appears to be more resistant even to allogeneic (donor lymphocyte infusion) when compared with other malignant diseases, such as CML (Verdonck et al. 1998) and Coscia et al. reported that the induction of peripheral anti-idiotype T cell responses in the skin through s.c. idiotype vaccination showed no effect on the residual tumor burden in MM patients (Coscia et al. 2004). This may be due to the fact that myeloma resides within a specialized and modified bone marrow microenvironment that strongly differs from peripheral sites. Indeed, in the presence of myeloma, plasmacytoid dendritic cells (pDCs) in the bone marrow (BM) microenvironment mediate immune deficiency and promote MM cell growth and drug resistance. Therefore, therapeutic modification of pDC function might be required for efficient myeloma immunotherapy. It was shown recently, that toll-like receptor activation on pDCs restored pDC immune function and abrogated pDC-induced MM cell growth (Chauhan et al. 2009).

Besides their inhibition of DC function, myeloma cells also directly inhibit T cell responses. Myeloma-derived TGFβ reduces T cell proliferation and activation through the inhibition of autocrine IL-2 pathways (Campbell et al. 2001). Such a mechanism may be responsible for alterations in the Vβ T cell repertoire after autologous bone marrow transplantation that have been reported in myeloma patients which were associated with reduced survival (Brown et al. 1997; Mariani et al. 2001). Therapeutic approaches to overcome these alterations involve the ex vivo activation of patient-derived T cells with anti-CD3 alone or together with anti-CD28 mAb-coated beads, eventually complemented by IL-15. Such treatment was able to restore the IL-2 autocrine pathways and T cell proliferation (Campbell et al. 2001) and to correct the skewing of the Vβ TCR repertoire (Brown et al. 1997). MM Ag-specific T cells circulating in the blood of MM patients could be isolated, expanded, and activated ex vivo for subsequent reinfusion.

5

5.5 Regulatory T Cells

CD4$^+$ regulatory T cells (Treg) play a critical role in the maintenance of peripheral self-tolerance but also in the suppression of tumor-reactive helper and cytotoxic T cells thereby representing a major tumor evasion strategy and an obstacle to successful tumor immunotherapy (Liyanage et al. 2002; Shevach 2002; Zou 2005). Treg cells can be distinguished from other T cell subsets by their constitutive expression of the interleukin (IL)-2 receptor alpha chain (CD25) and also by the expression of the transcription factor forkhead box P3 (FOXP3), a master regulator of Treg cell development. Treg secrete inhibitory cytokines such as IL-10 and TGFβ (Liyanage et al. 2002) and exert T cell suppressive activity (Curiel et al. 2004). Treg cells suppress both the induction of the immune response in the draining lymph nodes as well as T cell activity inside the target organ (Suri-Payer and Fritzsching 2006). Treg have been found to be expanded in the blood and tumors of many patients with different tumors and increased densities of tumor-infiltrating FoxP3$^+$ Tregs have been associated with poor prognosis in various solid tumors (Curiel et al. 2004; Hiraoka et al. 2006; Sato et al. 2005; Gao et al. 2007; Kobayashi et al. 2007). The depletion of Treg cells induced effective immunity in mice and spontaneous tumor rejection (Yu et al. 2005). In the past, there was a controversy as to whether Treg are increased or decreased in multiple myeloma and if they possess functional capacity or are rather dysfunctional (Prabhala et al. 2006; Joshua et al. 2008) but more recent studies favor the notion that Treg in myeloma patients are increased and functional and may contribute to myeloma immune escape. A potential role of Treg in the immune suppression in MM was initially suggested in 2004 (Prabhala et al. 2004), and more recently increased Treg frequencies in myeloma patients were interpreted as a response to the process of malignant transformation (Beyer et al. 2006; Laronne-Bar-On et al. 2008; Feyler et al. 2009). While an experimental evidence of functional relevance for myeloma-specific T-cell immunity is still missing, the current observations suggest that therapeutic targeting of Treg in multiple myeloma may provide an option to improve the immunological and clinical outcome of immunotherapeutic approaches.

5.6 Humoral Immunotherapy

B cell malignancies were the first to be efficiently treated by tumor-directed monoclonal antibodies, such as rituximab (anti-CD20). Since then, antibody-based therapy is clinically explored in many tumor diseases and multiple new therapeutic antibodies with a broad variety of specificities are being developed. Clinical efficiency of most therapeutic antibodies is based on their capacity to recruit and activate cytotoxic effector mechanisms of the innate immune system. This occurs either by engagement of activating Fc receptors expressed on NK cells or macrophages on the tumor cell surface leading to antibody-dependent cellular cytotoxicity (ADCC) or by activating the complement cascade through tumor cell–bound antibodies (CDCC).

One major issue of antibody therapy of MM is the selection of a suitable surface antigen. So far, various candidate molecules that were found to be overexpressed on malignant plasma cells have been suggested. These involve common plasma cell markers such as CD38, CD138 or CD74, VEGF, the unclustered surface type II transmembrane glycoprotein, HM1.24 (Yang et al. 2003), PSGL1, which is the major ligand of P-Selectin and a marker of plasmacytic differentiation expressed at high levels on normal and neoplastic plasma cells (Tripodo et al. 2009),

FGF receptor 3 (FGFR3), which plays a role in the development of t(4;14)-positive multiple myeloma (Qing et al. 2009), CD1d (Spanoudakis et al. 2009), IGF-1R (Descamps et al. 2009), CS1 (Tai et al. 2008) or OFA/iLR (Friedrichs et al. 2008). Spontaneous antibody responses against the latter antigen were capable of killing myeloma cells in ADCC assays and correlated with lower probability of disease progression (Siegel et al. 2008). Therapeutic, monoclonal antibodies against these myeloma-associated antigens have been generated and some of them, including antibodies directed against FGFR3 (Qing et al. 2009), CD74 (milatuzumab) (Stein et al. 2009), IGF-1R mAb (AVE1642) (Descamps et al. 2009), or CS1 (HuLuc63) (Hsi et al. 2008) exerted strong ADCC-mediated reactivity against human multiple myeloma in xenograft mouse models. Some therapeutic antibodies have been evaluated already in clinical trials. A CD20-directed phase II study with rituximab in combination with melphalan and prednisone failed to result in improved response rates or event-free survival (Baz et al. 2007). This might be due to the fact that less than 20% of fresh myeloma cells express CD20 (Treon et al. 2001; Musto et al. 2003; Lim et al. 2004). However, a phase I study targeting IGF-1R, which is highly expressed on myeloma cells, with the IGF-1R monoclonal antibody CP-751,871 showed clinical response in 9 out of 27 myeloma patients treated (Lacy et al. 2008). In the next future, a broad variety of therapeutic antibodies for immunotherapy of multiple myeloma will be developed and evaluated in early clinical trials.

5.7 Adoptive Cellular Therapy

The capacity of the immune system, particularly of T cells, to eradicate hematological tumors was discovered after the introduction of autologous stem cell transplantation in the late 1980s. At that time, it became apparent that allogeneic BMT resulted in lower relapse rates than autologous stem cell transplantation or T-cell-depleted allogeneic BMT. Similarly, allogeneic stem cell transplantation resulted in a higher rate of molecular remission in MM (Bensinger et al. 1996; Corradini et al. 1999). In 2007, Levenga et al. treated 24 MM patients with partial T cell-depleted myeloablative SCT and preemptive donor lymphocyte infusion. Seven of these patients (29%) achieved continuous CR (Levenga et al. 2007). Other investigators treated MM patients by DLI after high-dose therapy with autologous stem cell transplant (Ballester et al. 2004) with promising clinical results or by a combination of post-transplant immunotherapy with escalating DLI and novel agents (thalidomide, bortezomib, and lenalidomide) to target complete remission and reported improved 5-year progressive-free and overall survival (Kroger et al. 2009).

Due to the high rate of treatment-related morbidity/mortality after allogeneic BMT, new treatment approaches seek to combine donor lymphocyte infusion (DLI) with less toxic non-myeloablative conditioning regimen (Singhal et al. 2000; Garban et al. 2001; Perez-Simon et al. 2003; Crawley et al. 2005). Several studies aimed at inducing MM-specific T cell responses before DLI in the donors through idiotype vaccination and repeated i.d. vaccinations of the recipients after the transfer. These vaccinations induced donor i.d.-specific cellular and/or humoral immune responses (Neelapu et al. 2005).

Besides cytotoxic T cells, preclinical studies suggest that natural killer lymphocytes (NK cells) may possess therapeutic capacity against multiple myeloma. It was shown that myeloma cells are susceptible to NK cell lysis (Frohn et al. 2002) and that NK cells are involved in the control of malignant plasma cells in MM patients. NK cells belong to the innate immune system and possess an inherent cytotoxic capacity. They recognize ligands overexpressed on the surface of many tumor cells, including MM. Some drugs, such as thalidomide can further augment this cytotoxic effect (Gonzalez et al. 1992; Frohn et al. 2002; Zheng et al. 2002; EL-Sherbiny et al. 2003).

Recently, Shi et al. clinically challenged this approach by transfusing haplo-identical, T cell-depleted NK cells after conditioning therapy with melphalan and fludarabine to patients with advanced multiple myeloma (MM) who received afterward autologous stem-cell transplantation. Clinical remissions were observed in 50% of the patients (Shi et al. 2008).

5.8 Conclusion

Immunotherapy of multiple myeloma is a lively and growing field. Major progress of the past years in understanding interactions between the immune system and malignant cells will strongly augment the design of clinically more efficient study protocols in multiple myeloma. Multiple different approaches are currently evaluated in clinical trials and it appears a question of when rather than if tumor immunotherapy in multiple myeloma will proof clinical efficiency.

References

Azuma T, Otsuki T, Kuzushima K, Froelich CJ, Fujita S, Yasukawa M (2004) Myeloma cells are highly sensitive to the granule exocytosis pathway mediated by WT1-specific cytotoxic T lymphocytes. Clin Cancer Res 10(21):7402–7412

Ballester OF, Fang T, Raptis A, Ballester G, Wilcox P, Hiemenz J, Tan B (2004) Adoptive immunotherapy with donor lymphocyte infusions and interleukin-2 after high-dose therapy and autologous stem cell rescue for multiple myeloma. Bone Marrow Transplant 34(5):419–423

Baz R, Fanning S, Kunkel L, Gaballa S, Karam MA, Reed J, Kelly M, Hussein M (2007) Combination of rituximab and oral melphalan and prednisone in newly diagnosed multiple myeloma. Leuk Lymphoma 48(12):2338–2344

Bensinger WI, Buckner CD, Anasetti C, Clift R, Storb R, Barnett T, Chauncey T, Shulman H, Appelbaum FR (1996) Allogeneic marrow transplantation for multiple myeloma: an analysis of risk factors on outcome. Blood 88(7):2787–2793

Beyer M, Kochanek M, Giese T, Endl E, Weihrauch MR, Knolle PA, Classen S, Schultze JL (2006) In vivoperipheralexpansionofnaiveCD4+CD25high FoxP3+ regulatory T cells in patients with multiple myeloma. Blood 107(10):3940–3949

Borrello I, Biedrzycki B, Sheets N, George B, Racke F, Loper K, Noonan K, Donnelly A, Hege K, Levitski HI (2004) Autologous tumor combined with a GM-CSF-secreting cell line vaccine (GVAX®) following autologous stem cell transplant (ASCT) in multiple myeloma. Blood 104:Abstract no. 440

Brown RD, Yuen E, Nelson M, Gibson J, Joshua D (1997) The prognostic significance of T cell receptor beta gene rearrangements and idiotype-reactive T cells in multiple myeloma. Leukemia 11(8):1312–1317

Brown R, Murray A, Pope B, Sze DM, Gibson J, Ho PJ, Hart D, Joshua D (2004) Either interleukin-12 or interferon-gamma can correct the dendritic cell defect induced by transforming growth factor beta in patients with myeloma. Br J Haematol 125(6):743–748

Campbell JD, Cook G, Robertson SE, Fraser A, Boyd KS, Gracie JA, Franklin IM (2001) Suppression of IL-2-induced T cell proliferation and phosphorylation of STAT3 and STAT5 by tumor-derived TGF beta is reversed by IL-15. J Immunol 167(1):553–561

Chauhan D, Singh AV, Brahmandam M, Carrasco R, Bandi M, Hideshima T, Bianchi G, Podar K, Tai YT, Mitsiades C, Raje N, Jaye DL, Kumar SK, Richardson P, Munshi N, Anderson KC (2009) Functional interaction of plasmacytoid dendritic cells with multiple myeloma cells: a therapeutic target. Cancer Cell 16(4):309–323

Chiriva-Internati M, Liu Y, Weidanz JA, Grizzi F, You H, Zhou W, Bumm K, Barlogie B, Mehta JL, Hermonat PL (2003) Testing recombinant adeno-associated virus-gene loading of dendritic cells for generating potent cytotoxic T lymphocytes against a prototype self-antigen, multiple myeloma HM1.24. Blood 102(9):3100–3107

Choi C, Witzens M, Bucur M, Feuerer M, Sommerfeldt N, Trojan A, Ho A, Schirrmacher V, Goldschmidt H, Beckhove P (2005) Enrichment of functional CD8 memory T cells specific for MUC1 in bone marrow of patients with multiple myeloma. Blood 105(5):2132–2134

Cook G, Campbell JD (1999) Immune regulation in multiple myeloma: the host-tumour conflict. Blood Rev 13(3):151–162

Cook G, Campbell JD, Carr CE, Boyd KS, Franklin IM (1999) Transforming growth factor beta from multiple myeloma cells inhibits proliferation and IL-2 responsiveness in T lymphocytes. J Leukoc Biol 66(6):981–988

Corradini P, Voena C, Tarella C, Astolfi M, Ladetto M, Palumbo A, Van Lint MT, Bacigalupo A, Santoro A, Musso M, Majolino I, Boccadoro M, Pileri A (1999) Molecular and clinical remissions in multiple myeloma: role of autologous and allogeneic transplantation of hematopoietic cells. J Clin Oncol 17(1):208–215

Coscia M, Mariani S, Battaglio S, Di Bello C, Fiore F, Foglietta M, Pileri A, Boccadoro M, Massaia M (2004) Long-term follow-up of idiotype vaccination in human myeloma as a maintenance therapy after high-dose chemotherapy. Leukemia 18(1):139–145

Crawley C, Lalancette M, Szydlo R, Gilleece M, Peggs K, Mackinnon S, Juliusson G, Ahlberg L, Nagler A, Shimoni A, Sureda A, Boiron JM, Einsele H, Chopra R, Carella A, Cavenagh J, Gratwohl A, Garban F, Zander A, Bjorkstrand B, Niederwieser D, Gahrton G, Apperley JF (2005) Outcomes for reduced-intensity allogeneic transplantation for multiple myeloma: an analysis of prognostic factors from the Chronic Leukaemia Working Party of the EBMT. Blood 105(11): 4532–4539

Curiel TJ, Coukos G, Zou L, Alvarez X, Cheng P, Mottram P, Evdemon-Hogan M, Conejo-Garcia JR, Zhang L, Burow M, Zhu Y, Wei S, Kryczek I, Daniel B, Gordon A, Myers L, Lackner A, Disis ML, Knutson KL, Chen L, Zou W (2004) Specific recruitment of regulatory T cells in ovarian carcinoma fosters immune privilege and predicts reduced survival. Nat Med 10(9):942–949

Curti A, Tosi P, Comoli P, Terragna C, Ferri E, Cellini C, Massaia M, D'Addio A, Giudice V, Di Bello C, Cavo M, Conte R, Gugliotta G, Baccarani M, Lemoli RM (2007) Phase I/II clinical trial of sequential subcutaneous and intravenous delivery of dendritic cell vaccination for refractory multiple myeloma using patient-specific tumour idiotype protein or idiotype (VDJ)-derived class I-restricted peptides. Br J Haematol 139(3):415–424

Dabadghao S, Bergenbrant S, Anton D, He W, Holm G, Yi Q (1998) Anti-idiotypic T-cell activation in multiple myeloma induced by M-component fragments presented by dendritic cells. Br J Haematol 100(4):647–654

Descamps G, Gomez-Bougie P, Venot C, Moreau P, Bataille R, Amiot M (2009) A humanised anti-IGF-1R monoclonal antibody (AVE1642) enhances Bortezomib-induced apoptosis in myeloma cells lacking CD45. Br J Cancer 100(2):366–369

EL-Sherbiny YM, Davies FE, Cook G, Johnson RJ, Cullen MJ, Sah A, Rawstron AC, Richards SJ, Morgan GJ (2003) NK cell repertoire in myeloma and the impact of thalidomide. Blood 102:Abstract no. 1617

Feyler S, von Lilienfeld-Toal M, Jarmin S, Marles L, Rawstron A, Ashcroft AJ, Owen RG, Selby PJ, Cook G (2009) CD4(+)CD25(+)FoxP3(+) regulatory T cells are increased whilst CD3(+)CD4(-) CD8(-)alphabetaTCR(+) Double Negative T cells are decreased in the peripheral blood of patients with multiple myeloma which correlates with disease burden. Br J Haematol 144(5):686–695

Frank C, Hundemer M, Ho AD, Goldschmidt H, Witzens-Harig M (2008) Cellular immune responses against the cancer-testis antigen SPAN-XB in healthy donors and patients with multiple myeloma. Leuk Lymphoma 49(4): 779–785

Friedrichs B, Siegel S, Kloess M, Barsoum A, Coggin J Jr, Rohrer J, Jakob I, Tiemann M, Heidorn K, Schulte C, Kabelitz D, Steinmann J, Schmitz N, Zeis M (2008) Humoral immune responses against the immature laminin receptor protein show prognostic significance in patients with chronic lymphocytic leukemia. J Immunol 180(9):6374–6384

Frohn C, Hoppner M, Schlenke P, Kirchner H, Koritke P, Luhm J (2002) Anti-myeloma activity of natural killer lymphocytes. Br J Haematol 119(3):660–664

Gale RP, Horowitz MM, Bortin MM (1989) IBMTR analysis of bone marrow transplants in acute leukaemia. Advisory Committee of the International Bone Marrow Transplant Registry (IBMTR). Bone Marrow Transplant 4(Suppl 3):83–84

Gao Q, Qiu SJ, Fan J, Zhou J, Wang XY, Xiao YS, Xu Y, Li YW, Tang ZY (2007) Intratumoral balance of regulatory and cytotoxic T cells is associated with prognosis of hepatocellular carcinoma after resection. J Clin Oncol 25(18):2586–2593

Garban F, Attal M, Rossi JF, Payen C, Fegueux N, Sotto JJ (2001) Immunotherapy by non-myeloablative allogeneic stem cell transplantation in multiple myeloma: results of a pilot study as salvage therapy after autologous transplantation. Leukemia 15(4):642–646

Glenchur H, Zinneman HH, Hall WH (1959) A review of fifty-one cases of multiple myeloma; emphasis on pneumonia and other infections as complications. AMA Arch Intern Med 103(2): 173–183

Gonzalez M, San Miguel JF, Gascon A, Moro MJ, Hernandez JM, Ortega F, Jimenez R, Guerras L, Romero M, Casanova F et al (1992) Increased expression of natural-killer-associated and activation antigens in multiple myeloma. Am J Hematol 39(2):84–89

Hansson L, Abdalla AO, Moshfegh A, Choudhury A, Rabbani H, Nilsson B, Osterborg A, Mellstedt H (2007) Long-term idiotype vaccination combined with interleukin-12 (IL-12), or IL-12 and granulocyte macrophage colony-stimulating factor, in early-stage multiple myeloma patients. Clin Cancer Res 13(5):1503–1510

Hiraoka N, Onozato K, Kosuge T, Hirohashi S (2006) Prevalence of FOXP3+ regulatory T cells increases during the progression of pancreatic ductal adenocarcinoma and its premalignant lesions. Clin Cancer Res 12(18):5423–5434

Hsi ED, Steinle R, Balasa B, Szmania S, Draksharapu A, Shum BP, Huseni M, Powers D, Nanisetti A, Zhang Y, Rice AG, van Abbema A, Wong M, Liu G, Zhan F, Dillon M, Chen S, Rhodes S, Fuh F, Tsurushita N, Kumar S, Vexler V, Shaughnessy JD Jr, Barlogie B, van Rhee F, Hussein M, Afar DE, Williams MB (2008) CS1, a potential new therapeutic antibody target for the treatment of multiple myeloma. Clin Cancer Res 14(9):2775–2784

Hsu FJ, Caspar CB, Czerwinski D, Kwak LW, Liles TM, Syrengelas A, Taidi-Laskowski B, Levy R (1997) Tumor-specific idiotype vaccines in the treatment of patients with B-cell lymphoma–long-term results of a clinical trial. Blood 89(9): 3129–3135

Hughes TP, Economou K, Mackinnon S, Vlitos M, Arthur CK, Guo AP, Rassool F, Apperley JF, Hows J, Goldman JM (1989) Slow evolution of chronic myeloid leukaemia relapsing after BMT with T-cell depleted donor marrow. Br J Haematol 73(4):462–467

Hundemer M, Schmidt S, Condomines M, Lupu A, Hose D, Moos M, Cremer F, Kleist C, Terness P, Belle S, Ho AD, Goldschmidt H, Klein B, Christensen O (2006) Identification of a new HLA-A2-restricted T-cell epitope within HM1.24 as immunotherapy target for multiple myeloma. Exp Hematol 34(4):486–496

Joshua DE, Brown RD, Ho PJ, Gibson J (2008) Regulatory T cells and multiple myeloma. Clin Lymphoma Myeloma 8(5):283–286

King CA, Spellerberg MB, Zhu D, Rice J, Sahota SS, Thompsett AR, Hamblin TJ, Radl J, Stevenson FK (1998) DNA vaccines with single-chain Fv fused to fragment C of tetanus toxin induce protective immunity against lymphoma and myeloma. Nat Med 4(11):1281–1286

Kobayashi N, Hiraoka N, Yamagami W, Ojima H, Kanai Y, Kosuge T, Nakajima A, Hirohashi S (2007) FOXP3+ regulatory T cells affect the development and progression of hepatocarcinogenesis. Clin Cancer Res 13(3):902–911

Kroger N, Badbaran A, Lioznov M, Schwarz S, Zeschke S, Hildebrand Y, Ayuk F, Atanackovic D, Schilling G, Zabelina T, Bacher U, Klyuchnikov E, Shimoni A, Nagler A, Corradini P, Fehse B, Zander A (2009) Post-transplant immunotherapy with donor-lymphocyte infusion and novel agents to upgrade partial into complete and molecular remission in allografted patients with multiple myeloma. Exp Hematol 37(7):791–798

Lacy MQ, Alsina M, Fonseca R, Paccagnella ML, Melvin CL, Yin D, Sharma A, Enriquez Sarano M, Pollak M, Jagannath S, Richardson P, Gualberto A (2008) Phase I, pharmacokinetic and pharmacodynamic study of the anti-insulinlike growth factor type 1 Receptor monoclonal antibody CP-751, 871 in patients with multiple myeloma. J Clin Oncol 26(19):3196–3203

Laronne-Bar-On A, Zipori D, Haran-Ghera N (2008) Increased regulatory versus effector T cell development is associated with thymus atrophy in mouse models of multiple myeloma. J Immunol 181(5):3714–3724

Lendvai N, Gnjatic S, Ritter E, Mangone M, Austin W, Reyner K, Jayabalan D, Niesvizky R, Jagannath S, Bhardwaj N, Chen-Kiang S, Old LJ,

Cho HJ (2010) Cellular immune responses against CT7 (MAGE-C1) and humoral responses against other cancer-testis antigens in multiple myeloma patients. Cancer Immun 10:4
Levenga H, Levison-Keating S, Schattenberg AV, Dolstra H, Schaap N, Raymakers RA (2007) Multiple myeloma patients receiving pre-emptive donor lymphocyte infusion after partial T-cell-depleted allogeneic stem cell transplantation show a long progression-free survival. Bone Marrow Transplant 40(4):355–359
Li Y, Bendandi M, Deng Y, Dunbar C, Munshi N, Jagannath S, Kwak LW, Lyerly HK (2000) Tumor-specific recognition of human myeloma cells by idiotype-induced CD8(+) T cells. Blood 96(8):2828–2833
Lim SH, Bailey-Wood R (1999) Idiotypic protein-pulsed dendritic cell vaccination in multiple myeloma. Int J Cancer 83(2):215–222
Lim SH, Zhang Y, Wang Z, Varadarajan R, Periman P, Esler WV (2004) Rituximab administration following autologous stem cell transplantation for multiple myeloma is associated with severe IgM deficiency. Blood 103(5):1971–1972
Liso A, Stockerl-Goldstein KE, Auffermann-Gretzinger S, Benike CJ, Reichardt V, van Beckhoven A, Rajapaksa R, Engleman EG, Blume KG, Levy R (2000) Idiotype vaccination using dendritic cells after autologous peripheral blood progenitor cell transplantation for multiple myeloma. Biol Blood Marrow Transplant 6(6):621–627
Liyanage UK, Moore TT, Joo HG, Tanaka Y, Herrmann V, Doherty G, Drebin JA, Strasberg SM, Eberlein TJ, Goedegebuure PS, Linehan DC (2002) Prevalence of regulatory T cells is increased in peripheral blood and tumor microenvironment of patients with pancreas or breast adenocarcinoma. J Immunol 169(5):2756–2761
Mariani S, Coscia M, Even J, Peola S, Foglietta M, Boccadoro M, Sbaiz L, Restagno G, Pileri A, Massaia M (2001) Severe and long-lasting disruption of T-cell receptor diversity in human myeloma after high-dose chemotherapy and autologous peripheral blood progenitor cell infusion. Br J Haematol 113(4):1051–1059
Matsui W, Huff CA, Wang Q, Malehorn MT, Barber J, Tanhehco Y, Smith BD, Civin CI, Jones RJ (2004) Characterization of clonogenic multiple myeloma cells. Blood 103(6):2332–2336
Musto P, Carella AM Jr, Greco MM, Falcone A, Sanpaolo G, Bodenizza C, Cascavilla N, Melillo L, Carella AM (2003) Short progression-free survival in myeloma patients receiving rituximab as maintenance therapy after autologous transplantation. Br J Haematol 123(4):746–747
Neelapu SS, Munshi NC, Jagannath S, Watson TM, Pennington R, Reynolds C, Barlogie B, Kwak LW (2005) Tumor antigen immunization of sibling stem cell transplant donors in multiple myeloma. Bone Marrow Transplant 36(4):315–323
Osterborg A, Yi Q, Henriksson L, Fagerberg J, Bergenbrant S, Jeddi-Tehrani M, Ruden U, Lefvert AK, Holm G, Mellstedt H (1998) Idiotype immunization combined with granulocyte-macrophage colony-stimulating factor in myeloma patients induced type I, major histocompatibility complex-restricted, CD8- and CD4-specific T-cell responses. Blood 91(7):2459–2466
Oyama T, Ran S, Ishida T, Nadaf S, Kerr L, Carbone DP, Gabrilovich DI (1998) Vascular endothelial growth factor affects dendritic cell maturation through the inhibition of nuclear factor-kappa B activation in hemopoietic progenitor cells. J Immunol 160(3):1224–1232
Peinert S, Prince HM, Guru PM, Kershaw MH, Smyth MJ, Trapani JA, Gambell P, Harrison S, Scott AM, Smyth FE, Darcy PK, Tainton K, Neeson P, Ritchie DS, Honemann D (2010) Gene-modified T cells as immunotherapy for multiple myeloma and acute myeloid leukemia expressing the Lewis Y antigen. Gene Ther 17(5):678–686
Perez-Simon JA, Martino R, Alegre A, Tomas JF, De Leon A, Caballero D, Sureda A, Sierra J, San Miguel JF (2003) Chronic but not acute graft-versus-host disease improves outcome in multiple myeloma patients after non-myeloablative allogeneic transplantation. Br J Haematol 121(1): 104–108
Perri RT, Hebbel RP, Oken MM (1981) Influence of treatment and response status on infection risk in multiple myeloma. Am J Med 71(6):935–940
Prabhala R, Neri P, Tassone P, Shammas MA, Bae J, Cumming VM, Allam CK, Daley JF, Desarneud F, Chauhan D, Blanchard E, Anderson K, Munshi NC, (2004) Dysregulated CD4+ CD25+ T-regulatory cells and TLRs in myeloma. Blood 104:Abstract no. 2466
Prabhala RH, Neri P, Bae JE, Tassone P, Shammas MA, Allam CK, Daley JF, Chauhan D, Blanchard E, Thatte HS, Anderson KC, Munshi NC (2006) Dysfunctional T regulatory cells in multiple myeloma. Blood 107(1):301–304
Qian J, Xie J, Hong S, Yang J, Zhang L, Han X, Wang M, Zhan F, Shaughnessy JD Jr, Epstein J,

5

Kwak LW, Yi Q (2007) Dickkopf-1 (DKK1) is a widely expressed and potent tumor-associated antigen in multiple myeloma. Blood 110(5): 1587–1594

Qian J, Hong S, Wang S, Zhang L, Sun L, Wang M, Yang J, Kwak LW, Hou J, Yi Q (2009) Myeloma cell line-derived, pooled heat shock proteins as a universal vaccine for immunotherapy of multiple myeloma. Blood 114(18):3880–3889

Qing J, Du X, Chen Y, Chan P, Li H, Wu P, Marsters S, Stawicki S, Tien J, Totpal K, Ross S, Stinson S, Dornan D, French D, Wang QR, Stephan JP, Wu Y, Wiesmann C, Ashkenazi A (2009) Antibody-based targeting of FGFR3 in bladder carcinoma and t(4;14)-positive multiple myeloma in mice. J Clin Invest 119(5):1216–1229

Raitakari M, Brown RD, Gibson J, Joshua DE (2003) T cells in myeloma. Hematol Oncol 21(1):33–42

Rasmussen T, Hansson L, Osterborg A, Johnsen HE, Mellstedt H (2003) Idiotype vaccination in multiple myeloma induced a reduction of circulating clonal tumor B cells. Blood 101(11):4607–4610

Reichardt VL, Okada CY, Liso A, Benike CJ, Stockerl-Goldstein KE, Engleman EG, Blume KG, Levy R (1999) Idiotype vaccination using dendritic cells after autologous peripheral blood stem cell transplantation for multiple myeloma–a feasibility study. Blood 93(7):2411–2419

Reichardt VL, Milazzo C, Brugger W, Einsele H, Kanz L, Brossart P (2003) Idiotype vaccination of multiple myeloma patients using monocyte-derived dendritic cells. Haematologica 88(10): 1139–1149

Rew SB, Lopes L, Koishihara Y, Kosaka M, Ozaki S, Peggs K, Chain B, Yong KL (2009) Potent anti-tumour cytotoxic T lymphocytes directed against the myeloma antigen HM1.24. Blood 102: Abstract no. 380

Rice A, Hart D (2002) Technology evaluation: APC-80200, Dendreon. Curr Opin Mol Ther 4(5):523–527

Ridgway D (2003) The first 1000 dendritic cell vaccines. Cancer Invest 21(6):873–886

Sato E, Olson SH, Ahn J, Bundy B, Nishikawa H, Qian F, Jungbluth AA, Frosina D, Gnjatic S, Ambrosone C, Kepner J, Odunsi T, Ritter G, Lele S, Chen YT, Ohtani H, Old LJ, Odunsi K (2005) Intraepithelial CD8+ tumor-infiltrating lymphocytes and a high CD8+/regulatory T cell ratio are associated with favorable prognosis in ovarian cancer. Proc Natl Acad Sci USA 102(51):18538–18543

Schmitt M, Schmitt A, Rojewski MT, Chen J, Giannopoulos K, Fei F, Yu Y, Gotz M, Heyduk M, Ritter G, Speiser DE, Gnjatic S, Guillaume P, Ringhoffer M, Schlenk RF, Liebisch P, Bunjes D, Shiku H, Dohner H, Greiner J (2008) RHAMM-R3 peptide vaccination in patients with acute myeloid leukemia, myelodysplastic syndrome, and multiple myeloma elicits immunologic and clinical responses. Blood 111(3):1357–1365

Schuster SJ, Neelapu SS, Gause BL (2009) Idiotype vaccine therapy (BiovaxID) in follicular lymphoma in first complete remission: phase III clinical trial results. J Clin Oncol 27:18s

Shevach EM (2002) CD4+ CD25+ suppressor T cells: more questions than answers. Nat Rev Immunol 2(6):389–400

Shi J, Tricot G, Szmania S, Rosen N, Garg TK, Malaviarachchi PA, Moreno A, Dupont B, Hsu KC, Baxter-Lowe LA, Cottler-Fox M, Shaughnessy JD Jr, Barlogie B, van Rhee F (2008) Infusion of haplo-identical killer immunoglobulin-like receptor ligand mismatched NK cells for relapsed myeloma in the setting of autologous stem cell transplantation. Br J Haematol 143(5):641–653

Siegel S, Friedrichs B, Budde AK, Barsoum A, Coggin J Jr, Tiemann M, Kabelitz D, Zeis M (2008) In-vivo detectable antibodies directed against the oncofetal antigen/immature laminin receptor can recognize and control myeloma cells–clinical implications. Leukemia 22(11):2115–2118

Singhal S, Safdar A, Chiang KY, Godder K, van Rhee F, Garner F, Foster B, Dubovsky D, Henslee-Downey PJ, Mehta J (2000) Non-myeloablative allogeneic transplantation ('microallograft') for refractory myeloma after two preceding autografts: feasibility and efficacy in a patient with active aspergillosis. Bone Marrow Transplant 26(11):1231–1233

Spanoudakis E, Hu M, Naresh K, Terpos E, Melo V, Reid A, Kotsianidis I, Abdalla S, Rahemtulla A, Karadimitris A (2009) Regulation of multiple myeloma survival and progression by CD1d. Blood 113(11):2498–2507

Stein R, Smith MR, Chen S, Zalath M, Goldenberg DM (2009) Combining milatuzumab with bortezomib, doxorubicin, or dexamethasone improves responses in multiple myeloma cell lines. Clin Cancer Res 15(8):2808–2817

Stevenson FK, Ottensmeier CH, Johnson P, Zhu D, Buchan SL, McCann KJ, Roddick JS, King AT, McNicholl F, Savelyeva N, Rice J (2004) DNA vaccines to attack cancer. Proc Natl Acad Sci USA 101(Suppl 2):14646–14652

Stritzke J, Zunkel T, Steinmann J, Schmitz N, Uharek L, Zeis M (2003) Therapeutic effects of idiotype vaccination can be enhanced by the combination of granulocyte-macrophage colony-stimulating factor and interleukin 2 in a myeloma model. Br J Haematol 120(1):27–35

Suri-Payer E, Fritzsching B (2006) Regulatory T cells in experimental autoimmune disease. Springer Semin Immunopathol 28(1):3–16

Tai YT, Dillon M, Song W, Leiba M, Li XF, Burger P, Lee AI, Podar K, Hideshima T, Rice AG, van Abbema A, Jesaitis L, Caras I, Law D, Weller E, Xie W, Richardson P, Munshi NC, Mathiot C, Avet-Loiseau H, Afar DE, Anderson KC (2008) Anti-CS1 humanized monoclonal antibody HuLuc63 inhibits myeloma cell adhesion and induces antibody-dependent cellular cytotoxicity in the bone marrow milieu. Blood 112(4):1329–1337

Tarte K, Lu ZY, Fiol G, Legouffe E, Rossi JF, Klein B (1997) Generation of virtually pure and potentially proliferating dendritic cells from non-CD34 apheresis cells from patients with multiple myeloma. Blood 90(9):3482–3495

Titzer S, Christensen O, Manzke O, Tesch H, Wolf J, Emmerich B, Carsten C, Diehl V, Bohlen H (2000) Vaccination of multiple myeloma patients with idiotype-pulsed dendritic cells: immunological and clinical aspects. Br J Haematol 108(4):805–816

Treon SP, Agus TB, Link B, Rodrigues G, Molina A, Lacy MQ, Fisher DC, Emmanouilides C, Richards AI, Clark B, Lucas MS, Schlossman R, Schenkein D, Lin B, Kimby E, Anderson KC, Byrd JC (2001) CD20-directed antibody-mediated immunotherapy induces responses and facilitates hematologic recovery in patients with Waldenstrom's macroglobulinemia. J Immunother 24(3):272–279

Tripodo C, Florena AM, Macor P, Di Bernardo A, Porcasi R, Guarnotta C, Ingrao S, Zerilli M, Secco E, Todaro M, Tedesco F, Franco V (2009) P-selectin glycoprotein ligand-1 as a potential target for humoral immunotherapy of multiple myeloma. Curr Cancer Drug Targets 9(5):617–625

van Rhee F, Szmania SM, Zhan F, Gupta SK, Pomtree M, Lin P, Batchu RB, Moreno A, Spagnoli G, Shaughnessy J, Tricot G (2005) NY-ESO-1 is highly expressed in poor-prognosis multiple myeloma and induces spontaneous humoral and cellular immune responses. Blood 105(10):3939–3944

Verdonck LF, Petersen EJ, Lokhorst HM, Nieuwenhuis HK, Dekker AW, Tilanus MG, de Weger RA (1998) Donor leukocyte infusions for recurrent hematologic malignancies after allogeneic bone marrow transplantation: impact of infused and residual donor T cells. Bone Marrow Transplant 22(11):1057–1063

Wang S, Hong S, Yang J, Qian J, Zhang X, Shpall E, Kwak LW, Yi Q (2006) Optimizing immunotherapy in multiple myeloma: restoring the function of patients' monocyte-derived dendritic cells by inhibiting p38 or activating MEK/ERK MAPK and neutralizing interleukin-6 in progenitor cells. Blood 108(13):4071–4077

Wen YJ, Barlogie B, Yi Q (2001) Idiotype-specific cytotoxic T lymphocytes in multiple myeloma: evidence for their capacity to lyse autologous primary tumor cells. Blood 97(6):1750–1755

Yang JC, Haworth L, Sherry RM, Hwu P, Schwartzentruber DJ, Topalian SL, Steinberg SM, Chen HX, Rosenberg SA (2003) A randomized trial of bevacizumab, an anti-vascular endothelial growth factor antibody, for metastatic renal cancer. N Engl J Med 349(5):427–434

Yi Q, Osterborg A, Bergenbrant S, Mellstedt H, Holm G, Lefvert AK (1995) Idiotype-reactive T-cell subsets and tumor load in monoclonal gammopathies. Blood 86(8):3043–3049

Yi Q, Freeman ME, Szmania S, Rosen N, Cottler-Fox M, Barlogie B, Tricot G, Van Rhee F (2003) Intranodal vaccination with idiotype-pulsed dendritic cells induces potent and long-lasting cellular and humoral immune responses in myeloma patients. Blood 102:Abstract no. 5277

Yu P, Lee Y, Liu W, Krausz T, Chong A, Schreiber H, Fu YX (2005) Intratumor depletion of CD4+ cells unmasks tumor immunogenicity leading to the rejection of late-stage tumors. J Exp Med 201(5):779–791

Zeis M, Frenzke H, Uharek L, Glass B, Schmitz N, Kronke M, Steinmann J (1998) Dendritic cells pulsed with idiotypic determinants induce antitumour immunity against established multiple myeloma. Blood 92:4229

Zheng C, Ostad M, Andersson M, Celsing F, Holm G, Sundblad A (2002) Natural cytotoxicity to autologous antigen-pulsed dendritic cells in multiple myeloma. Br J Haematol 118(3):778–785

Zinneman HH, Hall WH (1954) Recurrent pneumonia in multiple myeloma and some observations on immunologic response. Ann Intern Med 41(6):1152–1163

Zou W (2005) Immunosuppressive networks in the tumour environment and their therapeutic relevance. Nat Rev Cancer 5(4):263–274

Part III

Clinical Features

Monoclonal Gammopathy and Smoldering Multiple Myeloma: Diagnosis, Staging, Prognosis, Management

6

Jens Hillengass, Thomas Moehler, and Michael Hundemer

Contents

Abstract Monoclonal gammopathy of unknown significance (MGUS) as one of the most common premalignant disorders and smoldering multiple myeloma (sMM) are both caused by a proliferation of monoclonal plasma cells leading to a detectable serum monoclonal protein and/or excess of plasma cells in the bone marrow. Prerequisite for the diagnosis is that plasma cell disease does not cause clinical symptoms. Cytogenetic aberrations are detectable in the majority of patient in the clonally expanded plasma cells. MGUS consistently proceeds symptomatic MM. The lifetime risk of progression into symptomatic multiple myeloma lies between 15% and 59% for patients with MGUS

J. Hillengass (✉)
Department of Medicine V,
University of Heidelberg,
Im Neuenheimer Feld 410, 69120
Heidelberg, Germany
e-mail: jens.hillengass@med.uni-heidelberg.de

T. Moehler and H. Goldschmidt (eds.), *Multiple Myeloma*,
Recent Results in Cancer Research 183, DOI: 10.1007/978-3-540-85772-3_6,

or sMM. Prognostic parameters for development of symptomatic multiple myeloma from MGUS or sMM are concentration of monoclonal protein, bone marrow plasmocytosis, a non-IgG subtype and an abnormal free-light chain ratio. Detection of more than 1 focal lesion in whole body MRI, 95% or more of bone marrow plasma cells displaying an aberrant phenotype in flow cytometry and an evolving clinical course in two consecutive follow-up visits are additional prognostic parameters for sMM. Currently there is no accepted secondary prevention strategy available for sMM and MGUS progression. Future studies are required to combine increasing knowledge on risk factors and molecular pathogenesis with targeted agents to prevent progression.

Table 6.1 Recommended work-up at baseline in patients with suspected monoclonal gammopathy of unknown significance/smoldering multiple myeloma

Medical history and physical examination
CBC
Serum calcium and creatinine
Protein studies
• Total serum protein and serum electrophoresis (serum M-protein quantitation)
• 24-h urine protein electrophoresis (urine M-protein quantitation)
• Serum and urine immunofixation
• Serum free-light-chain measurement (FLC ratio)
β2-microglobulin
Bone marrow aspirate
Skeletal survey
MRI of thoracic-lumbar spine and pelvis

FLC free-light-chain, *MRI* magnetic resonance imaging

6.1 Definition of Monoclonal Gammopathy of Undetermined Significance (MGUS) and Smoldering Multiple Myeloma (sMM)

Monoclonal gammopathy of undetermined significance (MGUS) is defined by the detection of a monoclonal protein in serum or urine at a concentration of 30 mg/l or below in protein electrophoresis or free-light-chain (FLC) assay, the presence of <10% of plasma cells in the bone marrow and no evidence of end organ damage (Kyle et al. 2010).

Smoldering (asymptomatic) multiple myeloma (sMM) is defined by the presence of a monoclonal protein level of 30 g/l or more or 10% or more of clonal plasma cells in the bone marrow but no end organ damage (Kyle et al. 2010; Blade et al. 2010) as summarized above and in Tables 6.1–6.3. The Mayo group has further clarified that for these criteria the monoclonal protein has to be of IgG or IgA and plasma cells need to be clonal (Kyle and Rajkumar 2009). Fifteen to twenty percent of newly diagnosed multiple myeloma patients are classified as sMM (Weber et al. 1997).

6.2 Prevalence of MGUS

MGUS is one of the most common premalignant disorders. Kyle et al. found an age-adjusted prevalence of MGUS in residents of Olmsted county in Minnesota (USA) of 4.0% in men versus 2.7% in women (Kyle et al. 2006). Other studies have clearly demonstrated that there are ethnic differences in the MGUS prevalence. The overall prevalence of MGUS in the Japanese population is lower than in western population with a prevalence of 2.8% in men versus 1.6% in women (Iwanaga et al. 2007). The highest overall prevalence reported so far was 5.84% among men in Ghana (Landgren et al. 2007). These results were confirmed by a comparative analysis of the MGUS prevalence among African Americans and white veterans in the

Table 6.2 Diagnostic criteria of smoldering multiple myeloma in different reported series

Study	M protein (g/dl)	Bone marrow plasma cells (%)
Kyle and Greipp (1980)	≥3	≥10
Alexanian et al. (1988)	>2	–
Wisloff et al. (1991)	IgA >1.5; IgG >3	–
Facon et al. (1995)	–	>15
Weber et al. (1997)	>2.5	–
Cesana et al. (2002)[a]	IgA 2.1–4.9; IgG 3.6–6.9; light chain proteinuria >1 g/24 h	>10
Rosinol et al. (2003)[b]	≥3	≥10
IMWG 200310[c]	≥3	≥10

Ig immunoglobulin, *IMWG* international myeloma working group
[a]Either diagnostic criterion is acceptable
[b]Both diagnostic criteria are required
[c]Either or both diagnostic criteria are acceptable

Table 6.3 Differential diagnosis for MGUS, SMM, and symptomatic MM

Feature	MGUS	SMM	Multiple myeloma
BMPC (%)	<10 and	≥10 and/or	≥10 and/or
Serum monoclonal protein (g/l)	<3	≥3	≥3
Clinical manifestation	Absent	Absent	Present[a]

From the International Myeloma Working Group
Clinical manifestations defining myeloma if other criteria (BMPC/monoclonal protein)
CRAB-criteria definition: C, Calcium conzentration in serum > 10.5 mg/dl; R, Renal impairment (serum creatinine > 2 mg/dl); A, Anemia (hemoglobin concentration < 10 g/dl or 2 g/dl below normal value; B, Signs of bone destruction (osteolyses and/or osteoporosis)
MGUS monoclonal gammopathy of undetermined significance, *SMM* smoldering (asymptomatic) multiple myeloma, *MM* multiple myeloma, *BMPC* bone marrow clonal plasma cells
[a]Clinical features may include increased serum calcium concentrations, renal failure, anemia, skeletal involvement (lytic lesions), recurrent bacterial infections, and/or extramedullary plasmacytomas

United States showing an age-adjusted prevalence ratio of 3.0 in African Americans compared to white veterans (Landgren et al. 2006).

Furthermore, there is a well-known correlation between age and the occurrence of MGUS. In the Japanese population, the prevalence increases with age in both sexes: from 1% in participants aged 42–49 years, 1.9% in those 50–59 years, 2.6% in those 60–69 years, 3% in those 70–79 years, and 4.4% in those 80 years and older (Iwanaga et al. 2007). Similar data with age related increase of incidence and prevalence are available from the United States (Olmsted county) with 5.3% in persons 70 years or older and 7.5% in those 85 years and older, respectively with a preference of men (Kyle et al. 2006).

Recently, Dispenzieri et al. have presented the most extensive investigation on the condition of light-chain MGUS by analyzing blood/serum samples from the Olmsted county cohort (Dispenzieri et al. 2010). Light-chain MGUS was defined as an abnormal protein electrophoresis with no IgH expression, plus increased concentration of the involved light chain. Whereas the overall prevalence of MGUS in this population was 3.3%, 0.8% of patients fulfilled the criteria for light-chain MGUS. Progression into plasma cell-disorders were approximately 1% per year for conventional and only 0.3% for light-chain MGUS. Of note, progression of light chain MGUS was always into light-chain myeloma. Importantly, the risk of renal diseases was increased in conventional and light-chain MGUS and 23% of light-chain MGUS had renal disease that was not recognized as being related to a plasma cell disorder.

6.3 Differential Diagnosis and Diagnostic Assessment

Monoclonal immunoglobulins can be associated with other lymphoproliferative disorders like AL-amyloidosis, Waldenström's disease (in case of a monoclonal IgM) or POEMS-syndrome, and patients should be evaluated for these entities. Figure 6.1 demonstrates the frequency of distinct monoclonal plasma cell-diseases in 1,684 consecutive cases of a Mayo Clinic population in 2006 (Kyle and Rajkumar 2007).

6.3.1 Initial Diagnostic Assessment

Recently expert panels have reviewed the initial diagnostic work-up of patients with monoclonal gammopathy (Kyle et al. 2010; Berenson et al. 2010; Blade et al. 2010). The first step is a complete medical history and physical examination. Laboratory assessment includes quantification of the M-protein in serum and urine by electrophoresis. Most experts recommend 24-h-urine collection and analysis of M-protein and total protein for all patients at initial diagnosis. Some experts consider it sufficient for patients with expected MGUS that presence of M-protein should initially be investigated in a regular urine specimen and – in case of positive result – have a follow-up investigation using a 24-h-urine specimen. Further recommended laboratory tests are serum electrolytes, blood count, and routine chemistry in particular to determine the renal function.

Finally serum FLC should be performed as an additional tool to assess risk for development of Multiple Myeloma (see below). Serum chemistry and hematology lab data particularly focus on the question if any of the "CRAB"-criteria relevant for the diagnosis of symptomatic multiple myeloma according to the International Myeloma Working Group are met (*C*alcium

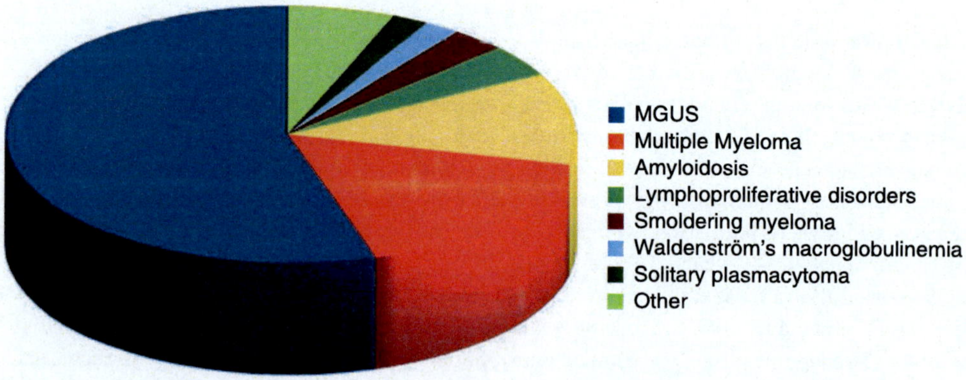

Fig. 6.1 Distribution of incidence of monoclonal plasma cell disorders (Kyle and Rajkumar 2007)

elevation (>2.75 mmol/l), *R*enal dysfunction (creatinine >173 μmol/l), *A*nemia (hemoglobin <100 g/l), and *B*one disease) (Kyle et al. 2010) (Tables 6.1–6.3).

Although some experts have questioned the relevance of bone evaluation for low-risk MGUS patients, the authors clearly recommend to assess bone disease at least with plain X-ray evaluation as part of the initial work-up (Berenson et al. 2010). For patients with bone pain or unclear results of the plain bone X-ray additional imaging techniques as MRI or CT are indicated (Bäuerle et al. 2009; Hillengass et al. 2010). Due to the prognostic impact and the possibility to recognize potentially clinical relevant lesions authors nowadays recommend a spine/pelvis MRI as part of initial work-up.

In addition, for initial work-up of IgM MGUS to investigate for lymphoproliferative disease an abdominal imaging technique is recommended at least as an abdominal ultrasound or CT of the abdomen (Weber et al. 2003).

Bäuerle et al. have demonstrated that 39% of MGUS and asymptomatic myeloma patients with normal bone skeletal survey had lesions in the axial skeleton and 37% in the extra-axial skeleton. Lesions in this group of patients can be clinically relevant as 13% of lesions violated the cortical bone implying an increased risk of fracture. Moreover MGUS patients in initial work-up need to be distinguished from solitary plasmocytoma which sometimes is difficult if the solitary plasmocytoma is not visible in the plain X-ray but produces an M-Protein sufficient to be detected by Immunofixation/protein electrophoresis. For these reasons, whole body MRI has to be considered superior to spinal MRI in initial work-up. The analysis by Bäuerle et al. did not reveal an alternative clinical or laboratory parameter that would predict the presence of lesions or even clinically relevant lesions in MGUS patients.

In summary, MRI of pelvis and spine are recommended in case of symptomatic MGUS/sMM patients. In addition, recent publications have recommended MRI of pelvis and spine for sMM and MGUS even in asymptomatic patients as MRI has overall prognostic implications and can reveal lesions that can lead to local clinical symptoms in the near future (e.g., fracture, extramedullary disease) (Blade et al. 2010; Kyle et al. 2010).

For patients with suspected osteopenia as per conventional X-ray skeletal status or in a CT a dual energy X-ray absorptiometry (DXA) scan is recommended. As described below (paragraph 6.5.5) in more detail MGUS and sMM patients with asymptomatic osteopenia can be considered for bisphosphonate treatment in case of significant osteopenia.

The plasma cell labeling index and flow-cytometric analysis of circulating plasma cells are possible additional investigations (Nowakowski et al. 2005). In the study by Perez-Persona a prognostic score for MGUS/sMM patients was developed using multicolor flow cytometry of bone marrow plasma cells to detect percentage of abnormal plasma cells. Immunoparesis and DNA ploidy status will be discussed later in this chapter in the sMM part (Perez-Persona et al. 2010).

Although cytogenetic evaluation has brought a wealth of data to support a sub-categorization of MGUS as described below, up to now there is no clear prognostic evidence for MGUS patients (Ross et al. 2010). Although cytogenetic investigation will be an important analysis in future clinical studies in MGUS, there is no general recommendation outside of clinical studies to perform those analyses using conventional cytogenetics or FISH (fluorescence in situ-hybridization) techniques.

6.3.2 Follow-up Recommendations

A first follow-up investigation should be performed 3–6 months after first diagnosis of MGUS/sMM. This visit should be focused on comparing the paraprotein in serum and urine with analysis obtained at first visit as well as renal function if no other clinical aspects occurred in the meantime. Further management of MGUS patients is dependent on the risk assessment.

Patients with low-risk MGUS (for risk factors see below) can be followed once a year and if stable in 2–3-year intervals. Patients with intermediate and high risk MGUS should receive follow-up investigation 3–6 months after first diagnosis and subsequently annually for lifetime. Bone marrow and imaging are not routinely performed on these follow-up visits but would be recommended if clinical evaluation or laboratory values indicate disease progression.

Bianchi et al. have recently investigated the relevance of regular long-term follow-up (Bianchi et al. 2010). Surprisingly, myeloma was diagnosed only in 16% of patients as a consequence of the routine follow-up whereas in 45% as a result of serious MM-related complication. In 25% MM was diagnosed as a result of less serious symptoms, during work-up of unrelated medical conditions (11%) or unknown (3%).

6.4 Risk Factors for Progression

6.4.1 Prognostic Factors for Progression for Patients with MGUS

In a prospective long-term study, Landgren et al. recently showed that among 77,469 Healthy donors 71 developed a MM and that in all cases a MGUS was present before, indicating that MM is consistently proceeded by MGUS (Landgren et al. 2009).

For monitoring the disease and future therapeutic options it is important to assess the risk of progression from MGUS into a clinical MM. The International Myeloma Working Group has summarized the existing research and identified five predictors to estimate the risk of progression into MM: (1) size of the M-protein; (2) type of paraprotein; (3) degree of plasma cell infiltration in bone marrow; (4) free-light-chain ratio in serum; and (5) flow-cytometric and cytogenetic characteristics.

Kyle et al. found that patients with a paraprotein level of 25 g/dl or higher had a risk of 49% to develop multiple myeloma or related disorder (Kyle et al. 2002). This related to a 14% risk of progression for patients with a paraprotein level lower than 5 g/dl. The relevance of paraprotein concentration as a strong predictor for progression was confirmed in subsequent studies. The type of immunoglobulin is relevant as IgM or IgA monoclonal protein is associated with a higher risk compared to IgG. The same group recently updated their recommendations and published relative risk according to the three risk factors M-Protein level, immunoglobulin subtype, and FLC ratio (Kyle et al. 2010) (Table 6.4). For IgA monoclonality this was shown earlier by Blade et al. (Blade et al. 1992). Regarding the bone marrow infiltration with plasma cells it was reported in 2002 that a percentage of more than 5% plasma cells in bone marrow is a risk factor for progression, but due to the introduction of the entity "smoldering myeloma" paticnt with more than 10% plasma cells in bone marrow are classified as smoldering myeloma anyway (Cesana et al. 2002). Rajkumar et al. showed that an abnormal free-light-chain ratio in serum predicts for a higher risk of progression as well as the presence of aberrant plasma cells in bone marrow (assessed by flow cytometry) in combination with their ploidity-status. Table 6.4 summarizes the risk-stratification model to

Table 6.4 Risk-stratification model to predict progression of monoclonal gammopathy of undetermined significance to myeloma or related disorders (Kyle et al. 2010)

Risk group	No. of patients	Relative risk	Absolute risk of progression at 20 years (%)	Absolute risk of progression at 20 years accounting for death as a competing risk (%)
Low-risk (serum M protein <1.5 gm/dl, IgG subtype, normal FLC ratio (0.26–1.65)	449	1	5	2
Low-intermediate-risk (any one factor abnormal)	420	5.4	21	10
High-intermediate-risk (any two factors abnormal)	226	10.1	37	18
High-risk (all three factors abnormal)	53	20.8	58	27

This table was originally published in Blood. Rajkumar et al. 2005 © The American Society of Hematology
MGUS monoclonal gammopathy of undetermined significance

predict progression of MGUS to multiple myeloma or related disorders.

6.4.2 Prognostic Factors for Progression of sMM

In the past 25 years, several authors have investigated risk factors for progression of sMM to myeloma. Initial publication contained "lytic bone lesions" as a strong risk factor but as nowadays osteolytic lesions are always considered a feature of symptomatic myeloma more recent publications excluded the group of asymptomatic patients with osteolyses from the analysis (Alexanian et al. 1988; Dimopoulos et al. 1993; Wisloff et al. 1991). Importantly, these publications already recognized additional risk factors that were confirmed subsequently as degree of infiltration by bone marrow plasma cells, concentration of M-protein and concentration of Bence–Jones proteinuria. More recently this important question was reevaluated as described in the following paragraph (Facon et al. 1995; Weber et al. 1997) (Table 6.5).

Kyle et al. investigated a cohort of 276 patients with sMM and 163 patients (59%) developed symptomatic multiple myeloma or AL-amyloidosis during follow-up (Kyle et al. 2007). For the first 5 years the risk of progression was 10% per year with approximately 3% per year for the next 5 years and 1% for the last 10 years of follow-up. The cumulative probability of progression into active multiple myeloma or AL-Amyloidosis was 51% at 5 years, 66% at 10 years and 73% at 15 years. The median time to progression was 4.8 years. Of the patients developing progressive disease 79% developed multiple myeloma. At diagnosis, significant risk factors for progression included the serum level and type of monoclonal protein, the presence of urinary light chains, the extent and pattern of bone marrow involvement and the reduction in uninvolved immunoglobulins. The concentration of serum monoclonal protein and percentage of plasma cells in bone marrow were the most important

6

Table 6.5 Milestone publications in the identification of factors for smoldering multiple myeloma associated with progression to symptomatic MM and risk groups

Study by	Risk factors	Risk group by factors		
		Low	Intermediate	High
Facon et al. (1995)	Hb <12 g/l; BMPC >20%; M protein >30 g/l (IgG); M protein >25 g/l (IgA) [median TTP in months]	0 [>50 mo]	1	2–3 [6 mo]
Weber et al. (1997)	M protein >30 g/l; IgA M–protein type; proteinuria >50 mg/24 h [median TTP in months]	0 [72 mo]	1 [39 mo]	2–3 [17 mo]
Rosinol et al. (2003)	Non-evolving vs. evolving [median TTP in years]	0 [45 mo]	–	1 [16 mo]
Kyle et al. (2007)	Low: M-Protein ≥3 g/dl, BMPC <10%; Intermediate: <3 g/dl, BMPC >10%; High: ≥3 g/dl, BMPC <10%; [cumulative probability of progression at 5 years]	[15%]	[43%]	[69%]
Dispenzieri et al. (2008)	FLC: <0.125 or >8; BMPC >10%; M-protein ≥3 g/dl [cumulative probability of progression at 5 years]	1 [25%]	2 [51%]	3 [76%]
Perez-Persona et al. (2010)	≥95% of BMPC with aberrant phenotype; decrease in ≥1 uninvolved immunoglobulin [cumulative probability of progression at 5 years]	0 [4%]	1 [46%]	2 [72%]
Hillengass et al. (2010)	Whole body MRI focal lesion (FL) (0 or 1 vs. >1 lesion) or diffuse MRI infiltration pattern [hazard ratio; median TTP]	0 (>43 mo, median not reached)		1 (HR: 4.05 FL/3.14 Diff; 14 mo)

BJ Bence-Jones, *MM* multiple myeloma, *BMPC* bone marrow plasma cells, *Hb* hemoglobin, *Ig* immunoglobulin, *TTP* time-to-progression, *FL* focal lesion as detected by MRI, *Diff* diffuse infiltration as detected by MRI

factors for progression. Therefore a predictive model with three groups was formed: group 1: BMPC <10%, M-Protein ≥3 g/dl, group 2: BMPC >10%, M-protein <3 g/dl, group 3: BMPC >10%, M-Protein ≥3 g/dl.

Subsequently, Dispenzieri described that the free-light-chain ratio is an independent additional risk factor for progression. Hemoglobin level, type of heavy chain and other factors were investigated as well but were not significant (Dispenzieri et al. 2008). Incorporating FLC ratio at a breakdown lower than 0.126 or higher than 8 resulted in an improvement of the prognostic classification with an even more balanced distribution (Table 6.5). The low (0–1 risk factor), intermediate (two risk factors), and high (three risk factors) risk group showed a probability of progression at 5 years of follow-up of 25%, 51%, and 71%, respectively (Table 6.5).

Rosinol et al. have confirmed in their study what is also clinical knowledge of many years and described that patients with progressive increase in the paraprotein ("evolving": increase of the M-protein in two of the consecutive follow-up visits) have a significant worse prognosis with a time to progression of 1.3 years compared to 3.9 years for the evolving and non-evolving types, respectively (Rosinol et al. 2003).

There are several different areas of research that add to the established risk factors as described above.

6.4.2.1 Immunophenotyping and Immunoparesis

Perez-Persona et al. have shown that the presence of an aberrant phenotype defined as the over expression of CD56 and CD19 with CD45 negativity and/or decreased CD38 reactivity in ≥95% of BMPC was a powerful predictor of early progression from sMM to active MM. The cumulative progression rate at 5 years was 64% versus 8% for the patients with ≥95% of aberrant BMPC or <95%, respectively. In this study the detection of immunoparesis as the decrease in one or two uninvolved immunoglobulins was also identified as a significant prognostic factor in multivariate analysis. Based on these two factors a prognostic stratification of sMM could be performed in three groups with a cumulative probability of progression at 5 years of 4%, 46%, and 72% when none, one, or two factors were present (Perez-Persona et al. 2010).

6.4.2.2 Role of Imaging in Prognostic Evaluation of sMM

Clinical studies investigating cross-section imaging as low dose computed tomography of the skeletal system, whole body or spinal MRI, and positron emission tomography have delivered data that have either revealed organ complications which were not detected with conventional staging procedures or revealed predictive (related to treatment indication) or prognostic relevance for symptomatic myeloma patients (Walker et al. 2007; Hillengass et al. 2010). Dimopolous et al. and Mariette et al. were among the first groups to describe the prognostic implication of MRI of the spine in asymptomatic myeloma/stage I Durie/Salmon (Dimopoulos et al. 1993; Mariette et al. 1999). More recently our group confirmed and extended on these earlier findings in 149 patients with asymptomatic multiple myeloma and found that 28% of patients with sMM had focal lesions (FL) typical for myeloma in whole body MRI. The presence of FL and more than one FL were strongest adverse prognostic factors for progression into MM in multivariate analysis. A diffuse infiltration pattern in MRI, a monoclonal protein of 40 g/l or greater, and bone marrow plasma cell infiltration of 20% or greater were other adverse prognostic factors for progression in univariate analysis.

It has been suggested to integrate MRI findings into the staging of multiple myeloma and the so-called Durie/Salmon PLUS classification was proposed (Table 6.6) (Baur et al. 2002; Durie Hematol J 2003). However, further prospective analysis of MRI is needed to find appropriate thresholds for the different stages of disease especially because rapid technical development leads to the possibility to perform total skeletal or whole body MRI. The imaging techniques and their application in multiple myeloma are also described in detail on page 133.

Table 6.6 Durie/Salmon PLUS staging-system (Baur et al. 2002, Durie et al. 2003)

Multiple myeloma stages	
IA	One focal myeloma lesion
IB	<5 focal lesion or mild diffuse infiltration
IIA/B	5–20 focal lesions or moderate diffuse infiltration
III/B	>20 focal lesions or severe diffuse infiltration

A serum creatinine <2.0 mg/dl, no extramedullary involvement

B serum creatinine >2.0 mg/dl, extramedullary involvement

6

6.4.3 Genetic Risk Stratification

The risk stratification of patients according to GEP profiles is an aim for future clinical studies. As the costs for this analysis are expected to substantially decrease and the standardization has greatly improved it is possible that in 5–10 years from now this technique will be available for routine work-up if prospective studies support the clinical value (Hose et al. 2009; Zhan et al. 2002).

6.5 Etiology and Pathogenesis of MGUS and sMM and Considerations Regarding Primary Prevention

6.5.1 Population-Based Studies

An important tool to further investigate the etiologic factors of MGUS and myeloma are population-based studies.

Large population-based prevalence studies were performed with the aim to assess the risk for MGUS and MM of relatives of patients with plasma cell-disorders. A study among Swedish residents showed that relatives of MGUS patients had increased risk for developing MGUS (RR = 2.8; 1.4–5.6), MM, lympho-plasmocytic lymphoma/Waldenström's macroglobulinemia and chronic lymphocytic leukemia. Vachon et al. confirmed, among residents of the Olmsted county, Minnesota, USA, that the risk of first-degree relatives from MGUS and MM patients to develop a plasma cell-disorder is increased by 2.6-fold. The prevalence of MGUS increased with age compared to patients from unaffected families starting with 1.6% in the age group of 40–49 up to 21% for the age group ≥81 years. Interestingly, the risk of MGUS or myeloma was seen among relatives of MM (RR, 2.0; 95% CI, 1.4–2.8) and MGUS patients (RR, 3.3; 95% CI, 2.1–4.8).

Genetic abnormalities were described that correlate with the risk of MGUS/MM: an analysis of germ line mutations in families with a high incidence showed that a mutation of CDKN2A increased the susceptibility for MM but also for melanoma and pancreatic cancer. Sandström et al. found in a family with congenital dyserythropoietic anemia type III an abnormal prevalence of MGUS and MM.

6.5.2 Concept of Chronic Antigenic Stimulation

Grass et al. recently demonstrated in sporadic and familial MGUS/MM that a frequent target of the paraprotein in MM and MGUS patients is a hyperphosphorylated form of paratarg-7, a protein with unknown function, which is expressed in all human tissues. Only sporadic or familial forms of myeloma with hyperphosphorylated paratarg-7 had a paratarg-7 specific paraprotein (Grass et al. 2010; Grass et al. 2009; Preuss et al. 2009). This finding suggests that hyperphosphorylation of paratarg-7 can cause autoimmunity and chronic antigenic stimulation leading to MGUS and multiple myeloma. Also Jego et al. have reported on mechanisms by which chronic antigen stimulation might contribute or lead to clonal proliferation (Jego et al. 2006). This research group demonstrated that an abnormal response to antigenic stimulation mediated by aberrant expression of Toll-like receptors and overexpression of interleukin 6 (IL-6) receptors can be a survival factor for myeloma cell lines and primary human myeloma cells.

These and other reports support the hypothesis that a proportion of MGUS and MM might arise from chronic (self) antigen stimulation. Removal of the antigen might therefore be one strategy to counteract MGUS while another consideration is to abort the abnormal immune response (Rajkumar 2009).

6.5.3 Molecular Genetics and Cytogenetics

Interestingly two types of primary cytogenetic abnormalities are detected in the majority of MGUS patients: hyperdiploidy (in approximately 50% of patients) or immunoglobulin heavy chain (IgH) translocations (in approximately 50% of patients) (Fig. 6.2). Only in a small proportion of MGUS patients hypodiploidy or no specific cytogenetic abnormality is found (Brousseau et al. 2007; Ross et al. 2010).

In the group of "IHT (IgH-translocation)-MGUS" IgH translocation commonly involve recurrent partner chromosome loci: 4p16.3 (FGF-R3 and MMSET), 6p21 [CCND3 (cyclin D3 gene)], 11q13 [CCND1 (cyclin D1)], 16q23 (c-maf) and 2βq11 (mafB) (Chng et al. 2007). Therefore at least six MGUS subentities: hyperdiploidy and the five most common primary IgH translocations have to be distinguished and considered for future primary intervention studies (Rajkumar 2009). It is likely that age, racial disparities, and environmental influences will have different impact on the various MGUS forms; therefore, future studies will need to examine the cytogenetic types separately. Importantly, cytogenetic abnormalities in MGUS do not necessarily have the same prognostic implications as the same translocation or abnormality in myeloma patients. Recently Ross and colleagues investigated cytogenetic abnormalities involving the MAF pathway in 2,207 patients with plasma cell dyscrasias

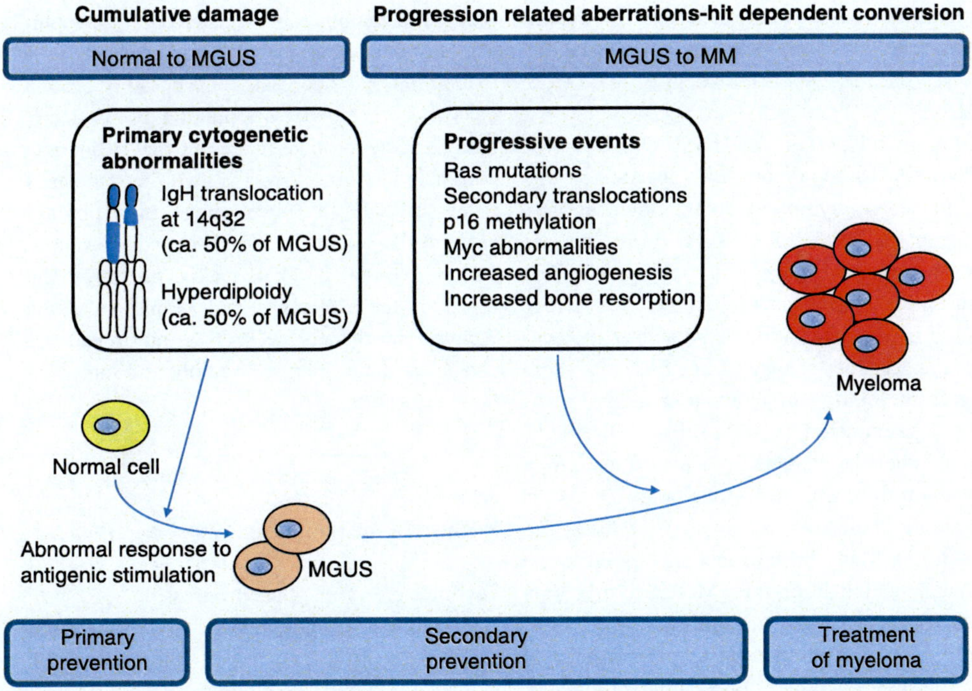

Fig. 6.2 Model of cytogenetic and molecular changes during progression of plasma cell disease

including 148 patients with sMM and 193 patients with MGUS. None of the investigated abnormalities (t14; 20) and t14; 16] predicted for a higher risk for progression (Ross et al. 2010).

From the above mentioned analysis and review age, hormonal factors, family history, immunosuppression, and exposure to certain pesticides have to be considered as risk factors for the development of MGUS and sMM.

6.5.4 Concepts for Secondary Prevention of Progression to Multiple Myeloma and Other Lymphoproliferative Diseases

Whereas the initiation of MGUS follows a cumulative damage model, the molecular pathogenesis leading from MGUS to MM has been a somewhat controversial topic. Research of several groups has demonstrated that overexpression or aberrant expression of cyclin-dependent kinases are hallmarks of plasma cell disease (Bergsagel and Kuehl 2003; Hose 2010).

Importantly, MGUS and sMM clonal plasma cells often harbor cytogenetic aberrations that are present in symptomatic myeloma as well (Magrangeas et al. 2005). Later during disease progression in MM additional cytogenetic and molecular changes occur (Cremer 2005) (Fig 6.2). It is currently undoubted that later molecular and genetic changes contribute to more aggressive multiple myeloma or increased resistance to therapy but it is not confirmed that additional molecular changes are a prerequisite for a transition from MGUS to myeloma (for details regarding molecular pathogenesis please see chapter 3). Many lines of evidence point to the concept that transition from MGUS to myeloma in the majority of patients could be the result of a progressive accumulation of plasma cells in the bone marrow with a consecutive remodeling of the bone marrow microenvironment including activation of osteoclasts.

Final confirmation of the time dependent "accumulation" model or the "second genetic hit" model could come from genome wide screening for myeloma specific mutations.

Several potentially pathogenetic genetic abnormalities have been described as "second hits": ras, p53, myc mutations, p16 methylation, and secondary translocations. The described genetic changes not only change the metabolism of the affected plasma cell clone but as a consequence induce paracrine loops involving IL-6 and other growth factors and a remodeling of the bone marrow microenvironment. The consequences including the increase of bone marrow angiogenesis are described in more detail in Chap. 4. The main regulator of IL-6 signaling in myeloma is the transducer and activator of transcription-3 (STAT3) (Bharti et al. 2004). Although an emerging ability of clonal plasma cells to induce osteolytic bone disease belongs to the stepwise process of malignancy. An increase in receptor activator of nuclear factor kB ligand (RANKL)-expression by osteoblasts (and possibly plasma cells) accompanied by reduction of its decoy receptor, osteoprotegerin are relevant (Roodman 2002). In addition, it was shown that increased levels of MIP-1a (macrophage inflammatory protein), IL-3, and IL-6 result in osteoclast activation (Lee et al. 2004; Tsubaki et al. 2007). The result of these changes and in particular the increase in the RANKL/OPG ratio leads to osteoclast maturation, activation, and increased bone resorption.

6.5.5 Summary of Clinical Studies to Halt Progression

To interfere with the progression of early asymptomatic plasma cell-disease MGUS and sMM have attracted a lot of interest and the evidence is summarized herein.

6.5.5.1
Bisphosphonates

The use of bisphosphonates in patients with MGUS but reduced bone density as determined by DXA scan was addressed in two clinical studies. Both studies could demonstrate that anti-resorptive therapy with intravenous zoledronate or oral alendronate improved the bone density. Neither study was powered to investigate fracture risk. Therefore, the use of bisphosphonates is finally an individual decision that can be justified in this situation.

Preclinical evidence of an anti-myeloma activity of bisphosphonates has led to clinical observations indicative of down-modulation of myeloma activity by bisphosphonate treatment (Corso et al. 2005). There are case reports describing a significant reduction of monoclonal protein in three patients with sMM (Dhodapkar et al. 1998). However, reduction of M-protein cannot be seen as regular response to bisphosphonates as a Spanish study investigating 12 patients with sMM treated with single agent pamidronate did not find any decrease in the M-protein level but could confirm a positive effect on bone formation (Martin et al. 2002). A large randomized Italian study showed a significantly reduced number of skeletal events but no prolongation of TTP or overall survival (Musto et al. 2003). While the potential toxicities of bisphosphonates as for example renal complications or osteonecrosis of the jaw have to be taken into consideration, treatment with bisphosphonates could be of benefit for patients with early bone disease such as MM-related osteopenia.

6.5.5.2
Alkylating Agents and Corticosteroids

Hjorth et al. performed a randomized study for sMM patients comparing immediate therapy with MP (melphalan/prednisone) versus observation until progression in a series of 50 patients (Hjorth et al. 1993, 1990; Hjorth et al. 1990). For the 25 patients allocated to the observation group the median time to progression was 12 months. The response rate to therapy in patient treated at diagnosis was similar to that of those who were observed initially and received therapy at the time of progression to active myeloma (52% vs. 55%). There was no significant difference in time to response or overall survival between the groups. Similar results were obtained in the studies by Grignani et al. and Riccardi et al. (Riccardi et al. 2000; Grignani et al. 1996).

6.5.5.3
Thalidomide

Up to now three studies have evaluated a potential role of Thalidomide in sMM. In a clinical phase II study with 29 patients initiated by Rajkumar et al., the rate of PR/CR was 34% and if minor responses were considered the ORR was 66% (Rajkumar et al. 2001, 2003). Three patients had progression while on treatment and the Kaplan–Meier estimates of progression-free survival were 80% at 1 year and 63% at 2 years follow-up. Similar results were reported by Weber et al. (Weber et al. 2003).

Recently Barlogie reported on the results of a study involving 76 sMM patients treated at an initial dose of 200 mg thalidomide per day. At 4 years of enrollment the ≥PR rate was 42% with a median time to response of 1–2 years. The median time to progression was 7 years (Barlogie et al. 2008). In all studies the thalidomide specific adverse events profile in particular the peripheral neuropathy was detected. All authors confirmed that Thalidomide can prolong the time-to-progression (TTP) but a clinical recommendation can only be made if a clinical benefit is confirmed in phase III randomized studies.

Based on the encouraging results regarding Thalidomide a Spanish group of investigators has started a phase III study comparing Lenalidomide/Dexamethasone (len/dex vs. observation) in high risk sMM patients. A similar study comparing Lenalidomide single agents with observation will be started by the ECOG (eastern cooperative oncology group). In addition, clinical studies using cyclooxygenase-2 inhibitors are currently underway.

6.5.5.4 Immunotherapy and Interference with Cytokine Network

Immunotherapy for MGUS/sMM has also raised interest as the immune system is intact for the majority of patients as a prerequisite to elicit an immune response against the plasma cell clone (Goodyear et al. 2008, 2005).

However, regarding the discouraging results for immunotherapy in patients with MM due to an impaired immune system and a large amount of malignant cells, patients with an early-stage plasma cell-disease might benefit from antitumor vaccination therapies before the MM-clone arises.

Hansson et al. vaccinated 28 patients with sMM (MM stage I/II) with autologous paraprotein combined with IL-12 or GM-CSF as adjuvants and were able to induce idiotype specific T-cell responses in a high proportion of patients (Hansson et al. 2007). This indicates that immunotherapy might be a promising approach to avoid a progression into MM. Furthermore, combination of vaccine strategies with immunomodulatory drugs as Thalidomide or Lenalidomide need to be considered as well to enhance the therapeutic effect of a specific immunotherapy.

A very interesting study was recently published by Lust et al., which was based on the earlier observation that serum levels of Interleukin-1 beta (IL1-beta) constitute a marker of progression in asymptomatic monoclonal gammopathies (Lust et al. 2009). In this trial, 47 patients with sMM were treated in this phase II study with an IL1-RA or observation. For patients with a submaximum IL6 suppression by IL1-RA alone dexamethasone was added to the therapy (53%). The median PFS for patients with a greater than 15% decrease in the 6-month high-sensitivity (hsCRP) level was 3 years ($n=35$) compared to 6 months for the group without change ($n=10$). In seven patients a decrease in plasma cell-labeling index paralleled the reduction in the hsCRP level. Further studies are therefore necessary to investigate this approach.

6.5.5.5 Summary and Brief Outlook Regarding Clinical Studies

Based on the improved knowledge about MGUS/sMM pathogenesis, the availability of novel agents and a better risk stratification concept, experts worldwide are currently reconsidering the concept of early therapeutic intervention.

The use of bisphosphonates for patients with decreased bone density on DXA scan is already an accepted approach. Furthermore therapeutic interventions with chemotherapeutic agents have not been successful to prevent progression or prolong OS survival of patients and therefore are in general not recommended. Ongoing and future studies will focus on patients at higher risk of progression including those patients for which evidence of progression becomes obvious because of consistently raising monoclonal protein level ("evolving type").

6.6 Summary and Conclusions

MGUS and sMM are the most prevalent premalignant conditions in worldwide population. Active myeloma for nearly all patients is preceded by MGUS/sMM. This observation as well as molecular and cytogenetic research support the two-hit genetic model of myeloma development starting with hyperdiploidy or IgH translocation followed by additional genetic alterations as ras, myc, or p53 mutations. Overall six or more subcategories can be defined based on genetic information in MGUS and sMM, although currently not relevant for clinical decision making.

Standard procedures for the diagnostic evaluation of MGUS are conventional X-ray techniques to assess impairment of the bone system, laboratory assessment in combination with bone marrow investigation to evaluate the influence on the hematopoietic system, and bone marrow involvement as well as renal function analysis. In addition, an MRI of spine and pelvis is recommended. Applying the results of these investigations to the IMWG staging system introduced in 2003 will lead to a distinction between MGUS, asymptomatic myeloma, and symptomatic myeloma based on the tumor mass and the presence or absence of end organ damage. For patients in whom categorization and indication for systemic therapy is unclear additional investigations as modern cross-section imaging can be helpful. In addition, symptoms as polyneuropathy and hyperviscosity may be the only symptoms of MM and may lead to a decision to start therapy in the absence of other myeloma related symptoms or organ damage.

Prognostic categorization of MGUS and sMM is considered important as high risk MGUS and sMM patients should be followed more frequently and might be candidates for early intervention clinical studies. Most important risk factors for MGUS are: BMPC>5%, M-Protein ≥1.5 g/dl, and abnormal FLC ratio. For sMM risk factors are: BMPC >10%, M-Protein>3 g/dl, and FLC<0.125/>8. Additional risk factors can be derived from quantification of BMPC with aberrant phenotype, analysis of decrease in uninvolved immunoglobulins, and follow-up information related to increase in tumor mass ("evolving course").

No primary prevention strategy is currently available for prevention of MGUS and sMM. The use of bisphosphonates for MGUS/sMM patients with decreased bone density on DXA scan is accepted. Interventional studies applying novel agents for secondary prophylaxis in MGUS and SMM focusing on the high risk patients are currently under way.

References

Alexanian R, Barlogie B, Dixon D (1988) Prognosis of asymptomatic multiple myeloma. Arch Intern Med 148:1963–1965

Barlogie B, van Rhee F, Shaughnessy JD Jr, Epstein J, Yaccoby S, Pineda-Roman M, Hollmig K, Alsayed Y, Hoering A, Szymonifka J, Anaissie E, Petty N, Kumar NS, Srivastava G, Jenkins B, Crowley J, Zeldis JB (2008) Seven-year median time to progression with thalidomide for smoldering myeloma: partial response identifies subset requiring earlier salvage therapy for symptomatic disease. Blood 112:3122–3125

Bauerle T, Hillengass J, Fechtner K, Zechmann CM, Grenacher L, Moehler TM, Christiane H, Wagner-Gund B, Neben K, Kauczor HU, Goldschmidt H, Delorme S (2009) Multiple myeloma and monoclonal gammopathy of undetermined significance: importance of whole-body versus spinal MR imaging. Radiology 252:477–485

Baur A, Stabler A, Nagel D, Lamerz R, Bartl R, Hiller E, Wendtner C, Bachner F, Reiser M (2002) Magnetic resonance imaging as a supplement for the clinical staging system of Durie and Salmon? Cancer 95:1334–1345

Berenson JR, Anderson KC, Audell RA, Boccia RV, Coleman M, Dimopoulos MA, Drake MT, Fonseca R, Harousseau JL, Joshua D, Lonial S, Niesvizky R, Palumbo A, Roodman GD, San-Miguel JF, Singhal S, Weber DM, Zangari M, Wirtschafter E, Yellin O, Kyle RA (2010) Monoclonal gammopathy of undetermined significance: a consensus statement. Br J Haematol 150:28–38

Bharti AC, Shishodia S, Reuben JM, Weber D, Alexanian R, Raj-Vadhan S, Estrov Z, Talpaz M, Aggarwal BB (2004) Nuclear factor-kappaB and

STAT3 are constitutively active in CD138+ cells derived from multiple myeloma patients, and suppression of these transcription factors leads to apoptosis. Blood 103:3175–3184

Bianchi G, Kyle RA, Colby CL, Larson DR, Kumar S, Katzmann JA, Dispenzieri A, Therneau TM, Cerhan JR, Melton LJ III, Rajkumar SV (2010) Impact of optimal follow-up of monoclonal gammopathy of undetermined significance (MGUS) on early diagnosis and prevention of myeloma-related complications. Blood 116(12):2019–2025

Blade J, Lopez-Guillermo A, Rozman C, Cervantes F, Salgado C, Aguilar JL, Vives-Corrons JL, Montserrat E (1992) Malignant transformation and life expectancy in monoclonal gammopathy of undetermined significance. Br J Haematol 81:391–394

Blade J, Dimopoulos M, Rosinol L, Rajkumar SV, Kyle RA (2010) Smoldering (asymptomatic) multiple myeloma: current diagnostic criteria, new predictors of outcome, and follow-up recommendations. J Clin Oncol 28:690–697

Brousseau M, Leleu X, Gerard J, Gastinne T, Godon A, Genevieve F, Dib M, Lai JL, Facon T, Zandecki M (2007) Hyperdiploidy is a common finding in monoclonal gammopathy of undetermined significance and monosomy 13 is restricted to these hyperdiploid patients. Clin Cancer Res 13:6026–6031

Cesana C, Klersy C, Barbarano L, Nosari AM, Crugnola M, Pungolino E, Gargantini L, Granata S, Valentini M, Morra E (2002) Prognostic factors for malignant transformation in monoclonal gammopathy of undetermined significance and smoldering multiple myeloma. J Clin Oncol 20:1625–1634

Chng WJ, Glebov O, Bergsagel PL, Kuehl WM (2007) Genetic events in the pathogenesis of multiple myeloma. Best Pract Res Clin Haematol 20:571–596

Corso A, Ferretti E, Lazzarino M (2005) Zoledronic acid exerts its antitumor effect in multiple myeloma interfering with the bone marrow microenvironment. Hematology 10:215–224

Dhodapkar MV, Singh J, Mehta J, Fassas A, Desikan KR, Perlman M, Munshi NC, Barlogie B (1998) Anti-myeloma activity of pamidronate in vivo. Br J Haematol 103:530–532

Dimopoulos MA, Moulopoulos A, Smith T, Delasalle KB, Alexanian R (1993) Risk of disease progression in asymptomatic multiple myeloma. Am J Med 94:57–61

Dispenzieri A, Kyle RA, Katzmann JA, Therneau TM, Larson D, Benson J, Clark RJ, Melton LJ III, Gertz MA, Kumar SK, Fonseca R, Jelinek DF, Rajkumar SV (2008) Immunoglobulin free light chain ratio is an independent risk factor for progression of smoldering (asymptomatic) multiple myeloma. Blood 111:785–789

Dispenzieri A, Katzmann JA, Kyle RA, Larson DR, Melton LJ III, Colby CL, Therneau TM, Clark R, Kumar SK, Bradwell A, Fonseca R, Jelinek DF, Rajkumar SV (2010) Prevalence and risk of progression of light-chain monoclonal gammopathy of undetermined significance: a retrospective population-based cohort study. Lancet 375:1721–1728

Durie BG, Kyle RA, Belch A, Bensinger W, Blade J, Boccadoro M, Child JA, Comenzo R, Djulbegovic B, Fantl D, Gahrton G, Harousseau JL, Hungria V, Joshua D, Ludwig H, Mehta J, Morales AR, Morgan G, Nouel A, Oken M, Powles R, Roodman D, San Miguel J, Shimizu K, Singhal S, Sirohi B, Sonneveld P, Tricot G, Van Ness B (2003) Scientific Advisors of the International Myeloma Foundation. Myeloma management guidelines: a consensus report from the Scientific Advisors of the International Myeloma Foundation. Hematol J. 4(6):379–398

Facon T, Menard JF, Michaux JL, Euller-Ziegler L, Bernard JF, Grosbois B, Daragon A, Azais I, Courouble Y, Kaplan G (1995) Prognostic factors in low tumour mass asymptomatic multiple myeloma: a report on 91 patients. The Groupe d'Etudes et de Recherche sur le Myelome (GERM). Am J Hematol 48:71–75

Goodyear O, Piper K, Khan N, Starczynski J, Mahendra P, Pratt G, Moss P (2005) CD8+ T cells specific for cancer germline gene antigens are found in many patients with multiple myeloma, and their frequency correlates with disease burden. Blood 106:4217–4224

Goodyear OC, Pratt G, McLarnon A, Cook M, Piper K, Moss P (2008) Differential pattern of CD4+ and CD8+ T-cell immunity to MAGE-A1/A2/A3 in patients with monoclonal gammopathy of undetermined significance (MGUS) and multiple myeloma. Blood 112:3362–3372

Grass S, Preuss KD, Ahlgrimm M, Fadle N, Regitz E, Pfoehler C, Murawski N, Pfreundschuh M (2009) Association of a dominantly inherited hyperphosphorylated paraprotein target with sporadic and familial multiple myeloma and monoclonal gammopathy of undetermined significance: a case-control study. Lancet Oncol 10:950–956

Grass S, Preuss KD, Pfreundschuh M (2010) Autosomal-dominant inheritance of hyperphosphorylated paratarg-7. Lancet Oncol 11:12

Grignani G, Gobbi PG, Formisano R, Pieresca C, Ucci G, Brugnatelli S, Riccardi A, Ascari E (1996) A prognostic index for multiple myeloma. Br J Cancer 73:1101–1107

Hansson L, Abdalla AO, Moshfegh A, Choudhury A, Rabbani H, Nilsson B, Osterborg A, Mellstedt H (2007) Long-term idiotype vaccination combined with interleukin-12 (IL-12), or IL-12 and granulocyte macrophage colony-stimulating factor, in early-stage multiple myeloma patients. Clin Cancer Res 13:1503–1510

Hillengass J, Fechtner K, Weber MA, Bauerle T, Ayyaz S, Heiss C, Hielscher T, Moehler TM, Egerer G, Neben K, Ho AD, Kauczor HU, Delorme S, Goldschmidt H (2010) Prognostic significance of focal lesions in whole-body magnetic resonance imaging in patients with asymptomatic multiple myeloma. J Clin Oncol 28:1606–1610

Hjorth M, Hellquist L, Holmberg E, Magnusson B, Rodjer S, Westin J (1990) Initial treatment in multiple myeloma: no advantage of multidrug chemotherapy over melphalan-prednisone. The Myeloma Group of Western Sweden. Br J Haematol 74:185–191

Hjorth M, Hellquist L, Holmberg E, Magnusson B, Rodjer S, Westin J (1993) Initial versus deferred melphalan-prednisone therapy for asymptomatic multiple myeloma stage I–a randomized study. Myeloma Group of Western Sweden. Eur J Haematol 50:95–102

Hose D, Moreaux J, Meissner T, Seckinger A, Goldschmidt H, Benner A, Mahtouk K, Hillengass J, Reme T, De VJ, Hundemer M, Condomines M, Bertsch U, Rossi JF, Jauch A, Klein B, Mohler T (2009) Induction of angiogenesis by normal and malignant plasma cells. Blood 114:128–143

Iwanaga M, Tagawa M, Tsukasaki K, Kamihira S, Tomonaga M (2007) Prevalence of monoclonal gammopathy of undetermined significance: study of 52, 802 persons in Nagasaki City, Japan. Mayo Clin Proc 82:1474–1479

Jego G, Bataille R, Geffroy-Luseau A, Descamps G, Pellat-Deceunynck C (2006) Pathogen-associated molecular patterns are growth and survival factors for human myeloma cells through Toll-like receptors. Leukemia 20:1130–1137

Kyle RA, Greipp PR (1980) Smoldering Multiple Myeloma.N Engl J Med 302:1347–1349

Kyle RA, Rajkumar SV (2007) Epidemiology of the plasma-cell disorders. Best Pract Res Clin Haematol 20:637–664

Kyle RA, Rajkumar SV (2009) Criteria for diagnosis, staging, risk stratification and response assessment of multiple myeloma. Leukemia 23: 3–9

Kyle RA, Therneau TM, Rajkumar SV, Offord JR, Larson DR, Plevak MF, Melton LJ III (2002) A long-term study of prognosis in monoclonal gammopathy of undetermined significance. N Engl J Med 346:564–569

Kyle RA, Therneau TM, Rajkumar SV, Larson DR, Plevak MF, Offord JR, Dispenzieri A, Katzmann JA, Melton LJ III (2006) Prevalence of monoclonal gammopathy of undetermined significance. N Engl J Med 354:1362–1369

Kyle RA, Remstein ED, Therneau TM, Dispenzieri A, Kurtin PJ, Hodnefield JM, Larson DR, Plevak MF, Jelinek DF, Fonseca R, Melton LJ III, Rajkumar SV (2007) Clinical course and prognosis of smoldering (asymptomatic) multiple myeloma. N Engl J Med 356:2582–2590

Kyle RA, Durie BG, Rajkumar SV, Landgren O, Blade J, Merlini G, Kroger N, Einsele H, Vesole DH, Dimopoulos M, San MJ, Avet-Loiseau H, Hajek R, Chen WM, Anderson KC, Ludwig H, Sonneveld P, Pavlovsky S, Palumbo A, Richardson PG, Barlogie B, Greipp P, Vescio R, Turesson I, Westin J, Boccadoro M (2010) Monoclonal gammopathy of undetermined significance (MGUS) and smoldering (asymptomatic) multiple myeloma: IMWG consensus perspectives risk factors for progression and guidelines for monitoring and management. Leukemia 24:1121–1127

Landgren O, Gridley G, Turesson I, Caporaso NE, Goldin LR, Baris D, Fears TR, Hoover RN, Linet MS (2006) Risk of monoclonal gammopathy of undetermined significance (MGUS) and subsequent multiple myeloma among African American and white veterans in the United States. Blood 107:904–906

Landgren O, Katzmann JA, Hsing AW, Pfeiffer RM, Kyle RA, Yeboah ED, Biritwum RB, Tettey Y, Adjei AA, Larson DR, Dispenzieri A, Melton LJ

6

III, Goldin LR, McMaster ML, Caporaso NE, Rajkumar SV (2007) Prevalence of monoclonal gammopathy of undetermined significance among men in Ghana. Mayo Clin Proc 82: 1468–1473

Landgren O, Kyle RA, Pfeiffer RM, Katzmann JA, Caporaso NE, Hayes RB, Dispenzieri A, Kumar S, Clark RJ, Baris D, Hoover R, Rajkumar SV (2009) Monoclonal gammopathy of undetermined significance (MGUS) consistently precedes multiple myeloma: a prospective study. Blood 113:5412–5417

Lee JW, Chung HY, Ehrlich LA, Jelinek DF, Callander NS, Roodman GD, Choi SJ (2004) IL-3 expression by myeloma cells increases both osteoclast formation and growth of myeloma cells. Blood 103:2308–2315

Lust JA, Lacy MQ, Zeldenrust SR, Dispenzieri A, Gertz MA, Witzig TE, Kumar S, Hayman SR, Russell SJ, Buadi FK, Geyer SM, Campbell ME, Kyle RA, Rajkumar SV, Greipp PR, Kline MP, Xiong Y, Moon-Tasson LL, Donovan KA (2009) Induction of a chronic disease state in patients with smoldering or indolent multiple myeloma by targeting interleukin 1{beta}-induced interleukin 6 production and the myeloma proliferative component. Mayo Clin Proc 84: 114–122

Mariette X, Zagdanski AM, Guermazi A, Bergot C, Arnould A, Frija J, Brouet JC, Fermand JP (1999) Prognostic value of vertebral lesions detected by magnetic resonance imaging in patients with stage I multiple myeloma. Br J Haematol 104:723–729

Martin A, Garcia-Sanz R, Hernandez J, Blade J, Suquia B, Fernandez-Calvo J, Gonzalez M, Mateo G, Orfao A, San Miguel JF (2002) Pamidronate induces bone formation in patients with smoldering or indolent myeloma, with no significant anti-tumour effect. Br J Haematol 118:239–242

Musto P, Falcone A, Sanpaolo G, Bodenizza C, Carella AM (2003) Pamidronate for early-stage, untreated myeloma. J Clin Oncol 21: 3177–3178

Nowakowski GS, Witzig TE, Dingli D, Tracz MJ, Gertz MA, Lacy MQ, Lust JA, Dispenzieri A, Greipp PR, Kyle RA, Rajkumar SV (2005) Circulating plasma cells detected by flow cytometry as a predictor of survival in 302 patients with newly diagnosed multiple myeloma. Blood 106:2276–2279

Perez-Persona E, Mateo G, Garcia-Sanz R, Mateos MV, de Las HN, de Coca AG, Hernandez JM, Galende J, Martin-Nunez G, Barez A, Alonso JM, Martin A, Lopez-Berges C, Orfao A, San Miguel JF, Vidriales MB (2010) Risk of progression in smoldering myeloma and monoclonal gammopathies of unknown significance: comparative analysis of the evolution of monoclonal component and multiparameter flow cytometry of bone marrow plasma cells. Br J Haematol 148:110–114

Preuss KD, Pfreundschuh M, Ahlgrimm M, Fadle N, Regitz E, Murawski N, Grass S (2009) A frequent target of paraproteins in the sera of patients with multiple myeloma and MGUS. Int J Cancer 125:656–661

Rajkumar SV (2009) Prevention of progression in monoclonal gammopathy of undetermined significance. Clin Cancer Res 15:5606–5608

Rajkumar SV, Dispenzieri A, Fonseca R, Lacy MQ, Geyer S, Lust JA, Kyle RA, Greipp PR, Gertz MA, Witzig TE (2001) Thalidomide for previously untreated indolent or smoldering multiple myeloma. Leukemia 15:1274–1276

Rajkumar SV, Gertz MA, Lacy MQ, Dispenzieri A, Fonseca R, Geyer SM, Iturria N, Kumar S, Lust JA, Kyle RA, Greipp PR, Witzig TE (2003) Thalidomide as initial therapy for early-stage myeloma. Leukemia 17:775–779

Rajkumar SV et al (2005) Serum free light chain ratio is an independent risk factor for progression in monoclonal gammopathy of undetermined significance (MGUS). Blood 106:812–817

Riccardi A, Mora O, Tinelli C, Valentini D, Brugnatelli S, Spanedda R, De PA, Barbarano L, Di SM, Giordano M, Delfini C, Nicoletti G, Bergonzi C, Rinaldi E, Piccinini L, Ascari E (2000) Long-term survival of stage I multiple myeloma given chemotherapy just after diagnosis or at progression of the disease: a multicentre randomized study. Cooperative Group of Study and Treatment of Multiple Myeloma. Br J Cancer 82:1254–1260

Roodman GD (2002) Role of the bone marrow microenvironment in multiple myeloma. J Bone Miner Res 17:1921–1925

Rosinol L, Blade J, Esteve J, Aymerich M, Rozman M, Montoto S, Gine E, Nadal E, Filella X, Queralt R, Carrio A, Montserrat E (2003) Smoldering multiple myeloma: natural history and recognition of an evolving type. Br J Haematol 123:631–636

Ross FM, Chiecchio L, Dagrada G, Protheroe RK, Stockley DM, Harrison CJ, Cross NC, Szubert AJ, Drayson MT, Morgan GJ (2010) The t(14;20) is a poor prognostic factor in myeloma but is associated with long-term stable disease in monoclonal gammopathies of undetermined significance. Haematologica 95:1221–1225

Tsubaki M, Kato C, Manno M, Ogaki M, Satou T, Itoh T, Kusunoki T, Tanimori Y, Fujiwara K, Matsuoka H, Nishida S (2007) Macrophage inflammatory protein-1alpha (MIP-1alpha) enhances a receptor activator of nuclear factor kappaB ligand (RANKL) expression in mouse bone marrow stromal cells and osteoblasts through MAPK and PI3K/Akt pathways. Mol Cell Biochem 304:53–60

Walker R, Barlogie B, Haessler J, Tricot G, Anaissie E, Shaughnessy JD Jr, Epstein J, van Hemert R, Erdem E, Hoering A, Crowley J, Ferris E, Hollmig K, van Rhee F, Zangari M, Pineda-Roman M, Mohiuddin A, Yaccoby S, Sawyer J, Angtuaco EJ (2007) Magnetic resonance imaging in multiple myeloma: diagnostic and clinical implications. J Clin Oncol 25:1121–1128

Weber DM, Dimopoulos MA, Moulopoulos LA, Delasalle KB, Smith T, Alexanian R (1997) Prognostic features of asymptomatic multiple myeloma. Br J Haematol 97:810–814

Weber D, Rankin K, Gavino M, Delasalle K, Alexanian R (2003) Thalidomide alone or with dexamethasone for previously untreated multiple myeloma. J Clin Oncol 21:16–19

Wisloff F, Andersen P, Andersson TR, Brandt E, Eika C, Fjaestad K, Gronvold T, Holm B, Lovasen K, Tjonnfjord GE (1991) Incidence and follow-up of asymptomatic multiple myeloma. The myeloma project of health region I in Norway. II. Eur J Haematol 47:338–341

Zhan F, Hardin J, Kordsmeier B, Bumm K, Zheng M, Tian E, Sanderson R, Yang Y, Wilson C, Zangari M, Anaissie E, Morris C, Muwalla F, van Rhee F, Fassas A, Crowley J, Tricot G, Barlogie B, Shaughnessy J Jr (2002) Global gene expression profiling of multiple myeloma, monoclonal gammopathy of undetermined significance, and normal bone marrow plasma cells. Blood 99:1745–1757

Imaging in Multiple Myeloma

7

Stefan Delorme and Andrea Baur-Melnyk

Contents

S. Delorme (✉)
Department of Radiology,
German Cancer Research Center,
Im Neuenheimer Feld 280, 69120
Heidelberg, Germany
e-mail: s.delorme@dkfz.de

Abstract In multiple myeloma, imaging is required to determine the stage of disease and to anticipate impending bone fractures. Whereas the traditionally used Durie and Salmon staging system includes lytic bone lesions in plain films as criteria, modern systems include MRI findings. MRI is most sensitive to both diffuse bone marrow involvement as well as solid plasma cell tumors. Whole-body low-dose CT (WBCT) may replace plain films in the near future, since it is quicker, more sensitive, and is better tolerated by patients. Intramedullary lesions are well seen as long as they are located in long bones where they are surrounded by fat. Diffuse bone marrow infiltration as well as intravertebral lesions, however, are difficult to detect with WBCT in the absence of frank destruction of cancellous bone. PET or PET-CT with 18-fluoro-deoxyglucose (FDG) are insensitive to diffuse bone marrow infiltration, but may help to assess treatment response in solitary or multiple solid plasma cell tumors which have a high FDG uptake before treatment.

7.1 Introduction

Multiple myeloma is a low-grade non-Hodgkin's B-cell lymphoma which is characterized by a proliferation of monoclonal, malignant plasma cells.

T. Moehler and H. Goldschmidt (eds.), *Multiple Myeloma*,
Recent Results in Cancer Research 183, DOI: 10.1007/978-3-540-85772-3_7,

It is a disease which usually originates in the bone marrow, and eventually extends into soft tissue or spreads into the peripheral blood (plasma cell leukemia). The main effects and causes of pain and disability are replacement of hematopoietic bone marrow (leading to anemia, leucopenia, and thrombocytopenia, and their sequelae), osteoporosis and bone destruction (leading to fractures and pain), renal damage by paraproteins, and systemic amyloidosis. The treatment consists of chemotherapy (often high-dose with stem cell rescue), thalidomide and its derivates, proteasome inhibitors, and bisphosphonates. Radiotherapy is used for local manifestations which are particularly painful, or where complications are imminent. Surgical stabilizations also have an important role for local disease. Vertebroplasty or kyphoplasty are used to prevent progressive vertebral collapse, and to treat pain. To date, however, there is no definite cure.

The term "*plasmacytoma*" denotes solitary plasma cell tumors without evidence of systemic spread – which has to be excluded by serum and bone marrow samples as well as imaging studies. They may also primarily arise outside the bone and are then termed "extraosseous soft-tissue myeloma." As a rule, soft-tissue involvement – either primary or secondary (by extension from a bone lesion) – indicates a dismal prognosis.

Monoclonal gammopathy of unclear significance (MGUS) has to be discriminated to overt multiple myeloma. Its criteria are a M-protein in serum <30 g/l, bone marrow plasma cells <10%, no evidence of any other B-cell proliferative disorders and no related organ or tissue impairment, such as renal damage or bone lesions (International myeloma working group 2003).

Multiple myeloma causes a wide variety of symptoms and complications, fractures and destruction of bones being the most painful and disabling ones. In osteoporotic bones, typically in the spine, fractures may occur with minimal trauma – or at least trauma insufficient to cause fracture in a normal bone. Fractures of tubular bones, whose stability relies mainly on cortical, not cancellous bone, are most commonly caused by focal solid myeloma nodules which erode the cortex from inside outward. Therefore, the radiologist is required to anticipate impending fractures and initiate referral for surgical stabilization or vertebroplasty. Furthermore, the presence or absence of focal destructions is an important criterion for initial staging (e.g., using the Durie and Salmon staging system) and for follow-up. Until today, the x-ray skeletal survey is standard for screening the skeleton for osteoporosis and bone destruction. Not surprisingly, whole-body CT is superior to plain x-ray films for finding focal bone destructions (Mahnken et al. 2002), and MRI is even more sensitive (Baur-Melnyk et al. 2008), particularly in the vertebral bone marrow, to show diffuse or focal involvement which has not or not yet caused destruction of mineralized bone.

7.2 Imaging Methods

7.2.1 Morphologic Imaging

We term plain x-ray, CT, and MRI "morphological" imaging techniques, as opposed to functional ones which measure microcirculation, diffusion, or metabolic processes. A plain x-ray skeletal survey is standard for staging and follow-up of bone involvement by multiple myeloma, and consists of a frontal and lateral view of the skull, the cervical, thoracic, and lumbar spine, a coned-down frontal image of the dens axis, as well as frontal views of the rib cage, humeri, femora, knees, and pelvis. The hallmark of neoplastic bone involvement is osteoporosis or focal destruction. CT, or whole-body CT (which requires state-of-the-art multidetector scanners) is reasonable alternative to x-ray films, for many reasons. Since the intrinsic contrast is high, the tube current can be lowered significantly (i.e., to 50–100 mAs, depending on the weight of the patient), resulting in an effective equivalent dose in the same range as that of a skeletal survey (4–5 mSv). The entire examination takes around 1 or 2 min, the patient lying comfortably on his or her back. Note that the varied positions required for x-ray films are painful and tiring for patients who are often elderly and disabled due to previous fractures. Iodine-containing contrast agents are contraindicated for patients with Bence-Jones proteinuria because of the risk of cast nephropathy and renal failure, and actually they are not needed for skeletal CT. Focal bone destruction is more easily seen than on plain films, and also easier to discriminate from normal sparing in trabecular bone, which will have fat and not soft-tissue density. Diffuse bone marrow involvement within preserved spongious bone, however, is difficult to detect with CT and better seen with MRI.

MRI of the spine, or whole-body MRI, is to date the most sensitive method for detecting diffuse and focal multiple myeloma in the spine as well as the extra-axial skeleton. Sequences commonly used are unenhanced and contrast-enhanced T1-weighted spin-echo sequences and T2-weighted sequences with fat suppression, either by spectral pre-saturation, or using STIR (short tau inversion recovery) techniques. If scanners with whole-body capabilities are available, the examination should include the entire skeleton, since most patients have axial as well as extra-axial bone lesions. If not, at least the spine should be scanned with MRI, because of the insensitivity of CT and plain x-ray films to intravertebral myeloma.

7.2.2 Functional Imaging

All of the above methods show the extent of tumor (or more specifically its damage to mineralized bone) but not its activity or viability, and have limitations when assessing treatment response or early progression. Patients with monoclonal gammopathy of unclear significance constitute a particular problem, because they have no measurable lesion at all which could be followed over time to anticipate progression. Functional imaging methods therefore measure microcirculation, diffusion of interstitial water molecules or glucose uptake as surrogates for tumor viability, and aggressiveness.

7.2.2.1 Dynamic Contrast-Enhanced MRI (DCE MRI)

The term DCE MRI denotes repeat scanning with high temporal resolution before, during, and after intravenous infusion of a Gadolinium-containing contrast agent, using fast T1-weighted sequences. The change in signal intensity (which depends on the concentration of contrast agent) over time in a given region is a function of local perfusion, relative blood volume, capillary surface exchange area, vessel permeability, and systemic elimination. To quantitatively describe such time-concentration curves, pharmacokinetic models are used, but the interpretation of parameters derived in this way with respect to pathophysiological processes has to be made with great caution. The parameter which is easiest to interpret is the maximal relative rise in intensity, since this is chiefly determined by the local, regional blood volume.

7.2.2.2 Diffusion-Weighted Imaging (DWI)

The freedom of interstitial water molecules to move depends on many factors, but cell density or the presence of organized structures (e.g., fibers) are of high influence. Studies, e.g., in brain tumors have shown that the diffusion is impaired within tumors, and that a decrease of diffusion may herald progression. Effective treatment may cause a transient decrease in diffusion, owing to toxic cell swelling, but thereafter, as the cellular load is reduced, diffusion increases significantly. DWI uses opposing phase gradients switched shortly after each other, which causes rephasing and thereby regain of signal in stationary water, but a signal loss in moving molecules. Within a certain range, such signal loss can be mainly attributed to diffusion rather than blood flow, and using varying gradient strengths and durations, the apparent diffusion coefficient (ADC) can be calculated. The experiences with multiple myeloma are still limited, and due to the presence of trabeculae, the conditions are more difficult than in the brain. However, it can be shown that a low ADC in fractured vertebrae indicates local tumor infiltration as a cause rather than osteoporosis. It is still unclear whether DWI may serve as a tool to monitor treatment or progression. Bone marrow in myeloma patients contains several components which may influence diffusion processes separately, such as hematopoietic cells, fatty marrow, and plasmacellular infiltrates, and it is unclear how changes in its composition will influence diffusion. Solid myeloma nodules will probably be more easily assessed since they lack hematopoietic and fatty components (Mulkern and Schwartz 2003).

7.2.2.3 Bone Scintigraphy and Positron Emission Tomography (PET)

Bone scintigraphy, using 99 m Tc-labeled bisphosphonates, is insensitive to diffuse or focal myeloma because there is no increased osteoblastic activity – unlike bone metastases from most other solid tumors. PET with 18-F-deoxyglucose (FDG) detects tumors according to their glucose demand, the glucose transport molecules expressed in the cell membrane, the local cell density, and the metabolic activity of the surrounding tissue. As a rule, multiple myeloma has a rather low metabolic activity, and is hardly detected when only a diffuse bone marrow involvement is present – simply because the local cell density is too low. Whenever myeloma is detected on PET scans – this is often the case in solid myeloma nodules – the standardized uptake value is a good parameter to monitor response, since after chemotherapy, the drop in glucose uptake clearly precedes the morphologically measurable response.

7.3 Radiological–Pathological Correlation

Three patterns of spread of multiple myeloma are relevant for imaging: diffuse bone marrow involvement, focal bone destructions by solid tumor nodules, and extraosseous manifestations. In diffuse bone marrow involvement, generalized or partial, hematopoietic and fatty marrow and plasmacellular infiltrates are found besides each other. In the beginning fat cell content might be even increased and hematopoiesis is still normal. As malignant plasma cells increase in number, they gradually replace normal marrow. Thus, there is a shift with an increase of cellular, and a decrease of fatty components. This process takes place within a preserved cancellous bone, which only gradually becomes eroded. Very typically, osteoporosis triggered by multiple myeloma progresses more rapidly than other forms, particularly senile or postmenopausal ones. Degradation of bone is mediated via osteoclast-activating factors (typically RANK-Ligand, Interleukin-2 and TNF) and amounts to frank focal destructions, where solid tumor nodules are present which contain almost no bony remnants. Such nodules contain malignant plasma cells and some tumor stroma, but neither hematopoietic fatty nor osseous components, and behave like any destructively growing solid tumor. Obviously, the loss of stability is much more severe than with diffuse bone marrow infiltration where the cancellous bone is at least partly preserved. Any destruction of cortical bone is by definition due to solid myeloma nodules.

Diffuse and focal bone involvement are commonly seen besides each other. Focal nodules may eventually extend beyond the confines of the bone and invade adjacent tissue, where they can cause symptoms like any other solid malignant tumor. Although the commonest cause of soft-tissue involvement is the extension of a primary bone lesion into adjacent tissue but primary soft-tissue lesions are also observed. Their pattern of spread does not usually follow the pathways commonly seen in carcinomas, but is often rather "atypical", like in melanoma or non-epithelial neoplasms (Zechmann et al. 2007).

By their nature, *x-ray films* only show the effects of myeloma on mineralized bone, namely, osteoporosis (Fig. 7.1a, b) and focal destructions (Fig. 7.2). The criteria of osteoporosis are the same as those used for postmenopausal or idiopathic forms, and it is the axial skeleton which is mainly involved. Rapid progression and an inhomogeneous, coarse and streaky appearance

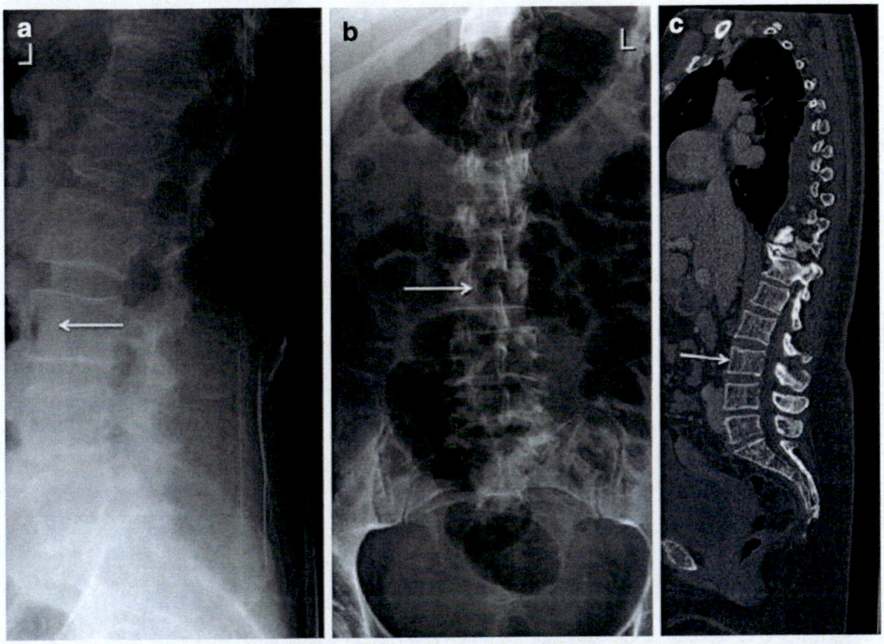

Fig. 7.1 Lateral (**a**) and frontal (**b**) lumbar spine x-ray films in a patient with multiple myeloma. Corresponding sagittal reconstruction from whole-body low-dose computed CT (WBCT) (**c**), sagittal T1-weighted (**d**) and fat-suppressed T2-weighted (**e**) MRI slices. Signs of osteoporosis are visible on the plain films as well as the reconstructed WBCT slices. There is a focal destruction in the third lumbar vertebra (*arrows*) which is visible on WBCT (c), and which corresponds to an area of low signal intensity in T1-weighted (d), and a slightly elevated signal intensity on fat-suppressed T2-weighted images (e). Without fat suppression, this area appears hypointense, due to the relatively high signal intensity of the surrounding. On the plain films, however (a, b), the corresponding region (*arrows*) appears innocent, and is also difficult to assess due to superimposition of bowel gas. The T1-weighted MRI also shows signs of diffuse bone marrow involvement, with a "salt-and-pepper" appearance in the not fat-suppressed T1- and T2-weighted images (d)

Fig. 7.1 (continued)

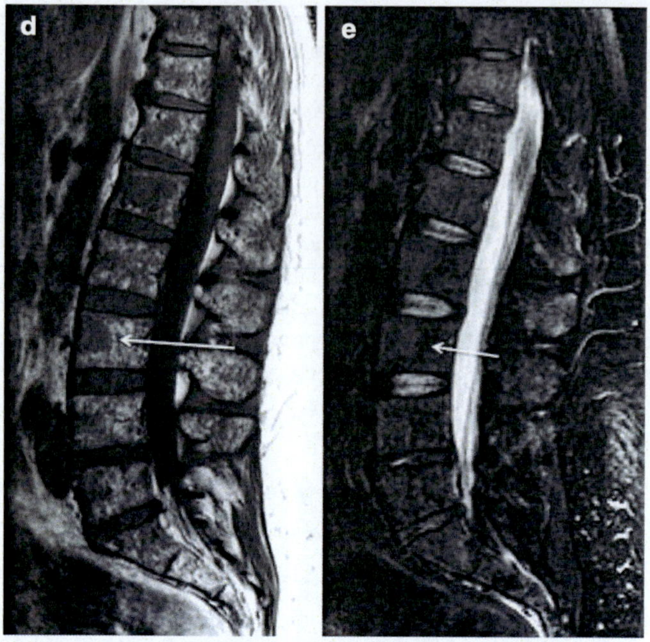

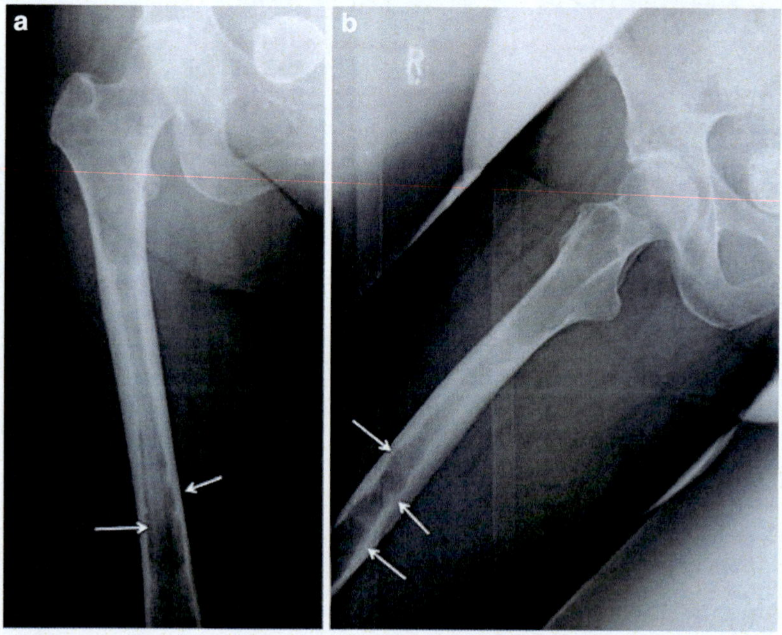

Fig. 7.2 Frontal (**a**) and lateral (**b**) x-ray of the femur showing multiple erosions (*arrows*) of the cortical bone, arising from the medullary space ("scalloping")

of the vertebral spongiosa are signs which may raise suspicion of a neoplastic cause in patients with osteoporosis, and so will osteoporosis in the young and in males. Otherwise only focal destructions will point more specifically at the true underlying cause. Notably, the presence of osteoporosis in patients with known plasma cell disorders does not prove a causal relationship. Due to its severity and rapid progression, osteoporosis due to myeloma frequently causes vertebral compression fractures, which are most often diagnosed on radiographs, but whose impact on stability should be assessed on CT.

Focal areas of destruction are by definition always due to solid myeloma nodules, which arise in the cancellous bone but then erode the cortical bone from the inside, causing the typical "scalloped" appearance (Fig. 7.2). In the skull, this occurs early, resulting in multiple, sharply delineated osteolytic lesions. As a rule, areas of focal, lytic bone destruction are more easily seen in cortical than in cancellous bone, because of the contrast between the defect and its surrounding. Areas of destruction inside the spongiosa of the vertebral bodies are almost invisible on radiographs (Fig. 7.1a, b), and the superimposition of soft tissue, air, or ribs makes the assessment even more difficult. In one study, half of the cases proven to have vertebral involvement on MRI were negative on x-ray films (Baur et al. 1996). Locations where trabeculae are "physiologically" rarefied, e.g., in the femoral neck, and which are common in the elderly, may be mistaken for lytic lesions. CT showing fatty density and MRI can rule out infiltration by myeloma.

Like x-ray films, *computed tomography (CT)* mainly shows alterations to mineralized bone, but there are no problems with superimposition. Pure bone marrow infiltrates may also be seen if they lie within fatty marrow, but are hardly visible in vertebral bodies (Fig. 7.3e), unless they are very osteoporotic. Furthermore, osteolytic areas in cancellous bone, which are occult to plain films, are easily detected. CT is the gold standard to assess the stability of bone and should be performed prior to vertebroplasty to ensure that the cortex is intact and the vertebral body will retain the injected material.

In *magnetic resonance imaging (MRI)*, the signal intensity of the spinal bone marrow on both T1- and T2-weighted images depends on the relation of fatty and cellular components, cellular ones being either hematopoietic marrow or plasmacellular infiltrates. In adults in the axial skeleton hematopoietic "red" marrow is present. In the periphery "yellow" fatty marrow is present. With age the fatty components within red marrow (usually 40–50%) increases. Typically, the vertebral bodies are T1-hyperintense (i.e., brighter than the intervertebral disk) and hypointense on fat-suppressed T2-weighted images (darker than normal disks). An increase in the cellular and decrease of the fatty component in the bone marrow will cause a decrease in T1 and an increase in signal on STIR images (Wasser et al. 2005). The best combination of sequences for imaging myeloma is a combination of T1-w SE and fat-suppressed sequences, e.g., STIR (Baur et al. 1998).

On T1- and T2-weighted images without fat suppression, one may also see a "salt-and-pepper" pattern, which is a mixture of small hypointense and hyperintense spots (Fig. 7.1d). This reflects an inhomogeneous composition of bone marrow with fatty islands and low-grade interstitial infiltration by myeloma cells. Those patients are usually stage I disease and do not require any treatment. Beware of pitfalls like young individuals with a high amount of hematopoiesis (thus low signal on T1-w SE images), or patients pre-treated with chemotherapy and possibly growth factors, in whom bone marrow reconversion may cause grossly misleading findings on MRI.

Since multiple myeloma is angiogenic, involved bone marrow shows enhancement on

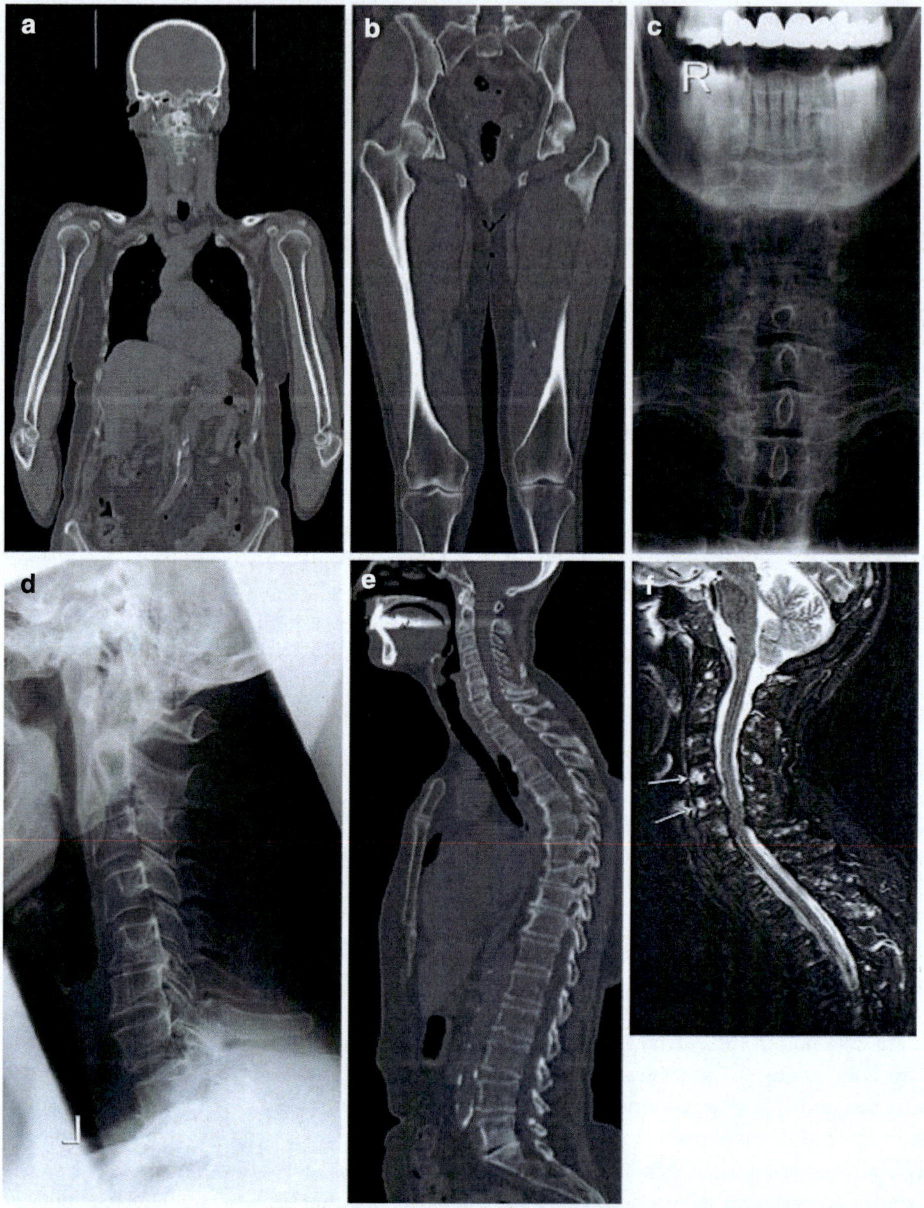

Fig. 7.3 Coronal reconstructions in WBCT over the long bones (**a**, **b**), frontal (**c**) and lateral (**d**) cervical x-ray films, sagittal WBCT reconstruction over the spine (**e**), and sagittal T2-weighted, fat-suppressed MRI (**f**) of the cervical spine in a patient with multiple myeloma. The long bones show no focal destructions. Note the low density in the CT of the medullary spaces of the long bones where any solid, intramedullary nodule would be frankly visible. The plain films of the cervical spine appear normal, and the sagittal reconstruction of WBCT shows osteoporosis, a fracture of the ninth thoracic vertebra, but no focal areas of destruction inside the vertebral bodies. The cervical MRI, however shows focal T2 hyperintense areas in the fourth and fifth cervical vertebra, along with disseminated tiny areas of signal elevation in all other vertebral bodies and spinous processes, typical of myeloma infiltration, and invisible with both plain x-rays and CT

fat-suppressed, contrast-enhanced T1-weighted images. The strength of enhancement has been histologically proven to depend on the degree of infiltration by myeloma cells, and also on vessel density (Baur et al. 2004; Nosas-Garcia 2004; Nosas-Garcia et al. 2005). Therefore, contrast-enhanced MRI may be used whenever unenhanced T1w or STIR images are inconclusive. Again, there is some age-dependence, but as a rule a signal increase by 40% or more is deemed pathological (Baur et al. 2004). Dynamic contrast-enhanced MRI may be used to better assess the kinetics of contrast enhancement (Fig. 7.4).

Solid myeloma nodules are homogeneously T1-hypointense and hyperintense on fat-suppressed images and show a strong enhancement on post-contrast images (Fig. 7.5). A breech of the cortical bone is easy to see, as the signal-free bone contour is interrupted, and the tumor extends beyond it. The distinction between diffuse and micronodular patterns is not sharp, and thus such discrimination is somewhat academic. In every area of bone destruction caused by myeloma a corresponding myeloma nodule should be found on MRI. A possible exception is the case of collapsed vertebrae in which compressed bone and reactive changes may cause the diagnosis to be difficult.

In *positron emission tomography* (PET or PET/CT, respectively), solid myeloma nodules have an increased uptake of 18 F-deoxyglucose (FDG), but their conspicuousness depends on the uptake of the surrounding tissue. The sensitivity of FDG-PET in vertebral bone marrow depends on the infiltration degree: in 30% of cases positive on MRI, PET was false negative, most frequently in diffuse infiltration patterns (Zamagni et al. 2007). It is more sensitive than the x-ray

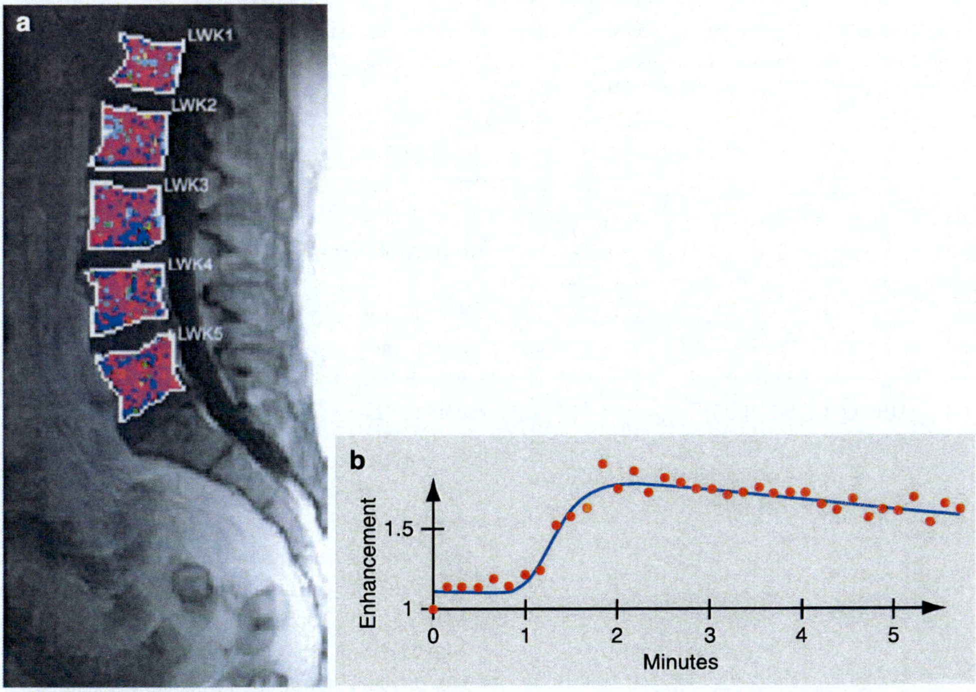

Fig. 7.4 Parameter maps from dynamic contrast-enhanced MRI (DCE MRI) (**a**) in a patient with multiple myeloma, showing diffuse and rather homogeneous contrast enhancement. A time-intensity curve obtained from these vertebrae (**b**) shows an early but nevertheless gradual rise in intensity during the first two minutes, followed by a "wash-out"

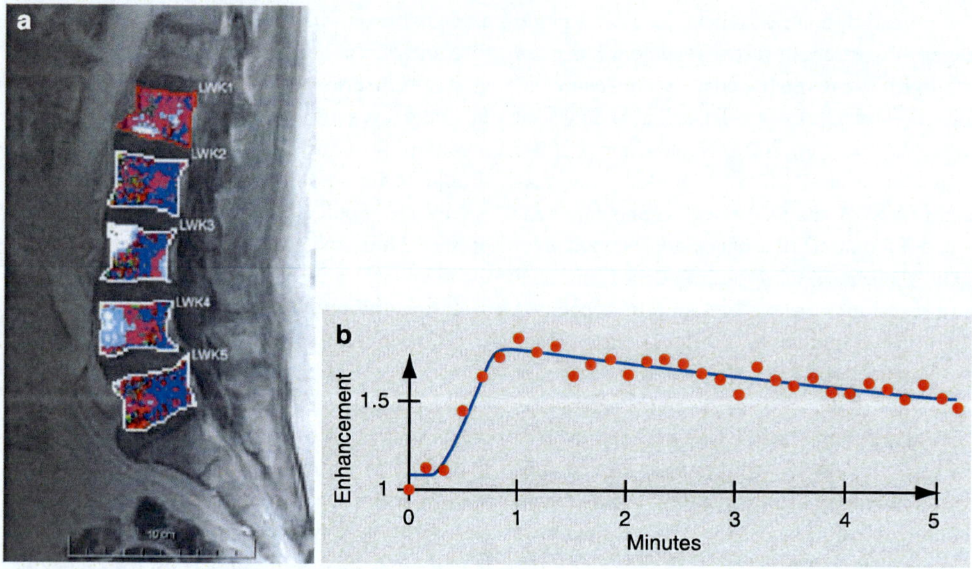

Fig. 7.5 Parameter maps from dynamic contrast-enhanced MRI (DCE MRI) (**a**) in a patient with multiple myeloma, showing markedly inhomogeneous enhancement and "hot spots" in the third and fourth vertebra, which on static images corresponded to solid plasma cell tumors. The time-intensity curve obtained from these areas (**b**) shows a marked and sharp rise with a maximum at one minute after injection, followed by a wash-out. Note the distinct difference between the curves in 7.4b (diffuse pattern) and 7.5b (focal pattern)

skeletal survey (Zamagni et al. 2007), but less sensitive than multidetector-CT (Hur et al. 2007). However, PET-CT is better, since new MDCT scanners allow for high resolution of bone in addition to FDG uptake as a marker for avid tumor tissue. Thereby PET-CT may play an increasing role for evaluation of success of therapy (Bredella et al. 2005).

Nevertheless, PET for staging and risk assessment is favored over MRI in the Anglo-American world, the rationale being that those myeloma foci which are clinically and prognostically relevant will also be positive on PET (Durie 2006; Durie et al. 2002). In Germany, conversely, PET is hardly used for multiple myeloma, since it has been almost generally excluded from reimbursement by the legal insurers.

7.4 Differential Diagnosis

Metastases due to solid tumors are far more common than is multiple myeloma, and they may be difficult to discriminate (Ooi et al. 2006). Features in favor of multiple myeloma are:

- Osteolytic lesions in the convexity of the skull and the diaphysis of long bones
- Nonreactive, sharply delineated, lytic lesions
- Scalloping (half-moon shaped erosions of cortical bone from its inward surface)
- Marked osteoporosis
- Negative bone scan or "cold lesions"
- No primary tumor as a possible cause of bone metastases

Osteosclerotic lesions are unlikely to be myeloma, although rare forms of sclerosing myeloma have been described.

Multiple myeloma affects mostly patients aged 50 or more – an age group in which osteoporosis is common and usually not caused by malignant disease. To tell whether osteoporosis in a given patient with known myeloma is independent of or rather caused by the disease can be difficult or impossible in x-rays or CT. However, in MRI diffuse infiltration can be depicted as the underlying cause.

Degenerative changes – particularly osteochondrosis with inflammatory bone reaction – may cause pain and also signal alterations in MRI like T2 hyperintensities and contrast uptake. However, there are some typical features of benign alterations:

- Hemispheric or triangular shape
- Abutting the upper or lower end plate
- Symmetric above and below one intervertebral disk
- Loss of height and T2 signal of the adjacent disk
- Osteosclerosis in CT

Fractured vertebrae may cause significant diagnostic problems. The lack of an overt destruction does not argue against a destruction as a cause, because the compression may have obscured it. In MRI, the features of fractures caused by either osteoporosis or myeloma may be also very similar, especially in severe collapse. Low T1 and high T2 signal intensity as well as marked contrast enhancement are signs in favor of malignant involvement as the underlying cause (Cuenod et al. 1996).

Diffusion-weighted MRI of fractured vertebrae may help in differential diagnosis showing a lower apparent diffusion coefficient when malignant involvement was the cause rather than when the fracture was due to trauma or osteoporosis (Raya et al. 2006).

7.5 Staging

The most widely used staging system – among more than ten systems – is the one proposed by Durie and Salmon in 1975, where the stages, ranging from one to three, rely on blood tests (e.g., hemoglobin, calcium, paraproteins) and the results of the x-ray skeletal survey (Durie and Salmon 1975). The latter are fallible, and their prognostic implications are very insecure because many lesions are missed. Most important is the discrimination between stage 1 and 2 without signs of disease progression, needing no treatment, and stages 2 or 3, both requiring chemotherapy. For current recommendations, see (Dispenzieri et al. 2007). A survival analysis demonstrated that the degree of skeletal involvement shown on MRI was pivotal for the patient's prognosis. Including MRI findings in a clinical staging system, such as the Durie & Salmon system, significantly improved the discrimination between the three groups concerning survival (Baur et al. 2002). Cross-section imaging with either MRI (or whole-body MRI where available) or CT is progressively replacing the skeletal survey. Durie did suggest a modified staging system ("Durie & Salmon PLUS") (Durie 2006). From what is known today, one would recommend performing whole-body MRI as a primary staging examination, and using x-ray films or CT for assessing bone stability where MRI is abnormal. If no scanners with whole-body capabilities are accessible, MRI should be performed for the entire spine, and the peripheral skeleton assessed with x-ray films or whole-body low-dose CT. Compared with whole-body MRI, however, CT appears to understage multiple myeloma (Baur-Melnyk et al. 2008). In addition, a baseline bone density measurement is always recommended.

7.6 Treatment Effects

MRI is without doubt the method of choice to monitor effects of chemotherapy, since it images the tumor directly, and not only its effects on mineralized bone, which may persist despite effective treatment. Chemotherapy will cause a reduction in T2 signal intensity and reduced contrast uptake in both diffusely involved bone marrow and solid nodules (Wasser et al. 2004). Although large studies are lacking, early results show that PET-CT might be a tool to show early effects of chemotherapy (Zamagni et al. 2007). In necrotic tumor a strong reduction of FDG uptake has been found (Bredella et al. 2002; Fonti et al. 2008).

7.7 Prognostic Factors

There are two events which are hard to predict: the progression into a stage needing treatment in patients with stage 1 multiple myeloma or monoclonal gammopathy of unclear significance (MGUS), and the occurrence of major complications – particularly fractures – in patients who already are in an advanced stage. Of patients with MGUS, e.g., 1% per year progress into myeloma (Kyle et al. 2002). Blood and bone marrow tests (albumin, paraproteins, β2-microglobulin, chromosomal and genetic factors) and the urine excretion of paraproteins are important factors, and so are the initial stage and the presence or absence of skeletal abnormalities (lytic lesions, osteoporosis with compression fractures). According to the criteria of the International Myeloma Working Group, the diagnosis of absence of bone involvement still relies on plain films, and CT or MRI are tools for clarification only (International myeloma working group 2003). However, a considerable proportion of MGUS patients do have abnormal findings at MRI – most frequently diffuse ones (T1 hypointensity, salt-and-pepper appearance), occasionally also focal lesions. Very probably, their classification as having MGUS rather than multiple myeloma is false, owing to the limited sensitivity of plain films, but there is no consensus as yet, when and how they should be "upstaged." In the new staging system of Durie & Salmon PLUS (Durie 2006), in patients with MGUS, whole-body MRI or PET-CT are required to exclude myeloma involvement (Table 7.1).

In patients, stage I disease according to the old staging system, abnormalities (focal or diffuse) in the skeletal MRI imply a significantly worse prognosis (time to progression, 10–16 months) than if the MRI were normal (32–43 months) (Baur-Melnyk et al. 2005; Moulopoulos et al. 1995; Vande Berg et al. 1996; Walker et al. 2007).

In stage 2 or 3, the relevant parameter is the time until the diseases progresses clinically, particularly until complications like fractures occur. Here also, besides serum markers, a pathological MRI is an independent bad prognostic sign, in particular the intensity of contrast agent uptake (Hillengass et al. 2007).

Table 7.1 Diagnostic criteria in the Durie & Salmon PLUS staging system (according to (Durie 2006))

Classification	Whole-body MRI and/ or FDG-PET
MGUS	All negative
Stage IA	Normal skeletal survey or single lesion (smoldering)
Stage IB	<5 focal lesions or mild diffuse disease
Stage IIA/B	5–20 focal lesions or moderate diffuse disease
Stage IIIA/B	>20 focal lesions or severe diffuse disease

Subclassification in stages II and III: A normal renal function/B abnormal renal function

7.8 The Radiologist's Tasks

Diagnosis and treatment monitoring rely on bone marrow histology and serum and urine tests, such as monoclonal immunoglobins, activity markers (e.g., β-microglobulin), enzymes, blood film, electrolytes, etc. Non-secreting myeloma may be difficult to monitor; here imaging plays an even more crucial role. Generally, imaging serves to:

- Verify the extent of skeletal and extraskeletal involvement
- Supply the information required by commonly used staging systems (e.g., Durie & Salmon (PLUS))
- Assess stability of involved bones
- Assess treatment response

The x-ray skeletal survey, until now standard for staging, will probably not remain for a longer period of time, given the higher sensitivities of both CT and MRI, and the additional information they provide on marrow infiltration, local bone stability, and soft-tissue extension. By using MDCT and/or MRI, 30–40% of patients will be upstaged. Some modified staging systems (Durie and Salmon PLUS) which include whole-body MRI and/or PET-CT have been suggested.

In long bones, x-ray films are usually sufficient to assess their stability, but in vertebrae and the pelvis this is best done with CT, at least in doubtful cases. CT is also best before vertebroplasty to ensure that the posterior cortex is intact.

For treatment monitoring and follow-up, MRI is clearly superior to x-ray films, for good reasons. Areas of destruction to mineralized bone, as seen on films, are simply the tip of the iceberg, the underlying tumor being invisible, and they usually show no reaction or sclerosis though the tumor itself does respond. To some extent, the same limitations also apply to CT, although CT is capable of demonstrating solid nodules (Horger et al. 2007). In vertebrae, however, it is clearly inferior to MRI.

References

Baur A, Stäbler A, Bartl R, Lamerz R, Reiser M (1996) Infiltrationsmuster des Plasmozytoms in der Magnetresonanztomographie. Fortschr Röntgenstr 164:457–463

Baur A, Stäbler A, Steinborn M, Schnarkowski P, Pistitsch C, Lamerz R, Bartl R, Reiser M (1998) Magnetresonanztomographie beim Plasmozytom: Wertigkeit verschiedener Sequenzen bei diffuser und fokaler Infiltrationsform. Fortschr Röntgenstr 168:323–329

Baur A, Stäbler A, Nagel D, Lamerz R, Bartl R, Hiller E, Wendtner C, Bachner F, Reiser M (2002) Magnetic resonance imaging as a supplement for the clinical staging system of Durie and Salmon? Cancer 95:1334–1345

Baur A, Bartl R, Pellengahr C, Baltin V, Reiser M (2004) Neovascularization of bone marrow in patients with diffuse multiple myeloma: a correlative study of magnetic resonance imaging and histopathologic findings. Cancer 101:2599–2604

Baur-Melnyk A, Buhmann S, Durr HR, Reiser M (2005) Role of MRI for the diagnosis and prognosis of multiple myeloma. Eur J Radiol 55:56–63

Baur-Melnyk A, Buhmann S, Becker C, Schoenberg SO, Lang N, Bartl R, Reiser MF (2008) Whole-body MRI versus whole-body MDCT for staging of multiple myeloma. Am J Roentgenol 190:1097–1104

Bredella MA, Caputo GR, Steinbach LS (2002) Value of FDG positron emission tomography in conjunction with MR imaging for evaluating therapy response in patients with musculoskeletal sarcomas. Am J Roentgenol 179: 1145–1150

Bredella MA, Steinbach L, Caputo G, Segall G, Hawkins R (2005) Value of FDG PET in the assessment of patients with multiple myeloma. Am J Roentgenol 184:1199–1204

Cuenod CA, Laredo JD, Chevret S, Hamze B, Naouri JF, Chapaux X, Bondeville JM, Tubiana JM (1996) Acute vertebral collapse due to osteoporosis or malignancy: appearance on unenhanced

7

and gadolinium-enhanced MR images. Radiology 199:541–549

Dispenzieri A, Rajkumar SV, Gertz MA, Fonseca R, Lacy MQ, Bergsagel PL, Kyle RA, Greipp PR, Witzig TE, Reeder CB, Lust JA, Russell SJ, Hayman SR, Roy V, Kumar S, Zeldenrust SR, Dalton RJ, Stewart AK (2007) Treatment of newly diagnosed multiple myeloma based on Mayo Stratification of Myeloma and Risk-adapted Therapy (mSMART): consensus statement. Mayo Clin Proc 82:323–341

Durie BG (2006) The role of anatomic and functional staging in myeloma: description of Durie/Salmon plus staging system. Eur J Cancer 42:1539–1543

Durie BG, Salmon SE (1975) A clinical staging system for multiple myeloma. Correlation of measured myeloma cell mass with presenting clinical features, response to treatment, and survival. Cancer 36(3):842–854

Durie BG, Waxman AD, D'Agnolo A, Williams CM (2002) Whole-body (18)F-FDG PET identifies high-risk myeloma. J Nucl Med 43:1457–1463

Fonti R, Salvatore B, Quarantelli M, Sirignano C, Segreto S, Petruzziello F, Catalano L, Liuzzi R, Rotoli B, Del Vecchio S, Pace L, Salvatore M (2008) 18 F-FDG PET/CT, 99mTc-MIBI, and MRI in evaluation of patients with multiple myeloma. J Nucl Med 49:195–200

Hillengass J, Wasser K, Delorme S, Kiessling F, Zechmann C, Benner A, Kauczor HU, Ho AD, Goldschmidt H, Moehler T (2007) Lumbar bone marrow microcirculation measurements from dynamic contrast-enhanced MRI is a predictor of event-free survival in progressive multiple myeloma. Clin Cancer Res 13:475–481

Horger M, Kanz L, Denecke B, Vonthein R, Pereira P, Claussen CD, Driessen C (2007) The benefit of using whole-body, low-dose, nonenhanced, multidetector computed tomography for follow-up and therapy response monitoring in patients with multiple myeloma. Cancer 109:1617–1626

Hur J, Yoon CS, Ryu YH, Yun MJ, Suh JS (2007) Efficacy of multidetector row computed tomography of the spine in patients with multiple myeloma: comparison with magnetic resonance imaging and fluorodeoxyglucose-positron emission tomography. J Comput Assist Tomogr 31:342–347

International myeloma working group (2003) Criteria for the classification of monoclonal gammopathies, multiple myeloma and related disorders: a report of the International Myeloma Working Group. Br J Haematol 121(5): 749–757

Kyle RA, Therneau TM, Rajkumar SV, Offord JR, Larson DR, Plevak MF, Melton LJ III (2002) A long-term study of prognosis in monoclonal gammopathy of undetermined significance. N Engl J Med 346:564–569

Mahnken AH, Wildberger JE, Gehbauer G, Schmitz-Rode T, Blaum M, Fabry U, Gunther RW (2002) Multidetector CT of the spine in multiple myeloma: comparison with MR imaging and radiography. Am J Roentgenol 178:1429–1436

Moulopoulos LA, Dimopoulos MA, Smith TL, Weber DM, Delasalle KB, Libshitz HI, Alexanian R (1995) Prognostic significance of magnetic resonance imaging in patients with asymptomatic multiple myeloma. J Clin Oncol 13:251–256

Mulkern RV, Schwartz RB (2003) In re: characterization of benign and metastatic vertebral compression fractures with quantitative diffusion MR imaging. Am J Neuroradiol 24(7):1489–1490; author reply 1490–1491

Nosas-Garcia S (2004) Dynamic contrast-enhanced MRI for assessing the disease activity of multiple myeloma: comparison with histological and clinical markers. Diss Med Fak University, Heidelberg

Nosas-Garcia S, Moehler T, Wasser K, Kiessling F, Bartl R, Zuna I, Hillengass J, Goldschmidt H, Kauczor HU, Delorme S (2005) Dynamic contrast-enhanced MRI for assessing the disease activity of multiple myeloma: a comparative study with histology and biochemical markers. J Magn Reson Imaging 22:154–162

Ooi GC, Chim JC, Au WY, Khong PL (2006) Radiologic manifestations of primary solitary extramedullary and multiple solitary plasmacytomas. Am J Roentgenol 186:821–827

Raya JG, Dietrich O, Reiser MF, Baur-Melnyk A (2006) Methods and applications of diffusion imaging of vertebral bone marrow. J Magn Reson Imaging 24:1207–1220

Vande Berg BC, Lecouvet FE, Michaux L, Labaisse M, Malghem J, Jamart J, Maldague BE, Ferrant A, Michaux JL (1996) Stage I multiple myeloma: value of MR imaging of the bone marrow in the determination of prognosis. Radiology 201:243–246

Walker R, Barlogie B, Haessler J, Tricot G, Anaissie E, Shaughnessy JD Jr, Epstein J, van Hemert R, Erdem E, Hoering A, Crowley J, Ferris E, Hollmig K, van Rhee F, Zangari M, Pineda-Roman M, Mohiuddin A, Yaccoby S, Sawyer J,

Angtuaco EJ (2007) Magnetic resonance imaging in multiple myeloma: diagnostic and clinical implications. J Clin Oncol 25:1121–1128

Wasser K, Moehler T, Neben K, Nosas S, Heiss J, Goldschmidt H, Hillengass J, Düber C, Kauczor HU, Delorme S (2004) Dynamische MRT des Knochenmarks zum Monitoring des Multiplen Myeloms unter Thalidomid-Monotherapie oder Kombination mit CED-Chemotherapie. Fortschr Röntgenstr 176:1285–1295

Wasser K, Moehler T, Nosas-Garcia S, Rehm C, Bartl R, Goldschmidt H, Düber C, Kauczor HU, Delorme S (2005) Korrelation zwischen MRT und Histopathologie des Knochenmarks bei Patienten mit Multiplem Myelom. Fortschr Röntgenstr 177:1116–1122

Zamagni E, Nanni C, Patriarca F, Englaro E, Castellucci P, Geatti O, Tosi P, Tacchetti P, Cangini D, Perrone G, Ceccolini M, Brioli A, Buttignol S, Fanin R, Salizzoni E, Baccarani M, Fanti S, Cavo M (2007) A prospective comparison of 18 F-fluorodeoxyglucose positron emission tomography-computed tomography, magnetic resonance imaging and whole-body planar radiographs in the assessment of bone disease in newly diagnosed multiple myeloma. Haematologica 92:50–55

Zechmann C, Giesel FL, Hillengass J, Mehndiratta A, Delorme S, Moehler M (2007) Where is the primary tumor? Lancet 370:1800

Part IV

Therapy

Novel Drugs in Myeloma: Harnessing Tumour Biology to Treat Myeloma

8

Kevin D. Boyd, Faith E. Davies, and Gareth J. Morgan

Contents

G.J. Morgan (✉)
Section of Haemato-Oncology,
The Institute of Cancer Research,
15 Cotswold Road, Sutton, Surrey,
SM2 5NG, United Kingdom
e-mail: gareth.morgan@icr.ac.uk

Abstract Steroids and alkylating agents have formed the backbone of myeloma therapy for decades with the result that patient outcomes improved very little over this period. The situation has changed recently with the advent of immunomodulatory agents and bortezomib, and patient outcomes are now improving. The introduction of bortezomib can be viewed as particularly successful as it was designed in the laboratory to fit a target that had been identified through biological research. As such, it has formed the template for new drug discovery in myeloma, with an increased understanding of the biology of the myeloma cell leading to the definition of upregulated pathways which are then targeted with a specific agent. This chapter will examine novel agents currently in development in the context of the abnormal biology of the myeloma cell and its microenvironment.

8.1 Introduction

Conventional chemotherapy, including high dose chemotherapy with autologous stem cell rescue, is successful in producing responses in the majority of patients with newly presenting multiple myeloma. However, relapse is almost universal

T. Moehler and H. Goldschmidt (eds.), *Multiple Myeloma*,
Recent Results in Cancer Research 183, DOI: 10.1007/978-3-540-85772-3_8,

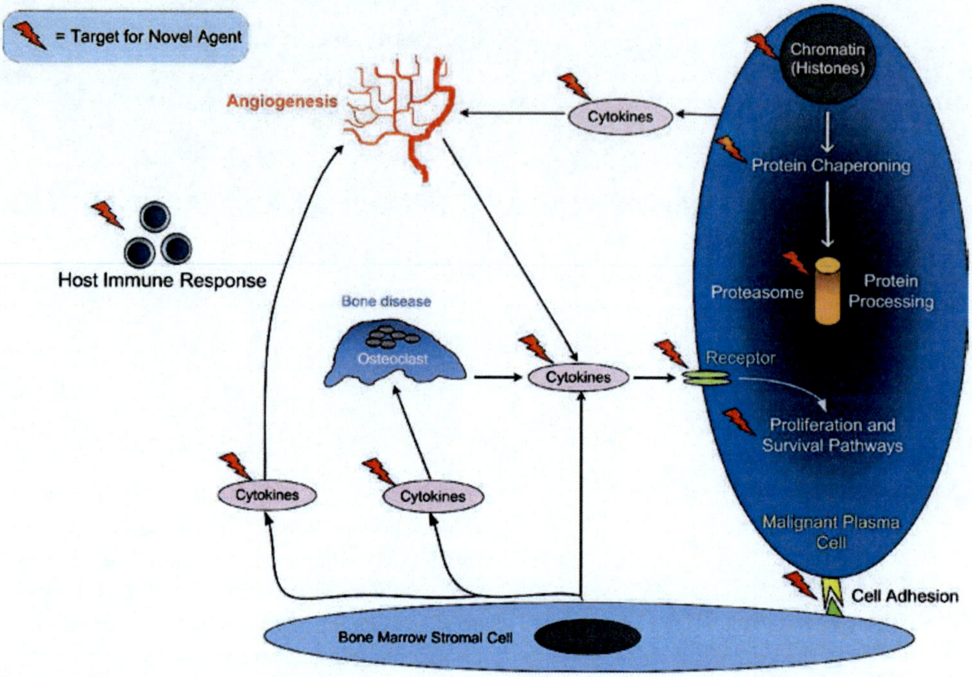

Fig. 8.1 Potential targets for novel agents within the myeloma cell and in the bone marrow microenvironment. Within the cell, drugs can target chromatin, protein chaperoning, protein processing, and intracellularsignalling pathways. Cell surface receptors and cell adhesion to stromal cells are also valid targets. In the bone marrow microenvironment, cytokines that stimulate the myeloma cell, and promote angiogenesis and bone disease can be targeted, whilst immunomodulatory drugs up-regulate the host immune system

and relapsed disease is more difficult to treat due to intrinsic or acquired drug resistance. Myeloma remains an incurable disease with a median survival of 4–5 years, and there is clearly a role for new drugs in its treatment. The development of novel agents has followed on from the huge expansion of knowledge of the biology of the myeloma cell and its interaction with the bone marrow milieu. Within the malignant plasma cell, constitutively activated signalling pathways resulting in cell growth, proliferation and avoidance of apoptosis have been defined. Within the bone marrow milieu, cytokines that stimulate angiogenesis and lytic bone disease and act as growth factors for the malignant clone have also been described. All of these pathways are potential targets for new drugs, and there are currently a raft of phase I and II trials of agents that target the myeloma cell and the cytokines and cells that make up its environment. This chapter will examine novel agents in the context of the biology of the tumour, first examining targets within the tumour cell, and then looking at targets within the bone marrow microenvironment (Fig. 8.1).

8.2 Intracellular Drug Targets

8.2.1 Targeting Signalling Pathways Within Myeloma Cells

External influences such as cytokine stimulation and physical interaction with bone marrow stromal cells trigger intracellular signalling

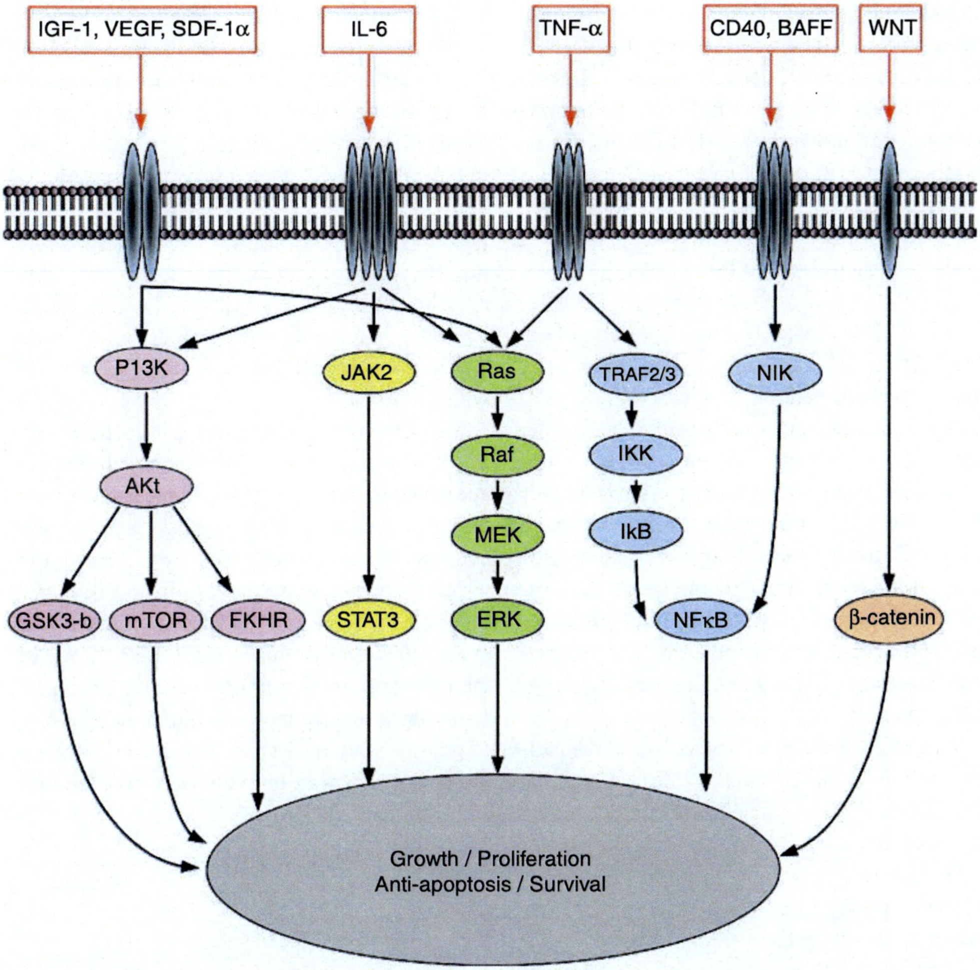

Fig. 8.2 Intracellular signalling pathways

cascades that contribute to the malignant phenotype of the myeloma cell, namely, avoidance of apoptosis, survival, growth and proliferation. Signalling pathways thought to be important in myeloma are the Ras/Raf/MEK/MAPK pathway, the JAK/STAT3 pathway, the P13K/Akt/mTOR pathway, the canonical and non-canonical NF-κB pathway and the Wnt/β-catenin pathway. In addition, the Wnt pathway has been identified as being important in osteolytic bone disease. Inhibition of any of these pathways has the potential to decrease the survival advantage of the myeloma cell and they all therefore constitute valid drug targets (Fig. 8.2).

8.2.1.1 The Ras/Raf/MEK/MAPK Pathway

The Mitogen-activated protein kinase (MAPK) cascade is a key signalling pathway involved in the regulation of cell differentiation, proliferation and survival. The pathway can be stimulated by many cytokines, including interleukin-6 (IL-6), insulin-like growth factor-1 (IGF-1), vascular endothelial growth factor (VEGF), tumour necrosis factor-α (TNFα), interleukin−21 (IL-21) and stromal cell derived factor-1 (SDF-1), which activate the Ras/Raf serine/threonine kinases. Raf activates the MAPK/ERK kinase (MEK) which in turn activates the extracellular signal-related kinase (ERK) (Roberts and Der 2007). ERK causes autocrine upregulation of the pathway, essential for the malignant phenotype. Mutations of the oncoprotein Ras were found in 23% of patients with myeloma in one case series, which makes it the most commonly mutated gene in myeloma (Chng et al. 2008b). Mutated cases had features associated with greater tumour burden such as higher plasma cell percentage on bone marrow biopsy, higher beta-2-microglobulin (β2m) and more advanced International Staging System (ISS) stage. Moreover, although mutated cases had similar response rates to non-mutated cases, responses were short-lived with shorter progression-free survival (PFS) and overall survival (OS) times.

One of the first steps of signalling in the pathway involves the transfer of farnesyl groups from farnesyl diphosphate to Ras, which allows Ras to be attached to the intracellular membrane. This step is targeted by *farnesyl transferase inhibitors* (FTIs), three of which have been demonstrated to have anti-myeloma activity. *Perillic acid* and *FTI-277* have induced apoptosis and inhibited the growth of myeloma cell lines (Beaupre et al. 2003; Bolick et al. 2003). *Tipifarnib (R115777)* has undergone a phase II trial involving 43 myeloma patients that showed it to be well tolerated and associated with disease stabilisation in 64% of patients (Alsina et al. 2004). This trial showed treatment with Tipifarnib to be associated with decreased levels of phosphorylated Akt and Signal Transducer and Activator of Transcription 3 (STAT3) but not ERK, suggesting that it may act through Ras-independent pathways. This has been borne out in research showing that Tipifarnib's in vitro efficacy does not correlate with Ras mutation status or inhibition of farnesyl transferase (Beaupre et al. 2004; Buzzeo et al. 2005; Armand et al. 2007). FTIs can potentially inhibit multiple farnesylated protein substrates involved in tumour proliferation, so although the initial rationale for their use was based on the knowledge of the importance of Ras in myeloma, they may work primarily through pathways other than the MAPK cascade. The pathway can, however, be targeted at other points. *Sorafenib (BAY 43-9006)* is a multikinase inhibitor that targets Raf and is being used in trials including patients with myeloma.

MEK has been targeted by the drug *AZD6244*. In vitro studies of this drug show it to trigger apoptosis in myeloma cell lines, sensitise cells to other chemotherapy agents, and inhibit cytokine-induced activation of osteoclasts which have an important role in the development of myeloma associated bone disease (Tai et al. 2007). Activation of MEK/ERK is one of the mechanisms of acquired steroid resistance, so combination regimens that involve blockade of this pathway may show synergism or sensitise previously drug-resistant tumours (Tsitoura and Rothman 2004).

8.2.1.2 The Janus Kinase (JAK)/STAT Pathway

The Janus Kinase (JAK)/STAT3 pathway is stimulated by cytokines such as IL-6 and IL-21 and has been shown to be constitutively activated in ~50% of primary myeloma samples, whilst suppression of STAT3 in these samples with curcumin leads to apoptosis (Bharti et al. 2004). Several other agents have been used to block STAT3 activity in myeloma cells, including the JAK 2 inhibitor *AG490* (De Vos et al. 2000), the pan-JAK inhibitor *pyridine 6* (Pedranzini et al. 2006) and *atiprimod* (Amit-Vazina et al. 2005), with similar results of decreased tumour cell viability and increased apoptosis. However, if myeloma cells are in the presence of bone marrow stromal cells, simultaneous inhibition of the MEK/ERK pathway and the JAK/STAT pathway is required in order to induce apoptosis (Chatterjee et al. 2004). This may be a consideration in the design of future drug trials. Currently atiprimod is the only agent targeting this pathway that has been moved forward into phase I/II patient trials. Preclinical studies have shown this anti-inflammatory agent to inhibit STAT3 activation, reducing the proliferative cytokine IL-6 and down-regulating the anti-apoptotic proteins bcl-2, bcl-X(L) and mcl-1 leading to cell death (Amit-Vazina et al. 2005). Mouse models have confirmed the potential utility of this drug (Neri et al. 2007).

8.2.1.3 The Phosphatidylinositol-3 Kinase (PI3-K)/Akt Pathway

IL-6 and IGF-1 have been shown to mediate proliferation and drug resistance through this pathway (Tu et al. 2000). Activation of Akt has been identified in ~50% of primary myeloma samples (Zollinger et al. 2008). IL-6 induces Akt phosphorylation, which in turn phosphorylates several downstream targets including mammalian target of rapamycin (mTOR), GSK-3B and forkhead transcription factor (FKHR). Upregulation of this pathway has been shown to inactivate FKHR, leading to G1/S phase transition. mTOR, a serine/threonine protein kinase, also regulates the G1/S phase gateway, up-regulating expression of downstream targets such as the D-Cyclins resulting in cellular proliferation. Akt activation has also been linked to resistance to dexamethasone-mediated apoptosis, mediated through inactivation of capsase-9(Hideshima et al. 2001). Blockade of this pathway should therefore lead to G1 growth arrest, and sensitization to steroid-induced apoptosis, and when Akt is down-regulated by siRNA constructs in activated samples, apoptosis is induced.

The pathway has been targeted at several points. P13-K has four class I isoforms (p110α, p110β, p110δ, p110γ), all of which can be inhibited in the laboratory with agents such as LY294002 which have poor solubility. *SF1126* is a soluble conjugate of this agent and retains its efficacy against all class I P13-K isoenzymes. It has demonstrated synergy with bortezomib, vincristine, steroids and alkylating agents and is currently in phase I trials (David et al. 2008). Pichromene is another drug capable of inhibiting all four P13-K enzymatic activities, leading to reduced expression of cyclins D1, D2 and D3 (Mao et al. 2008) Inhibitors of the individual enzymatic isoforms are also in development, including *CAL-101*, which has been shown to induce apoptosis in cell lines even in the presence of bone marrow stromal cells (Ikeda et al. 2008b). Downstream from P13-K, Akt has been targeted by *Perifosine*, a synthetic alkylphospholipid that inhibits phosphorylation, and therefore activation, of Akt. It has been shown to be cytotoxic to myeloma cell lines both when they are in isolation and when they are in the presence of bone marrow stromal cells, to show synergism to MEK inhibitors, dexamethasone and doxorubicin, and to have anti-myeloma activity in a mouse model (Hideshima et al. 2006a). A clinical trial using perifosine monotherapy in 48 patients induced a minor response in one patient, with stable disease in 22 patients. Perifosine with dexamethasone was used in the same trial by 31 patients with progressive disease, with four showing a partial response, eight a minor response and 15 with stable disease (Richardson et al. 2007c). It has also been used in combination with bortezomib with an overall response rate (ORR) of 40%, and with lenalidomide + dexamethasone with an ORR of 50% (Richardson et al. 2007b; Jakubowiak et al. 2008). These response rates are similar to those obtained with their respective partner drugs without perifosine, so it is difficult from these small trials to assess if any benefit is derived from the addition of perifosine. In the bortezomib trial, a 37% response rate was reported in patients classed as previously resistant to bortezomib, so its role may lie in sensitising chemotherapy-resistant myeloma. Other Akt inhibitors have been developed such as phosphatidylinositol ether lipid analogues (PIAs) and API-2, but these have not been characterised in myeloma yet.

Rapamycin is an antifungal compound produced naturally by *Streptomyces hygroscopicus* which has been discovered to be a specific inhibitor of mTOR, inducing G0/G1 arrest, and sensitising myeloma cells to dexamethasone-induced apoptosis (Stromberg et al. 2004). In vitro studies suggest that it may be synergistic with both bortezomib and lenalidomide (Raje et al. 2004; O'Sullivan et al. 2006). Two rapamycin analogues, *temsirolimus (CCI-779)* and *RAD-001*, have been developed which work by binding to the FK506 binding protein FKBP-12 which then binds to and inhibits mTOR (LoPiccolo et al. 2008). Temsirolimus has demonstrated induction of apoptosis and inhibition of proliferation in a myeloma mouse model (Frost et al. 2004), and also down-regulation of VEGF thereby reducing angiogenesis (Frost et al. 2007). A phase I trial combining temsirolimus with bortezomib showed a tolerable side-effect profile with an overall response rate (ORR) of 33%, and phase II studies are ongoing (Ghobrial et al. 2008). The use of RAD-001 has yet to be reported in myeloma. It has been suggested that inhibition of mTOR may feedback to produce upregulation of upstream elements of the pathway such as Akt, and that P13-K and Akt may be better targets within this pathway (Yap et al. 2008). This will need to be examined in further experimental work.

8.2.1.4 The Nuclear Factor-Kappa B (NF-κB) Pathway and the Ubiquitin Proteasome System

NF-κB is a transcription factor which has been found to be upregulated in both tumour and stromal cells of patients with myeloma. The constitutive activation of NF-κB in myeloma cells deregulates cell cycle and apoptotic pathways, whilst in the stromal cells it triggers the production of cytokines such as IL-6 and B-Cell Activating Factor (BAFF) which cause paracrine stimulation of the myeloma cells, including upregulation of the NF-κB pathway itself (Chauhan et al. 1996; Tai et al. 2006). Within the tumour cells, there are two NF-κB pathways, the canonical and non-canonical, both of which involve the proteasome. In the canonical pathway, an inhibitor of IκB kinase β (IKKβ) phosphorylates the inhibitory IκB proteins which are then processed by the proteasome leading to their inactivation. In the non-canonical pathway, IKKα phosphorylates p100/NFκB2, leading to the removal of an inhibitory C-terminal by the proteasome. The end result of both pathways is accumulation of NFκB in the nucleus. Constitutive activation of both pathways has been linked to mutations of multiple genes such as *TRAF3* and *CYLD* in myeloma (Annunziata et al. 2007; Keats et al. 2007).

The ubiquitin proteasome system (UPS) is responsible for intracellular protein degradation. Proteins are conjugated with a polypeptide, ubiquitin, and are then processed by the 26S proteasome, which consists of 19S flanking units controlling entrance to the 20S core (Peters et al. 1991). Within the 20S core proteolysis occurs by three activities; chymotrypsin-like (CT-L), trypsin-like (T-L) and caspase-like (C-L) (Chauhan et al. 2008). The proteasome is involved in processing many proteins involved in progression through cell cycle and survival. Pharmacological inhibition of the proteasome causes a build-up of mis-folded and unwanted proteins, including the inhibitory NF-κB proteins such as IκB, resulting in apoptosis.

Bortezomib (PS-341) is a boronic acid dipeptide which inhibits the 26S Proteasome, specifically the CT-L and C-L proteasomal activities. Although inhibition of IκB degradation appears to be the major target of bortezomib, it has been shown to affect other pathways through inhibition of ubiquitinated proteins other than those of the NF-κB pathway and through other direct mechanisms. For example, it may indirectly downregulate both the JAK/STAT and P13-K/Akt pathways via downregulation of gp130 (Hideshima et al. 2003a). It may also affect DNA repair by cleavage of DNA repair enzymes, and phosphorylate p53 causing its activation (Hideshima et al. 2003b). The APEX study showed bortezomib monotherapy to be superior to dexamethasone in patients with relapsed myeloma (Richardson et al. 2005b). OR rates were 43% in the bortezomib group versus 17% in the dexamethasone group, which resulted in a superior overall survival (OS) of 29.8 months versus 23.7 months, despite 62% of the steroid group crossing over to the bortezomib arm (Richardson et al. 2007). Although it remains the only single-agent to show a survival benefit in relapsed myeloma patients, the fact that the majority of relapsed patients fail to respond to monotherapy has lead to a multitude of clinical trials incorporating bortezomib with other agents in order to improve response rates. The combination of bortezomib and liposomal doxorubicin has been shown to lead to improved time to progression and improved survival compared to bortezomib monotherapy (Orlowski et al. 2007b). Bortezomib has been shown to improve progression free survival (PFS) when combined with melphalan+prednisolone in a large phase III trial in newly presenting patients not suitable for auto-transplantation (San Miguel et al. 2008). Bortezomib has therefore been demonstrated to show synergism with conventional chemotherapy and novel agents, and to improve outcome in newly presenting and relapsed patients. Its current place in the treatment of myeloma, both in terms of optimal partner drugs and sequence of treatment, remains to be defined and is likely to change as newer agents become available.

Based on the success of bortezomib, other proteasome inhibitors have been developed with a view to increasing efficacy, altering the side-effect profile and providing more convenient dosing. *Carfilzomib (PR-171)* is an intravenous preparation that blocks CT-L activity but differs from bortezomib in that it shows minimal cross-reactivity with other catalytic sites within the proteasome or with other proteasome classes and may therefore have a more favourable side-effect profile. It activates apoptosis via caspase 8 and 9 in a similar fashion to bortezomib, but is more potent. Two phase II trials have been reported using carfilzomib as monotherapy in relapsed patients. One demonstrated an ORR of 54% in bortezomib naïve patients, which dropped to 19% in patients previously exposed to bortezomib. Deterioration in renal function was seen in five patients, two of which were related to tumour lysis syndrome which may be evidence of potency of the drug (Orlowski et al. 2007; Vij et al. 2009). A second was in a particularly treatment refractory group of patients which may account for the disappointing response rate of 14%. Increases in creatinine were again seen in this trial, although there was no study discontinuation due renal failure (Jagannath et al. 2009). More recent patient assessments have suggested that concurrently administering intravenous fluids with carfilzomib resolves this issue. Neurotoxicity was reported at low rates in these two trials, and chronic administration of carfilzomib in experimental animals does not result in neurotoxicity, raising the possibility that bortezomib-associated peripheral neuropathy may not be a class effect (Demo et al. 2009). A new approach to improving the side-effect profile of proteasome inhibitors is to target the immunoproteasome, a proteasomal variant that is only found in haemopoietic cells. *NPI0052* differs from bortezomib in several ways, not least of which is that it is orally active in animal models. It blocks all three proteasomal activities (CT-L, T-L and C-L) compared to the CT-L and T-L inhibition of bortezomib, and irreversibly binds to the proteasome whereas bortezomib is a reversible inhibitor. It also appears to induce apoptosis via different signalling pathways, with NPI0052 apoptosis mediated via caspase 8, whereas bortezomib requires activation of both caspase 8 and caspase 9 (Chauhan et al. 2005). It is a more potent inhibitor of the NF-κB pathway. Whether these biological differences translate into improved efficacy needs to be evaluated in clinical trials. The compound *IPSI-001* has been identified as a potent immunoproteasome inhibitor that is effective at inhibiting the proliferation of patient myeloma samples, and is able to overcome drug resistance including bortezomib resistance (Kuhn et al. 2008). Carfilzomib also has some anti-immunoproteasomal activity.

Although NF-κB pathway inhibition appears to be central to the mechanism of action of proteasome inhibitors, their effects are broader than this and attempts have therefore been made to specifically target the pathway. Kinase inhibitors of IκB have been developed and shown to have anti-myeloma efficacy in vitro and in mouse models (Hideshima et al. 2006b), and other novel inhibitors are in development (Meinel et al. 2008). However, no clinical trials have been reported to date, so it is not clear whether inhibiting the pathway through targets other than the proteosome will provide any advantage.

8.2.1.5 The Wingless/int (Wnt)/β-Catenin Pathway

Wnts are a family of glycoproteins that bind to frizzled transmembrane receptors on the myeloma cell, leading to intracellular accumulation of unphosphorylated β-catenin which is normally degraded by the proteasome. Stimulation of myeloma cell lines with Wnt-3a has been shown to lead to cytoplasmic accumulation and nuclear localization of β-catenin, which then binds to T-cell factor transcriptional factors to activate downstream targets such as c-myc and Cyclin D2 resulting in cellular proliferation (Derksen et al. 2004). It has been suggested that the pathway is constitutively activated in myeloma due to hypermethylation (and therefore suppression) of genes acting as negative regulators of the pathway (Chim et al. 2007). A small molecule inhibitor of the nuclear binding of β-catenin to its transcriptional factor, *PKF115-584*, has been shown to be cytotoxic to myeloma cell lines and patient myeloma cells (Sukhdeo et al. 2007). There are no clinical trials at present, and the effect of any Wnt pathway inhibitor on osteolytic bone disease, which is thought to be largely mediated by the Wnt-signalling antagonist dickkopf1, would need to be carefully monitored, as our current understanding of this pathway suggests that its inhibition may result in decreased myeloma cellular proliferation, but a paradoxical increase in osteolytic activity that may exacerbate destructive bone disease.

8.2.2 Targeting the Unfolded Protein Response

The endoplasmic reticulum is responsible for post-translational modification and folding of proteins. This system is placed under stress in myeloma cells, where there is overproduction of secretary proteins, triggering a complex pathway known as the Unfolded Protein Response (UPR) which aims to prevent the accumulation of misfolded proteins. If this system fails, proteins are eliminated by ubiquitination and proteasomal digestion, or alternatively by the aggresome.

The UPR is complex, initiated by three transmembrane receptors which diverge into several pathways. The protein chaperone heat shock protein 90 (HSP90) is involved in the functioning of all three endoplasmic reticulum bound receptor pathways. HSP90 overexpression is seen in myeloma tumour cells, but not in normal plasma cells (Chatterjee et al. 2007). HSP90 inhibition should be a promising treatment as, although it only targets a single biological function, the number of chaperone client proteins affected is large and includes IGFR1 and FGFR3 as well as key proteins of the NF-κB pathway such as NIK and IKK (Qing et al. 2006). Upregulation of HSP90, HSP70 and HSP27 is seen in myeloma cells treated with bortezomib, suggesting a protective effect to the stress induced on the cell by proteasome inhibition, and providing the rationale for combining proteasome inhibition with HSP inhibition in clinical trials.

The antibiotic geldanamycin binds to HSP90, interfering with its chaperone function, and treatment of cell lines with analogues of geldanamycin causes myeloma cell death due to the unfolded protein response death pathway (Davenport et al. 2007). The first anti-cancer agents directed against HSP90 were therefore analogues of geldanamycin. *Tanespimycin* (*KOS-953*) showed some activity in phase I trials with two partial responses (PRs), one minimal response (MR) and six stable diseases (SDs) recorded in 22 patients so was moved into a phase II trial combined with bortezomib (Richardson et al. 2005a). Preliminary data from this showed three responses in bortezomib refractory patients, and responses of>PR in 7/19 bortezomib naïve patients (Richardson et al. 2007d), and there is now a phase III trial underway of bortezomib+tanespimycin versus bortezomib. More recently, several HSP90 inhibitors that are not derived from geldanamycin have been developed with some evidence that they may have unique properties and actions relative to geldanamycin (Okawa et al. 2008). *NVP-AUY922* is a diarylisoxazole-based drug that has been shown to effectively induce apoptosis in some myeloma cell lines (Stuhmer et al. 2008). A phase I trial is underway in solid tumours, and this agent warrants further attention in myeloma. A phase I trial of another non-geldanamycin derived HSP 90 inhibitor, *KW2478*, is underway and to date has demonstrated tolerability, but no significant clinical responses at the doses used (Cavenagh et al. 2008). However, the maximum tolerated dose has not been reached in this study and dose escalation is ongoing. There is some evidence that inhibition of HSP90 leads to upregulation of the HSP70 family of heat-shock proteins, which may be a mechanism of resistance to this class of drug. Simultaneous inhibition of HSP90 and HSP72 may therefore be required for maximum anti-tumour effect (Davenport et al. 2008).

Another way of targeting the cell protein handling system is through inhibition of the aminopeptidase enzyme system that catalyses the hydrolysis of amino acids from the N terminus of proteins. The aminopeptidase inhibitor *CHR-2797* has been demonstrated to induce apoptosis in a panel of myeloma cell lines and patient samples, and to show synergy with dexamethasone (Davies et al. 2007a). A Phase I trial of patients with haematological malignancies demonstrated efficacy in acute myeloid leukaemia but only enrolled two patients with myeloma, but based on the encouraging in vitro data, further clinical trials in myeloma are warranted (Davies et al. 2007b).

8.2.3 Targeting Chromatin

Epigenetic changes constitute alterations in the gene expression pattern not attributable to the primary base sequence, and include the way that our DNA is packaged by histones and abnormal DNA methylation. Histones are the protein spools around which DNA is wound, without which it would not be possible to package the genome into the nucleus. For mRNA transcription to occur, the tight histone coils need to relax and open, so the histones act as transcription regulators. Histone deacetylation by histone deacetylase (HDAC) results in a closed chromatin pattern to which transcription factors cannot bind, leading to gene silencing, whereas acetylation by histone acetyltransferase (HAT) opens up the chromatin structure to allow transcription. Haematological malignancies have been shown to mediate transcriptional repression of tumour suppressor genes through recruitment of HDAC (Marks et al. 2001) and

HDAC inhibition of myeloma cells has been shown to result in apoptosis (Catley et al. 2003). HDAC inhibitors also act on a number of non-histone proteins that are associated with oncogenesis such as p53, HSP90 and α-tubulin. α-tubulin is deacetyated by HDAC6 and is part of the aggresome system, a protein disposal system analogous to the proteasome where misfolded proteins are transported to lysosomes by the microtubule organising centre (MTOC) to be degraded by autophagy. Inhibition of α-tubulin by tubacin produces synergy with bortezomib, providing some evidence that inhibiting both of the cell's protein disposal mechanisms is beneficial (Hideshima et al. 2005). Some of these compounds may therefore simultaneously relax the chromatin structure to allow transcription of tumour suppressor genes, inhibit the aggresomal pathway and inhibit HSP90. HDAC inhibitors are divided into six classes based on their structure, and several have been shown to have anti-myeloma efficacy.

8.2.3.1 Histone Deacetylase (HDAC) Inhibitors

Suberoylanilide hydroxamic acid (SAHA) (vorinostat) has been shown to upregulate $p21^{WAF1}$ and p53 expression and dephosphorylate Rb via inhibition of HDAC (Mitsiades et al. 2003). It has been used as a single agent in a phase I trial involving ten patients, when it was well tolerated orally and induced one MR (Richardson et al. 2007e). It has been shown to decrease proteasomic activity, so may act synergistically with bortezomib. Two phase I studies and a case series of the combination of SAHA and bortezomib have been reported. In the first study of 16 relapsed patients, eight achieved a PR or near complete response (nCR) (Badros et al. 2007). In the second two-centre study, a 26% PR rate was reported in 34 patients at one centre, and 9/22 patients showed a response at the second centre (Weber et al. 2009), whilst in the small series of six patients, one VGPR and four MRs were seen (Mazumder et al. 2008).It has also been used in a phase I trial in combination with lenalidomide + dexamethasone in nine patients and demonstrated tolerability (Siegel et al. 2009). A phase III study of SAHA + bortezomib versus bortezomib is underway.

The **depsipeptide** FK228 (Romidepsin, FR901288) was demonstrated to induce apoptosis was demonstrated to induce apoptosis in myeloma cell lines and patient tumour cells (Khan et al. 2004) and has recently been reported to show encouraging activity in a small phase II trial when given in combination with bortezomib and dexamethasone. A 67% ORR + 28% MR were seen in 18 relapsed patients, including a response in two patients who were progressing on a bortezomib maintenance programme. It is impossible to know whether the addition of depsipeptide or dexamethasone overcame the drug resistance in these cases.

LBH589 (Panobinostat) has shown potent anti-myeloma activity in vitro and potentiates the effects of other drugs such as dexamethasone, bortezomib and melphalan (Maiso et al. 2006). As well as upregulating $p21^{WAF1}$ and p53, it has been shown to control cell proliferation and survival through HSP90 and induce apoptosis through the aggresome pathway. A phase II study of panobinostat monotherapy has been reported which showed good oral tolerability, a VGPR on one patient who had previously received five lines of therapy, and a MR in one patient post ten lines of treatment (Wolf et al. 2008). Phase I trials combining panobinostat with bortezomib (Siegel et al. 2008) and lenalidomide (Spencer et al. 2009) have demonstrated the safety of these combinations.

PXD101 has demonstrated antiproliferative activity in cell lines and shows additive/synergistic effects with other agents. Its use has been reported in a phase II trial where it was given as monotherapy for two courses, and then with dexamethasone if progressive disease was reported. Twenty-four patients were enrolled, with no objective responses reported in patients exposed to monotherapy, although some stable disease was seen. A minimal response was seen with the addition of dexamethasone (Sullivan et al. 2006). *ITF2357* has been given to 15 patients with myeloma, inducing one PR (Galli et al. 2007). *SRT501 (resveratrol)* is a naturally occurring polyphenol found in red wine and is one of the sirtuin family of NAD-dependant histone deacetylases. It has been shown to induce apoptosis in myeloma cell lines by down-regulating anti-apoptotic proteins such as cyclin D1, cIAP, XIAP, survivin and bcl-2 and up-regulating pro-apoptotic gene products such as Bax and apoptosis proteasome activating factor-1 (Apaf-1), resulting in suppression of the NF-κB and STAT3 pathways and activation of apoptosis via caspase 3. A phase II trial is underway in myeloma patients starting with resveratrol monotherapy with bortezomib being added for progressive disease. *NVP-LAQ824* has been shown in vitro to inhibit the growth of tumour cells at a much lower concentration than SAHA, so may be a more potent drug (Atadja et al. 2004). It has been shown to induce apoptosis in myeloma cells and to have efficacy in a myeloma murine model, but no clinical trial data has been reported to date (Catley et al. 2003). Multiple other HDAC inhibitors are in development, including *KD5170* and *tubacin*.

8.2.3.2 Hypomethylating Agents

Hypermethylation of the 5′ gene promoter region of genes is an epigenetic mechanism of tumour suppressor gene silencing that has been shown to be present in myeloma (Takahashi et al. 2004). Inhibition of this process may therefore allow increased expression of tumour suppressor genes so constitutes a valid drug target. The DNA methyltransferase inhibitor *5-azacytidine* has been shown to induce apoptosis in myeloma cells, to overcome the survival advantage conferred by IL-6, IGF-1 and adherence to bone marrow stromal cells, and to enhance the activity of doxorubicin and bortezomib (Kiziltepe et al. 2007). It has been stated that the kinetics of its action suggests that its effect may not be mediated via DNA hypomethylation, but by protein synthesis inhibition (Khong et al. 2008). There is extensive clinical data on the use of these agents in other haematological conditions such as myelodysplasia and acute myeloid leukaemia, but none in myeloma to date.

8.2.3.3 New Alkylators

Bendamustine was synthesised in the former East German Democratic Republic in the 1960s and was used in East Germany for 30 years before German unification for the treatment of lymphoma, myeloma and breast cancer, although there were few validated studies from this time to support its use. It has structural similarities to both alkylating agents and purine analogues, and has been demonstrated to have a substance specific interaction with DNA, resulting in minimal cross resistance with other alkylators (Strumberg et al. 1996). A phase III trial has been conducted comparing melphalan + prednisolone with bendamustine + prednisolone in 131 newly presenting patients (Ponisch et al. 2006). Overall response rates were 75% in the bendamustine group and 70% in the melphalan group, with CR rates of 32% in the bendamustine group and 13% in the melphalan group. It has also demonstrated efficacy when used in combination with novel agents in the relapsed patient setting. A phase I trial of bendamustine, prednisolone and thalidomide showed a response in 24/28 patients (Ponisch et al. 2008), whilst it has been used in two phase I trials in combination with bortezomib and dexamethasone and shown impressive response rates of 84% and 88% respectively (Hrusovsky and Heidtmann 2005; Fenk et al. 2007).

8.2.4 Targeting Intracellular Cell Cycle Regulatory Proteins

8.2.4.1 Cyclin D Kinases

Cyclin D dysregulation is central to myeloma pathogenesis, and a classification system has been proposed which shows dysregulation of cyclin D pathways to be a unifying result of at least seven different disease initiating events (Bergsagel et al. 2005). D Cyclins are involved in progression through the G1/S stage of the cell cycle, and their over-expression therefore allows for uncontrolled cellular proliferation without the normal pause that allows for cells with genetic defects to be detected and undergo apoptosis. As cyclin D dysregulation is seen in virtually all myeloma samples, they make an attractive drug target, and several companies have compounds with preclinical data. *P276-00* inhibits CDK4/cyclin D1 and has been shown to inhibit cell growth and induce apoptosis through regulation of cell cycle progression, as well as overcoming the proliferative stimuli of cytokines such as IL-6 and IGF-1. Its in vitro efficacy was borne out in a myeloma mouse model, and a phase I trial is underway (Raje et al. 2009). Similar preclinical efficacy has been demonstrated for the plant cytokinin *kinetin riboside* which inhibits transactivation of *CCND2*, reducing levels of Cyclin D1 and D2 proteins, resulting in cell cycle arrest in vitro and tumour growth inhibition in xenografted mice (Tiedemann et al. 2008). Some of the novel agents seem to have narrow specificity, such as *Purvalanol* against CDK1 and *NVP-LCQ195/AT9311* against CDK1/2, whilst others are broad antagonists of cyclin D pathways with *AT7519* having activity against CDK1,2,4,5,9 and glycogen synthase (GSK) 3b, *SNS-032* inhibiting CDK2,7 and 9 and *RGB286638* having broad activity (McMillin et al. 2007; Cirstea et al. 2008; Santo et al. 2008; Wierda et al. 2008; Zeng et al. 2008). As the initial classification system suggests that either CDK1, 2 or 3 is dysregulated, it would appear that this is an example of an area where, in the future, it may be possible to tailor the drug to the patient based on genetic abnormalities detected in their myeloma clone. Before technology allows that approach, broad spectrum cyclin inhibitors may be more likely to have efficacy in any individual patient, but they may be found to have broader side effects. Clinical data are available from a Phase I trial of SNS-032 (a CDK2, 3 and 9 inhibitor) where patients with myeloma and Chronic Lymphocytic Leukemia (CLL) were treated with a once weekly infusion. Dose-limiting toxicity and tumour lysis were seen in CLL patients, but not in patients with myeloma. No objective responses were recorded, but this remains an exciting therapeutic area (Wierda et al. 2008).

8.2.4.2 Aurora Kinases

The three aurora kinases (aurora A, B and C) regulate the G2 cell cycle checkpoint and as such are intimately involved in centrosome and spindle formation. Targeting these kinases should allow for the arrest of cells at the G2 checkpoint to allow for the recognition of genomic abnormalities that would normally result in apoptosis. Over-expression of *RHAMM*, a centrosome associated gene, has been demonstrated to correlate with the degree of centrosome amplification, whilst centrosome amplification correlates with poor prognosis (Shi et al. 2007; Chng et al. 2008a). Recent data has shown that the presence of aurora A over-expression is an independent poor prognostic factor (Hose et al. 2009). It may therefore be possible to target these new agents to patients with centrosomal amplification of aurora kinase over-expression and thus improve the outlook for a group of patients who have a poor prognosis with current therapies. Data have been published on multiple aurora kinase inhibitors, including *VX-680, ZK, ADZ 1152, VE-465, ENMD-2076* and *MLN8237*, showing that they are effective in inducing apoptosis of myeloma cell lines and patient samples (Shi et al. 2007; Evans et al. 2008a, b; Gorgun et al. 2008; Wang et al. 2008b). Some of these have isoenzymatic specificities, whilst others such as *ENMD-981693* are multikinase inhibitors which also have activity against proteins such as FGFR3 (Hembrough et al. 2007). Several of these compounds have been taken forward into phase I trials, but no clinical data is available in a myeloma cohort.

8.2.4.3
Pim Kinases

The three Pim kinases are a recently described family of serine/threonine kinases which are potent inhibitors of apoptosis. They mediate this via phosphorylation of the cyclin-dependant kinase inhibitor p27(Kip1) which overcomes G1 arrest thereby allowing cell cycle progression, promoting cellular proliferation (Morishita et al. 2008). Pim-2 has been found to be transciptionally upregulated in myeloma cell lines, and its over-expression is increased by cytokine such as IL-6, BAFF and TNF-α (Asano et al. 2007). Down-regulation of Pim by inhibitory short inhibitory RNAs (siRNAs) has been shown to decrease the proliferation induced by stimulatory cytokines, and to augment the effect of dexamethasone and mTOR inhibitors. On this basis, Pim inhibitors are being taken into phase I trials.

8.2.4.4
Inhibitor of Apoptosis Proteins

Inhibitors of Apoptosis Proteins (IAPs) are a family of proteins that inhibit caspases 8 and 9 and thereby act as regulators of programmed cell death. IAPs include X-chromosome linked IAP (XIAP or BIRC4), cellular IAP 1 (c-IAP1 or BIRC2), c-IAP2 (BIRC3) and survivin, of which XIAP is the best described and possibly the most potent suppressor of apoptosis (Vucic and Fairbrother 2007). XIAP has been found at high levels in patient samples, and has been demonstrated to fall following successful treatment with both conventional chemotherapy and bortezomib (Gaponova et al. 2008). IAP inhibitors are in development and have demonstrated in vitro efficacy against a number of myeloma cell lines, as well as synergy with a range of conventional and novel agents (Khong and Spencer 2007).

8.3
Extracellular Drug Targets

Conditions outside the myeloma cell are essential to its survival. Physical interaction with bone marrow stromal cells trigger the release of cytokines from the stromal cells that mediate destructive bone disease and angiogenesis as well as directly stimulating growth and survival pathways within the tumour cells via the pathways discussed previously such as JAK/STAT3 and NF-κB. Drug resistance also seems to be mediated by cell adhesion to stromal cells.

8.3.1
Targeting Cytokines or Their Receptors

A possible advantage of abrogating upstream targets such as IL-6 and IGF-1 compared to components of the intracellular signalling pathways that they induce is the ability to affect several pathways simultaneously. Myeloma cells show a remarkable capacity to adapt and escape drug toxicity by upregulation of alternative pathways, so blockade of IL-6, which stimulates the JAK/STAT, Ras/Raf/MEK/MAPK and P13K/Akt, may be more efficacious than targeting any one of the individual downstream targets.

8.3.1.1 Interleukin-6 (IL-6)

IL-6 is possibly the most important, and certainly the most studied, of the cytokines known to be important in myeloma cell survival. High levels of IL-6 or soluble IL-6 receptor have been shown to be associated with adverse prognosis in myeloma, acting as surrogate markers of disease bulk much in the same way as β2m (Bataille et al. 1989; Pulkki et al. 1996). A proportion of tumour cells show autocrine IL-6 production, and patients with higher autocrine production have more advanced disease, whilst their tumour cells are more resistant to apoptosis (Frassanito et al. 2001). However, the major site of IL-6 production in the myeloma bone marrow appears to be stromal cells, with secretion being triggered by tumour/stromal cell binding or by secretion of cytokines such as TNFα from the tumour. Activation of the IL-6 receptor on myeloma cells triggers three signalling pathways; Ras/Raf/MEK/MAPK which appears to mediate cellular proliferation, JAK/STAT3 which mediates survival and P13K/Akt which has been shown to be important in drug resistance (Ogata et al. 1997; Catlett-Falcone et al. 1999; Hideshima et al. 2001). However, some myeloma cell lines show proliferation and survival independent of the presence of Il-6 in the growing medium, so although IL-6 does appear to be important in myeloma pathogenesis, it is not the *sine qua non* of the myeloma cell. This is reflected in disappointing results reported of clinical trials of IL-6 blockade. The IFM 99-03 trial randomised 166 patients to receive a murine anti-IL-6 monoclonal antibody (*BE-8*) or placebo as part of a tandem transplant trial in patients defined as high risk(Moreau et al. 2006). No difference was seen in OS or EFS, although this may have been due to the efficiency of the IL-6 inhibition with this particular agent. Another monoclonal antibody directed against IL-6 (*CNTO 328*) has been produced which, when used as monotherapy in relapsed patients, produced a PR in 3/13 patients (Kurzrock et al. 2008). As with the majority of novel agents, synergy with existing agents is likely to be where any clinical utility lies, and augmentation of bortezomib's effect has been demonstrated in vitro. Preliminary results of the combination of CNTO 328 and bortezomib demonstrated a 57% response rate in 21 relapsed patients (Rossi et al. 2008), and on this basis, a phase III study randomising to bortezomib +/– CNTO 328 is underway.

8.3.1.2 Insulin-Like Growth Factor-1 (IGF-1)

Binding of IGF-1 to its receptor on the myeloma cell induces activation of the Ras/Raf/MEK/MAPK, P13K/Akt pathways, and indirectly the NF-κB pathway, contributing to proliferative and anti-apoptotic cell signalling (Qiang et al. 2002). It has also been shown to inhibit the anti-myeloma activity of dexamethasone, cytotoxic chemotherapy and bortezomib providing the rationale for antagonism of IGF-1 to augment the response to these agents (Mitsiades et al. 2002, 2004). IGF-1 has been suggested to be a prognostic factor with low levels (<13 nmol/l) being associated with a median prognosis that has not been reached at 80 months (Standal et al. 2002). There is good evidence that it plays a role in myeloma pathogenesis and is therefore a valid drug target. Inhibition of the IGF-1 receptor has been achieved with monoclonal antibodies that block IGF-1 binding, and by tyrosine kinase inhibitors, with both approaches showing in vitro activity (Maiso et al. 2008). Clinical data is available on two monoclonal antibodies; *AVE1642* was administered to 14 patients with relapsed disease and was well tolerated, although no objective responses were recorded (Moreau et al. 2007). *CP-751,871* was given to 47 patients either as monotherapy, or with dexamethasone or rapamycin. Of the 27 patients that received the combination of the antibody and steroids, 2CRs and 4PRs were recorded. Interestingly, the patients with the CRs had previously been classified as refractory to dexamethasone which may provide some evidence for uncoupling of cell adhesion-mediated drug resistance (CAMDR) pathways through IGF-1 inhibition (M Lacy et al 2007).

8.3.1.3
Fibroblast Growth Factor (FGFR3)

Fifteen percent of primary myeloma samples have the t(4;14) which results in the dysregulation of two genes; fibroblast growth receptor 3 (*FGFR3*) and *MMSET*, and leads to ectopic expression of the FGFR3 tyrosine kinase receptor. This cytogenetic subgroup has a particularly poor prognosis, so finding a treatment that specifically targets this group is attractive. βFGF has been shown to be secreted by myeloma cells and is important in tumour angiogenesis. It upregulates production of IL-6 by bone marrow stromal cells, so will feed back to augment the growth and survival pathways in the tumour. Similarly, IL-6 has been shown to increase βFGF production, so there is a paracrine mutual stimulatory circuit in place (Bisping et al. 2003). Multiple tyrosine kinase inhibitors active against the FGFR3 receptor have been shown to be active against myeloma cells in vitro and in murine myeloma models, including *PRO-001, TKI 258 (CHIR-258), PKC-412, ENMD-981693* and *XL999* (Chen et al. 2004; Trudel et al. 2005, 2006, 2007; Hembrough et al. 2007). Clinical data is available on only one molecule, *AB1010*, which produced two responses in 19 patients (Arnulf et al. 2007).

8.3.1.4
Vascular Endothelial Growth Factor (VEGF)

As well as its role in tumour angiogenesis, VEGF has been demonstrated to be involved in cell migration via the P13K/AKT pathway, proliferation via the MEK/ERK pathway and survival through upregulation of mcl-1 (Podar and Anderson 2005). Increased bone marrow angiogenesis has been linked to poor outcome in myeloma, and although VEGF has not been directly linked to prognosis, it makes an attractive therapeutic target. Tyrosine kinase inhibitors that block the VEGF receptor, and anti-VEGF antibodies have both demonstrated efficacy in cell line experiments and mouse models of myeloma (Podar et al. 2004, 2006; Campbell et al. 2006). One of these molecules, *pazopanib (GW786034)*, was shown to be ineffective as monotherapy in relapsed myeloma patients (Prince et al. 2007). A humanised monoclonal antibody targeting VEGF (*Bevacizumab*) has been used in two small phase II trials, combined with lenalidomide and dexamethasone with responses reported in 7 out of 10 patients (Raschko et al. 2007) and in combination with thalidomide (Somlo et al. 2005). Larger trials will be needed to ascertain if inhibition of VEGF adds value to existing immunomodulatory drug regimens.

8.3.1.5
Platelet Derived Growth Factor Receptor β (PDGFRβ)

Dasatinib is a tyrosine kinase inhibitor that has activity against a number of receptor and non-receptor kinases, including bcr-abl, Src family kinases, c-KIT, PDGFRβ and FGFR3. FGFR3 is known to be of relevance in the t(4;14) group of patients, whilst PDGFRβ and c-Src have recently been identified as being constitutively activated in the plasma cells and endothelial cells of myeloma patients, and to mediate the release of pro-angiogenic factors such as VEGF (Coluccia et al. 2008). Dasatinib may target myeloma primarily through these receptor kinases, and it has been shown to inhibit tumour growth and angiogenesis in vitro and in myeloma mouse models. Early results of a phase II trial using dasatinib at the same dose as is used in chronic phase chronic myeloid leukaemia (70 mg BD) showed that it was reasonably well tolerated. No responses were reported at that dose, although the trial was ongoing with a planned dose increase (Wildes et al. 2007).

8.3.1.6 CD40 Ligand

Binding of CD40 ligand to its receptor triggers myeloma cell proliferation via p53-dependant pathways and migration via P13K/Akt and NF-κB signalling (Tai et al. 2003). CD40 also mediates cell binding to fibronectin, and therefore drug resistance mechanisms, in a similar way to SDF-1. Blockade of CD40 ligand binding with a monoclonal antibody (*SGN40*) has been shown to induce apoptosis in cell line experiments, to inhibit proliferation stimulated by IL-6 but not IGF-1 and to be augmented by lenalidomide (Tai et al. 2004, 2005). A second monoclonal antibody, *XmAb5485*, has been shown to induce potent antibody-dependant cell-mediated cytotoxicity against myeloma both in vitro and in mouse tumour models (Zhukovsky et al. 2008).

8.3.1.7 B-Cell Activating Factor (BAFF) and a Proliferation-Inducing Ligand (APRIL)

These two TNF family members have a similar structure and share receptor targets, BAFF interacting with transmembrane activator and calcium modulating cyclophilin ligand interactor (TACI), B-cell maturation antigen (BCMA) and B-cell activating factor receptor (BAFF-R), whilst APRIL can only bind to TACI and BCMA. Through these receptors, they stimulate Ras/Raf/MEK/MAPK, P13K/Akt and NF-κB signalling and have been shown to mediate steroid resistance in this way (Moreaux et al. 2004). They constitute possible drug targets.

8.3.1.8 TNF-Related Apoptosis-Inducing Ligand (TRAIL)

TRAIL ligands induce apoptosis in myeloma cells. This effect is inhibited by osteoprotegerin produced by osteoblasts, another example of pro-survival pathways mediated by the bone marrow milieu. However, this effect has been overcome by stimulating the TRAIL death receptor with agonists of DR4 or 5, and stimulation of this pathway has potential therapeutic implications (Locklin et al. 2007). Monoclonal TRAIL agonists such as *LBY135* exist and have shown synergy with other agents (Khong and Spencer 2007).

8.3.1.9 Fas

The stimulation of Fas receptor by Fas Ligand promotes caspase-dependant apoptotic signalling. *APO010* is a recombinant form of Fas ligand which has been shown to have preclinical anti-myeloma activity against cell lines, and to inhibit tumour growth in mouse models (Ocio et al. 2007). It has been taken forward into phase I clinical trials.

8.3.1.10 p38 mitogen-activated protein kinase (MAPK)

p38 MAPK mediates the production of multiple cytokines including IL-1, IL-6, TNFalpha, VEGF and MIP-1alpha. p38 MAPK has been targeted by the agent *SCIO-469* which decreases constitutive p38a MAPK phosphorylation, with downstream effects of inhibition of HSP27 and upregulation of p53 (Navas et al. 2006; Vanderkerken et al. 2007). In cell line experiments, it has been shown to augment bortezomib activity, whilst in myeloma mouse models, it reduced tumour size and paraprotein levels whilst reducing angiogenesis and having a beneficial effect on destructive bone disease (Hideshima et al. 2004). A phase II trial has been reported which started relapsed refractory patients on SCIO-469 monotherapy and then instituted bortezomib for patients with no response (Siegel et al. 2006). Of 62 patients treated, the best responses to monotherapy were stable disease in 24%. Combination therapy produced a PR in 26% of patients, including 4 who had previously been classed as bortezomib refractory. Preliminary work has been done on a second agent, *LY2228820*, which showed similar effects of decreased HSP27 activation, modest cytotoxicity as monotherapy but synergism with bortezomib, and inhibition of tumour growth and osteoclastogenesis in mouse models, suggesting that this class of drug may have a beneficial effect on skeletal disease (Ishitsuka et al. 2008).

8.3.2 Targeting Myeloma Cell Adhesion Molecules

8.3.2.1 Stromal Cell Derived Factor-1 (SDF-1)

SDF-1α is produced by both myeloma and stromal cells, and through binding to its receptor CXCR4 (CD184), it plays a critical role in up-regulating binding of myeloma cells to stromal cells and fibronectin. An inhibitor to CXCR4 has been developed which has been used to enhance the mobilisation of CD34+ cells for harvesting prior to autologous transplant. *AMD3100* has been shown to effectively mobilise stem cells from 71% of myeloma patients who have previously failed peripheral stem cell harvesting with chemotherapy and growth factor stimulation, thus giving the option of the proven benefit of autologous transplantation to a significant number of patients who would previously have been denied this treatment (Calandra et al. 2008). However, of equal interest may be the role of this agent in sensitising myeloma cells to other chemotherapy agents by disrupting their interaction with the protective environment of the bone marrow milieu. AMD3100 does not induce apoptosis of tumour cells by itself. However, cell lines that are resistant to bortezomib, dexamethasone, melphalan and doxorubicin in the presence of stromal cells become sensitised to these agents in the presence of AMD3100. In a murine model, mice treated with the combination of AMD3100 and bortezomib show a higher rate of tumour regression than those treated with bortezomib alone, with circulating apoptotic myeloma cells present in the circulation (Azab et al. 2009). There is one report of AMD3100 stimulating plasma cell proliferation (Kim et al. 2008) so careful evaluation of this agent will be required in clinical trials, but it has promise as an agent to overcome CAMDR.

8.3.2.2 Cell Surface 1 Surface Antigen (CS1)

CS1, a member of the immunoglobulin gene superfamily, is universally and highly expressed on myeloma cells, where it has been shown to function as a cell adhesion molecule. A humanised monoclonal antibody (*Elotuzumab (HuLuc63)*) with CS1 specificity has been produced and has been shown in preclinical trials to decrease bone marrow stromal adherence and to induce antibody-dependant cell cytotoxicty (Tai et al. 2008). This effect was augmented by dexamethasone and other chemotherapies in dexamethasone resistant cell lines, suggesting a possible role in sensitisation of tumours to other agents. In mouse xenograft models, it showed significant anti-tumour activity. Early results of a phase I trial showed no clinical responses at the first dose level, although pharmacokinetic investigations suggested that higher doses will be needed to maintain the drug concentration at the minimal biological activity level defined in the mouse models (Bensinger et al. 2007). Dose finding studies are also exploring the feasibility of its combination with lenalidomide and dexamethasone (Singhal et al. 2009) and with bortezomib (Jakubowiak et al. 2009). A concern for this drug, and anti-CD56 treatments, is that the NK cell cytotoxic anti-tumour effect may be inhibited as both of these markers are present in high numbers on NK cells.

8.3.2.3 CD56

CD56 (neural cell adhesion molecule) is present on the surface of the plasma cells of ~70% of patients with myeloma. It has a role in myeloma cell adhesion to the bone marrow stroma, and lack of expression of CD56 has previously been linked to extramedullary disease, plasma cell leukaemia and an aggressive clinical phenotype (Pellat-Deceunynck et al. 1998). However, recent analysis of a large series of myeloma patients showed that the presence or absence of CD56 had no effect on overall survival. (Mateo et al. 2008). There are two approaches to targeting cell surface molecules such as CD56 with monoclonal antibodies. One is to use the antibody to block binding of the surface receptor to its ligand to make the cell more immunogenic and therefore trigger antibody dependant cell cytotoxicity (ADCC). The second is to use the monoclonal antibody as a vehicle for delivery of toxins to the cell, in which case the cell surface marker should be chosen on the basis of being highly expressed in the malignant clone, but present in small numbers in the surface of normal cells in the haemopoietic compartment and in other tissues. This approach is taken by *IMGN901* (*huN901-DM1*) which is a humanised monoclonal antibody conjugated with the cytotoxic agent maytansinoid. Once bound to CD56, the antibody is internalised to release the cytotoxic agent within the cell. Eighteen patients with CD56+ disease have received the antibody in a phase I trial, with three MRs recorded (Chanan-Khan et al. 2008).

8.3.2.4 CD38

CD38 is a transmembrane glycoprotein involved in cell adhesion and calcium mobilisation. It is almost universally present on the surface of myeloma cells and is present in much lower numbers on other haemopoietic cells so is therefore an obvious targets for the delivery of immunotoxins. Indeed, an anti-CD38 monoclonal antibody conjugated to an analogue of ricin was one of the earliest attempts at delivering targeted treatment to the myeloma cell (Goldmacher et al. 1994). Although preclinical data looked promising with effective killing of myeloma cells with minimal cross-reactivity with haemopoietic cells, it did not lead on to clinical applications. More recently newer antibodies have been produced with the aim of instigating ADCC, and although limited preclinical data is available on these agents, one (*SAR650984*) has been shown to have an effect in mouse xenograft models (Stevenson 2006; Park et al. 2008).

8.3.2.5 CD138

CD138 is another cell surface molecule that is almost universally expressed on myeloma cells. There is recent preclinical data on *nBT062*, a monoclonal antibody conjugated to maytansinoid, with promising in vitro results and efficacy in mouse xenograft models (Ikeda et al. 2008).

8.3.2.6 CD66

CD66 has been shown to be co-expressed with CD38 in nearly all patients with myeloma (Richardson et al. 2008). It has been used in a novel way to deliver targeted radiotherapy to patients before stem cell transplantation. A monoclonal antibody conjugated to yttrium-90 has been infused as part of the conditioning therapy prior to high dose melphalan in a phase I study and was shown to be well tolerated with no significant increase in time to engraftment (Orchard et al. 2008). Focal uptake of the antibody was seen in two patients suggesting that in vivo tumour targeting was occurring. This is a novel method of delivering up to 25 Gy of radiotherapy to the bone marrow with minimal additional toxicity.

8.3.3 Targeting the Host Immune System

8.3.3.1 Immunomodulatory Drugs (IMiDs)

Thalidomide and its analogues lenalidomide and pomalidomide are collectively known as the immunomodulatory agents. They share similar mechanisms of action, although they have differing potencies and slightly different side effect profiles. Firstly, they directly activate apoptotic signalling in the myeloma cell. This is primarily achieved through capsase 8 mediated pathways, but the IMiDs also affect the cell at the mitochondrial level, causing c-jun terminal kinase (JNK) dependant release of cytochrome-c and Smac into the cytoplasm, where they regulate other cell survival pathways to mediate apoptosis (Anderson 2005). Secondly, they increase NK cell number and function to augment the host immune response against the tumour. Thalidomide has been shown not to stimulate T cells alone, but to act as a co-stimulator to trigger proliferation of anti-CD3 stimulated T cells. They cause nuclear factor of activated T-cells 2 and activator protein 1 to translocate to the nucleus via activation of P13K signalling pathways, resulting in increased IL-2 and IF-γ secretion. The end result is increased NK cell numbers, and increased antibody-dependant cell cytotoxicity (Davies et al. 2001; Hayashi et al. 2005). Thirdly, they decrease the secretion of key cytokines such as IL-6, TNF-a, VEGF and IGF-1 from bone marrow stromal cells, and in this way affect multiple downstream signalling pathways including NF-κB. The net result of these mechanisms is decreased angiogenesis, a decrease in the supportive and protective effect of the bone marrow milieu including reduced cell adhesion-mediated drug resistance, a decrease in multiple intracellular growth and proliferation pathways, a direct triggering of apoptosis and augmentation of the host cell-mediated anti-tumour immune response.

Thalidomide

Since it was withdrawn from the market in 1961 following its implication as the causative factor in phocomelia, thalidomide has enjoyed a revival based on the same anti-angiogenic properties that cause its most serious side effect, first as a treatment for erythema nodosum associated with leprosy, and more recently as an effective treatment for myeloma. The seminal study of thalidomide in myeloma treated 84 relapsed/refractory patients with a dose starting at 200 mg/day and increasing to 800 mg/day, a higher dose than that employed in most regimens today. A 32% response rate was observed (Singhal et al. 1999). A recent 10 year update on this study, which was expanded to include 169 patients, showed that 17 are still alive with ten remaining event free (van Rhee et al. 2008). Subsequent trials have demonstrated superior response rates when used with dexamethasone and highlighted some potentially serious side effects such as peripheral motor and sensory neuropathy and deep vein thrombosis (Rajkumar et al. 2006). The addition of thalidomide to the commonly used regimen of melphalan and prednisolone for patients not deemed suitable for autologous transplantation has been demonstrated to prolong progression free and overall survival in a large randomised phase III trial (Palumbo et al.

2006). Based on this data, thalidomide, usually in combination a steroid and an alkylator, has become a commonly used regimen both as induction prior to autotransplantation and as therapy for elderly patients, based on proven improved response rates in the former and proven improved survival in the latter. However, in an attempt to increase potency and to reduce side effects, analogues have been produced which may eventually supersede thalidomide.

Lenalidomide (CC-5013)

Structurally, lenalidomide has the same backbone as thalidomide, but with the addition of an amino (NH_2) group and the removal of a carbonyl (C=O) group from the phthaloyl ring. It has good oral bioavailability when administered as a once daily dose, with renal drug excretion of the unmetabolised drug. Care is therefore needed in administering lenalidomide to patients with severe renal impairment to avoid drug accumulation and toxicity, and a recommended dosing system for patients with severe renal impairment based on pharmacodynamic studies has been proposed (Chen et al. 2007). The main potential side effects of this drug are similar to thalidomide, but it has more of a propensity for causing bone marrow suppression with resulting neutropenia, so is generally administered for 21 days followed by a rest week in order to allow for recovery of blood counts.

The evidence for efficacy of lenalidomide in relapsed myeloma patients comes from two large phase III trials of essentially identical design involving 705 patients in total (MM-009 and MM-010) which were reported in the same issue of the New England Journal of Medicine (Dimopoulos et al. 2007; Weber et al. 2007). Both trials involved the administration of dexamethasone 40 mg once daily, initially for D1–4, 9–12, 17–20 for 4 months and then D1–4 only. To this was added either lenalidomide 25 mg for 21/28 or placebo. Both trials had very similar results with significantly increased overall response rates in the lenalidomide group (MM-009:61% vs 20%, $p<0.001$; MM-010: 60% vs 24%, $p<0.001$), increased time to progression (MM-009 and MM-010: 11 months vs 5 months, $p<0.001$) and improved OS (MM-009: 30 months vs 20 months, $p<0.001$; MM-010: not reached vs 20 months, $p=0.03$). The high rates of thromboembolism in this and subsequent trials containing the combination of lenalidomide and dexamethasone mean that some form of thromboprophylaxis is considered mandatory. Taken together, these trials were proof that lenalidomide improves response and survival rates in relapsed myeloma patients when used with dexamethasone. Several subgroup analyses from these trials have been reported. Given the similar structures of thalidomide and lenalidomide, it was important to establish whether patients who had previously received thalidomide derived benefit from subsequently being treated with lenalidomide. Of the 704 patients in the two pooled trials, 39% had previous exposure to thalidomide. The thalidomide naïve group had experienced less lines of therapy and a shorter duration of living with myeloma. Thalidomide exposed patients treated with lenalidomide showed higher response rates and longer PFS compared to the placebo group, although the PFS was less than in those treated with lenalidomide who were thalidomide naïve. There was no difference in survival based on previous thalidomide exposure (Wang et al. 2008a). Another interesting subgroup analysis suggested that patients who required a steroid reduction had superior response and survival rates compared to those who continued on dexamethasone 40 mg (San-Miguel et al. 2007).

Further trials have since been carried out combining lenalidomide with a variety of other agents in the relapsed setting including alkylating agents, anthracyclines and bortezomib, with various response rates (Baz et al. 2006; Morgan et al. 2007; Richardson et al. 2007a). Its use has also been reported in newly presenting patients with promising results. Used in combination with dexamethasone in an early phase II trial a

91% response rate was reported in 34 patients (Rajkumar et al. 2005). The same group is conducting a larger, randomised trial comparing lenalidomide in combination with high or low dose dexamethasone. The final results of this are not available, but preliminary results were published that showed a significantly higher OS in the low dose steroid group at 18 months follow-up (91% vs. 80% in 445 randomised patients) (Rajkumar et al. 2007). This is the second large trial to show a poorer outcome with high dose steroids in combination with lenalidomide than with low dose steroids, an effect probably attributable to increased infection rates in the high dose group. A large trial combining lenalidomide with melphalan and prednisolone in elderly patients is also underway, the preliminary results of which were encouraging (Palumbo et al. 2007). Like all novel agents, lenalidomide's role in new and relapsed patients requires further elucidation by well-conducted randomised trials, buts its potential efficacy in both these setting is proven.

Pomalidomide (CC4047)

Although there are several other IMiDs in development, pomalidomide is the only one with published clinical trial data at present. It has been shown to have efficacy in phase I trials, with a 50% response rate being reported in 20 relapsed patients treated with oral pomalidomide monotherapy (Streetly et al. 2008). A phase II trial using pomalidomide in combination with high-dose dexamethasone showed a 62% response rate in 37 relapsed patients. Neutropenia was the most common serious adverse event. Of interest, four patients who had previously been classed as refractory to lenalidomide showed responses (Lacy et al. 2008). Also reported are responses to thalidomide in patients who have progressed on pomalidomide therapy, supporting the notion that cross-resistance between the IMiDs is not absolute (Mughal et al. 2009).

8.3.4 Targeting Bone Disease

Myeloma bone disease is due to an imbalance between bone resorption by osteoclasts and new bone formation by osteoblasts. Myeloma cells produce osteoclast activating factors such as receptor activator of nuclear factor-kappa B ligand (RANKL), macrophage inflammatory protein-1α (MIP-1α) and IL-6. Conversely, osteoblast activity is suppressed by cytokines such as dikkopf-1 (DKK1), frizzled-related protein 2, IL-7 and IL-3 (Roodman 2008). This tips the balance towards bone resorption, resulting in the osteoporosis and lytic lesions that characterise destructive myeloma bone disease, but it also provides several targets whose manipulation may alter this balance. There is some evidence that novel agents such as proteasome inhibitors and IMiDs have a direct effect on bone disease that is supplementary to the beneficial effect of tumour bulk reduction. Bortezomib has been shown to induce the differentiation of mesenchymal stem cells into osteoblasts (Mukherjee et al. 2008), and responding patients in the APEX trial were shown to have increases in their serum alkaline phosphatase levels as a marker of increased osteoblastic activation (Zangari et al. 2007). The new IMiDs such as lenalidomide and CC-4047 have been shown to alter the balance of bone resorption by inhibiting osteoclast formation (Anderson et al. 2006; Breitkreutz et al. 2008). The effects of these new drugs on bone disease are welcome side effects of drugs whose primary role is to reduce tumour burden, whilst bisphosphonate therapy is currently the standard of care for prevention of bone lesions. However, although bisphosphonates have been proven to reduce skeletal events, primarily vertebral crush fractures, these events still occur at a higher rate than in an age-matched population, which will become more relevant as myeloma patients live for longer with improved therapies. This fact, and concern over bisphosphonate side effects such as osteonecrosis of the jaw, means that there remains a role for novel agents to specifically target myelomatous bone disease. Agents that disrupt the abnormal osteoclast/osteoblast balance in myeloma have the potential to make the bone marrow niche a less conducive place for myeloma cells to thrive, and there is hope that these agents could inhibit myeloma cell growth and there is hope that these agents could inhibit myeloma cell growth as well as improving rates of skeletal related events. Evidence of this effect comes from the MRC Myeloma IX trial, where patients were randomised to an oral bisphosphonate, clodronic acid, or an intravenous bisphosphonate, zoledronic acid. Zoledronic acid decreased skeletal events, but also reduced mortality by 16%, resulting in an extension of median OS by 5.5 months (p=0.04) Morgan GJ et al. 2007. It is likely that in the future the treatment of myelomatous skeletal disease may involve combination therapy, incorporating a bisphosphonate with one of the agents mentioned below.

8.3.4.1 Receptor Activator of NF-κB Ligand (RANKL)

RANKL is a potent stimulator of osteoclastogenesis, but in the normal bone marrow milieu, its effects are largely blocked by its decoy receptor osteoprotegrin (OPG) which is present in higher numbers than RANKL. This balance is upset in myeloma as OPG is decreased which tips the balance in favour of osteoclast mediated bone resorption. *Denosumab* (*AMG162*) is a humanised monoclonal antibody that binds to RANKL and neutralises it in a similar way to endogenous OPG, tipping the balance back in favour of osteoblastic bone formation. It has been shown to increase bone mineral density in osteopenic post-menopausal women in a large phase III trial, where it was given either 3 monthly or 6 monthly (McClung et al. 2006). There is some thought that bone destruction leads to the release of factors that promote myeloma cell growth, and animals treated with denosumab have shown decreased paraprotein levels and prolonged survival. However, preliminary data from a phase II study of denosumab in plateau phase or relapsed myeloma showed no impact on disease burden, (Vij et al. 2007). A phase III trial in myeloma patients is underway, the results of which are likely to be available within a year.

8.3.4.2 Dickkopf-1 (DKK1) and Wingless/int (Wnt)

Wnt/b-catenin signalling plays a central role in bone homeostasis through promotion of osteoblast differentiation. It may also regulate OPG expression and therefore impact on RANKL mediated osteoclastogenesis. DKK1 inhibits Wnt by binding to its co-receptor lipoprotein-related protein 5 (LRP5). Plasma cells from patients without myeloma, and from patients with MGUS do not express DKK1, whereas it is found in high levels in myeloma bone marrow samples, making it likely to be a key player in the development of myeloma bone lesions (Yaccoby et al. 2007). Treating mice with an anti-DKK1 antibody (*BHQ880*) was shown to prevent the normal inhibition of osteoblasts seen in myeloma, although no change in osteoclast numbers was seen. Treatment resulted in decreased numbers of osteolytic bone lesions and a 25% increase in new bone formation (Yaccoby et al. 2007; Heath et al. 2009). This agent is in trials in osteoporosis, and a trial in myeloma is being planned.

8.3.4.3 Macrophage Inflammatory Protein 1-α (MIP-1α)

MIP-1α (also known as chemokine-chemokine ligand 3 (CCL3)) is another inflammatory cytokine released by myeloma cells that upregulates the number and function of osteoclasts. It is present in high levels in patients with significant myeloma bone disease, and its production has been shown to be upregulated by interactions between myeloma cells and stromal cells via VCAM-1 (Hashimoto et al. 2004; Abe et al. 2009). Binding of MIP-1a to its receptor CCR1 has been shown to stimulate osteoclast formation independently of RANKL, and to induce myeloma cell migration and proliferation via the Akt pathway. MLN3897 is a specific antagonist of CCR1 which has demonstrated in preclinical data a 40% decrease in osteoclast number and a 70% decrease in osteoclast function, as well as affecting myeloma cell migration and adhesion (Vallet et al. 2007). It is currently in phase II trials in rheumatoid arthritis and multiple sclerosis, and warrants further examination in myeloma bone disease.

8.3.4.4 Activin A

Activin A is a member of the TNF-α superfamily. It is produced by bone marrow stromal cells and its expression has been found to be increased fourfold in myeloma patients with multiple bone lesions compared to those with one or less lesions (Vallet et al. 2008). *ACE-011* is a clinical grade Activin A inhibitor that has been shown to stimulate osteoblast differentiation and inhibit osteoclastogenesis in vitro, and to inhibit myeloma cell growth in vivo. A single dose reduced markers of bone resorption in postmenopausal women (Ruckle et al. 2008).

8.4 Conclusion

Steroids and alkylating agents have formed the backbone of myeloma therapy for decades, with other conventional agents such as anthracyclines, platinum drugs and vincristine adding minimal additional benefit. As a result, patient outcomes showed little real improvement until recently, with the most important breakthrough being proof of dose escalation as opposed to drug discovery. This has changed in the last decade with the advent of the IMiDs and bortezomib. These drugs came to be used in myeloma through very different routes, thalidomide having been in existence for over 50 years and utilised for myeloma because of its known antiangiogenic properties, whilst bortezomib was designed in the laboratory specifically to target myeloma through inhibition of the proteasome. Thalidomide, lenalidomide and bortezomib have widened the treatment options for both the newly presenting and the relapsed patient. All these drugs have been proven to improve responses in both newly presenting and relapsed patients. Optimum combinations of these agents within regimens, and optimum sequencing of regimens are points for debate and will be covered in other chapters.

Bortezomib could be viewed as especially successful as it arose directly from laboratory research into myeloma cell biology, being designed to fit a specific target. As such it has formed a template for the design of other novel agents, with upregulated pathways being defined within the plasma cell and then targeted with a specific agent. There has been a huge expansion in research in myeloma molecular biology in the last decade which has led to a long list of potential drug targets within the cell. Increasing understanding of the role that the bone marrow microenvironment plays in promoting myeloma cell survival and drug resistance has also led to the definition of targets outside the myeloma cell. As a result of this expansion in knowledge of cell biology, there are now a huge number of novel agents in phase I and phase II trials. The current challenge in myeloma therapy is to build on the success of IMiDs and proteasome inhibitors and fit some of these promising new agents into current treatment paradigms.

The best results in these early phase trials have been seen with new analogues of existing drugs, i.e. new proteasome inhibitors and new IMiDs. Other truly new agents have so far been relatively disappointing when used as monotherapy. This is maybe not surprising given the specific nature of some of these drugs. Myeloma is a biologically heterogeneous disease and is the end product of dysregulation of multiple different pathways in individual patients. It is currently drugs that have quite a broad spectrum of action that are the most effective, such as proteasome inhibitors which affect not only the NF-κB pathway but also all other proteins that are degraded by the proteasome. Until we have better technology to define dysregulated pathways within the individual patient, drugs which have multiple targets such as HSP90 inhibitors are most likely be clinically effective in a group of patients. Novel agents that do find their way into clinical practise are likely to do so because they demonstrate synergism with existing agents or uncouple drug resistance mechanisms to existing agents. Because these new drugs are not conventionally cytotoxic, they are likely to have non-overlapping side effects so may be suited to being used in combination regimens. To put things into context, one has to remember that both thalidomide and bortezomib showed response rates of 30–40% when used as monotherapy in relapsed patients, which is the context that most new drugs are introduced. However, when combined with steroids and alkylating agents the response rates double. There is often in vitro evidence of synergy for these new agents and existing agents that provide rationale for certain combinations. Treatment of a myeloma cell with bortezomib, for example, is known to result in activation of the unfolded protein response; blocking this escape mechanism with heat shock protein inhibitors may therefore augment response to bortezomib. This, and other combinations of novel agents, will need careful evaluation in well-designed randomised trials with the addition of novel agent or placebo to existing gold standard treatments.

References

Abe M, Hiura K, Ozaki S, Kido S, Matsumoto T (2009) Vicious cycle between myeloma cell binding to bone marrow stromal cells via VLA-4-VCAM-1 adhesion and macrophage inflammatory protein-1alpha and MIP-1beta production. J Bone Miner Metab 27(1):16–23

Alsina M, Fonseca R, Wilson EF, Belle AN, Gerbino E, Price-Troska T, Overton RM, Ahmann G, Bruzek LM, Adjei AA, Kaufmann SH, Wright JJ, Sullivan D, Djulbegovic B, Cantor AB, Greipp PR, Dalton WS, Sebti SM (2004) Farnesyltransferase inhibitor tipifarnib is well tolerated, induces stabilization of disease, and inhibits farnesylation and oncogenic/tumor survival pathways in patients with advanced multiple myeloma. Blood 103(9): 3271–3277

Amit-Vazina M, Shishodia S, Harris D, Van Q, Wang M, Weber D, Alexanian R, Talpaz M, Aggarwal BB, Estrov Z (2005) Atiprimod blocks STAT3 phosphorylation and induces apoptosis in multiple myeloma cells. Br J Cancer 93(1):70–80

Anderson KC (2005) Lenalidomide and thalidomide: mechanisms of action–similarities and differences. Semin Hematol 42(4 suppl 4):S3–S8

Anderson G, Gries M, Kurihara N, Honjo T, Anderson J, Donnenberg V, Donnenberg A, Ghobrial I, Mapara MY, Stirling D, Roodman D, Lentzsch S (2006) Thalidomide derivative CC-4047 inhibits osteoclast formation by down-regulation of PU.1. Blood 107(8):3098–3105

Annunziata CM, Davis RE, Demchenko Y, Bellamy W, Gabrea A, Zhan F, Lenz G, Hanamura I, Wright G, Xiao W, Dave S, Hurt EM, Tan B, Zhao H, Stephens O, Santra M, Williams DR, Dang L, Barlogie B, Shaughnessy JD Jr et al (2007) Frequent engagement of the classical and alternative NF-kappaB pathways by diverse genetic abnormalities in multiple myeloma. Cancer Cell 12(2): 115–130

Armand JP, Burnett AK, Drach J, Harousseau JL, Lowenberg B, San Miguel J (2007) The emerging role of targeted therapy for hematologic malignancies: update on bortezomib and tipifarnib. Oncologist 12(3):281–290

Asano J, Abe M, Fujii S, Tanaka O, Mihara A, Nakamura S, Miki K, Kagawa K, Takeuchi K, Yata K, Hashimoto T, Ozaki S, Hiasa M, Matsumoto T (2007) The serine/threonine kinase pim-2 is a novel anti apoptotic mediator in myeloma cells. Blood 110:Abstract 243

Atadja P, Gao L, Kwon P, Trogani N, Walker H, Hsu M, Yeleswarapu L, Chandramouli N, Perez L, Versace R, Wu A, Sambucetti L, Lassota P, Cohen D, Bair K, Wood A, Remiszewski S (2004) Selective growth inhibition of tumor cells by a novel histone deacetylase inhibitor, NVP-LAQ824. Cancer Res 64(2):689–695

Azab AK, Runnels JM, Pitsillides C, Moreau AS, Azab F, Leleu X, Jia X, Wright R, Ospina B, Carlson AL, Alt C, Burwick N, Roccaro AM, Ngo HT, Farag M, Melhem MR, Sacco A, Munshi NC, Hideshima T, Rollins BJ et al (2009) The CXCR4 inhibitor AMD3100 disrupts the interaction of multiple myeloma cells with the bone marrow microenvironment and enhances their sensitivity to therapy. Blood 113(18): 4341–4351

Badros A, Philip S, Niesvizky R, Goloubeva O, Harris C, Zweibel J, Wright J, Burger A, Grant S, Baer MR, Egorin MJ (2007) Phase I trial of suberoylanilide hydroxamic acid (SAHA)+bortezomib (bort) in relapsed multiple myeloma (MM) patients. Blood 110:Abstract 1168

Bataille R, Jourdan M, Zhang XG, Klein B (1989) Serum levels of interleukin 6, a potent myeloma cell growth factor, as a reflect of disease severity in plasma cell dyscrasias. J Clin Invest 84(6): 2008–2011

Baz R, Walker E, Karam MA, Choueiri TK, Jawde RA, Bruening K, Reed J, Faiman B, Ellis Y, Brand C, Srkalovic G, Andresen S, Knight R, Zeldis J, Hussein MA (2006) Lenalidomide and pegylated liposomal doxorubicin-based chemotherapy for relapsed or refractory multiple myeloma: safety and efficacy. Ann Oncol 17(12):1766–1771

Beaupre DM, McCafferty-Grad J, Bahlis NJ, Boise LH, Lichtenheld MG (2003) Farnesyl transferase inhibitors enhance death receptor signals and induce apoptosis in multiple myeloma cells. Leuk Lymphoma 44(12):2123–2134

Beaupre DM, Cepero E, Obeng EA, Boise LH, Lichtenheld MG (2004) R115777 induces Ras-independent apoptosis of myeloma cells via multiple intrinsic pathways. Mol Cancer Ther 3(2):179–186

Bensinger W, Zonder J, Singhal S (2007) Phase I trial of huLuc63 in multiple myeloma. Blood 110:Abstract 1180

Bergsagel PL, Kuehl WM, Zhan F, Sawyer J, Barlogie B, Shaughnessy J Jr (2005) Cyclin D dysregulation: an early and unifying pathogenic event in multiple myeloma. Blood 106(1):296–303

Bharti AC, Shishodia S, Reuben JM, Weber D, Alexanian R, Raj-Vadhan S, Estrov Z, Talpaz M, Aggarwal BB (2004) Nuclear factor-kappaB and STAT3 are constitutively active in CD138+ cells derived from multiple myeloma patients, and suppression of these transcription factors leads to apoptosis. Blood 103(8):3175–3184

Bisping G, Leo R, Wenning D, Dankbar B, Padro T, Kropff M, Scheffold C, Kroger M, Mesters RM, Berdel WE, Kienast J (2003) Paracrine interactions of basic fibroblast growth factor and interleukin-6 in multiple myeloma. Blood 101(7):2775–2783

Bolick SC, Landowski TH, Boulware D, Oshiro MM, Ohkanda J, Hamilton AD, Sebti SM, Dalton WS (2003) The farnesyl transferase inhibitor, FTI-277, inhibits growth and induces apoptosis in drug-resistant myeloma tumor cells. Leukemia 17(2):451–457

Breitkreutz I, Raab MS, Vallet S, Hideshima T, Raje N, Mitsiades C, Chauhan D, Okawa Y, Munshi NC, Richardson PG, Anderson KC (2008) Lenalidomide inhibits osteoclastogenesis, survival factors and bone-remodeling markers in multiple myeloma. Leukemia 22(10): 1925–1932

Buzzeo R, Enkemann S, Nimmanapalli R, Alsina M, Lichtenheld MG, Dalton WS, Beaupre DM (2005) Characterization of a R115777-resistant human multiple myeloma cell line with cross-resistance to PS-341. Clin Cancer Res 11(16):6057–6064

Calandra G, McCarty J, McGuirk J, Tricot G, Crocker SA, Badel K, Grove B, Dye A, Bridger G (2008) AMD3100 plus G-CSF can successfully mobilize CD34+ cells from non-Hodgkin's lymphoma, Hodgkin's disease and multiple myeloma patients previously failing mobilization with chemotherapy and/or cytokine treatment: compassionate use data. Bone Marrow Transplant 41(4):331–338

Campbell RA, Sanchez E, Chen H, Turker L, Trac O, Li M, Shalitin D, Gordon M, Pang S, Bonavida B, Said J, Plowman GD, Fuh G, Berenson J (2006)

Anti-VEGF antibody treatment markedly inhibits tumor growth in SCID-hu models of human multiple myeloma. Blood 108:Abstract 846

Catlett-Falcone R, Landowski TH, Oshiro MM, Turkson J, Levitzki A, Savino R, Ciliberto G, Moscinski L, Fernandez-Luna JL, Nunez G, Dalton WS, Jove R (1999) Constitutive activation of Stat3 signaling confers resistance to apoptosis in human U266 myeloma cells. Immunity 10(1):105–115

Catley L, Weisberg E, Tai YT, Atadja P, Remiszewski S, Hideshima T, Mitsiades N, Shringarpure R, LeBlanc R, Chauhan D, Munshi NC, Schlossman R, Richardson P, Griffin J, Anderson KC (2003) NVP-LAQ824 is a potent novel histone deacetylase inhibitor with significant activity against multiple myeloma. Blood 102(7):2615–2622

Cavenagh JD, Yong J, Byrne J, Cavet J, Johnson P, Morgan G, Williams C, Akinaga S, Francis G, Kilborn J (2008) The safety, pharmacokinetics and pharmacodynamics of KW-2478, a novel Hsp90 antagonist, inpatients with B-cell malignancies: a first-in-man, phase I, multicentre, open-label, dose escalation study. Blood 112: Abstract 2777

Chanan-Khan A, Gharibo M, Jagannath S, Munshi N, Anderson KC, DePaolo D, P. Lee K, Miller K, Guild R, Zildjian S, Qin A (2008) Phase I study of IMGN901 in patients with relapsed and relapsed/refractory CD56-positive multiple myeloma. Blood 112:Abstract 3689

Chatterjee M, Stuhmer T, Herrmann P, Bommert K, Dorken B, Bargou RC (2004) Combined disruption of both the MEK/ERK and the IL-6R/STAT3 pathways is required to induce apoptosis of multiple myeloma cells in the presence of bone marrow stromal cells. Blood 104(12):3712–3721

Chatterjee M, Jain S, Stuhmer T, Andrulis M, Ungethum U, Kuban RJ, Lorentz H, Bommert K, Topp M, Kramer D, Muller-Hermelink HK, Einsele H, Greiner A, Bargou RC (2007) STAT3 and MAPK signaling maintain overexpression of heat shock proteins 90alpha and beta in multiple myeloma cells, which critically contribute to tumor-cell survival. Blood 109(2):720–728

Chauhan D, Uchiyama H, Akbarali Y, Urashima M, Yamamoto K, Libermann TA, Anderson KC (1996) Multiple myeloma cell adhesion-induced interleukin-6 expression in bone marrow stromal cells involves activation of NF-kappa B. Blood 87(3):1104–1112

Chauhan D, Catley L, Li G, Podar K, Hideshima T, Velankar M, Mitsiades C, Mitsiades N, Yasui H, Letai A, Ovaa H, Berkers C, Nicholson B, Chao TH, Neuteboom ST, Richardson P, Palladino MA, Anderson KC (2005) A novel orally active proteasome inhibitor induces apoptosis in multiple myeloma cells with mechanisms distinct from Bortezomib. Cancer Cell 8(5):407–419

Chauhan D, Bianchi G, Anderson KC (2008) Targeting the UPS as therapy in multiple myeloma. BMC Biochem 9 suppl 1:S1

Chen J, Lee BH, Williams IR, Gilliland DG (2004) PKC412 effectively inhibits constitutively activated FGFR3 mutants in murine leukemia models and t(4;14) myeloma cell lines. Blood 104:Abstract 2448

Chen N, Lau H, Kong L, Kumar G, Zeldis JB, Knight R, Laskin OL (2007) Pharmacokinetics of lenalidomide in subjects with various degrees of renal impairment and in subjects on hemodialysis. J Clin Pharmacol 47(12):1466–1475

Chim CS, Pang R, Fung TK, Choi CL, Liang R (2007) Epigenetic dysregulation of Wnt signaling pathway in multiple myeloma. Leukemia 21(12):2527–2536

Chng WJ, Braggio E, Mulligan G, Bryant B, Remstein E, Valdez R, Dogan A, Fonseca R (2008a) The centrosome index is a powerful prognostic marker in myeloma and identifies a cohort of patients that might benefit from aurora kinase inhibition. Blood 111(3):1603–1609

Chng WJ, Gonzalez-Paz N, Price-Troska T, Jacobus S, Rajkumar SV, Oken MM, Kyle RA, Henderson KJ, Van Wier S, Greipp P, Van Ness B, Fonseca R (2008b) Clinical and biological significance of RAS mutations in multiple myeloma. Leukemia 22(12):2280–2284

Cirstea D, Hideshima T, Pozzi S, Vallet S, Ikeda H, Santo L, Loferer H, Vaghela N, Okawa Y, Perrone G, Gorgun G, Calabrese E, Munshi NC, Anderson KC, Raje N (2008) RGB 286638, a novel multi-targeted small molecule inhibitor, induces multiple myeloma (MM) cell death through abrogation of CDKDependent and independent survival mechanisms. Blood 112: Abstract 2759

Coluccia AM, Cirulli T, Neri P, Mangieri D, Colanardi MC, Gnoni A, Di Renzo N, Dammacco F, Tassone P, Ribatti D, Gambacorti-Passerini C, Vacca A (2008) Validation of PDGFRbeta and c-Src tyrosine kinases as tumor/vessel targets in patients with multiple myeloma: preclinical efficacy of the novel, orally available inhibitor dasatinib. Blood 112(4):1346–1356

Davenport EL, Moore HE, Dunlop AS, Sharp SY, Workman P, Morgan GJ, Davies FE (2007) Heat shock protein inhibition is associated with activation of the unfolded protein response pathway in myeloma plasma cells. Blood 110(7):2641–2649

Davenport E, Zeisig A, Wiseglass L, Moore HE, Hockley SL, Gonzalez D, Smith E, Sharp S, Workman P, Morgan GJ, Davies F (2008) Inhibitors of heat shock protein 72 induction enhance apoptosis induced by HSP90 inhibitors. Blood 112:Abstract 2625

David E, Peng X, Barwick BG, Kaufman JL, Garlich JR, Lonial S (2008) SF1126, a novel P13K inhibitor results in downstream inhibition of the P13K axis and displays sequence specific synergy when combined with bortezomib in multiple myeloma cells. Blood 112:Abstract 5167

Davies FE, Raje N, Hideshima T, Lentzsch S, Young G, Tai YT, Lin B, Podar K, Gupta D, Chauhan D, Treon SP, Richardson PG, Schlossman RL, Morgan GJ, Muller GW, Stirling DI, Anderson KC (2001) Thalidomide and immunomodulatory derivatives augment natural killer cell cytotoxicity in multiple myeloma. Blood 98(1):210–216

Davies F, Moore H, Davenport E (2007a) Aminopeptidase inhibition as a targeted treatment strategy in myeloma. Blood 110:Abstract 2505

Davies F, Ossenkopple G, Zachee P (2007b) A Phase I study of CHR-2797, an orally active aminopeptidase inhibitor in elderly and/or treatment refractory patients with acute myeloid leukaemia or multiple myeloma. Blood 110:Abstract 443

De Vos J, Jourdan M, Tarte K, Jasmin C, Klein B (2000) JAK2 tyrosine kinase inhibitor tyrphostin AG490 downregulates the mitogen-activated protein kinase (MAPK) and signal transducer and activator of transcription (STAT) pathways and induces apoptosis in myeloma cells. Br J Haematol 109(4):823–828

Demo SD, Aujay MA, Bennett MK, Lewis ER, Molineaux CJ, Kirk CJ (2009) Chronic administration of carfilzomib in experimental animals does not cause neurotoxicity. Clin Lymphoma Myeloma 8(7):Abstract 178

Derksen PW, Tjin E, Meijer HP, Klok MD, MacGillavry HD, van Oers MH, Lokhorst HM, Bloem AC, Clevers H, Nusse R, van der Neut R, Spaargaren M, Pals ST (2004) Illegitimate WNT signaling promotes proliferation of multiple myeloma cells. Proc Natl Acad Sci USA 101(16):6122–6127

Dimopoulos M, Spencer A, Attal M, Prince HM, Harousseau JL, Dmoszynska A, San Miguel J, Hellmann A, Facon T, Foa R, Corso A, Masliak Z, Olesnyckyj M, Yu Z, Patin J, Zeldis JB, Knight RD (2007) Lenalidomide plus dexamethasone for relapsed or refractory multiple myeloma. N Engl J Med 357(21):2123–2132

Evans R, Naber C, Steffler T, Checkland T, Keats J, Maxwell C, Perry T, Chau H, Belch A, Pilarski L, Reiman T (2008a) Aurora A kinase RNAi and small molecule inhibition of Aurora kinases with VE-465 induce apoptotic death in multiple myeloma cells. Leuk Lymphoma 49(3):559–569

Evans RP, Naber C, Steffler T, Checkland T, Maxwell CA, Keats JJ, Belch AR, Pilarski LM, Lai R, Reiman T (2008b) The selective Aurora B kinase inhibitor AZD1152 is a potential new treatment for multiple myeloma. Br J Haematol 140(3):295–302

Fenk R, Michael M, Zohren F, Graef T, Czibere A, Bruns I, Neumann F, Fenk B, Haas R, Kobbe G (2007) Escalation therapy with bortezomib, dexamethasone and bendamustine for patients with relapsed or refractory multiple myeloma. Leuk Lymphoma 48(12):2345–2351

Frassanito MA, Cusmai A, Iodice G, Dammacco F (2001) Autocrine interleukin-6 production and highly malignant multiple myeloma: relation with resistance to drug-induced apoptosis. Blood 97(2):483–489

Frost P, Moatamed F, Hoang B, Shi Y, Gera J, Yan H, Frost P, Gibbons J, Lichtenstein A (2004) In vivo antitumor effects of the mTOR inhibitor CCI-779 against human multiple myeloma cells in a xenograft model. Blood 104(13):4181–4187

Frost P, Shi Y, Hoang B, Lichtenstein A (2007) AKT activity regulates the ability of mTOR inhibitors to prevent angiogenesis and VEGF expression in multiple myeloma cells. Oncogene 26(16):2255–2262

Galli M, Salmoiraghi S, Golay J, Gozzini A, Bosi A, Crippa C, Rossi G, Pescosta N, Cortelazzo S, Sechi A, Oldoni T, Rambaldi A (2007) A phase II multiple dose clinical trial of histone deacetylase inhibitor ITF2357 in patients with relapsed or progressive multiple myeloma: preliminary results. Blood 110:Abstract 1175

Gaponova T, Misurin A, Mendeleeva L, Varlamova E, Parovichnikova E, Savchenko V (2008)

Expression of XIAP in Multiple Myeloma Patients. Blood 112:Abstract 5118

Ghobrial I, Munshi N, Schlossman R (2008) Phase I trial of CCI-779 (temsirolimus) and weekly bortezomib in relapsed and/or refractory multiple myeloma. Blood 112:Abstract 3696

Goldmacher VS, Bourret LA, Levine BA, Rasmussen RA, Pourshadi M, Lambert JM, Anderson KC (1994) Anti-CD38-blocked ricin: an immunotoxin for the treatment of multiple myeloma. Blood 84(9):3017–3025

Gorgun G, Calabrese E, Mani M, Hideshima T, Ikeda H, Perrone G, Santo L, Cirstea D, Blotta S, Richardson PG, Ecsedy J, Anderson KC (2008). A novel aurora-a kinase inhibitor MLN8237 induces cytotoxicity and cell cycle arrest in experimental multiple myeloma models. Blood 112:Abstract 1719

Hashimoto T, Abe M, Oshima T, Shibata H, Ozaki S, Inoue D, Matsumoto T (2004) Ability of myeloma cells to secrete macrophage inflammatory protein (MIP)-1alpha and MIP-1beta correlates with lytic bone lesions in patients with multiple myeloma. Br J Haematol 125(1): 38–41

Hayashi T, Hideshima T, Akiyama M, Podar K, Yasui H, Raje N, Kumar S, Chauhan D, Treon SP, Richardson P, Anderson KC (2005) Molecular mechanisms whereby immunomodulatory drugs activate natural killer cells: clinical application. Br J Haematol 128(2):192–203

Heath DJ, Chantry AD, Buckle CH, Coulton L, Shaughnessy JD Jr, Evans HR, Snowden JA, Stover DR, Vanderkerken K, Croucher PI (2009) Inhibiting Dickkopf-1 (Dkk1) removes suppression of bone formation and prevents the development of osteolytic bone disease in multiple myeloma. J Bone Miner Res 24(3):425–436

Hembrough TA, Chen X, Burke PA, Swartz GM, Bengali K, Brokx R, LaVallee TM, Bray MR (2007) Inhibition of multiple myeloma tumor growth and FGFR3 by the aurora-angiogenesis inhibitor ENMD-981693. Blood 110:Abstract 1209

Hideshima T, Nakamura N, Chauhan D, Anderson KC (2001) Biologic sequelae of interleukin-6 induced PI3-K/Akt signaling in multiple myeloma. Oncogene 20(42):5991–6000

Hideshima T, Chauhan D, Hayashi T, Akiyama M, Mitsiades N, Mitsiades C, Podar K, Munshi NC, Richardson PG, Anderson KC (2003a) Proteasome inhibitor PS-341 abrogates IL-6 triggered signaling cascades via caspase-dependent downregulation of gp130 in multiple myeloma. Oncogene 22(52):8386–8393

Hideshima T, Mitsiades C, Akiyama M, Hayashi T, Chauhan D, Richardson P, Schlossman R, Podar K, Munshi NC, Mitsiades N, Anderson KC (2003b) Molecular mechanisms mediating antimyeloma activity of proteasome inhibitor PS-341. Blood 101(4):1530–1534

Hideshima T, Podar K, Chauhan D, Ishitsuka K, Mitsiades C, Tai YT, Hamasaki M, Raje N, Hideshima H, Schreiner G, Nguyen AN, Navas T, Munshi NC, Richardson PG, Higgins LS, Anderson KC (2004) p38 MAPK inhibition enhances PS-341 (bortezomib)-induced cytotoxicity against multiple myeloma cells. Oncogene 23(54):8766–8776

Hideshima T, Bradner JE, Wong J, Chauhan D, Richardson P, Schreiber SL, Anderson KC (2005) Small-molecule inhibition of proteasome and aggresome function induces synergistic antitumor activity in multiple myeloma. Proc Natl Acad Sci USA 102(24):8567–8572

Hideshima T, Catley L, Yasui H, Ishitsuka K, Raje N, Mitsiades C, Podar K, Munshi NC, Chauhan D, Richardson PG, Anderson KC (2006a) Perifosine, an oral bioactive novel alkylphospholipid, inhibits Akt and induces in vitro and in vivo cytotoxicity in human multiple myeloma cells. Blood 107(10):4053–4062

Hideshima T, Neri P, Tassone P, Yasui H, Ishitsuka K, Raje N, Chauhan D, Podar K, Mitsiades C, Dang L, Munshi N, Richardson P, Schenkein D, Anderson KC (2006b) MLN120B, a novel IkappaB kinase beta inhibitor, blocks multiple myeloma cell growth in vitro and in vivo. Clin Cancer Res 12(19):5887–5894

Hose D, Reme T, Meissner T, Moreaux J, Seckinger A, Lewis J, Benes V, Benner A, Hundemer M, Hielscher T, Shaughnessy JD Jr, Barlogie B, Neben K, Kramer A, Hillengass J, Bertsch U, Jauch A, De Vos J, Rossi JF, Mohler T et al (2009) Inhibition of aurora-kinases for tailored risk adapted treatment of multiple myeloma. Blood 113(18):4331–4340

Hrusovsky I, Heidtmann H (2005) Combination therapy of bortezomib with low-dose bendamustine in elderly patients with advanced multiple myeloma. Blood 106:Abstract 5122

Ikeda H, Hideshima T, Lutz R, Vallet S, Pozzi S, Santo L, Calabrese E, Dälken B, Uherek C, Aigner S, Osterroth F, Fultiniti M, Okawa Y, Perrone G, Gorgun G, Yasui H, Cristia D, Raje N, Munshi N,

Richardson P, et al. (2008a) The monoclonal antibody nBT062 conjugated to cytotoxic maytansinoids has potent and selective cytotoxicity against CD138 positive multiple myeloma cells in vitro and in vivo. Blood 112:Abstract 1716

Ikeda H, Hideshima T, Okawa Y, Vallet S, Pozzi S, Santo L, Gorgun G, Fulciniti M, Raje NS, Perrone G, Munshi N, Richardson P, Lannutti BJ, Puri KD, Giese NA, Anderson KC (2008b) CAL-101, a specific inhibitor of the p110 isoform of phosphatidylinositide 3-kinase induces cytotoxicity in multiple myeloma (MM). Blood 112: Abstarct 2753

Ishitsuka K, Hideshima T, Neri P, Vallet S, Shiraishi N, Okawa Y, Shen Z, Raje N, Kiziltepe T, Ocio EM, Chauhan D, Tassone P, Munshi N, Campbell RM, Dios AD, Shih C, Starling JJ, Tamura K, Anderson KC (2008) p38 mitogen-activated protein kinase inhibitor LY2228820 enhances bortezomib-induced cytotoxicity and inhibits osteoclastogenesis in multiple myeloma; therapeutic implications. Br J Haematol 141(5):598–606

Jagannath S, Vij R, Stewart AK, Somlo G, Jakubowiak A, Reiman T, Trudel S, Taylor J, Fuhrman D, Cruickshank S, Schwartz R, Kunkel L, Siegel D, Consortium TMMR (2009) Phase II study of carfilzomib in patients with relapsed and refractory myeloma (PX-171-003). Clin Lymphoma Myeloma 8(7):Abstract 377

Jakubowiak A, Richardson P, Zimmerman T (2008) Phase I results of perifosine (KRX-0401) in combination with lenalidomide and dexamethasone in patients with relapsed or refractory multiple myeloma (MM). Blood 112:Abstract 3691

Jakubowiak AJ, Bensinger W, Zimmerman T, Chanan-Khan A, Singhal A, Siegel D, Anderson K (2009) Phase I study of Elotuzumab (HuLuc63) in combination wuth bortezomib in relapsed multiple myeloma. Clin Lymphoma Myeloma 8(7):Abstract 264

Keats JJ, Fonseca R, Chesi M, Schop R, Baker A, Chng WJ, Van Wier S, Tiedemann R, Shi CX, Sebag M, Braggio E, Henry T, Zhu YX, Fogle H, Price-Troska T, Ahmann G, Mancini C, Brents LA, Kumar S, Greipp P et al (2007) Promiscuous mutations activate the noncanonical NF-kappaB pathway in multiple myeloma. Cancer Cell 12(2):131–144

Khan SB, Maududi T, Barton K, Ayers J, Alkan S (2004) Analysis of histone deacetylase inhibitor, depsipeptide (FR901228), effect on multiple myeloma. Br J Haematol 125(2):156–161

Khong T, Spencer A (2007) A new generation XIAP inhibitor induces apoptosis of human myeloma cells and synergises with conventional and novel anti-myeloma therapeutics. Blood 110:Abstract 4787

Khong T, Sharkey J, Spencer A (2008) The effect of azacitidine on interleukin-6 signaling and nuclear factor-kappaB activation and its in vitro and in vivo activity against multiple myeloma. Haematologica 93(6):860–869

Kim H-Y, Kim S-W, Lee H-J (2008) The CXCR4 antagonist AMD3100 stimulates the proliferation of plasma cells. Blood 112:Abstract 1701

Kiziltepe T, Hideshima T, Catley L, Raje N, Yasui H, Shiraishi N, Okawa Y, Ikeda H, Vallet S, Pozzi S, Ishitsuka K, Ocio EM, Chauhan D, Anderson KC (2007) 5-Azacytidine, a DNA methyltransferase inhibitor, induces ATR-mediated DNA double-strand break responses, apoptosis, and synergistic cytotoxicity with doxorubicin and bortezomib against multiple myeloma cells. Mol Cancer Ther 6(6):1718–1727

Kuhn DJ, Hunsucker SA, Chen Q, Voorhees PM, Orlowski M, Orlowski RZ (2008) Targeted inhibition of the immunoproteasome is a potent strategy against models of multiple myeloma that overcomes resistance to conventional drugs and non-specific proteasome inhibitors. Blood 113:4667–4676

Kurzrock R, Fayad L, Voorhees P, Furman RR, Lonial S, Borghaei H, Jagannath S, Sokol L, Cornfeld M, Qi M, Jiao T, Herring J, Qin X, van Rhee F (2008) A phase I study of CNTO 328, an anti-interleukin-6 monoclonal antibody in patients with B-cell non-hodgkin's lymphoma, multiple myeloma, or ccastleman's disease. Blood 112:Abstract 1009

Lacy MQ, Hayman SR, Gertz MA (2008) Pomalidomide (CC4047) plus low-dose dexamethasone (Pom/dex) is highly effective therapy in relapsed multiple myeloma. Blood 112:Abstract 866

Locklin RM, Croucher PI, Russell RG, Edwards CM (2007) Agonists of TRAIL death receptors induce myeloma cell apoptosis that is not prevented by cells of the bone marrow microenvironment. Leukemia 21(4):805–812

LoPiccolo J, Blumenthal GM, Bernstein WB, Dennis PA (2008) Targeting the PI3K/Akt/mTOR pathway: effective combinations and clinical considerations. Drug Resist Updat 11(1–2):32–50

Lacy M, Alsina M, Roberts L (2007) Phase I dose escalation study of the monoclonal antibody against the insulin like growth factor I receptor CP-751,871 in patients with multiple myeloma. Blood 110:Abstract 1171

Maiso P, Carvajal-Vergara X, Ocio EM, Lopez-Perez R, Mateo G, Gutierrez N, Atadja P, Pandiella A, San Miguel JF (2006) The histone deacetylase inhibitor LBH589 is a potent anti-myeloma agent that overcomes drug resistance. Cancer Res 66(11):5781–5789

Maiso P, Ocio EM, Garayoa M, Montero JC, Hofmann F, Garcia-Echeverria C, Zimmermann J, Pandiella A, San Miguel JF (2008) The insulin-like growth factor-I receptor inhibitor NVP-AEW541 provokes cell cycle arrest and apoptosis in multiple myeloma cells. Br J Haematol 141(4):470–482

Mao X, Wood TW, Wang X, St-Germain J, Moran MF, Datti A, Wrana J, Batey RA, Schimmer AD (2008) A novel chromene-based pan-P13 kinase inhibitor displays perclinical activity in leukemia and myeloma. Blood 112:Abstract 1605

Marks P, Rifkind RA, Richon VM, Breslow R, Miller T, Kelly WK (2001) Histone deacetylases and cancer: causes and therapies. Nat Rev Cancer 1(3):194–202

Mateo G, Montalban MA, Vidriales MB, Lahuerta JJ, Mateos MV, Gutierrez N, Rosinol L, Montejano L, Blade J, Martinez R, de la Rubia J, Diaz-Mediavilla J, Sureda A, Ribera JM, Ojanguren JM, de Arriba F, Palomera L, Terol MJ, Orfao A, San Miguel JF (2008) Prognostic value of immunophenotyping in multiple myeloma: a study by the PETHEMA/GEM cooperative study groups on patients uniformly treated with high-dose therapy. J Clin Oncol 26(16):2737–2744

Mazumder A, Jagannath S, Vesole DH (2008) Treatment of multiple myeloma with vorinstat in combination with bortezomib: a case series. Blood 112:Abstract 5213

McClung MR, Lewiecki EM, Cohen SB, Bolognese MA, Woodson GC, Moffett AH, Peacock M, Miller PD, Lederman SN, Chesnut CH, Lain D, Kivitz AJ, Holloway DL, Zhang C, Peterson MC, Bekker PJ (2006) Denosumab in postmenopausal women with low bone mineral density. N Engl J Med 354(8):821–831

McMillin DW, Delmore J, Negri JM, Hayden P, Mitsiades N, Richardson PG, Schlossman R, Munshi NC, Anderson KC, Mitsiades CS (2007) Activity of CDK1/2 inhibitor LCQ195 against multiple myeloma cells. Blood 110:Abstract 1519

Meinel F, Mandl-Weber S, Baumann P (2008) The novel NFkB inhibitor V1810 induces apoptosis and cell cycle arrest in multiple myeloma cells and overcomes NFkB mediated drug resistance. Blood 2008:Abstract 1715

Mitsiades CS, Mitsiades N, Poulaki V, Schlossman R, Akiyama M, Chauhan D, Hideshima T, Treon SP, Munshi NC, Richardson PG, Anderson KC (2002) Activation of NF-kappaB and upregulation of intracellular anti-apoptotic proteins via the IGF-1/Akt signaling in human multiple myeloma cells: therapeutic implications. Oncogene 21(37):5673–5683

Mitsiades N, Mitsiades CS, Richardson PG, McMullan C, Poulaki V, Fanourakis G, Schlossman R, Chauhan D, Munshi NC, Hideshima T, Richon VM, Marks PA, Anderson KC (2003) Molecular sequelae of histone deacetylase inhibition in human malignant B cells. Blood 101(10):4055–4062

Mitsiades CS, Mitsiades NS, McMullan CJ, Poulaki V, Shringarpure R, Akiyama M, Hideshima T, Chauhan D, Joseph M, Libermann TA, Garcia-Echeverria C, Pearson MA, Hofmann F, Anderson KC, Kung AL (2004) Inhibition of the insulin-like growth factor receptor-1 tyrosine kinase activity as a therapeutic strategy for multiple myeloma, other hematologic malignancies, and solid tumors. Cancer Cell 5(3):221–230

Moreau P, Hullin C, Garban F, Yakoub-Agha I, Benboubker L, Attal M, Marit G, Fuzibet JG, Doyen C, Voillat L, Berthou C, Ketterer N, Casassus P, Monconduit M, Michallet M, Najman A, Sotto JJ, Bataille R, Harousseau JL (2006) Tandem autologous stem cell transplantation in high-risk de novo multiple myeloma: final results of the prospective and randomized IFM 99-04 protocol. Blood 107(1): 397–403

Moreau P, Hulin C, Facon T (2007) Phase I study of AVE1642 anti-IGF-1R monoclonal antibody in patients with advanced multiple myeloma. Blood 110:Abstract 1171

Moreaux J, Legouffe E, Jourdan E, Quittet P, Reme T, Lugagne C, Moine P, Rossi JF, Klein B, Tarte K (2004) BAFF and APRIL protect myeloma cells from apoptosis induced by interleukin 6 deprivation and dexamethasone. Blood 103(8): 3148–3157

Morgan GJ, Davies FE, Gregory WM, Cocks K, Bell SE, Szubert AJ, Navarro-Coy N, Drayson MT, Owen RG, Feyler S, Ashcroft AJ, Ross F, Byrne J, Roddie H, Rudin C, Cook G, Jackson GH, Child JA (2007) National Cancer Research

Institute Haematological Oncology Clinical Study Group. First -line treatment with zoledronic acid as compared with clodronic acid in multiple myeloma (MRC Myeloma IX): a randomised controlled trial. Lancet 376 (9757): 1989–1999

Morgan GJ, Schey SA, Wu P, Srikanth M, Phekoo KJ, Jenner M, Davies FE (2007) Lenalidomide (Revlimid), in combination with cyclophosphamide and dexamethasone (RCD), is an effective and tolerated regimen for myeloma patients. Br J Haematol 137(3):268–269

Morishita D, Katayama R, Sekimizu K, Tsuruo T, Fujita N (2008) Pim kinases promote cell cycle progression by phosphorylating and down-regulating p27Kip1 at the transcriptional and post-transcriptional levels. Cancer Res 68(13): 5076–5085

Mughal T, Streetly MJ, Kazmi M, Smith M (2009) Response to thalidomide in patients with MM following disease progression with pomalidomide. Clin Lymphoma Myeloma 8(7):Abstract 616

Mukherjee S, Raje N, Schoonmaker JA, Liu JC, Hideshima T, Wein MN, Jones DC, Vallet S, Bouxsein ML, Pozzi S, Chhetri S, Seo YD, Aronson JP, Patel C, Fulciniti M, Purton LE, Glimcher LH, Lian JB, Stein G, Anderson KC et al (2008) Pharmacologic targeting of a stem/progenitor population in vivo is associated with enhanced bone regeneration in mice. J Clin Invest 118(2):491–504

Navas TA, Nguyen AN, Hideshima T, Reddy M, Ma JY, Haghnazari E, Henson M, Stebbins EG, Kerr I, O'Young G, Kapoun AM, Chakravarty S, Mavunkel B, Perumattam J, Luedtke G, Dugar S, Medicherla S, Protter AA, Schreiner GF, Anderson KC et al (2006) Inhibition of p38alpha MAPK enhances proteasome inhibitor-induced apoptosis of myeloma cells by modulating Hsp27, Bcl-X(L), Mcl-1 and p53 levels in vitro and inhibits tumor growth in vivo. Leukemia 20(6):1017–1027

Neri P, Tassone P, Shammas M, Yasui H, Schipani E, Batchu RB, Blotta S, Prabhala R, Catley L, Hamasaki M, Hideshima T, Chauhan D, Jacob GS, Picker D, Venuta S, Anderson KC, Munshi NC (2007) Biological pathways and in vivo antitumor activity induced by atiprimod in myeloma. Leukemia 21(12):2519–2526

Ocio E, Maiso P, Garayoa M, Dupuis M, Pandieua A, San Miguel JF (2007) The activation of Fas receptor by APO010, a recombinant form of Fas ligand, induces in vitro and in vivo antimyeloma activity. Blood 120:Abstract 1515

O'Sullivan G, Leleu X, Jia X (2006) The combination of the mTOR inhibitor rapamycin and proteasome inhibitor bortezomib is synergistic in vitro in multiple myeloma. Blood 108:Abstract 3495

Ogata A, Chauhan D, Teoh G, Treon SP, Urashima M, Schlossman RL, Anderson KC (1997) IL-6 triggers cell growth via the Ras-dependent mitogen-activated protein kinase cascade. J Immunol 159(5):2212–2221

Okawa Y, Hideshima T, Steed P, Vallet S, Hall S, Huang K, Rice J, Barabasz A, Foley B, Ikeda H, Raje N, Kiziltepe T, Yasui H, Enatsu S, Anderson KC (2008) SNX-2112, a selective Hsp90 inhibitor, potently inhibits tumor cell growth, angiogenesis, and osteoclastogenesis in multiple myeloma and other hematological tumors by abrogating signaling via Akt and ERK. Blood 113(4):846–855

Orchard K, Cooper M, Lewington V, Tristram M, Zivanovic M, Thom J, Quadri S, Richardson D, Causer L, Johnson P (2008) Targeted radiotherapy in the conditioning prior to haematopoietic stem cell transplantation: results of a phase I radiation dose escalation study using yttrium-90-labelled anti-CD66 monoclonal antibody demonstrating high BM uptake of radiation. Blood 112:Abstract 2189

Orlowski R, Stewart K, Vallone M (2007a) Safety and antitumour efficacy of the proteasome inhibitor carfilzomib (PR-171) dosed for five consecutive days in hematological malignancies: phase I results. Blood 110:Abstract 409

Orlowski RZ, Nagler A, Sonneveld P, Blade J, Hajek R, Spencer A, San Miguel J, Robak T, Dmoszynska A, Horvath N, Spicka I, Sutherland HJ, Suvorov AN, Zhuang SH, Parekh T, Xiu L, Yuan Z, Rackoff W, Harousseau JL (2007b) Randomized phase III study of pegylated liposomal doxorubicin plus bortezomib compared with bortezomib alone in relapsed or refractory multiple myeloma: combination therapy improves time to progression. J Clin Oncol 25(25):3892–3901

Palumbo A, Bringhen S, Caravita T, Merla E, Capparella V, Callea V, Cangialosi C, Grasso M, Rossini F, Galli M, Catalano L, Zamagni E, Petrucci MT, De Stefano V, Ceccarelli M, Ambrosini MT, Avonto I, Falco P, Ciccone G, Liberati AM et al (2006) Oral melphalan and prednisone chemotherapy plus thalidomide compared with melphalan and prednisone alone in elderly patients with multiple myeloma: randomised controlled trial. Lancet 367(9513): 825–831

Palumbo A, Falco P, Corradini P, Falcone A, Di Raimondo F, Giuliani N, Crippa C, Ciccone G, Omede P, Ambrosini MT, Gay F, Bringhen S, Musto P, Foa R, Knight R, Zeldis JB, Boccadoro M, Petrucci MT (2007) Melphalan, prednisone, and lenalidomide treatment for newly diagnosed myeloma: a report from the GIMEMA–Italian multiple myeloma network. J Clin Oncol 25(28):4459–4465

Park PU, Blanc V, Deckert J, Lejeune P, Bartle LM, Skaletskaya A, Mayo MF, Zhang C, Wetzel M-C, Tavares DJ, Lutz RJ, Chittenden T, Bissery M-C, Lambert JM, Goldmacher VS (2008) SAR650984: a potent anti-CD38 therapeutic antibody with three mechanisms of action (Apoptosis, ADCC, CDC) for hematological malignancies. Blood 112:Abstract 2756

Pedranzini L, Dechow T, Berishaj M, Comenzo R, Zhou P, Azare J, Bornmann W, Bromberg J (2006) Pyridone 6, a pan-Janus-activated kinase inhibitor, induces growth inhibition of multiple myeloma cells. Cancer Res 66(19):9714–9721

Pellat-Deceunynck C, Barille S, Jego G, Puthier D, Robillard N, Pineau D, Rapp MJ, Harousseau JL, Amiot M, Bataille R (1998) The absence of CD56 (NCAM) on malignant plasma cells is a hallmark of plasma cell leukemia and of a special subset of multiple myeloma. Leukemia 12(12): 1977–1982

Peters JM, Harris JR, Kleinschmidt JA (1991) Ultrastructure of the approximately 26 S complex containing the approximately 20 S cylinder particle (multicatalytic proteinase/proteasome). Eur J Cell Biol 56(2):422–432

Podar K, Anderson KC (2005) The pathophysiologic role of VEGF in hematologic malignancies: therapeutic implications. Blood 105(4):1383–1395

Podar K, Catley LP, Tai YT, Shringarpure R, Carvalho P, Hayashi T, Burger R, Schlossman RL, Richardson PG, Pandite LN, Kumar R, Hideshima T, Chauhan D, Anderson KC (2004) GW654652, the pan-inhibitor of VEGF receptors, blocks the growth and migration of multiple myeloma cells in the bone marrow microenvironment. Blood 103(9):3474–3479

Podar K, Tonon G, Sattler M, Tai YT, Legouill S, Yasui H, Ishitsuka K, Kumar S, Kumar R, Pandite LN, Hideshima T, Chauhan D, Anderson KC (2006) The small-molecule VEGF receptor inhibitor pazopanib (GW786034B) targets both tumor and endothelial cells in multiple myeloma. Proc Natl Acad Sci USA 103(51):19478–19483

Ponisch W, Mitrou PS, Merkle K, Herold M, Assmann M, Wilhelm G, Dachselt K, Richter P, Schirmer V, Schulze A, Subert R, Harksel B, Grobe N, Stelzer E, Schulze M, Bittrich A, Freund M, Pasold R, Friedrich T, Helbig W et al (2006) Treatment of bendamustine and prednisone in patients with newly diagnosed multiple myeloma results in superior complete response rate, prolonged time to treatment failure and improved quality of life compared to treatment with melphalan and prednisone–a randomized phase III study of the East German study group of hematology and oncology (OSHO). J Cancer Res Clin Oncol 132(4):205–212

Ponisch W, Rozanski M, Goldschmidt H, Hoffmann FA, Boldt T, Schwarzer A, Ritter U, Rohrberg R, Schwalbe E, Uhlig J, Zehrfeld T, Schirmer V, Haas A, Kreibich U, Niederwieser D (2008) Combined bendamustine, prednisolone and thalidomide for refractory or relapsed multiple myeloma after autologous stem-cell transplantation or conventional chemotherapy: results of a phase I clinical trial. Br J Haematol 143(2):191–200

Prince HM, Honemann D, Spencer A (2007) VEGF-R inhibition with pazopanib (GW786034) is ineffective in pretreated myeloma. Haematologica 92(Suppl 2):Abstract 602

Pulkki K, Pelliniemi TT, Rajamaki A, Tienhaara A, Laakso M, Lahtinen R (1996) Soluble interleukin-6 receptor as a prognostic factor in multiple myeloma. Finnish leukaemia group. Br J Haematol 92(2):370–374

Qiang YW, Kopantzev E, Rudikoff S (2002) Insulinlike growth factor-I signaling in multiple myeloma: downstream elements, functional correlates, and pathway cross-talk. Blood 99(11): 4138–4146

Qing G, Yan P, Xiao G (2006) Hsp90 inhibition results in autophagy-mediated proteasome-independent degradation of IkappaB kinase (IKK). Cell Res 16(11):895–901

Raje N, Kumar S, Hideshima T (2004) Combination of the mTOR inhibitor rapamycin and revlimid (CC-5013) has synergistic activity in multiple myeloma. Blood 104:Abstract 1492

Raje N, Hideshima T, Mukherjee S, Raab M, Vallet S, Chhetri S, Cirstea D, Pozzi S, Mitsiades C,

Rooney M, Kiziltepe T, Podar K, Okawa Y, Ikeda H, Carrasco R, Richardson PG, Chauhan D, Munshi NC, Sharma S, Parikh H et al (2009) Preclinical activity of P276-00, a novel small-molecule cyclin-dependent kinase inhibitor in the therapy of multiple myeloma. Leukemia 23(5):961–970

Rajkumar SV, Hayman SR, Lacy MQ, Dispenzieri A, Geyer SM, Kabat B, Zeldenrust SR, Kumar S, Greipp PR, Fonseca R, Lust JA, Russell SJ, Kyle RA, Witzig TE, Gertz MA (2005) Combination therapy with lenalidomide plus dexamethasone (Rev/Dex) for newly diagnosed myeloma. Blood 106(13):4050–4053

Rajkumar SV, Blood E, Vesole D, Fonseca R, Greipp PR (2006) Phase III clinical trial of thalidomide plus dexamethasone compared with dexamethasone alone in newly diagnosed multiple myeloma: a clinical trial coordinated by the Eastern cooperative oncology group. J Clin Oncol 24(3): 431–436

Rajkumar SV, Jacobus S, Callander N, Fonseca R, Vesole D, Williams M, Abonour R, Siegel D, Greipp P (2007) A randomized trial of lenalidomide plus high-dose dexamethasone (RD) versus lenalidomide plus low-dose dexamethasone (Rd) in newly diagnosed multiple myeloma (E4A03): a trial coordinated by the eastern cooperative oncology group. Blood 110:Abstract 74

Raschko M, Markovina S, Miyamoto S (2007) Phase II trial of bevacizumab combined with low dose dexamethasone and lenalidomide (Bev/Rev/Dex) for relapsed or refractory myeloma. Blood 110:Abstract 1173

Richardson PG, Chanan-Khan AA, Alsina M, Doss D, Landrigan B, Kettner D, Albitar M, Mitsiades C, Cropp GF, Johnson RG, Hannah AL, Anderson KC (2005a) Safety and activity of KOS-953 in patients with relapsed refractory multiple myeloma (MM): interim results of a phase 1 trial. Blood 106:Abstract 361

Richardson PG, Sonneveld P, Schuster MW, Irwin D, Stadtmauer EA, Facon T, Harousseau JL, Ben-Yehuda D, Lonial S, Goldschmidt H, Reece D, San-Miguel JF, Blade J, Boccadoro M, Cavenagh J, Dalton WS, Boral AL, Esseltine DL, Porter JB, Schenkein D et al (2005b) Bortezomib or high-dose dexamethasone for relapsed multiple myeloma. N Engl J Med 352(24):2487–2498

Richardson P, Jagannath S, Raje N (2007a) Lenalidomide, bortezomib, and dexamethasone (Rev/Vel/Dex) in patients with relapsed or relapsed/refractory multiple myeloma (MM): preliminary results of a phase II study. Blood 110:Abstract 2714

Richardson P, Jakubowiak A, Wolf J (2007b) Phase I/II report from a multicenter trial of perifosine (KRX-0401)+bortezomib in patients with relapsed or relapsed/refractory multiple myeloma previously treated with bortezomib. Blood 110:Abstract 1170

Richardson P, Lonial S, Jakubowiak A, Krishnan A, Wolf J, Densmore J, Singhal S, Ghobrial I, Stephenson J, Mehta J, Colson K, Francis D, Kendall T, Obadike N, Sullivan K, Martin J, Hideshima T, Lai L, Sportelli P, Gardner L et al (2007c) Multicenter phase II study of perifosine (KRX-0401) alone and in combination with dexamethasone (dex) for patients with relapsed or relapsed/ refractory multiple myeloma (MM): promising activity as combination therapy with manageable toxicity. Blood 2007: Abstract 1164

Richardson PG, Chanan-Khan A, Lonial S, Krishman A, Carroll M, Cropp GF, Kersey K, Abitar M, Johnson RG, Hannah AL, Anderson KC (2007d). Tanespimycin (T)+bortezomib (BZ) in multiple myeloma (MM): confirmation of the recommended dose using a novel formula. Blood 110:Abstract 1165

Richardson PG, Mitsiades CS, Colson K, Reilly E, McBride L, Chiao J, Sun L, Ricker JL, Rizvi S, Oerth C, Atkins B, Fearen I, Anderson KC, Siegel DS (2007e) Final results of a phase I trial of oral vorinostat (suberoylanilide hydroxamic acid, SAHA) in patients with advanced multiple myeloma. Blood 110:Abstract 1179

Richardson PG, Sonneveld P, Schuster M, Irwin D, Stadtmauer E, Facon T, Harousseau JL, Ben-Yehuda D, Lonial S, Goldschmidt H, Reece D, Miguel JS, Blade J, Boccadoro M, Cavenagh J, Alsina M, Rajkumar SV, Lacy M, Jakubowiak A, Dalton W et al (2007f) Extended follow-up of a phase 3 trial in relapsed multiple myeloma: final time-to-event results of the APEX trial. Blood 110(10):3557–3560

Richardson D, Hodges E, Mani A, Orchard K (2008) CD66 expression on malignant and normal plasma cells: a potential target for therapy. Blood 112:Abstract 5073

Roberts PJ, Der CJ (2007) Targeting the Raf-MEK-ERK mitogen-activated protein kinase cascade for the treatment of cancer. Oncogene 26(22):3291–3310

Roodman GD (2008) Bone building with bortezomib. J Clin Invest 118(2):462–464

Rossi J-F, Manges RF, Sutherland HJ, Jagannath S, Voorhees P, Sonneveld P, Delforge M, Pegourie B, Alegre A, Rubia J, Police D, Bandekar R, Xie H, Orlowski RZ (2008) Preliminary results of CNTO 328, an anti-interleukin-6 monoclonal antibody, in combination with bortezomib in the treatment of relapsed or refractory myeloma. Blood 112:Abstract 867

Ruckle J, Jacobs M, Kramer W, Pearsall AE, Kumar R, Underwood KW, Seehra J, Yang Y, Condon CH, Sherman ML (2008) A single-dose, randomized, double-blind, placebo-controlled study of ACE-011 (ActRIIA-IgG1) in postmenopausal women. J Bone Miner Res 24(4):744–752

San Miguel JF, Schlag R, Khuageva NK, Dimopoulos MA, Shpilberg O, Kropff M, Spicka I, Petrucci MT, Palumbo A, Samoilova OS, Dmoszynska A, Abdulkadyrov KM, Schots R, Jiang B, Mateos MV, Anderson KC, Esseltine DL, Liu K, Cakana A, van de Velde H et al (2008) Bortezomib plus melphalan and prednisone for initial treatment of multiple myeloma. N Engl J Med 359(9):906–917

San-Miguel JF, Dimopoulos M, Weber D (2007) Dexamethasone dose adjustments seem to result in better efficacy and improved tolerability in patients with relapsed/refractory multiple myeloma who are treated with lenalidomide/dexamethasone (MM009/010 sub-analysis). Blood 110:Abstract 2712

Santo L, Vallet S, Hideshima T, Cirstea D, Pozzi S, Vaghela N, Ikeda H, Okawa Y, Gorgun G, Perrone G, Calabrese E, Squires MS, Ladetto M, Munshi NC, Boccadoro M, Anderson KC, Raje N (2008) AT7519, a novel small molecule multicyclin dependent kinase inhibitor, induces apoptosis in multiple myeloma VIA GSK3β. Blood 112:Abstract 251

Shi Y, Reiman T, Li W, Maxwell CA, Sen S, Pilarski L, Daniels TR, Penichet ML, Feldman R, Lichtenstein A (2007) Targeting aurora kinases as therapy in multiple myeloma. Blood 109(9): 3915–3921

Siegel DS, Krishnan A, Lonial S, Chatta G, Alsina M, Jagannath S, Richardson P, Hohl RJ, Lust JA, Bensinger W, Carrum G, Moreb J, Simic A, Barlogie B, Maziarz RT, Anderson KC, Lin J, Lowe A, Vetticaden S, Zhu J (2006) Phase II trial of SCIO-469 as monotherapy (M) or in combination with bortezomib (MB) in relapsed refractory multiple myeloma (MM). Blood 108: Abstract 3580

Siegel D, Sezer O, San Miguel JF, Mateos M, Prosser I, Cavo M, Jalaluddin M, Hazell K, Bourquelot PM, Anderson KC (2008) A phase IB, multi-center, open-label, dose-escalation study of oral panobinostat (LBH589) and I.V. bortezomib in patients with relapsed multiple myeloma. Blood 112:Abstract 2781

Siegel DS, Weber DM, Mitsiades C, Rizvi S, Howe J, Reiser D, Anderson KC, Richardson PG (2009) Vorinostat/lenalidomide/dexamethasone: a phase I study. Clin Lymphoma Myeloma 8(7):Abstract 241

Singhal S, Mehta J, Desikan R, Ayers D, Roberson P, Eddlemon P, Munshi N, Anaissie E, Wilson C, Dhodapkar M, Zeddis J, Barlogie B (1999) Antitumor activity of thalidomide in refractory multiple myeloma. N Engl J Med 341(21): 1565–1571

Singhal A, Jagannath S, Vij R, Lonial S (2009) Phase 1b study of elotuzumab (HuLuc63) in combination with lenalidomide in relapsed multiple myeloma. Clin Lymphoma Myeloma 8(7):Abstract 129

Somlo G, Bellamy W, Zimmerman T (2005) Phase II randomized trial of bevacizumab versus bevacizumab and thalidomide for relapsed/ refractory multiple myeloma. Blood 106:Abstract 2571

Spencer A, Lomial S, Taylor K, Jalaluddin M, Hazell K, Bourquelot PM, San Miguel JF (2009) Panobinostat and lenalidomide combination phase I trial in myeloma. Clin Lymphoma Myeloma 8(7):Abstract 329

Standal T, Borset M, Lenhoff S, Wisloff F, Stordal B, Sundan A, Waage A, Seidel C (2002) Serum insulinlike growth factor is not elevated in patients with multiple myeloma but is still a prognostic factor. Blood 100(12):3925–3929

Stevenson GT (2006) CD38 as a therapeutic target. Mol Med 12(11–12):345–346

Streetly MJ, Gyertson K, Daniel Y, Zeldis JB, Kazmi M, Schey SA (2008) Alternate day pomalidomide retains anti-myeloma effect with reduced adverse events and evidence of in vivo immunomodulation. Br J Haematol 141(1):41–51

Stromberg T, Dimberg A, Hammarberg A, Carlson K, Osterborg A, Nilsson K, Jernberg-Wiklund H

(2004) Rapamycin sensitizes multiple myeloma cells to apoptosis induced by dexamethasone. Blood 103(8):3138–3147

Strumberg D, Harstrick A, Doll K, Hoffmann B, Seeber S (1996) Bendamustine hydrochloride activity against doxorubicin-resistant human breast carcinoma cell lines. Anticancer Drugs 7(4):415–421

Stuhmer T, Zollinger A, Siegmund D, Chatterjee M, Grella E, Knop S, Kortum M, Unzicker C, Jensen MR, Quadt C, Chene P, Schoepfer J, Garcia-Echeverria C, Einsele H, Wajant H, Bargou RC (2008) Signalling profile and antitumour activity of the novel Hsp90 inhibitor NVP-AUY922 in multiple myeloma. Leukemia 22(8):1604–1612

Sukhdeo K, Mani M, Zhang Y, Dutta J, Yasui H, Rooney MD, Carrasco DE, Zheng M, He H, Tai YT, Mitsiades C, Anderson KC, Carrasco DR (2007) Targeting the beta-catenin/TCF transcriptional complex in the treatment of multiple myeloma. Proc Natl Acad Sci USA 104(18): 7516–7521

Sullivan D, Singhal S, Schuster M, Berenson J, Gimsing P, Wislöff F, Waage A, Alsina M, Gerwien R, Clarke A, Moller K, Ooi CE (2006) A phase II study of PXD101 in advanced multiple myeloma. Blood 108:Abstract 3583

Tai YT, Podar K, Mitsiades N, Lin B, Mitsiades C, Gupta D, Akiyama M, Catley L, Hideshima T, Munshi NC, Treon SP, Anderson KC (2003) CD40 induces human multiple myeloma cell migration via phosphatidylinositol 3-kinase/AKT/NF-kappa B signaling. Blood 101(7):2762–2769

Tai YT, Catley LP, Mitsiades CS, Burger R, Podar K, Shringpaure R, Hideshima T, Chauhan D, Hamasaki M, Ishitsuka K, Richardson P, Treon SP, Munshi NC, Anderson KC (2004) Mechanisms by which SGN-40, a humanized anti-CD40 antibody, induces cytotoxicity in human multiple myeloma cells: clinical implications. Cancer Res 64(8):2846–2852

Tai YT, Li XF, Catley L, Coffey R, Breitkreutz I, Bae J, Song W, Podar K, Hideshima T, Chauhan D, Schlossman R, Richardson P, Treon SP, Grewal IS, Munshi NC, Anderson KC (2005) Immunomodulatory drug lenalidomide (CC-5013, IMiD3) augments anti-CD40 SGN-40-induced cytotoxicity in human multiple myeloma: clinical implications. Cancer Res 65(24):11712–11720

Tai YT, Li XF, Breitkreutz I, Song W, Neri P, Catley L, Podar K, Hideshima T, Chauhan D, Raje N, Schlossman R, Richardson P, Munshi NC, Anderson KC (2006) Role of B-cell-activating factor in adhesion and growth of human multiple myeloma cells in the bone marrow microenvironment. Cancer Res 66(13):6675–6682

Tai YT, Fulciniti M, Hideshima T, Song W, Leiba M, Li XF, Rumizen M, Burger P, Morrison A, Podar K, Chauhan D, Tassone P, Richardson P, Munshi NC, Ghobrial IM, Anderson KC (2007) Targeting MEK induces myeloma-cell cytotoxicity and inhibits osteoclastogenesis. Blood 110(5): 1656–1663

Tai YT, Dillon M, Song W, Leiba M, Li XF, Burger P, Lee AI, Podar K, Hideshima T, Rice AG, van Abbema A, Jesaitis L, Caras I, Law D, Weller E, Xie W, Richardson P, Munshi NC, Mathiot C, Avet-Loiseau H et al (2008) Anti-CS1 humanized monoclonal antibody HuLuc63 inhibits myeloma cell adhesion and induces antibody-dependent cellular cytotoxicity in the bone marrow milieu. Blood 112(4):1329–1337

Takahashi T, Shivapurkar N, Reddy J, Shigematsu H, Miyajima K, Suzuki M, Toyooka S, Zochbauer-Muller S, Drach J, Parikh G, Zheng Y, Feng Z, Kroft SH, Timmons C, McKenna RW, Gazdar AF (2004) DNA methylation profiles of lymphoid and hematopoietic malignancies. Clin Cancer Res 10(9):2928–2935

Tiedemann RE, Mao X, Shi CX, Zhu YX, Palmer SE, Sebag M, Marler R, Chesi M, Fonseca R, Bergsagel PL, Schimmer AD, Stewart AK (2008) Identification of kinetin riboside as a repressor of CCND1 and CCND2 with preclinical antimyeloma activity. J Clin Invest 118(5): 1750–1764

Trudel S, Li ZH, Wei E, Wiesmann M, Chang H, Chen C, Reece D, Heise C, Stewart AK (2005) CHIR-258, a novel, multitargeted tyrosine kinase inhibitor for the potential treatment of t(4;14) multiple myeloma. Blood 105(7):2941–2948

Trudel S, Stewart AK, Rom E, Wei E, Li ZH, Kotzer S, Chumakov I, Singer Y, Chang H, Liang SB, Yayon A (2006) The inhibitory anti-FGFR3 antibody, PRO-001, is cytotoxic to t(4;14) multiple myeloma cells. Blood 107(10):4039–4046

Trudel S, Yang XZ, Li ZH, Liang S-B, Aftab DT (2007) Evaluation of XL999, a potent inhibitor of FGFR3, for the potential treatment of t(4;14) positive multiple myeloma. Blood 110:Abstract 2515

8

Tsitoura DC, Rothman PB (2004) Enhancement of MEK/ERK signaling promotes glucocorticoid resistance in CD4+ T cells. J Clin Invest 113(4): 619–627

Tu Y, Gardner A, Lichtenstein A (2000) The phosphatidylinositol 3-kinase/AKT kinase pathway in multiple myeloma plasma cells: roles in cytokine-dependent survival and proliferative responses. Cancer Res 60(23):6763–6770

Vallet S, Raje N, Ishitsuka K, Hideshima T, Podar K, Chhetri S, Pozzi S, Breitkreutz I, Kiziltepe T, Yasui H, Ocio EM, Shiraishi N, Jin J, Okawa Y, Ikeda H, Mukherjee S, Vaghela N, Cirstea D, Ladetto M, Boccadoro M et al (2007) MLN3897, a novel CCR1 inhibitor, impairs osteoclastogenesis and inhibits the interaction of multiple myeloma cells and osteoclasts. Blood 110(10):3744–3752

Vallet S, Mukherjee S, Vaghela N, Pozzi S, Santo L, Cirstea D, Fulciniti M, Rahemtullah A, Attar E, Guimaraes A, Xie W, Patel C, Schoonmaker J, Weller E, Hideshima T, Munshi NC, Seehra J, Scadden D, Anderson KC, Raje N (2008) Restoration of bone balance via activin a inhibition results in anti-myeloma activity. Blood 112:Abstract 645

van Rhee F, Dhodapkar M, Shaughnessy JD Jr, Anaissie E, Siegel D, Hoering A, Zeldis J, Jenkins B, Singhal S, Mehta J, Crowley J, Jagannath S, Barlogie B (2008) First thalidomide clinical trial in multiple myeloma: a decade. Blood 112(4):1035–1038

Vanderkerken K, Medicherla S, Coulton L, De Raeve H, Willems A, Lawson M, Van Camp B, Protter AA, Higgins LS, Menu E, Croucher PI (2007) Inhibition of p38alpha mitogen-activated protein kinase prevents the development of osteolytic bone disease, reduces tumor burden, and increases survival in murine models of multiple myeloma. Cancer Res 67(10):4572–4577

Vij R, Horvath N, Spencer A, Taylor K, Vadhan-Raj S, Smith J, Qian Y, Jun S (2007) An open-label, phase 2 trial of denosumab in the treatment of relapsed (R) or plateau-phase (PP) multiple myeloma (MM). Blood 110:Abstract 3604

Vij R, Orlowski R, Stewart AK, Jagannath S, Kukreti V, Taylor J, Fuhrman D, Cruickshank S, Schwartz R, Kunkel L, Siegel D, (MMRC) TMMRc (2009) Phase II study of carfilzomib in patients with relapsed myeloma (PX-171-004). Clin Lymphoma Myeloma 8(7):Abstract 493

Vucic D, Fairbrother WJ (2007) The inhibitor of apoptosis proteins as therapeutic targets in cancer. Clin Cancer Res 13(20):5995–6000

Wang M, Dimopoulos MA, Chen C, Cibeira MT, Attal M, Spencer A, Rajkumar SV, Yu Z, Olesnyckyj M, Zeldis JB, Knight RD, Weber DM (2008a) Lenalidomide plus dexamethasone is more effective than dexamethasone alone in patients with relapsed or refractory multiple myeloma regardless of prior thalidomide exposure. Blood 112(12):4445–4451

Wang X, Sinn AL, Suvannasankha A, Crean CD, Chen L, Zhang S, Liang J, Zhang G, Pollok KE, Abonour R, Sidor C, Bray MR, Farag SS (2008b) The novel aurora kinase inhibitor ENMD-2076 has potent single agent activity against multiple myeloma (MM) in vitro and in vivo, and shows synergistic activity in combination with lenalidomide. Blood 112:Abstract 3660

Weber DM, Chen C, Niesvizky R, Wang M, Belch A, Stadtmauer EA, Siegel D, Borrello I, Rajkumar SV, Chanan-Khan AA, Lonial S, Yu Z, Patin J, Olesnyckyj M, Zeldis JB, Knight RD (2007) Lenalidomide plus dexamethasone for relapsed multiple myeloma in North America. N Engl J Med 357(21):2133–2142

Weber DM, Badros A, Jagannath S, Siegel D, Richon V, Rizvi S, Garvia-Vargas J, Reiser D, Anderson KC (2009) Vorinostat and bortezomib in relpased/refractory MM. Clin Lymphoma Myeloma 8(7):Abstract 242

Wierda WG, Chen R, Plunkett W, Coutre S, Badros AZ, Popplewell L, Siegel D, Sinha R, Harvey D, Fox J, Mahadocon K, Kegley P, M.G. Bolton (2008) A phase 1 trial of SNS-032, a potent and specific CDK 2, 7 and 9 inhibitor, in chronic lymphocytic leukemia and multiple myeloma. Blood 112:Abstract 3178

Wildes TM, Ruddell A, Gao F, Uy G, Cashen A, Abboud C, Westervelt P, Dipersio JF, Vij R (2007) The activity and toxicity of dasatinib in relapsed or plateau-phase multiple myeloma. Blood 110:Abstract 1182

Wolf JL, Siegel D, Matous J, Lonial S, Goldschmidt H, Schmitt S, Vij R, Malgalhaes-Silverman M, Abonour R, Jalaluddin M, Li M, Hazell K, Bourquelot PM, Mateos M-V, Anderson KC, Spencer A, Harousseau J-L, Bladé J (2008) A phase II study of oral panobinostat (LBH589) in adult patients with advnced refractory multiple myeloma. Blood 112:Abstract 2774

Yaccoby S, Ling W, Zhan F, Walker R, Barlogie B, Shaughnessy JD Jr (2007) Antibody-based inhibition of DKK1 suppresses tumor-induced bone resorption and multiple myeloma growth in vivo. Blood 109(5):2106–2111

Yap TA, Garrett MD, Walton MI, Raynaud F, de Bono JS, Workman P (2008) Targeting the PI3K-AKT-mTOR pathway: progress, pitfalls, and promises. Curr Opin Pharmacol 8(4):393–412

Zangari M, Esseltine D, Cavallo F, Neuwirth R, Elice F, Burns MJ, Yaccoby S, Richardson P, Sonneveld P, Tricot G (2007) Predictive value of alkaline phosphatase for response and time to progression in bortezomib-treated multiple myeloma patients. Am J Hematol 82(9):831–833

Zeng S, Li ZH, Chesi M, Leung-Hagesteijn C, Liang S, Bergsagel PL, Trudel S (2008) Pre-clinical evaluation of a small molecule inhibitor of CDK1 as potential therapy for MYC expressing mutiple myeloma tumors. Blood 112:Abstract 3667

Zhukovsky EA, Horton H, Peipp M, Pong E, Bernett M, Karki S, Richards J, Chu S, Repp R, Desjarlais J (2008) An Fc-engineered humanized anti-CD40 monoclonal antibody, XmAb5485, exhibits potent activity in vitro and in vivo against non-hodgkin lymphoma, chronic lymphocytic leukemia and multiple myeloma. Blood 112:Abstract 881

Zollinger A, Stuhmer T, Chatterjee M, Gattenlohner S, Haralambieva E, Muller-Hermelink HK, Andrulis M, Greiner A, Wesemeier C, Rath JC, Einsele H, Bargou RC (2008) Combined functional and molecular analysis of tumor cell signaling defines 2 distinct myeloma subgroups: Akt-dependent and Akt-independent multiple myeloma. Blood 112(8):3403–3411

Firstline Treatment and Maintenance in Newly Diagnosed Multiple Myeloma Patients

9

Murielle Roussel, Thierry Facon, Philippe Moreau, Jean-Luc Harousseau, and Michel Attal

Contents

M. Roussel (✉)
Hématologie Clinique, CHU Purpan,
Place du Docteur Baylac,
31059 Toulouse, Cedex 9, France
e-mail: roussel.m@chu-toulouse.fr

Abstract High dose therapy (HDT) with autologous stem cell transplantation (ASCT) is the standard of care for eligible newly diagnosed MM patients. Several randomized studies demonstrated a survival advantage for patients undergoing transplantation, compared with conventional chemotherapy. Introduction of new drugs in this setting have markedly increased survival rates within the last 10 years. Efforts to further improve response rates and survival in those patients are still needed, mainly by increasing the depth of tumor reduction and the duration of response through more effective induction, consolidation and maintenance therapies. Nevertheless, this approach is currently challenged by the promising results of long-term treatment with novel agents. Recent data suggest that the upfront combination of a proteasome inhibitor plus one immunomodulatory drug (IMiD) is highly effective. The most promising 3-drug association might be Bortezomib, Lenalidomide and dexamethasone (VRD). Adjunction of a 4th drug is not proven to be more efficient. Consolidation and maintenance therapies are emerging in all trials with great results. For elderly patients, or not eligible for ASCT, the introduction of novel agents has also changed the management of the disease. Melphalan-prednisone-thalidomide and bortezomib-melphalan-prednisone are the two standards of care. Current trials are challenging the role

T. Moehler and H. Goldschmidt (eds.), *Multiple Myeloma*,
Recent Results in Cancer Research 183, DOI: 10.1007/978-3-540-85772-3_9,

of alkylators in the frontline setting. Maintenance therapy is also undergoing evaluation.

The treatment of newly diagnosed multiple myeloma (MM) patients has been highly modified during the last decade. The availability of the novel agents like thalidomide, bortezomib, and lenalidomide has expanded treatment options and has improved the outcome of patients with MM. Following the introduction of these agents in the relapsed/refractory setting, they reached the initial treatment of MM. A number of phase II and III trials have demonstrated the efficacy of novel agent combinations both in the transplant and non transplant settings, and based on these results standard frontline regimens are being challenged and modified.

Patients with symptomatic MM require treatment (International Myeloma Working Group 2003). The choice of initial therapy depends on eligibility for high-dose therapy (HDT) and autologous stem cell transplantation (ASCT), determined by age, performance status, and coexisting comorbidities. All patients under 65 years of age should be evaluated at diagnosis for transplant eligibility. Melphalan-containing regimens should be avoided as induction therapy in transplant candidates in order to preserve hematopoietic stem cells. For others, melphalan-prednisone-thalidomide (MPT) and melphalan-prednisone-bortezomib (MPV) currently appear to be the treatments of choice, but other combinations without alkylating agents could provide good options.

9.1 Frontline Treatment in MM Patients Eligible for High-Dose Therapy

HDT with ASCT is the standard of care for eligible newly diagnosed MM patients following the results of several randomized studies that demonstrated a survival advantage for patients undergoing transplantation, compared with conventional chemotherapy (Attal et al. 1996; Child et al. 2003; Blade et al. 2005; Fermand et al. 2005; Barlogie et al. 2006a). Introduction of new drugs in this setting has markedly increased survival rates within the last 10 years. Efforts to further improve response rates and survival in those patients are still needed, mainly by increasing the depth of tumor reduction and the duration of response through more effective induction, consolidation, and maintenance therapies. Nevertheless, this approach is currently challenged by the promising results of long-term treatment merely with novel agents.

This chapter will focus on the current issues concerning the treatment of newly diagnosed young MM patients. Three main points will be discussed:

1. What is the best induction regimen: two, three, or four-drug combination?
2. Should HDT be performed upfront or at time of relapse?
3. Can consolidation and/or maintenance therapies increase the depth of responses and prolong duration of responses and survival?

9.1.1 Induction Treatment: What Combination of New Drugs?

For many years, vincristine, doxorubicin, and dexamethasone (VAD) was the standard induction therapy in upfront patients who were candidates for HDT (Alexanian et al. 1990; Lane et al. 2005). However, overall response rate (ORR) was only in the range of 55–60%, and complete responses (CRs) were achieved in only a small number of patients. Moreover, the response to VAD induction had no impact on the outcome after ASCT. In the last 10 years, induction regimens dramatically changed following the onset of thalidomide, bortezomib, and lenalidomide. Therefore, various combinations of drugs are now available with high response rates. New drug-based induction regimens decrease the tumor burden before HDT but also offer high and deep response rates after HDT. All these agents demonstrated significant superiority over VAD, and, as a result, VAD is no longer recommended as initial therapy.

9.1.1.1 Two-Drug Induction Regimens

Thalidomide-Based Induction Regimens

Thalidomide was the first "novel" agent to be tested in frontline setting. The use of thalidomide plus dexamethasone (Thal-Dex) has been studied in four randomized trials and has emerged as one of the most commonly used induction regimens, at least in United States (Cavo et al. 2005; Macro et al. 2006; Rajkumar et al. 2006, 2008). All studies have demonstrated that Thal-Dex regimen was superior to VAD with good response rates (63–76% ORR). Thal-Dex had the advantage of oral administration but the limitation of high rate of non-hematological toxicities, mainly peripheral neuropathy (PN) and thrombotic events. In the French MAG study (Macro et al. 2006), which compared Thal-Dex to VAD, the initial response rate improvement (35% vs. 13%) was not persistent after ASCT (44% vs. 42%). This Thal-Dex induction regimen might therefore be not good enough and, with the availability of lenalidomide, is less prescribed to newly diagnosed MM patients.

Bortezomib-Based Induction Regimens

In the last 5 years, bortezomib also reached the frontline setting and various phase II and phase III clinical trials were conducted (Harousseau et al. 2006, 2008; Rosinol et al. 2007). The ORR ranges from 60% to 85% with 15% to 20% CRs. In all the studies, the CR markedly increased after transplant (30–40%). The IFM phase III trial 2005-01 compared bortezomib plus dexamethasone (Vel-Dex) to VAD. After four cycles of induction, the ORR with Vel-Dex was significantly higher than that with VAD (82% vs. 65%, including 39% vs. 16% very good partial response (VGPR) or better) and this benefit remained after HDT (≥VGPR 68% vs. 47%). With a median follow-up of 32 months, an improvement of progression-free survival (PFS) had already been observed for Vel-Dex relative to the VAD arm (36 vs. 30 months, respectively; $p=0.057$). Predictive factors for prolonged PFS were: VGPR before and after HDT. Superiority of Vel-Dex over VAD induction therapy was also observed for high-risk patients (ISS 2 or 3 and t(4;14) or del 17p) (Harousseau et al. 2009).

Lenalidomide-Based Induction Regimens

Lenalidomide (Rev) is also undergoing first-line evaluation. Rev-Dex regimen was studied in attempt to improve the Thal-Dex regimen, based on the assumption that lenalidomide is more effective and less neurotoxic than thalidomide. Two large randomized trials, one conducted by ECOG (Rajkumar et al. 2010) and the other by SWOG (Zonder et al. 2007), have shown that the majority of patients respond to induction with Rev/Dex (ORR of 82 and 85% with a CR rate of 4–22%, respectively). In the ECOG trial, 90 of the initial 431 patients went off therapy after the initial four cycles and received HDT followed by ASCT; the 2-year PFS in these patients is 65% and the 3-year OS 92%.

9.1.1.2 Three-Drug Regimens

As all new drugs have shown excellent feasibility and efficacy combined with Dex as induction therapy before intensification, several investigators postulated that this high response rate could be further increased with adjunction of a third drug without a burden of toxicities.

Anthracyclins or Cyclophosphamide in Combination with Thalidomide, Bortezomib, or Lenalidomide

Two randomized trials, conducted by the HOVON group, showed that the addition of adriamycin to Thal-Dex (TAD) (Lokhorst et al. 2010) or Vel-Dex (PAD) (Sonneveld et al. 2008) resulted in an increase in the ORR (71% and 80%, respectively). The CR plus VGPR was 37% and 41%, respectively, which are twice higher values than those obtained with VAD. In the study of TAD vs. VAD, the benefit in favor of TAD remained after ASCT when considering the VGPR rate (54% vs. 44%; $p=0.03$). This translates into a superior PFS for TAD compared with VAD-treated patients (34 vs. 25 months, respectively; $p<0.001$) but a similar OS (59 vs. 62 months). In the PAD vs. VAD trial, the bortezomib arm induced a significantly higher VGPR rate (41% vs. 17%) but few CRs (5% vs. 1%); nevertheless, the CR significantly increased after transplant (15% vs. 4% $p<0.001$).

The British group, in the MRC IX myeloma trial, compared cyclophosphamide + Thal-Dex (CTD) with cyclophosphamide + VAD (CVAD) as induction regimen before transplant, and found the CTD arm to be significantly superior, with ORR of 91% and 82%, including 21% and 14% CR, respectively (Morgan et al. 2009). The CR rate after transplant also remained favorable for the thalidomide arm (65% vs. 48% for CTD vs. CVAD, respectively; $p=0.08$).

In the same way, cyclophosphamide was combined to Vel-Dex (VelCD or Cybor-D) as induction regimen before HDT in two trials conducted by the German group and by the Mayo Clinic, respectively (Knop et al. 2009; Khan et al. 2010; Reeder et al. 2009, Reeder et al. 2010). In the German DSMM XIa Trial, 414 patients were included. Data from the first completed 200 pts were analyzed as intend-to-treat (ITT) population: 84% of patients achieved partial response (PR) or better after three cycles with 12% of CR.

The CyBor-D regimen efficacy was evaluated after four cycles in 63 newly diagnosed MM patients (bortezomib 1.3 mg/m^2 intravenously on days 1, 4, 8, and 11; cyclophosphamide 300 mg/m^2 orally on days 1, 8, 15, and 22; and dexamethasone 40 mg orally on days 1–4, 9–12, and 17–20 on a 28-day cycle). The ORR was impressive with 67% of VGPR or better and 47% of CR/near CR.

Finally, Khan et al. reported the results from a phase II trial combining lenalidomide and low-dose dexamethasone with cyclophosphamide (RCd) as initial therapy for newly diagnosed MM (Khan et al. 2010). Fifty three patients were enrolled. The median number of cycles was 5 (range: 1–20). The best response based on all enrolled patients on an ITT basis was 83%, including CR: 2%, VGPR: 38%, PR: 43%, and less than PR: 17%. Hematological toxicity was the most common with grade 4 toxicity seen in eight patients. Non-hematological toxicities included neuropathy, diarrhea, cystitis, and thrombosis. Thirteen patients had dose adjustments, most commonly due to hematological toxicity attributed to lenalidomide or cyclophosphamide.

Bortezomib in Combination with Thalidomide or Lenalidomide

Several phase II studies have explored the feasibility and efficacy of the combination of bortezomib with thalidomide in untreated MM patients. The high and rapid ORR (90% = PR, with 20% CR) prompted the design of phase III trials.

Thus, the Italian group compared bortezomib plus Thal-Dex (VTD) with Thal-Dex (Cavo et al. 2009). Four hundred and seventy four patients were randomized to the VTD ($n=236$) or Thal-Dex ($n=238$) arm. VTD was significantly superior after induction (VGPR or better: 61% vs. 28%) and after consolidation (82% vs. 67%). Superiority of the VTD vs. Thal-Dex arm in terms of CR rate was confirmed in patients with high-risk cytogenetics, as defined by the presence of t(4;14) and/or del(17p) (58% vs. 33%, respectively; $p=0.004$). In addition, this translated into a significantly longer PFS (76% vs. 58% at 30 months for VTD vs. Thal-Dex, respectively), but no significant differences in OS have yet been observed.

The Spanish group has performed a similar comparison (VTD vs. Thal-Dex), with in addition a third arm, based on chemotherapy (VBCMP/VBAD plus bortezomib) (Rosinol et al. 2009). Two hundred and ninety nine patients were evaluable for response and toxicity to induction therapy and 177 to ASCT. Results presented at last ASH meeting indicate that the VTD arm was superior in terms of response rates (VGPR or better=59% before and 78% after ASCT), time to progression (TTP) and PFS.

The IFM also recently reported on a phase III trial (IFM 2007-02) comparing Vel-Dex to vTD (with low doses of bortezomib=1 mg/m^2 and =100 mg/day) (Harousseau et al. 2010). Hundred and ninety one patients were evaluable for response after four cycles. vTD induced significantly higher VGPR rates (50% vs. 36%, $p=0.047$) but identical CR rates (14% vs. 12%). It is important to note that dose reduction of bortezomib significantly decreased grade 2 or more PN incidence in the vTD arm without reduced response rates. This superiority was persistent after HDT (VGPR or better: 66% vs. 54%, $p=0.044$).

The most promising three-drug induction regimen might be the combination of bortezomib with Rev/Dex (VRD) (Richardson et al. 2010). VRD has been investigated in a phase I/II trial in which 66 patients were enrolled. All patients responded, including 67%≥VGPR and 39% CR/nCR. Moreover, responses were independent of cytogenetics. Most common toxicities included sensory neuropathy (80%) and fatigue (64%), with only 27%/2% grade 2/3 neuropathy (PN). Additionally, 32% reported neuropathic pain (11%/3% grade 2/3). Thrombosis was rare (6% overall) and no treatment-related mortality was seen. With median follow-up of 21 months, estimated 18-month PFS and OS for the combination treatment with/without transplant was 75% and 97%, respectively.

The IFM finished last year the accrual of a phase II study investigating three cycles of VRD before HDT followed by ASCT. Results will be available at the next ASH meeting.

9.1.1.3 Four-Drug Induction Regimens

The EVOLUTION 2 trial have explored the combination of cyclophosphamide with VRD (VDCR) in 43 patients (Kumar et al. 2009); 33 patients were evaluable for response. ORR was 94% with 57% of VGPR or better. Response rates in the VDCR arm appeared somewhat higher than in the other arms at this early time point, although there also appeared to be higher rates of serious AEs, including possible treatment-related mortality in the VDCR arm.

The HOVON group (Ludwig et al. 2010) has investigated, for its part, the cyclophosphamide+VTD (VTDC) regimen. Response rates were of great value but toxicities were also increased. Forty nine patients were randomized to each arm. One patient (VTDC arm) was not evaluable for response. Response rates following induction were ORR: 100%/96% and CR+nCR: 51%/44%, respectively. At data cutoff, 47 VTD and 35 VTDC patients had undergone ASCT; response rates post ASCT in 38 and 27 evaluable patients were similar within the two arms with ORR: 100% and CR+nCR 39%/33%, respectively. PN was reported in 35% (VTD) and 29% (VTDC) of patients, including 8% grade 3 in each arm and 2% grade

4 in the VTD arm. Both VTD and VTDC are highly active induction regimens; the efficacy profiles were similar between the arms, but there were higher rates of toxicity in the VTDC arm compared with the VTD arm.

Taken together, these data suggest that the upfront combination of a proteasome inhibitor plus one immunomodulatory drug (IMiD) is highly effective. These data lead us to conclude that VAD is no longer the gold-standard induction regimen. Thal-Dex can be an option with the addition of another chemotherapy agent, such as cyclophosphamide or an anthracyclin. A similar possibility may exist for lenalidomide-based induction regimens. VTD has proved to be highly effective as a frontline treatment and is significantly superior to VAD or Thal-Dex before and after ASCT with a very manageable toxic pattern. The most promising three-drug association might be VRD. Adjunction of a fourth drug is not proven to be more efficient but is definitely more toxic.

9.1.2 Autologous Stem Cell Transplantation Upfront or at the Time of Relapse?

In the 1990s, several randomized trials demonstrated the superiority of HDT with ASCT compared to conventional chemotherapy in terms of prolonged PFS, OS, and time without symptoms or treatment toxicities (TwiSTT) (Attal et al. 1996; Fermand et al. 1998; Child et al. 2003; Blade et al. 2005; Fermand et al. 2005; Barlogie et al. 2006). HDT (usually based on melphalan 200 mg/m^2) followed by ASCT prolonged OS as compared with chemotherapy in prospective randomized trials conducted by the French (IFM) and English (MRC) groups and has provided evidence for longer than 10-year survivorship in at least a subset of patients. Nevertheless, the US (SWOG 9,321) and French (MAG91) studies and the Spanish (PETHEMA-94) trial, though confirming the benefit of ASCT in terms of ORR and event-free survival (EFS), found no greater OS than with chemotherapy.

ASCT is currently considered to be the standard care for younger patients with MM, mainly because of its low treatment mortality rate (1–2%), the benefit in response rate, and survival. In the setting of new drug-containing regimen, it is important to assess whether ASCT enhances the quality and depth of response. Several randomized trials indicated an improved CR rate following ASCT, which already translates into prolonged PFS. These data imply that induction with novel agents and ASCT are complementary rather than alternative treatment approaches. Nevertheless, the favorable results obtained with long-term treatment with these novel combinations, in patients who are not candidate for HDT, are challenging the role of upfront ASCT. Some investigators already stated that HDT should no longer be used in frontline therapy. Stem cell collection should be performed within the first months of therapy with novel agents and reserve the HDT at time of relapse. But a lot of arguments could favor HDT in frontline patients. HDT is no more toxic and expensive (arguments that can be opposed to novel agents). Quality of life is only impaired for a short period of time after HDT and it has been already demonstrated that time without symptoms and treatment toxicity was improve if HDT was preformed upfront. Furthermore, the strategy of delayed HDT is reasonable only if the feasibility of ASCT at time of relapse is good. It could be a major concern for patients aged between 60 and 65 years at time of diagnosis. The IFM in association with the Dana Farber Cancer Institute (DFCI) will soon assess this issue in a large joint phase III trial. Patients will be randomly assigned to receive HDT upfront or at time of relapse. Induction and consolidation therapies will be based on the DFCI RVD regimen. The Italian GIMEMA cooperative group is currently conducting a similar trial. Preliminary data have been presented in the last ASCO congress. Patients, in a 2 × 2 factorial plan, will receive either a tandem ASCT with melphalan 200 mg/m^2 or six cycles of melphalan, prednisone, and lenalidomide (MPR). 117 pts received three cycles of MPR and 122 pts underwent their first ASCT. Response rates are similar in the two groups with 13% vs. 16% of CR, and 55% vs. 53% of VGPR or better, respectively (Palumbo et al. 2010b).

9.1.3 Maintenance/Consolidation Treatment

Although HDT with ASCT improves CR rates and PFS, almost all patients ultimately relapse. An optimal maintenance treatment should prolong PFS with acceptable toxicity, not compromise treatment at time of relapse, and, furthermore, prolong OS. The impact of maintenance therapy with chemotherapy after HDT has always failed to prolong PFS and OS.

In the 1980s, maintenance treatment with corticosteroids (Berenson et al. 2002) and/or interferon has been a first choice. Following the initial randomized study showing prolonged remissions with α-interferon maintenance in patients responding to conventional induction therapy (Mandelli et al. 1990), a number of randomized trials were performed but their results were controversial. Two meta-analyses of randomized trials showed that with interferon maintenance, time to PFS and OS was increased by 4–7 months (Fritz and Ludwig 2000; Myeloma Trialists' Collaborative Group 2001). However, most investigators considered that the benefit was small and needed balancing against cost and potential toxicity of prolonged treatment with α-interferon. In addition, α-interferon has been used after ASCT, with the hypothesis that it might be more effective in patients with minimal residual disease. In a retrospective analysis of the European Bone Marrow and Blood Transplant Registry, interferon maintenance was associated with improved PFS and OS in patients responding to high-dose therapy (Bjorkstrand et al. 2001). However, two randomized trials failed to confirm this result (Cunningham et al. 1998; Barlogie et al. 2006).

The availability of novel agents (particularly oral thalidomide and lenalidomide) has renewed the concept of maintenance. Five randomized studies with thalidomide have been completed (Attal et al. 2006; Barlogie et al. 2006; Morgan et al. 2009; Spencer et al. 2009; Lokhorst et al. 2010). The IFM group, in the IFM 9,902 trial, was the first to show that thalidomide as maintenance after tandem ASCT was superior to no maintenance or pamidronate alone. Thalidomide increased the CR+VGPR rate (67 vs. 55 and 57%, respectively), the 3-year PFS (52 vs. 36 and 37%, respectively), and the 4-year OS (87 vs. 77 and 74%, respectively). The Australian group obtained similar results upon comparing thalidomide (for 12 months) plus prednisone (until progression) with prednisone alone. Within the Total Therapy 2 program, the Arkansas group tested also the impact of thalidomide as maintenance. In the initial report, CR rate and 5-year PFS were significantly better in the thalidomide arm (62 vs. 43% and 56 vs. 44%, respectively) but there was no OS improvement. However, in an updated analysis, with a median follow-up of 72 months, the prolonged OS was confirmed in a subgroup of patients with poor-risk cytogenetics. In total, four of five randomized trials showed a benefit in PFS and OS with thalidomide maintenance. But what group of patients will really benefit of thalidomide? In the IFM trial, only patients who failed to achieve at least VGPR had significantly longer PFS in the thalidomide arm. The shorter OS duration observed in several studies appears to be a result of a shorter survival time after relapse, which may be caused by different factors, such as the duration of maintenance treatment, the possible selection of more resistant clones, the age of patients, toxicities from previous treatments, and the availability of salvage treatments. Future studies should be aimed at identifying patients who may benefit from thalidomide maintenance and establishing the appropriate dose and optimal duration of therapy. The Australian trial showed that maintenance for only 1 year did not adversely affect the outcome after relapse, but two studies (from the MRC and the Arkansas group) suggested that the long-term use of thalidomide may induce more resistant relapses. Finally, the incidence of thalidomide induced PN is cumulative and related to the time of exposure. Long-term treatment with thalidomide is actually impossible.

The more favorable toxicity profile of lenalidomide makes it an ideal maintenance agent and has prompted several ongoing trials designed to compare continuous treatment until relapse with non-maintenance or treatment for only a short period after ASCT. Two large randomized phase III trials, one conducted by the IFM (Attal et al. 2010), the second by the CALGB (McCarthy et al. 2010), were presented in the last ASCO meeting. Lenalidomide was given orally after HDT at 10–15 mg/day up to progression. Results were similar with an improvement of PFS (around 24 months in the placebo arm versus not reached in the lenalidomide arm). The safety profile was good and subgroup analysis showed that the benefice of maintenance therapy was seen irrespective of response after HDT and initial prognostic factors. With a median follow-up of 24 months for the IFM trial, there is no difference in the OS.

Bortezomib was investigated in the consolidation setting. Consolidation with VTD may induce molecular remission in a number of patients (Ladetto et al. 2010). Ongoing randomized studies by several European study groups are further investigating bortezomib as consolidation and maintenance therapy. For example, the DSMM is investigating the use of bortezomib as consolidation treatment following induction therapy with VCD plus high-dose therapy. The phase III GIMEMA trial also includes a consolidation randomization. Following induction treatment with VTD or TD and tandem transplantation, patients are randomized to receive VTD or TD consolidation therapy. In the HOVON 65 MM/GMMG-HD four trial, bortezomib versus thalidomide maintenance therapy is being examined following initial randomization between PAD and VAD induction.

9.2 Frontline Treatment in Elderly MM Patients

Treatment with melphalan (or cyclophosphamide) and prednisone (MP) has been used since the 1960s. Despite poor CR rates and 40% overall response rates, MP was the most widely accepted treatment option for elderly patients ineligible for HDT (Alexanian et al. 1969; Bataille and Harousseau 1997). Long-term outcomes were disappointing, with a median PFS duration of about 18 months and a median OS time of about 3 years. More complex combinations with alkylating agents have been substituted but often with added toxicity and no survival advantage (Myeloma Trialists' Collaborative Group 1998).

High-dose dexamethasone (Dex) alone or Dex-based regimens have provided other options. Although Dex gives better response rates, its use among patients over 65 is cautious because of greater toxicities, mainly infectious, and lack of benefit in terms of overall survival (Alexanian et al. 1992; Hernandez et al. 2004; Facon et al. 2006).

Introduction of highly active new drugs in this setting has markedly increased survival rates within the last decade. Overall, two "backbones" have been used for the development of combinations with new agents: MP (or C), in Europe, and Dex, in North America.

This chapter will discuss the current issues concerning the treatment of newly diagnosed elderly MM patients. Four main points will be reviewed:

1. What is the best partner for MP or alkylators: thalidomide, bortezomib, and/or lenalidomide?
2. Can new drugs replace alkylating agents?
3. Can we reduce new drugs toxicities, especially for the elderly patients?
4. Can maintenance therapies prolong duration of responses and survival?

9.2.1 What Is the Best Combination with Alkylating Agents?

Alkylating agents with prednisone, at least in Europe, are the core of treatment for frontline elderly patients. Several trials evaluated the role of new agents combined to melphalan or cyclophosphamide in this setting.

9.2.1.1 Thalidomide

Recently, a number of studies have investigated the addition of novel agents to the traditional MP regimen. The combination of MP plus thalidomide has been investigated in five randomized phase III trials (Palumbo et al. 2005; Facon et al. 2007; Wijermans et al. 2008; Hulin et al. 2009; Waage et al. 2010a). In the three first published trials (GIMEMA, IFM 99-06, and IFM 01-01), the superiority of MPT over MP or MP plus placebo was clearly demonstrated. These results were very concordant within the three studies. The addition of thalidomide to MP resulted in a significantly greater ORR, as well as a longer TTP, PFS time, or EFS time. Of note, 30–50% of the patients achieved at least a VGPR. In the IFM 01-01 study, response results were slightly inferior but still significantly superior to those of MP plus placebo, with a 62% ORR and a 7% CR rate. Median PFS times with MPT were similar in all three studies, ranging from 24 to 29 months. In both IFM studies, but not in the GIMEMA study, the PFS advantage observed with MPT translated into a significant OS advantage. There were some substantial differences in study design, such as the dose of thalidomide and duration of treatment, which included maintenance thalidomide in all except the two IFM studies. In the Nordic Study, the addition of thalidomide to MP resulted in a significant advantage in terms of RR and time to progression compared with MP. However, these favorable results did not translate into an OS advantage. The study was hampered by a high proportion of patients with a poor performance status and used higher doses of melphalan and thalidomide. These characteristics likely contributed to more frequent early deaths in the MPT group, especially in the oldest patients. Regarding toxicities, MPT was associated with a significantly increased risk of complications, especially somnolence or fatigue, constipation, PN, and deep venous thrombosis (DVT). Thrombo-embolic events usually occurred early in therapy (90% within 4 months). Anticoagulation prophylaxis is able to reduce thrombosis/embolism, and recommendations have been recently published by the International Myeloma Working Group. PN occurred after prolonged administration of thalidomide and was a frequent cause of discontinuation. More than 50% of patients treated for 12 months suffered from PN, although in most patients it was of grade 1/2. The incidence of grade 3/4 PN varied from 2% to 9%. Neurotoxicity will probably be reduced by thalidomide treatment of shorter durations and at lower doses. These results led to the approval of thalidomide in 2008 for previously untreated MM patients by the European Medicines Agency (EMEA). In a recent meta-analysis on survival of 1682 individual patients treated with MPT or MP in six different randomized studies, including the trials previously reported, the addition of thalidomide to MP significantly improved progression-free survival and overall survival (Waage et al. 2010). Similar data have been presented in a meta-analysis of published data (Kapoor et al. 2009)

Other combinations have been examined in an attempt to improve outcomes in the elderly patient group. For example, the combination CTD was investigated in a large phase III randomized study by the MRC (Myeloma IX) comparing, in patients ineligible for transplantation, MP to CTD with an attenuated Dex dose (CTDa: cyclophosphamide 500 mg orally weekly, thalidomide 200 mg daily, Dex 20 mg on days 1–4 and 15–16 of a 28-day cycle) (Morgan et al. 2007). This first randomization was followed by a maintenance randomization comparing thalidomide 100 mg daily to relapse to no thalidomide. In this group of 854 less fit patients (median age, 73 years; range, 57–89 years), CTDa achieved a significantly higher RR (82.5% vs. 49%), including VGPR (47.5% vs. 9.5%) and CR (22.5% vs. 6%) rates. Patients induced with CTDa seem to survive for approximately a year longer than patients induced with MP (Morgan et al. 2009). CTDa survival results seem comparable to those achieved in the IFM MPT studies, and CTDa response rates are comparable to those achieved in IFM 99-06.

9.2.1.2
Bortezomib

In vitro studies have shown a synergistic effect between bortezomib and melphalan plus corticosteroids. Based on these promising findings, bortezomib was added to the standard MP (MPV regimen) in elderly untreated MM patients in a phase I/II trial conducted by the Spanish Myeloma Group (GEM/PETHEMA) (Mateos et al. 2006). Sixty patients were enrolled in this trial and, after a median of seven cycles, the ORR was 89% with a 32% CR rate. MPV was generally well tolerated and the majority of adverse events occurred during the first two cycles of treatment. These results led to a large, randomized, phase III VISTA trial (Velcade as Initial Standard Treatment: Assessment with melphalan and prednisone), in which 682 patients were included and randomized to receive either MP alone or in combination with bortezomib (San Miguel et al. 2008). MPV was found to be significantly superior to MP for all efficacy endpoints: CR rate, ORR, PFS, TTP, time to next therapy (TNT), and OS. 30% of patients in the MPV arm achieved CRs, compared with only 4% in the MP arm. Median time to achieve CR was 4 months. Patients who achieved CR had a median duration of response of 24 months. The primary endpoint of the trial was TTP, and MPV resulted in a 52% reduced risk of progression compared with MP, with a median TTP of 24 months for MPV and 16 months for MP. With an updated median follow-up of 26 months, the OS analysis showed a 36% reduced risk of death for MPV and the 3-year OS is 72% for MPV and 59% for MP, despite 45% of MP patients having received treatment with bortezomib upon progression. The efficacy of bortezomib was also evaluated in subgroups of patients who had a poor prognosis. In 107 patients who were 75 years of age or older, as compared with 237 younger patients, the median TTP was identical, the rate of CR (according to EBMT criteria) was slightly lower (26% vs. 32%), and the median OS was not significantly shorter. The 26 patients with high-risk cytogenetic profiles – including the presence of a t(4;14),t(14;16) translocation or a 17p deletion – and the 142 patients with standard cytogenetic profiles had the same rate of CR(28%), with similar TTP and OS. Fewer patients in the MPV versus MP arm required subsequent therapy (38% vs. 57%, respectively). Re-treatment with bortezomib was effective in the MPV arm (6% of CRs) at the moment of relapse, as were the IMiDs (4% of CRs with thalidomide and lenalidomide-based combinations). Regarding toxicity, the frequency of serious adverse events was higher in the MPV arm (46% vs. 36%). No significant differences were reported in the incidence of hematologic toxicity and the most divergent grade 3/4 toxicities between MPV and MP were gastrointestinal events (20% vs. 6%) and PN (13% vs. 0%). In addition, 17% and 14% of patients experienced grade 2 and grade 1 PN, respectively, for a total incidence of 44%. However, it was reversible in most patients; 79% of PN events improved (by at least one grade) in a median of 2 months and 60% of PN events completely resolved in a median of 6 months. Herpes zoster was more frequent with MPV (13% vs. 4%), but the rate with MPV decreased to 3% among patients receiving antiviral prophylaxis. Thrombo-embolic events were very low and the same in both arms (1%). Upon analyzing the tolerability by treatment cycle it was found that the major incidence of adverse events in the MPV arm occurred during the first four cycles. These results led to the approval in 2008 of bortezomib for previously untreated MM patients by the US Food Drug Administration (FDA) and the EMEA.

9.2.1.3 Lenalidomide

Lenalidomide has also been examined for the treatment of elderly patients with newly diagnosed MM. In a phase I/II trial, the combination of lenalidomide with MP (MPR) was found to result in an ORR of 81% and a 24% CR rate (Palumbo et al. 2007). With a median follow-up of 29.5 months, the median TTP and PFS times were 28.5 months and the 2-year OS rate was 90.5%. The main AEs included neutropenia, thrombocytopenia, and thromboembolism. Following these promising results, an international phase III study, MM 015, was conducted comparing MP with MPR (with or without lenalidomide maintenance) (Palumbo et al. 2010). Four hundred and fifty nine patients were enrolled in the study. Twenty-five percent of patients were older than 75 years. Patients were randomly assigned to receive either nine cycles of MP or MPR or MPR+R maintenance. The ORR was 50%, 68%, and 77%, respectively. Four percent of patients achieved CR within the MP arm compared to 11% in the MPR arm and 16% in the MPR+R arm. The primary objective was PFS between MP vs. MPR+R. Median follow-up at time of reporting was 21 months. Although median PFS was not reached in the MPR+R, PFS was only 13 months for the MP and 14 months for the MPR patients. The most common grade 3/4 adverse events were neutropenia and thrombocytopenia (70% and 38%, respectively in the MPR arm). More than 60% of patients required growth factor support. This hematological toxic pattern, especially in the older patients, could explain the disappointing results of this regimen. Results of the ongoing ECOG E1A06 study comparing MPT with MPR will be of great interest. The HOVON and the Nordic Myeloma Study Group are also conducting a phase III trial in elderly patients comparing MPT plus maintenance thalidomide with MPR followed by maintenance with lenalidomide. This trial will further clarify the role of lenalidomide in the nontransplant setting.

9.2.1.4 Combinations of New Agents Plus MP

VMPT

In the Italian GIMEMA trial, MPV was compared with bortezomib, melphalan, prednisone, and thalidomide (VMPT) followed by maintenance with VT (Palumbo et al. 2010). Initially, patients received a scheme similar to that previously reported in the VISTA trial (bortezomib administered twice per week), adding thalidomide (50 mg/day) in the VMPT arm. The protocol was subsequently amended: both VMPT and MPV schedules were changed to nine 5-week cycles and the bortezomib schedule was modified to weekly administration. Five hundred and eleven patients were included. The VGPR rate was significantly higher in the VMPT group (59% vs. 50%), including a CR rate of 38% in the VMPT group and 24% in the MPV group. Maintenance therapy did not further enhance response rates. The incidence of grade 3/4 adverse events was similar in both groups except for neutropenia (37% vs. 28%), noting that the weekly infusion of bortezomib significantly decreased the incidence of grade 3/4 PN (9% for VMPT and 8% for MPV). With a median follow-up of 26.5 months, 3-year PFS is 54% in the VMPT + VT arm vs. 40% in the MPV arm ($p=0.006$).

9.2.2 Firstline Treatment: Can New Agents Replace Alkylators?

9.2.2.1 Thalidomide

Two studies conducted in the United States were designed to compare thalidomide plus dexamethasone (Thal-Dex) versus Dex as primary therapy for newly diagnosed patients (Rajkumar et al. 2006, 2008). These studies enrolled a total of 677 young and elderly patients but primarily targeted patients unable or unwilling to undergo upfront ASCT. Thal-Dex resulted in significantly higher response rates (63% vs. 41%) and prolonged TTP compared to Dex (22.6 vs. 6.5 months), leading to FDA approval in 2006. However, the toxicity of dexamethasone was significant and the combination had an even greater toxicity (hyperglycemia, fatigue, insomnia and muscle weakness). In the ECOG study, there were 5% treatment-related deaths. Similar toxicities were noted in the other Thal-Dex study. A further confirmation of high level of toxicity was provided by the Central European phase III study in elderly patients ($n=289$) comparing Thal-Dex with MP (Ludwig et al. 2009). Patients were randomized to either thalidomide 50–400 mg daily plus Dex 40 mg on days 1–4 and days 15–18 on even cycles and on days 1–4 on odd cycles, during a 28-day cycle, or to melphalan 0.25 mg/kg and prednisone 2 mg/kg orally on days 1–4 during a 28–42-day cycle. For maintenance, patients achieving stable disease or better were randomized to receive 3 MU interferon-α2b three times per week with or without thalidomide 100 mg daily. The study reported significantly higher CR and VGPR rates (26% vs. 13%) as well as RR (68% vs. 50%) for patients receiving Thal-Dex. PFS was similar in both groups (median, 21 and 17 months for MP and Thal-Dex, respectively), but significantly shorter OS was observed in the Thal-Dex group (median, 49 and 42 months for MP and Thal-Dex, respectively). The population was very elderly, especially in the Thal-Dex group, with 60% of patients between the ages 70 and 79 and 10% ≥80 years. Patients received a high-dose Dex regimen and thalidomide dosing was up to 400 mg/day. Thus, the very elderly patient population and the higher doses of thalidomide and Dex used likely contributed to a higher mortality rate in Thal-Dex-treated patients during the first year of study, especially in patients with a poorer performance status.

Overall, when considering all of these Thal-Dex experiences, in terms of both efficacy and toxicity, there is evidence that this combination is not superior to MPT and may not be optimal for elderly patients.

9.2.2.2 Lenalidomide

A subanalysis of the phase III ECOG trial examined the efficacy of lenalidomide-Dex (RD) versus lenalidomide-low dose Dex (Rd) in patients ≥65 years old (Rajkumar et al. 2010). The 1-year survival rate was found to be significantly better for patients receiving Rd than for those receiving RD (94% vs. 83%, respectively; $p < 0.004$). High-dose Dex in a community-setting seems more toxic than low-dose Dex, with more early deaths in the first 4 months, increased risk of thrombo-embolic complications, and higher overall risk of serious adverse events, particularly in patients older than 65 years.

9.2.2.3 Combinations of New Agents

Bortezomib and Thalidomide

In an attempt to optimize the treatment of elderly untreated MM patients, the Spanish myeloma trial (GEMO5) was designed to compare six cycles of induction therapy with MPV versus bortezomib, thalidomide, and prednisone (VTP) (Mateos et al. 2009). The MPV regimen was based on one intensive "VISTA" 6-week cycle followed by five adapted 5-week cycles (bortezomib was given as a weekly dose on days 1, 8, 15, and 22). The VTP arm was the same as MPV, but substituting the melphalan with thalidomide at 100 mg/day. A total of 260 patients have been recruited so far and preliminary results show no significant differences in efficacy (RR of 81% in both arms, with CR rates of 22% and 27% for MPV and VTP, respectively). The VTP arm was found to be cardiotoxic. After induction therapy, patients were randomized to receive maintenance therapy for 3 years with thalidomide (50 mg daily) plus bortezomib (VT) or prednisone plus bortezomib (VP); bortezomib is given on a conventional schedule (days 1, 4, 8, and 11) every 3 months. Maintenance increased response rates.

9.2.3 Can We Reduce Toxicities of New Drugs-Incorporating Regimens?

9.2.3.1 Bortezomib in a Weekly Schedule

As already mentioned, a reduced frequency of administration of bortezomib in combination with MP was investigated in two European studies in patients ≥65 years old. In the Spanish myeloma group trial, patients were randomized to receive six cycles of MPV or bortezomib plus thalidomide plus prednisone (VTP) (Mateos et al. 2009). During cycle 1 of the induction treatment, bortezomib was administered twice weekly, and in subsequent cycles bortezomib was only administered once weekly. The results indicate that efficacy was similar between the two regimens, whereas differences were observed in toxicities. Notably, the rate of grade 3 or 4 PN was only 5% with the reduced-dose MPV regimen, and only 12% of patients discontinued treatment. The Italian myeloma group also investigated a reduced frequency of administration of bortezomib in a trial designed to compare bortezomib, melphalan, prednisone, and thalidomide (VMPT) with MPV in elderly patients (Palumbo et al. 2009). Bortezomib was initially administered twice weekly in a proportion of patients; however, following a protocol amendment, all patients received bortezomib once weekly at 1.3 mg/m^2. A comparison of efficacy and toxicity in patients receiving twice-weekly or once-weekly bortezomib in the MPV arm revealed that a shift from twice weekly to once-weekly bortezomib dosing reduced the rate of CR from 27% to 20%, but that it also substantially reduced the incidence of sensory neuropathy (14% vs. 2%) and rate of treatment discontinuation (15% vs. 4%).

The results of these two studies suggest that a reduction in bortezomib administration from twice weekly to once weekly leads to a reduction in toxicity of the MPV regimen while retaining significant efficacy, although not at the same level as reported in the original VISTA trial. Longer follow-up is needed to assess the impact on PFS and OS.

9.2.3.2 Low-Dose Dexamethasone

Along with the frequent and serious Dex side effects, there were also data suggesting that high doses of Dex were possibly not necessary in combination with novel agents, such as thalidomide or lenalidomide. The ECOG group proceeded recently with the E4A03 study comparing lenalidomide plus high-dose Dex (40 mg daily on days 1–4, 9–12, and 17–20) with lenalidomide plus low-dose Dex (40 mg daily on days 1, 8, 15, and 22) (Rajkumar et al. 2010). A total of 445 patients (median age, 66 years; aged up to 88 years) were treated, including 233 over the age of 65 years. The significant toxicity of the high-dose Dex regimen was fully confirmed, but the good news was the modest toxicity of the low-dose Dex regimen. Infection/pneumonia, fatigue, hyperglycemia, deep venous thrombosis, and cardiac ischemia were significantly less frequent with the low-dose Dex schedule. Overall, nonhematologic toxicity grade ≥3 was found in 52% of patients receiving RD compared to 34% of patients receiving Rd. Early deaths were also significantly less frequent in the low-dose Dex arm (1.4% vs. 4.5%). In patients aged over 65 years, the 2-year survival was significantly superior in the group of patients receiving the low-dose Dex regimen (82% vs. 67%). In patients receiving primary therapy beyond four cycles with Rd, the ORR was 89% with a 22% CR rate, and a 56% VGPR rate. Overall, and even though the study was not designed to test efficacy of long-term lenalidomide plus Dex (median durations on treatment were only 4 months in the high-dose Dex arm and 6 months in the low-dose Dex arm), Rd was found to be highly active in newly diagnosed elderly patients. There is no doubt that these results will be of major importance in the future and will influence the fate of other Dex-based combinations.

9.2.3.3 Prevention of IMiDs-Associated Venous Thromboembolism (VTE)

The International Myeloma Working Group has provided in 2008 detailed guidelines on the appropriate thromboprophylaxis for patients in patients treated with thalidomide or lenalidomide (Palumbo et al. 2008). The panel recommended aspirin for patients with low risk factor for VTE. LMWH (equivalent to enoxaparin 40 mg/day) is recommended for those with intermediate or high-risk factors. LMWH is also recommended for all patients receiving concurrent high-dose dexamethasone or doxorubicin. Full-dose warfarin targeting a therapeutic INR of 2–3 is an alternative to LMWH, although there are limited data in the literature with this strategy and it might not be recommended for cancer patients. In the absence of clear data from randomized studies as a foundation for recommendations, many of the following proposed strategies are the results of common sense or derive from the extrapolation of data from many studies not specifically designed to answer these questions.

9.2.4 Maintenance Therapy in Elderly

Results from the MRC Myeloma IX maintenance study indicate that thalidomide maintenance has a non significant effect in improving PFS in non-intensively treated patients (Morgan et al. 2009). Lenalidomide and bortezomib are still under investigation and a longer follow-up is needed for confirming their role as maintenance treatment.

The Spanish myeloma group investigated a 3 years maintenance with VT or VP (bortezomib: 1.3 mg/m^2/day 1, 4, 8, 11/3 months; Thalidomide: 50 mg/day; Prednisone: 50 mg alternating days) (Mateos et al. 2009). This maintenance regimen increased the CR from 25% to 42% with a low toxicity profile. VT was superior in terms of TTEvents. Despite these good results, considering their toxicity profile, first of all peripheral neuropathy, and, in case of thalidomide, the lack of correlation between cumulative dose and outcome, a limited administration is suggested. In contrast, lenalidomide showed a benefit from prolonged treatment, making the drug one of the best choices for long-term maintenance treatment. Several trials are also ongoing with lenalidomide maintenance. In the MM 015, at time of data cut-off (December 1, 2009) most of patients had continued onto maintenance therapy phase (Palumbo et al. 2010). Only 8% of patients receiving lenalidomide maintenance required dose reduction suggesting continued treatment is well tolerated. Median PFS and OS are not reached in this arm.

References

Alexanian R et al (1969) Treatment for multiple myeloma. Combination chemotherapy with different melphalan dose regimens. JAMA 208(9): 1680–1685

Alexanian R et al (1990) VAD-based regimens as primary treatment for multiple myeloma. Am J Hematol 33(2):86–89

Alexanian R et al (1992) Primary dexamethasone treatment of multiple myeloma. Blood 80(4): 887–890

Attal M et al (1996) A prospective, randomized trial of autologous bone marrow transplantation and chemotherapy in multiple myeloma Intergroupe Francais du Myelome. N Engl J Med 335(2):91–97

Attal M et al (2006) Maintenance therapy with thalidomide improves survival in patients with multiple myeloma. Blood 108(10):3289–3294

Attal M et al (2010) Lenalidomide maintenance after transplantation for myeloma. ASCO Meeting Abstracts 28:8018

Barlogie B et al (2006a) Standard chemotherapy compared with high-dose chemoradiotherapy for multiple myeloma: final results of phase III US Intergroup Trial S9321. J Clin Oncol 24(6):929–936

Barlogie B et al (2006b) Thalidomide and hematopoietic-cell transplantation for multiple myeloma. N Engl J Med 354(10):1021–1030

Bataille R, Harousseau JL (1997) Multiple myeloma. N Engl J Med 336(23):1657–1664

Berenson JR et al (2002) Maintenance therapy with alternate-day prednisone improves survival in multiple myeloma patients. Blood 99(9): 3163–3168

Bjorkstrand B et al (2001) Alpha-interferon maintenance treatment is associated with improved survival after high-dose treatment and autologous stem cell transplantation in patients with multiple myeloma: a retrospective registry study from the European Group for Blood and Marrow Transplantation (EBMT). Bone Marrow Transplant 27(5):511–515

Blade J et al (2005) High-dose therapy intensification compared with continued standard chemotherapy in multiple myeloma patients responding to the initial chemotherapy: long-term results from a prospective randomized trial from the Spanish cooperative group PETHEMA. Blood 106(12):3755–3759

Cavo M et al (2005) Superiority of thalidomide and dexamethasone over vincristine-doxorubicin-dexamethasone (VAD) as primary therapy in preparation for autologous transplantation for multiple myeloma. Blood 106(1):35–39

Cavo M et al (2009) A phase III study of double autotransplantation incorporating bortezomib-thalidomide-dexamethasone (VTD) or thalidomide-dexamethasone (TD) for multiple myeloma: superior clinical outcomes with VTD compared to TD. ASH Annual Meeting Abstracts 114(22):351

Child JA et al (2003) High-dose chemotherapy with hematopoietic stem-cell rescue for multiple myeloma. N Engl J Med 348(19):1875–1883

Cunningham D et al (1998) A randomized trial of maintenance interferon following high-dose chemotherapy in multiple myeloma: long-term follow-up results. Br J Haematol 102(2): 495–502

Facon T et al (2006) Dexamethasone-based regimens versus melphalan-prednisone for elderly multiple myeloma patients ineligible for high-dose therapy. Blood 107(4):1292–1298

Facon T et al (2007) Melphalan and prednisone plus thalidomide versus melphalan and prednisone alone or reduced-intensity autologous stem cell transplantation in elderly patients with multiple myeloma (IFM 99-06): a randomised trial. Lancet 370(9594):1209–1218

Fermand JP et al (1998) High-dose therapy and autologous peripheral blood stem cell transplantation in multiple myeloma: up-front or rescue treatment? Results of a multicenter sequential randomized clinical trial. Blood 92(9): 3131–3136

Fermand JP et al (2005) High-dose therapy and autologous blood stem-cell transplantation compared with conventional treatment in myeloma patients

9

aged 55–65 years: long-term results of a randomized control trial from the Group Myelome-Autogreffe. J Clin Oncol 23(36):9227–9233

Fritz E, Ludwig H (2000) Interferon-alpha treatment in multiple myeloma: meta-analysis of 30 randomised trials among 3948 patients. Ann Oncol 11(11):1427–1436

Harousseau JL et al (2006) Bortezomib plus dexamethasone as induction treatment prior to autologous stem cell transplantation in patients with newly diagnosed multiple myeloma: results of an IFM phase II study. Haematologica 91(11): 1498–1505

Harousseau JL et al (2008) Bortezomib/dexamethasone versus VAD as induction prior to autologous stem cell transplantion (ASCT) in previously untreated multiple myeloma (MM): updated data from IFM 2005/01 trial. J Clin Oncol (Meeting Abstracts) 26(15 suppl):8505

Harousseau JL et al (2009) High complete and very good partial response rates with bortezomib – dexamethasone as induction prior to ASCT in newly diagnosed patients with high-risk myeloma: results of the IFM2005-01 phase 3 trial. ASH Annual Meeting Abstracts 114(22):353

Harousseau JL et al (2010) Comparison of reduced-dose bortezomib plus thalidomide plus dexamethasone (vTD) to bortezomib plus dexamethasone (VD) as induction treatment prior to ASCT in de novo multiple myeloma (MM): results of IFM2007-02 study. ASCO Meeting Abstracts 28:8014

Hernandez JM et al (2004) Randomized comparison of dexamethasone combined with melphalan versus melphalan with prednisone in the treatment of elderly patients with multiple myeloma. Br J Haematol 127(2):159–164

Hulin C et al (2009) Efficacy of melphalan and prednisone plus thalidomide in patients older than 75 years with newly diagnosed multiple myeloma: IFM 01/01 trial. J Clin Oncol 27(22): 3664–3670

International Myeloma Working Group (2003) Criteria for the classification of monoclonal gammopathies, multiple myeloma and related disorders: a report of the International Myeloma Working Group. Br J Haematol 121(5):749–757

Kapoor P et al (2009) Melphalan and prednisone (MP) versus melphalan, prednisone and thalidomide (MPT) as initial therapy for previously untreated elderly and/or transplant ineligible patients with multiple myeloma: a meta-analysis of randomized controlled trials. ASH Annual Meeting Abstracts 114(22):615

Khan ML et al (2010) A comparison of lenalidomide/dexamethasone (RD) versus cyclophosphamide/lenalidomide/dexamethasone (CRD) versus cyclophosphamide/bortezomib/dexamethasone (CyborD) in newly diagnosed multiple myeloma. ASCO Meeting Abstracts 28:8131

Knop S et al (2009) Bortezomib, IV cyclophosphamide, and dexamethasone (VelCD) as induction therapy in newly diagnosed multiple myeloma: results of an interim analysis of the German DSMM Xia trial. J Clin Oncol (Meeting Abstracts) 27(15S):8516

Kumar S et al (2009) Novel three- and four-drug combinations of bortezomib, dexamethasone, cyclophosphamide, and lenalidomide, for newly diagnosed multiple myeloma: encouraging results from the multi-center, randomized, Phase 2 EVOLUTION study. ASH Annual Meeting Abstracts 114(22):127

Ladetto M et al (2010) Major tumor shrinking and persistent molecular remissions after consolidation with bortezomib, thalidomide, and dexamethasone in patients with autografted myeloma. J Clin Oncol 28(12):2077–2084

Lane SW et al (2005) Role of VAD in the initial treatment of multiple myeloma. Blood 106(10): 3674; author reply 3674–3675

Lokhorst HM et al (2010) A randomized phase 3 study on the effect of thalidomide combined with adriamycin, dexamethasone, and high-dose melphalan, followed by thalidomide maintenance in patients with multiple myeloma. Blood 115(6):1113–1120

Ludwig H et al (2009) Thalidomide-dexamethasone compared with melphalan-prednisolone in elderly patients with multiple myeloma. Blood 113(15): 3435–3442

Ludwig H et al (2010) Phase II study of bortezomib, thalidomide, and dexamethasone +/- cyclophosphamide as induction therapy in previously untreated multiple myeloma (MM): safety and activity including evaluation of MRD EHA Meeting Abstracts 0371

McCarthy PL et al (2010) Phase III intergroup study of lenalidomide versus placebo maintenance therapy following single autologous stem cell transplant (ASCT) for multiple myeloma (MM): CALGB 100104. ASCO Meeting Abstracts 28:8017

Macro M et al (2006) Dexamethasone + Thalidomide (Dex/Thal) Compared to VAD as a pre-transplant treatment in newly diagnosed multiple myeloma (MM): a randomized trial. ASH Annual Meeting Abstracts 108(11):57

Mandelli F et al (1990) Maintenance treatment with recombinant interferon alfa-2b in patients with multiple myeloma responding to conventional induction chemotherapy. N Engl J Med 322(20): 1430–1434

Mateos MV et al (2006) Bortezomib plus melphalan and prednisone in elderly untreated patients with multiple myeloma: results of a multicenter phase 1/2 study. Blood 108(7):2165–2172

Mateos M-V et al (2009) A prospective, multicenter, randomized, trial of bortezomib/melphalan/prednisone (VMP) versus bortezomib/thalidomide/prednisone (VTP) as induction therapy followed by maintenance treatment with bortezomib/thalidomide (VT) versus bortezomib/prednisone (VP) in elderly untreated patients with multiple myeloma older than 65 years. ASH Annual Meeting Abstracts 114(22):3

Morgan GJ et al (2007) Thalidomide combinations improve response rates; results from the MRC IX study. ASH Annual Meeting Abstracts 110(11):3593

Morgan GJ et al (2009) The addition of thalidomide to the induction treatment of newly presenting myeloma patients increases the CR rate which is likely to translate into improved PFS and OS. ASH Annual Meeting Abstracts 114(22):352

Myeloma Trialists' Collaborative Group (1998) Combination chemotherapy versus melphalan plus prednisone as treatment for multiple myeloma: an overview of 6,633 patients from 27 randomized trials. J Clin Oncol 16(12):3832–3842

Myeloma Trialists' Collaborative Group (2001) Interferon as therapy for multiple myeloma: an individual patient data overview of 24 randomized trials and 4012 patients. Br J Haematol 113(4):1020–1034

Palumbo A et al (2005) Oral melphalan, prednisone, and thalidomide for newly diagnosed patients with myeloma. Cancer 104(7):1428–1433

Palumbo A et al (2007) Melphalan, prednisone, and lenalidomide treatment for newly diagnosed myeloma: a report from the GIMEMA–Italian Multiple Myeloma Network. J Clin Oncol 25(28): 4459–4465

Palumbo A et al (2008) Prevention of thalidomide- and lenalidomide-associated thrombosis in myeloma. Leukemia 22(2):414–423

Palumbo A et al (2009) Bortezomib, melphalan, prednisone and thalidomide (VMPT) followed by maintenance with bortezomib and thalidomide for initial treatment of elderly multiple myeloma patients. ASH Annual Meeting Abstracts 114(22):128

Palumbo A et al (2010a) A phase III study to determine the efficacy and safety of lenalidomide in combination with melphalan and prednisone (MPR) in elderly patients with newly diagnosed multiple myeloma. EHA Meeting Abstract 2010:566

Palumbo A et al (2010b) A phase III trial of melphalan/prednisone/lenalidomide (MPR) versus melphalan (200 mg/m^2) and autologous transplantation (MEL200) in newly diagnosed myeloma patients. ASCO Meeting Abstracts 28:8015

Rajkumar SV et al (2006) Phase III clinical trial of thalidomide plus dexamethasone compared with dexamethasone alone in newly diagnosed multiple myeloma: a clinical trial coordinated by the Eastern Cooperative Oncology Group. J Clin Oncol 24(3):431–436

Rajkumar SV et al (2008) Multicenter, randomized, double-blind, placebo-controlled study of thalidomide plus dexamethasone compared with dexamethasone as initial therapy for newly diagnosed multiple myeloma. J Clin Oncol 26(13): 2171–2177

Rajkumar SV et al (2010) Lenalidomide plus high-dose dexamethasone versus lenalidomide plus low-dose dexamethasone as initial therapy for newly diagnosed multiple myeloma: an open-label randomised controlled trial. Lancet Oncol 11(1):29–37

Reeder CB et al (2009) Cyclophosphamide, bortezomib and dexamethasone induction for newly diagnosed multiple myeloma: high response rates in a phase II clinical trial. Leukemia 23(7):1337–1341

Reeder CB et al (2010) Once- versus twice-weekly bortezomib induction therapy with CyBorD in newly diagnosed multiple myeloma. Blood 115(16):3416–3417

Richardson PG et al (2010) Lenalidomide, bortezomib, and dexamethasone combination therapy in patients with newly diagnosed multiple myeloma. Blood 116(5):679–686

Rosinol L et al (2007) Phase II PETHEMA trial of alternating bortezomib and dexamethasone as induction regimen before autologous stem-cell transplantation in younger patients with multiple myeloma: efficacy and clinical implications of tumor response kinetics. J Clin Oncol 25(28): 4452–4458

Rosinol L et al (2009). Thalidomide/dexamethasone (TD) vs. bortezomib (Velcade)a/thalidomide/dexamethasone (VTD) vs. VBMCP/VBAD/Velcadea as induction regimens prior autologous stem cell transplantation (ASCT) in multiple myeloma (MM): results of a phase III PETHEMA/GEM trial. ASH Annual Meeting Abstracts 114(22):130

San Miguel JF et al (2008) Bortezomib plus melphalan and prednisone for initial treatment of multiple myeloma. N Engl J Med 359(9):906–917

Sonneveld P et al (2008) First analysis of HOVON-65/GMMG-HD4 randomized Phase III trial comparing bortezomib, adriamycine, dexamethasone (PAD) vs VAD as induction treatment prior to high dose melphalan (HDM) in patients with newly diagnosed multiple myeloma (MM). ASH Annual Meeting Abstracts 112(11):653

Spencer A et al (2009) Consolidation therapy with low-dose thalidomide and prednisolone prolongs the survival of multiple myeloma patients undergoing a single autologous stem-cell transplantation procedure. J Clin Oncol 27(11):1788–1793

Waage A et al (2010a) MP versus MPT for previously untreated elderly patients with multiple myeloma: a meta-analysis of 1,682 individual patient data from six randomized clinical trials. ASCO Meeting Abstracts 28:8130

Waage A et al (2010b) Melphalan and prednisone plus thalidomide or placebo in elderly patients with multiple myeloma. Blood 116(9):1405–1412

Wijermans P et al (2008) Melphalan + prednisone versus melphalan + prednisone + thalidomide in induction therapy for multiple myeloma in elderly patients: final analysis of the Dutch Cooperative Group HOVON 49 Study. ASH Annual Meeting Abstracts 112(11):649

Zonder JA et al (2007) Superiority of lenalidomide (Len) plus high-dose dexamethasone (HD) compared to HD alone as treatment of newly-diagnosed multiple myeloma (NDMM): results of the randomized, double-blinded, placebo-controlled SWOG trial S0232. ASH Annual Meeting Abstracts 110(11):77

High-Dose Therapy and Autologous Peripheral Blood Stem Cell Transplantation in Patients with Multiple Myeloma

10

Rainer Haas, Ingmar Bruns, Guido Kobbe, and Roland Fenk

Contents

Abstract Since its introduction in 1983, high-dose therapy followed by autologous peripheral blood stem cell transplantation is a pillar of the treatment of patients with multiple myeloma. In the last decades, a multitude of clinical trials helped to improve strategies based on high-dose therapy and autologous stem cell transplantation resulting in a continuously prolongation of overall survival of patients. In this chapter we will review the progress, which has been made in order to enhance the mobilisation of autologous stem cells and increase the effectiveness of this treatment.

R. Haas (✉)
Department of Hematology, Oncology and Clinical Immunology, Heinrich-Heine-University, Moorenstr. 5, 40225 Düsseldorf, Germany
e-mail: haas@med.uni-duesseldorf.de

T. Moehler and H. Goldschmidt (eds.), *Multiple Myeloma*,
Recent Results in Cancer Research 183, DOI: 10.1007/978-3-540-85772-3_10,

10.1 Introduction

High-dose chemotherapy (HDT) and autologous peripheral blood stem cell transplantation (SCT) has improved response rates and duration of survival in patients with multiple myeloma (MM) (Bensinger 2008). Recent research concentrating on the pathogenesis and the molecular basis of the disease has led to the development of novel agents, which are not only targeting tumor cells but also stromal cells supporting tumor cell growth. Three of these novel agents, thalidomide (Glasmacher et al. 2006), lenalidomide (Dimopoulos et al. 2007; Weber et al. 2007), and bortezomib (Richardson et al. 2005) are remarkably effective in reducing the malignant cell clone. This had led to the incorporation of these novel agents not only in salvage, but also into first-line protocols resulting in an improvement of treatment outcome. In the following, we will review the clinical trials that are based on high-dose therapy and autologous peripheral blood SCT in patients with MM.

10.2 Peripheral Blood Stem Cell Mobilization

10.2.1 The Role of Adhesion Molecules

Whereas in the beginning of HDT and autologous SCT bone marrow was the main source for blood stem cell transplantation, blood-derived stem cell grafts have replaced bone marrow. Before we present the various methods used for the mobilization of peripheral blood stems cells, a few remarks are necessary concerning our current understanding of the bone marrow's stem cell niche as first proposed by Schofield and colleagues (Schofield 1983). This niche is a very special place within the bone marrow microenvironment as it guarantees the lifelong maintenance of the most primitive hematopoietic stem cell (HSC) population. The various components of the niche regulate the finely tuned balance between self-renewal and differentiation along the respective hematopoietic lineages. Apart from osteoblast and endothelial cells, the bone marrow contains a broad variety of different stromal cells, including fibroblasts and adipocytes, which form a highly specialized micro architecture as it is needed for the differentiation of the various hematopoietic progenitor and precursor cells. Apart from the production of hematopoietic growth factors and cytokines by the stromal cells of the bone marrow microenvironment, they mediate adhesive interactions essential for migration, circulation, and proliferation of HSC (Verfaillie et al. 1994; Prosper et al. 1998; Whetton and Graham 1999). The receptor and ligands involved include members of the ß1 and ß2 integrin family, selectins and super immunoglobulin families (Fig. 10.1) (Soligo et al. 1990; Verfaillie et al. 1991; Simmons et al. 1992; Teixido et al. 1992; Liesveld et al. 1993; Kinashi and Springer 1994). Some of their natural ligands are expressed on endothelial cells or other stromal cells. The binding partners may also represent compounds of the extracellular matrix of the bone marrow microenvironment.

In the following, we will present some of the receptors and ligands of the bone marrow microenvironment, which are involved in migration and mobilization of HSC. There is an L-selectin (CD62L) recognizing carbohydrate residue on endothelial cells. This interaction mediates the initial attachment of leukocytes to endothelial cells, a process termed as tethering. L-selectin is highly expressed on circulating $CD34^+$ stem and progenitor cells implying an essential role for homing of stem cells following transplantation (Mohle et al. 1995). The ß1 integrins very late antigen 4 ([VLA-4] CD29/CD49d) and VLA-5 (CD29/CD49e) are heterodimers permitting adhesion of hematopoietic progenitor cells to different

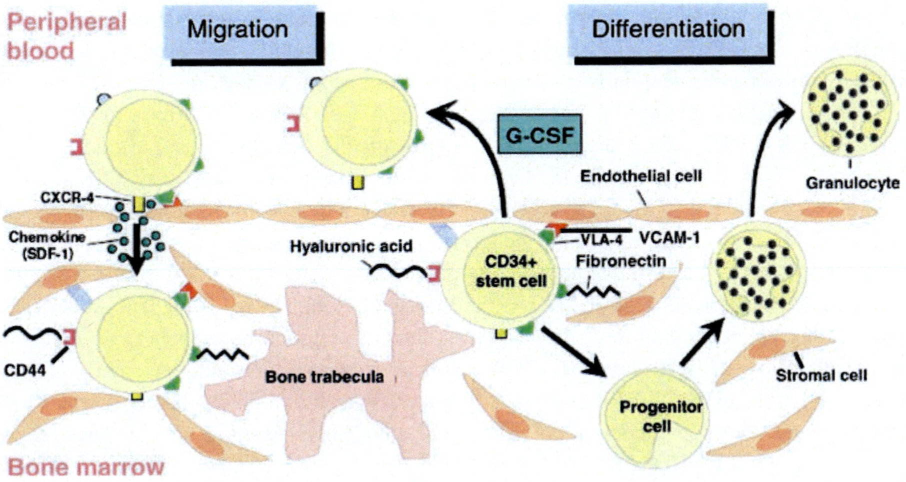

Fig. 10.1 Role of adhesion molecules and their ligands for mobilization of CD34⁺ hematopoietic stem cells

compounds of the bone marrow stroma. In particular, the VLA-4-mediated interaction between hematopoietic stem cells and bone marrow stroma is of functional relevance for hematopoiesis as well as for mobilization and homing of $CD34^+$ cells (Prosper et al. 1998; Miyake et al. 1991; Yanai et al. 1994; Hamamura et al. 1996). We observed that circulating $CD34^+$ cells express VLA-4 at a lower level in comparison to $CD34^+$ cells in the bone marrow. The release of $CD34^+$ cells and their migratory capacity is apparently related to the expression level of VLA-4 (Prosper et al. 1998; Mohle et al. 1995; Leavesley et al. 1994; Yamaguchi et al. 1998; Bellucci et al. 1999; Lichterfeld et al. 2000). Looking at circulating $CD34^+$ cells from peripheral blood during G-CSF-enhanced marrow recovery in comparison to $CD34^+$ cells from steady-state bone marrow we found a significantly reduced functional state of the VLA-4 receptor (Lichterfeld et al. 2000). Moreover, the number of circulating $CD34^+$ cells during marrow recovery was inversely related to the activation state and not to the expression level of VLA-4. This observation clearly suggests that the functional state of VLA-4 in circulating $CD34^+$ cells is different from that in bone marrow $CD34^+$ cells.

Besides VLA-4, the ß2 integrin leukocyte function-associated molecule-1 ([LFA-1], CD18/CD11a) mediates interactions between $CD34^+$ hematopoietic progenitor cells and bone marrow stroma. On circulating $CD34^+$ cells, LFA-1 had a lower expression level than on bone marrow-derived $CD34^+$ cells (Mohle et al. 1995). Functionally, the adhesion to and migration through an endothelial cell layer could be inhibited using LFA-1-directed blocking monoclonal antibodies (Mohle et al. 1995, 1997). There is also a relationship between cell adhesion and signal transduction pathways, which are activated by cytokines (Hughes and Pfaff 1998). Other adhesion molecules relevant in the context of mobilization and homing are the platelet endothelial cell adhesion molecule-1 (PECAM, CD31) and CD44. It is also strongly expressed on $CD34^+$ hematopoietic stem and progenitor cells. The ligands of CD44, hyaluronic acid, and osteopontin are components of the stromal microenvironment. Monoclonal antibodies directed against CD44 lower the adhesion of $CD34^+$ cells to bone marrow stroma, induce the mobilization of progenitor cells in mice, and prevent hematopoiesis in long-term bone marrow cultures (Miyake et al. 1990; Khaldoyanidi et al. 1996, 1997; Oostendorp et al.

1998; Rosel et al. 1999). Beside growth factors and adhesion molecules, the alpha chemokine CXCL12 also known as stromal-derived factor 1 (SDF-1) plays a relevant role in blood stem cell migration (Aiuti et al. 1997). The cellular receptor of SDF-1 is CXCR-4, which functions as coreceptor for T cell-tropic HIV-1 strains (Bleul et al. 1996). CXCR-4 is expressed in $CD34^+$ cells dependent on the degree of differentiation. The subset of $CD34^+/CD38^{low}$ and $CD34^+$/HLA-DR^{low} cells representing a population of more immature progenitor cells stain brightly positive for CXCR-4, whereas a lower level of CXCR-4 expression was observed on the population of $CD34^+/CD38^{bright}$ and $CD34^+$/HLA-DR^{bright} cells (Deichmann et al. 1997; Viardot et al. 1998). SDF-1 acts as chemoattractant for hematopoietic stem cells (Aiuti et al. 1997; Mohle et al. 1998; Voermans et al. 1999).

10.2.2 The Role of Hematopoietic Growth Factors

In the vast majority of patients and normal donors hematopoietic growth factors are used for the mobilization of peripheral blood stem cell and progenitor cells. Our first studies addressing the mobilizing ability of hematopoietic growth factors were carried using granulocyte macrophage colony-stimulating factor (GM-CSF). In a group of 11 patients with different types of hematological malignancies and a history of extensive previous cytotoxic chemotherapy, an approximately 18-fold increase of circulating colony-forming units granulocyte macrophage (CFU-GM) in comparison to baseline values was observed (Socinski et al. 1988). An even fivefold greater enhancement was observed when GM-CSF was administered following cytotoxic chemotherapy to increase the natural rebound of circulating $CD34^+$ cell during hematopoietic recovery (Socinski et al. 1988). Looking at the mobilizing capacity of G-CSF in comparison to GM-CSF, no significant difference became apparent between these two growth factors (Winter et al. 1996; Hohaus et al. 1998). In the following studies, peripheral blood stem cell mobilization was performed in the context of a cytotoxic chemotherapy. This kind of peripheral blood stem cell mobilization is generally associated with a lower likelihood of harvesting malignant cells, particularly if the malignancy proved to be chemosensitive (Hohaus et al. 1993; Haas et al. 1992, 1994a, 1997). The advantage of a chemotherapy-based peripheral blood stem cell mobilization is best reflected by the data of a study with an intraindividual comparison (Mohle et al. 1994). In that setting, we observed a sevenfold greater yield of $CD34^+$ cells per leukapheresis after G-CSF-supported chemotherapy compared with steady-state administration of G-CSF at a dose of 5 μg/kg/day.

In order to get a better understanding of the processes underlying peripheral blood mobilization, we and other groups looked for differences between $CD34^+$ cells from bone marrow and peripheral blood during G-CSF-enhanced marrow recovery and found a 3.7-fold greater peak concentration of $CD34^+$ cells in the peripheral blood during G-CSF-supported recovery in comparison with bone marrow samples from steady-state hematopoiesis (Haas et al. 1995). Independent of the method used for peripheral blood stem cell mobilization the vast majority of circulating $CD34^+$ cells were found to be in the G_0/G_1 phase, including a greater proportion of more primitive $CD34^+$ cells. This could be concluded from the results of functional assays enumerating the long-term culture-initiating cells and pre-CFU-GM (Tarella et al. 1995). The functional data were in line with findings made by immunophenotyping demonstrating that a greater proportion of mobilized peripheral blood stem cells expressed the early stem cell-associated antigen Thy-1 in comparison with bone marrow (Fig. 10.2) (Haas et al. 1995).

We addressed this aspect on a molecular level and assessed the gene expression of 1,185 genes in highly enriched bone marrow

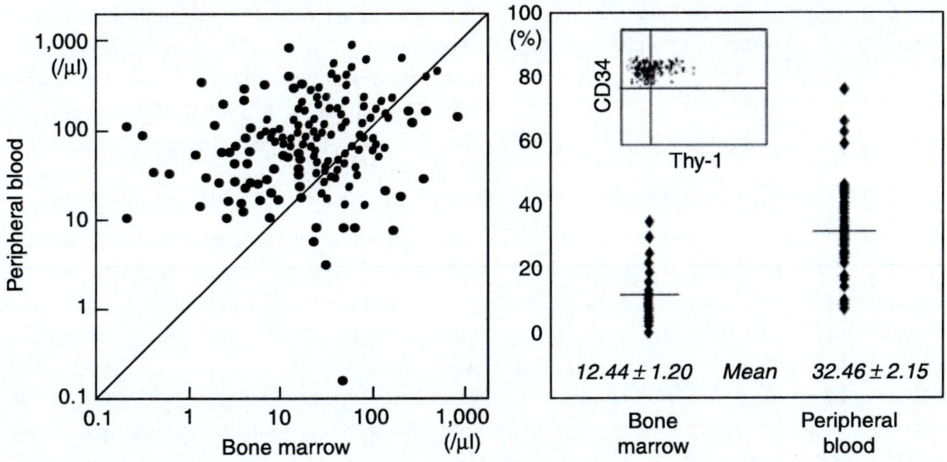

Fig. 10.2 Intraindividual comparison between CD34⁺ cells from peripheral blood and bone marrow. *Left*: Concentration of CD34⁺ cells in bone marrow samples before the start of cytotoxic chemotherapy and in peripheral blood (peak level) obtained during cytokine-enhanced marrow recovery. The mean concentration of CD34⁺ cells was 2.3-fold greater in peripheral blood compared to bone marrow samples. *Right*: Proportion of CD34⁺/Thy-1⁺ cells in bone marrow samples from 20 patients before mobilization and 48 leukapheresis products collected during G-CSF-enhanced marrow recovery post-chemothreapy

CD34⁺ or G-CSF-mobilized peripheral blood CD34⁺. Using cDNA array technology we found that 65 genes were significantly differentially expressed. These data molecularly confirmed and explained the finding that CD34⁺ cells residing in the bone marrow cycle more rapidly, whereas circulating CD34⁺ cells consist of a higher number of quiescent stem and progenitor cells. All together, these results are a strong basis for the preferential use of blood-derived progenitor cells rather than bone marrow for autologous or allogeneic transplantation since the more primitive hematopoietic progenitor cells or even stem cells are particularly relevant for sustained long-term hematopoiesis following myeloablative conditioning therapy (Haas et al. 1995; Dercksen et al. 1995).

The composition of the various CD34⁺ cell subsets also depends on whether G-CSF is administered during steady-state hematopoiesis or following cytotoxic chemotherapy. In a study including patients with acute leukemia, Hodgkin's disease, non-Hodgkin's lymphoma, or MM, the amount of CD34⁺ cells collected post-chemotherapy was 5.7-fold greater in comparison with a peripheral blood stem cell harvest obtained during steady state (Haas et al. 1995). In particular, the mean proportion of more primitive CD34⁺ progenitors lacking HLA-DR or CD38 expression was smaller in patients with peripheral blood stem cell collection following G-CSF-supported chemotherapy than during steady-state mobilization. Considering the greater number of CD34⁺ cells mobilized in total, the absolute amount of CD34⁺/HLA-DR⁻ cells was still 2.3-fold greater post-chemotherapy. On the other hand, the proportion of lineage-committed CD34⁺/CD33⁺ cells was significantly enhanced post-chemotherapy in comparison with steady-state mobilization. These data are in line with findings of another group showing that CD34⁺ cells, mobilized following G-CSF during steady state, contained a greater proportion of CD38$^-$ cells than CD34$^+$ cells mobilized by other regimens (To et al. 1994).

10.2.3 The Role of Cytotoxic Stem Cell Mobilization

Irrespective of the growth factor used and the particular mode of application, there is always a wide variation in the mobilization efficacy between normal volunteers as well as among patients (Roberts et al. 1995). Individual factors or characteristics associated with peripheral blood stem cell mobilization in patients are essentially the dose of cytotoxic chemotherapy administered for mobilization, the underlying disease and the cumulative amount of previous cytotoxic treatment, as well as previous radiotherapy. For instance, administration of 7 g/m^2 cyclophosphamide in comparison with 4 g/m^2 resulted in significantly greater peak levels of CD34$^+$ cells in the peripheral blood of patients with MM (Goldschmidt et al. 1996). Goldschmidt et al. treated 103 myeloma patients with 7 g/m^2 cyclophosphamide followed by daily 300 µg G-CSF to harvest peripheral blood progenitor cells (Goldschmidt et al. 1997). Peripheral blood stem cell autografts containing >2.0 × 10^6 CD34$^+$ cells per kg body weight were obtained at the first attempt from 90 of 100 evaluable patients. The most significant factor predicting impairment of peripheral blood stem cell collection was the duration of previous melphalan treatment. In multivariate discriminate analysis, treatment with melphalan during the most recent chemotherapy cycles prior to mobilization and previous radiotherapy had a marginally significant negative influence on the efficacy of peripheral blood stem cell collection. The functional capacity of CD34$^+$ cells to restore hematopoiesis after myeloablative treatment was not reduced related to the duration of melphalan exposure. At the time of best response to conventional treatment, a median paraprotein reduction of 21% was achieved following high-dose cyclophosphamide. Two heavily pre-treated patients died, and one patient developed pulmonary toxicity WHO grade IV following high-dose cyclophosphamide. Potential transplant candidates should undergo mobilization and harvesting of PBPC before melphalan-containing treatment. Combinations of hematopoietic growth factors and their dose-modifications should be investigated to improve PBPC collection and to allow a dose reduction of the mobilization chemotherapy. Another study reported on the G-CSF-related mobilization efficiency in 120 patients with MM who received cytotoxic chemotherapy (Martin-Murea et al. 1998). Three schedules of G-CSF administration starting 24 h after the end of chemotherapy were used: (a) a standard dose of 300 µg/day until the completion of peripheral blood stem cell collection, (b) dose escalation from 300 to 600–1,200 µg/day during marrow recovery, (c) 600 or 1,200 µg/day starting 24 h after cytotoxic chemotherapy. As a result, the individual dose per kg bodyweight varied between 2.83 and 23.08 µg. No relationship was found between the dose of G-CSF administered and the peak level of circulating CD34$^+$ cells or the CD34$^+$ cell counts recorded over the entire collection period. In another retrospective study, including 61 patients with lymphoma, we looked for patient-associated factors that may influence the yield of CD34$^+$ cells following G-CSF-supported cytotoxic chemotherapy (Haas et al. 1994a). We found that previous cytotoxic chemotherapy and irradiation adversely affected the yield of CD34$^+$ cells. As consequence, we proposed to harvest peripheral blood stem cells as early as possible during the course of the disease to ensure a yield sufficient to support HDT.

The minimum quantity of CD34$^+$ cells needed for transplantation is generally accepted to lie between 2.5 and 5.0 × 10^6/kg body weight (Hohaus et al. 1993; Haas et al. 1994b; Reiffers et al. 1994). In the context of these analyses, a relationship was found between the number of CD34$^+$ cells transplanted and the time required for hematological reconstitution. Not surprisingly, patients who received a greater number of $CD34^+$ cells/kg needed shorter recovery times than patients grafted with a smaller number of $CD34^+$ progenitor cells (Hohaus et al. 1993; Bensinger et al. 1994; Weaver et al. 1995; Ketterer et al. 1998). Following the successful experience made with peripheral blood stem cells in the context of autografting, this source of hematopoietic stem and progenitor cells also serves for allogeneic transplantation (Dreger et al. 1994; Bensinger et al. 1995; Korbling et al. 1995; Schmitz et al. 1995).

In the following, we will address the aspect of contamination of the autograft with malignant cells. Gene-marking studies in patients with acute myeloid leukemia and neuroblastoma have shown that malignant cells reinfused along with leukapheresis products may contribute to relapse. Thus, a reduction in the number of malignant cells in autografts is desirable. Cremer et al. analyzed the percentage of malignant cells and the number of $CD34^+$ peripheral blood stem cells in leukapheresis products mobilized by G-CSF alone compared with high-dose cyclophosphamide plus G-CSF in patients with MM (Cremer et al. 1998). A quantitative polymerase chain reaction assay involving CDR3-specific primers based on the method of limiting dilutions was used to determine the tumor loads of leukapheresis products. Sixteen autografts from eight patients with MM were analyzed intraindividually in matched pairs. The percentage of malignant cells was lower in leukapheresis products obtained after cyclophosphamide administration ($p=0.017$; median 0.0067 vs 0.009%), whereas the number of $CD34^+$ cells was higher ($p=0.012$; median 0.3 vs 0.095%). The calculated number of malignant cells per $CD34^+$ cell was significantly lower in leukapheresis products after cytotoxic mobilization as well ($p=0.017$). We conclude that mobilization by cyclophosphamide plus G-CSF leads to a lower number of malignant cells per $CD34^+$ cell in LPs compared with G-CSF alone.

10.2.4 The Role of Pegfilgrastim for Stem Cell Mobilization

Progress in the field of peripheral blood stem cell mobilization has been made by a chemical modification of G-CSF, i.e., the pegylation of filgrastim. Different from the original compound PEG-filgrastim is characterized by a significantly longer half-life because of a substantially reduced renal elimination (Zamboni 2003). In the first study including patients with different types of hematological malignancies, we could demonstrate safety and efficacy of this new compound in mobilizing a sufficient number of $CD34^+$ cells required for at least one autologous transplantation (Steidl et al. 2005). In a subsequent study, pegfilgrastim was given at two different dose levels for PBPC mobilization in patients with stage II or III MM (Bruns et al. 2006). Four days after cytotoxic therapy with cyclophosphamide (4 g/m^2), a single dose of either 6 mg pegfilgrastim or 12 mg pegfilgrastim or daily doses of 8 μg/kg unconjugated G-CSF were administered. Pegfilgrastim was equally potent at 6 and 12 mg with regard to mobilization and yield of $CD34^+$ cells. Pegfilgrastim in either dose was associated with a more rapid white blood count recovery ($p=0.03$) and an earlier performance of the first apheresis procedure ($p<0.05$) in comparison to unconjugated G-CSF. There was no difference regarding $CD34^+$ cell maximum and yield. We therefore concluded that a single dose of 6 mg pegfilgrastim is equally potent as 12 mg for mobilization and harvest of peripheral blood stem cells in patients with MM. In the context of pegfilgrastim, it was interesting to note that the pegfilgrastim-exposed $CD34^+$ cells had a subset composition different from that of filgrastim-mobilized $CD34^+$ cells, i.e., a greater proportion of more primitive $CD34^+$ cells as characterized by the lack of CD38 expression (Fig. 10.3) (Bruns et al. 2008). The different subset composition was accompanied by a significantly different gene expression profile reflecting the

10

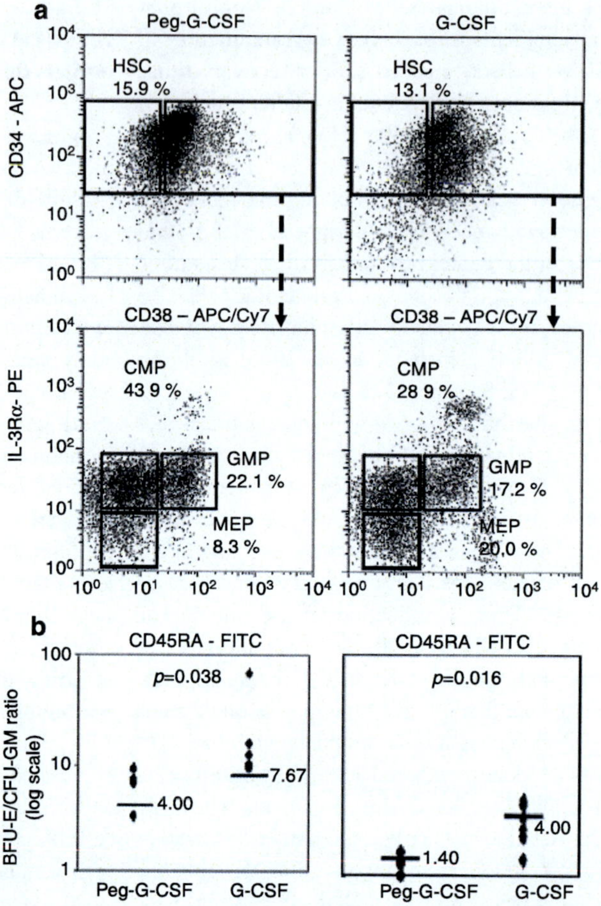

Fig. 10.3 (**a**) Different patterns of hematopoietic stem and progenitor cells in the peripheral blood of patients stimulated with either Peg-G-CSF (*left*) or G-CSF (*right*). Immunomagnetic selection of CD34⁺ cells followed by multicolor flow cytometry was utilized to analyze hematopoietic stem and progenitor cell subsets. After gating on viable cells and lineage-depletion subfractions of hematopoietic stem cells (Lin^-, $CD34^+$, $CD38^-$), common myeloid progenitors (Lin^-, $CD34^+$, $CD38^+$, $IL\text{-}3Ra^+$, $CD45RA^-$), granulocyte monocyte progenitors (Lin^-, $CD34^+$, $CD38^+$, $IL\text{-}3Ra^+$, $CD45RA^+$), and megakaryocyte erythrocyte progenitors (Lin^-, $CD34^+$, $CD38^+$, $IL\text{-}3Ra^-$, $CD45RA^-$) were determined. (**b**) Clonogenic assays of mononuclear cells (*left*) and purified $CD34^+$ cells (*right*) of patients mobilized by either Peg-G-CSF or G-CSF. Mononuclear cells from apheresis products of patients mobilized with either Peg-G-CSF or G-CSF were seeded in semisolid growth medium containing stem cell factor, GM-CSF, colony-stimulating factor, interleukin-3, interleukin-6, and erythropoietin.

preponderance of a more immature $CD34^+$ cell subset on the level of the transcriptome. For instance, the $CD34^+$ cells mobilized by pegylated G-CSF had higher expression levels of genes indicative of early hematopoiesis, including HOXA9, MEIS1, and GATA3. We found lower expression of genes characteristic of erythroid and later stages of myeloid differentiation and a lower functional burst-forming unit erythroid/colony-forming unit-granulocyte-macrophage ratio. Consistently, greater numbers of hematopoietic stem cells and common myeloid progenitors and fewer megakaryocyte-erthrocyte progenitors were found in the pegylated-G-CSF-mobilized $CD34^+$ cells. Additionally, sorted pegylated-G-CSF-mobilized hematopoietic stem cells displayed higher expression of HOXA9 in comparison to G-CSF-mobilized hematopoietic stem cells. In line with the gene expression data, $CD34^+$ cells mobilized by pegylated G-CSF, as well as sorted hematopoietic stem cells, showed a significantly greater cell cycle activity. Thus, stimulation with pegylated-G-CSF or G-CSF results in different expression of key regulatory genes and different functional properties of mobilized hematopoietic stem cells as well as their progeny, a finding that might be relevant for the application of these cells in blood stem cell transplantation.

This can be concluded from the results of a recent clinical trial in which the authors found significantly greater leukocyte, reticulocyte, and platelet counts on day 100 after initial engraftment following transplantation of pegfilgrastim-mobilized autografts compared to grafts mobilized by unconjugated G-CSF (Vanstraelen et al. 2006). Of interest, the number of pegfilgrastim mobilized CD34$^+$ cells transplanted was even smaller than the number of G-CSF-mobilized cells ($p=0.0575$). Hence, it was assumed that different biological functions of pegfilgrastim-mobilized cells may have accounted for these observations (Vanstraelen et al. 2006). Searching for the underlying mechanism that may explain the different transcriptional and functional phenotypes of pegfilgrastim-mobilized cells, it has been previously shown in a murine G-CSF receptor knock-out model that pegfilgrastim and G-CSF exert their pharmacological effects via the same G-CSF receptor (Kotto-Kome et al. 2004). Thus, the different effects of G-CSF and pegfilgrastim are apparently not related to activation of different receptors. Interestingly, in a recent randomized clinical trial, the effect of continuous intravenous administration versus daily single subcutaneous doses of G-CSF on CD34$^+$ cell mobilization was examined (Lee et al. 2005). The authors found that CD34$^+$ cell peak concentrations were reached 2 days earlier following continuous intravenous G-CSF administration compared to daily subcutaneous injections. These findings and the mobilization kinetics observed following the administration of pegfilgrastim suggest that the time-course of stimulation (pulsatile vs. continuous), rather than a dose-related mechanism, might account for the distinct effects of pegfilgrastim and G-CSF on hematopoietic stem and progenitor cells.

10.3 High-Dose Therapy and Autologous Stem Cell Transplantation

10.3.1 The Beginning of High-Dose Therapy in the 1980

Dr. Solly published the first well-documented case of a patient with MM in 1844, and treatment consisted of rhubarb and orange peel (Solly 1844). Dr. Thomas Watson used an alternative treatment 1 year later, who prescribed steel and quinine after application of phlebotomy in a similar patient (Macintyre 1850). It was nearly 100 years later that Blokhin et al. (1958) reported the effective application of melphalan in a small series of patients, and this was the beginning of modern chemotherapy as treatment in patients with MM (Fig. 10.4). Another

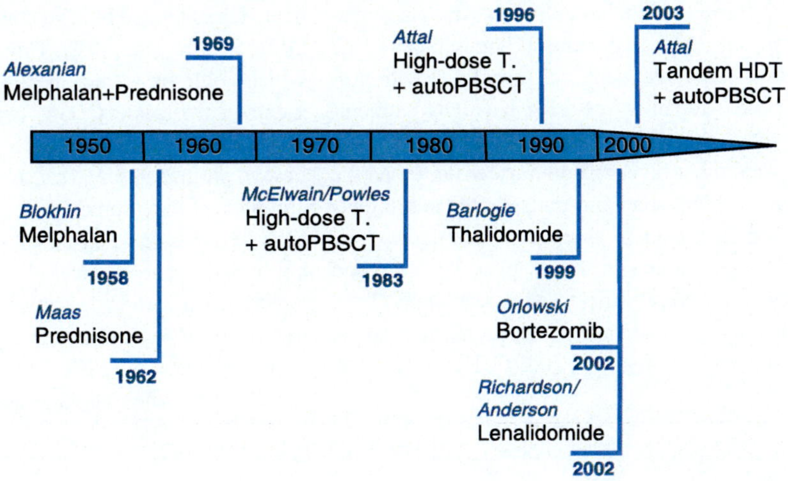

Fig. 10.4 Timeline of the treatment of patients with multiple myeloma

important step was the introduction of steroids (Maas 2008). Taken together, the combination of melphalan and prednisone was established by Alexanian et al. in 1969 (Alexanian et al. 1969). In a randomized trial of 183 patients with MM, a survival benefit of 6 months could be observed with melphalan and prednisone in comparison to melphalan alone. Based on this study, the classic Alexanian protocol became the standard of care for patients with MM for nearly 30 years. Several trials compared different combination chemotherapies to melphalan and prednisone in a randomized fashion, and various combinations were associated with higher response rates or a more rapid induction of remission (Myeloma Trialists' Collaborative Group 1998). Still, no combination could show a survival advantage, and thus melphalan and prednisone remained the gold standard of myeloma therapy for decades. Median overall survival in this time was approximately 3 years.

The change in treatment standards began when Mc Elwain and Powles (1983) reported on a patient with plasma cell leukemia who achieved a complete remission after treatment with 140 mg/m^2 melphalan. In the following, the group from the Royal Marsden Hospital showed a dose-effect of melphalan in patients with MM. While a complete remission could only be observed in 5% of patients following conventional chemotherapy, administration of 140 mg/m^2 melphalan induced complete remissions in 35% of patients (Cunningham et al. 1994). This treatment was associated with prolonged cytopenias, resulting in a high treatment-related mortality. Despite this experience, several other investigators further increased the dose of melphalan and transplanted autologous blood stem cells in order to reduce the toxicity of the procedure. In that respect, Barlogie and coworkers were pioneers, who developed "Total Therapy," an intensive treatment regimen using HDT and autologous PBSCT (Barlogie et al. 1999).

10.3.2 The Role of Purging of the Autograft

MM is characterized by a various degree of peripheral blood and bone marrow involvement with malignant plasma cells. Therefore, hematopoietic stem cell grafts often contain tumor cells. Using qualitative IgH PCR, it has been shown that almost all unselected leukapheresis products contained cells belonging to the myeloma clone (Corradini et al. 1995, 1999; Martinelli et al. 2000). As a consequence, several groups tried to reduce the number of tumor cells in autografts (Vescio et al. 1999; Lemoli et al. 1999; Stewart et al. 2001). The most widely used in vitro purging method is the positive selection of $CD34^+$ progenitor cells using immunomagnetic beads. Still, clone-specific IgH rearrangements were detectable in most $CD34^+$-enriched leukapheresis products (Bird et al. 1994; Abonour et al. 1998; Lemoli et al. 1996; Johnson et al. 1996) as well as in autografts obtained after negative selection of lineage-positive cells, even despite the combined use of positive selection of $CD34^+$ cells and depletion (Lemoli et al. 1999; Barbui et al. 2002; Tricot et al. 1998). The use of quantitative IgH PCR on samples from blood stem cell harvests has provided the means to accurately quantify the success of in vitro purging procedures. A reduction of three log of contaminating myeloma cells has been demonstrated in most studies (Barbui et al. 2002; Schiller et al. 1995; Thunberg et al. 1999), which could be further increased using experimental small-scale $CD34^+$ separation systems (Voena et al. 2002; Cremer et al. 1997). Different in vivo purging strategies also did not result in a complete elimination of clonotypic cells in stem cells harvests. It could be shown that the number of malignant cells was significantly lower in leukapheresis products obtained after cytotoxic mobilization than after steady-state mobilization (Cremer et al. 1998). Repeated courses of mobilization chemotherapy led to a median reduction of myeloma cells of 0.2 log per cycle (Ladetto et al. 2002). There were no differences in the number of myeloma cells in leukapheresis products obtained at different days during the harvesting period (Ladetto et al. 2002; Zhou et al. 2003; Kiel et al. 1998; Lincz et al. 2001). A median 15-fold higher proportion of tumor cells was found in bone marrow harvests than in peripheral blood leukapheresis products (Ladetto et al. 2002; Vescio et al. 1996), which resulted in equal total clonotypic cell numbers in BM or PB autografts, because of the increased total number of required cells for peripheral blood SCT.

The prognostic value of IgH PCR of stem cell harvests is questionable. In one study, patients, who received leukapheresis products with no evidence of residual myeloma cells as assessed by IgH PCR, were more likely to obtain a CR following transplantation and had a borderline significant longer progression-free and overall survival (Lopez-Perez et al. 2000, 2001). Others could not consequently reproduce this finding (Mitterer et al. 2001; Galimberti et al. 2003). It is conceivable, that the possibility to purge an autograft to PCR negativity is a reflection of a lower tumor burden in vivo and therefore associated with a better prognosis, while the tumor cells infused in patients with PCR positive autografts per se are not of relevance. This is in line with clinical findings showing, that the use of selected autografts did not have a significant benefit regarding the event-free or overall-survival of patients in three randomized multicenter trials (Vescio et al. 1999; Stewart et al. 2001; Lemoli et al. 2000; Bourhis et al. 2007). Moreover, the incidence of infections and delayed engraftment is greater in patients receiving $CD34^+$ selected PB stem cell grafts in comparison to those who autografted using unselected leukapheresis products. Because of these results and the high costs of the selection procedure, today $CD34^+$ cell selection of autografts has been abandoned in case of MM.

10.3.3 The Role of the Conditioning Regimen

The reason, why a reduction of graft contamination by myeloma cells does not improve disease control, most probably is the failure of HDT to eradicate the malignant cells in patients to a level below the number of reinfused tumor cells. Thus, great effort has been undertaken to further improve the conditioning regimen of HDT and autologous SCT.

Melphalan has been given as monotherapy, in combination with total body irradiation (TBI) and in combination with other chemotherapeutic agents. TBI was used in analogue to regimen in patients with leukemia because MM is a radiosensitive malignancy. In a retrospective study, we evaluated the efficacy and toxicity of a high-dose melphalan-based therapy with or without TBI followed by peripheral blood SCT in patients with MM (Goldschmidt et al. 1998). Between June 1992 and June 1996, 104 patients with a median age of 51 years underwent transplantation at the University of Heidelberg. Fifty patients were treated with TBI plus melphalan 140 mg/m^2 while 54 patients received melphalan 200 mg/m^2. Following peripheral blood stem cell autografting, the median time to attainment of platelets $\geq 20 \times 10^9$/L and neutrophils $\geq 0.5 \times 10^9$/L was 11 and 14 days, with no difference between the treatment groups. In the TBI group significantly longer periods of total parenteral nutrition were required due to the occurrence of severe mucositis. Two patients from the TBI group died of transplantation-related complications. Following high-dose treatment, remission state improved in 43 out of 102 patients. No statistically significant advantage in reaching complete or partial remission was observed with TBI and high-dose melphalan compared to the treatment with high-dose melphalan alone. The optimal high-dose treatment, with particular reference to the inclusion or omission of TBI, should be prospectively investigated. These findings were confirmed by a prospective randomized study (Moreau et al. 2002). Patients randomly assigned to melphalan 200 mg/m^2 in this study had significantly faster hematologic recovery, less transfusion requirements, a lower incidence of severe mucositis, and had to stay a shorter period of time in hospital. While the median duration of event-free survival was similar in both arms, the 4 years estimate for overall survival was significantly better in patients receiving melphalan 200 mg/m^2 with 66% versus 46%. In accordance to this result, the EBMT presented registry data on 2,404 patients with an autologous transplantation for MM showing that patients, who had received preparative regimen without TBI, had a significantly longer overall survival (Bjorkstrand 2001). As a consequence, preparative regimens including TBI are not recommended.

Hypothesizing a positive dose-response relationship several groups tried to further increase the dose of HDT regimen. Several groups obtained dose intensification by a more intensive chemotherapeutic regimen (Fenk et al. 2005a; Anagnostopoulos et al. 2004; Abraham et al. 1999; Martinelli et al. 2003). So, patients with advanced myeloma were included in a pilot study and received idarubicin 60 mg/m^2, melphalan 200 mg/m^2, and cyclophosphamide 120 mg/kg (Heyll et al. 1997). Seven of eight patients in the pilot study achieved a near complete remission, and the toxicity observed appeared to be acceptable. There was no toxic death, but severe mucositis and fever of unknown origin were observed in all patients. However, when this regimen was compared to melphalan 200 mg/m^2 in a randomized trial for previously untreated patients, the rate of near complete remissions was higher with the dose intense regimen with 30% versus 10%, but did not translate in a better event-free or overall survival (Fenk et al. 2005a). Moreover, the intensive regimen was associated with a significantly increased toxicity in terms of severe mucositis followed by infectious complications associated with a treatment-related mortality of 20%. In line with this finding, other studies using different dose-escalated conditioning regimen have also shown an increased mortality without improvement of event- free or overall survival (Anagnostopoulos et al. 2004; Abraham et al. 1999; Martinelli et al. 2003). In the light of these data, the generally accepted high-dose therapy for patients with MM in our days is melphalan 200 mg/m^2.

Currently studies are under way, which combine bortezomib with melphalan as part of the high-dose therapy. Promising results with high CR rates in relapsing and refractory patients have been reported so far (Roussel et al. 2008), but further randomized studies have to confirm this preliminary data in the future.

10.3.4 Supportive Care During High-Dose Chemotherapy

With melphalan 200 mg/m^2 treatment-related mortality of HDT is relatively low and mainly related to hematological toxicity associated with febrile neutropenia and mucositis. The majority of severe infectious complications result from grade IV neutropenia. Without administering hematopoietic growth factors, increased levels of G-CSF have been observed in patients during the early phase of marrow aplasia following HDT and autologous SCT (Haas et al. 1993). During later periods of marrow reconstitution after HDT, the use of recombinant human G-CSF has been shown to accelerate neutrophil engraftment and to decrease the duration of febrile neutropenia, which resulted in a reduced risk of treatment-related infections (Valteau-Couanet et al. 2005; Olivieri et al. 2004).

Pegfilgrastim, a pegylated derivate of filgrastim is characterized by a prolonged plasma half-life in vivo due to decreased renal clearance. It has a similar effect on neutrophil recovery as the usual filgrastim in patients receiving conventional chemotherapy (Holmes et al. 2002; Johnston et al. 2000). Pegfilgrastim is given only once following the end of cytotoxic chemotherapy, which is obviously advantageous and more convenient for the patient. Pegfilgrastim administration following HDT with autologous transplantation leads to elevated plasma levels of pegfilgrastim, which are inversely related to the number of neutrophils (Fig. 10.5) (Fenk et al. 2006). Pegfilgrastim levels are more than 100-fold higher than physiological G-CSF levels observed after HDT with autologous SCT (Haas et al. 1993) and approximately tenfold higher than G-CSF levels after daily G-CSF application (Piccirillo et al. 1999). The duration of severe neutropenia is 5 days shorter in patients receiving pegfilgrastim compared to those without growth factor. The susceptibility to pegfilgrastim stimulation is reflected by an approximately fivefold rise of the absolute neutrophil count on the day following the administration of pegfilgrastim. Patients showing this kind of response to pegfilgrastim have a particularly short period of neutropenia. Our findings are in line with other groups (Vanstraelen et al. 2006; Staber et al. 2005; Jagasia et al. 2005). In addition, they showed that there is no difference between the daily administrations of G-CSF versus the single injection of pegfilgrastim with regard to the time needed for neutrophil recovery. Despite the shortened duration of neutropenia, the duration of the stay in hospital is not shortened since there is no difference with respect to platelet recovery, infectious complications, mucositis, and the need for parenteral nutrition between the patients receiving pegfilgrastim and those without. The rate and severity of mucositis can be reduced by the addition of human recombinant keratinocyte growth factor, which is a stimulator of the mucosal stem cells (Kobbe et al. 2006).

10.3.5 High-Dose Chemotherapy Is Superior to Conventional Chemotherapy

Since the introduction of HDT up to now, at least 20,000 patients with MM were treated with HDT and autologous SCT according to a European Blood and Marrow Transplant (EBMT) registry study (Bjorkstrand and Gahrton 2007). The first randomized study to demonstrate the superiority of HDT in comparison to conventional chemotherapy was from the French "intergroupe francophone de myelome" (IFM) and included 200 untreated patients, who were younger than 65 years without severe renal impairment (Attal et al. 1996). In this trial, the rate of complete remissions was significantly enhanced from 5% with conventional chemotherapy to 22% with HDT and autologous SCT. The improved response rate translated into a significantly longer median event-free survival of 44 months following HDT versus 18 months in the control arm. There was also a significantly longer median overall survival of 57 versus 44 months. The British Medical Research Council (MRC) (Child et al. 2003) published similar results 7 years later. Therefore, HDT supported by autologous PBSCT became the standard therapy for young patients with multiple myeloma and normal renal function. Later, there were five other studies comparing single HDT and autologous PBSCT with conventional chemotherapy (Fermand et al. 1998, 2005; Palumbo et al. 2004; Blade et al. 2005; Barlogie et al. 2006a). These studies were confirmatory with regard to the two studies from France and the UK. Still there were some concerns because of the lack of a significant survival benefit. Looking at the results of all randomized trials a greater rate of complete remissions in the patients receiving HDT could be observed in six of seven studies (Attal et al. 1996; Child et al. 2003; Fermand et al. 1998, 2005; Palumbo et al. 2004; Blade et al. 2005). In contrast, a longer event-free survival was found in five of seven studies (Attal et al. 1996; Child et al. 2003; Fermand et al. 1998, 2005; Palumbo et al. 2004), while a longer overall survival was noted in three of seven studies (Attal et al. 1996; Child et al. 2003; Palumbo et al. 2004). In a meta-analysis of

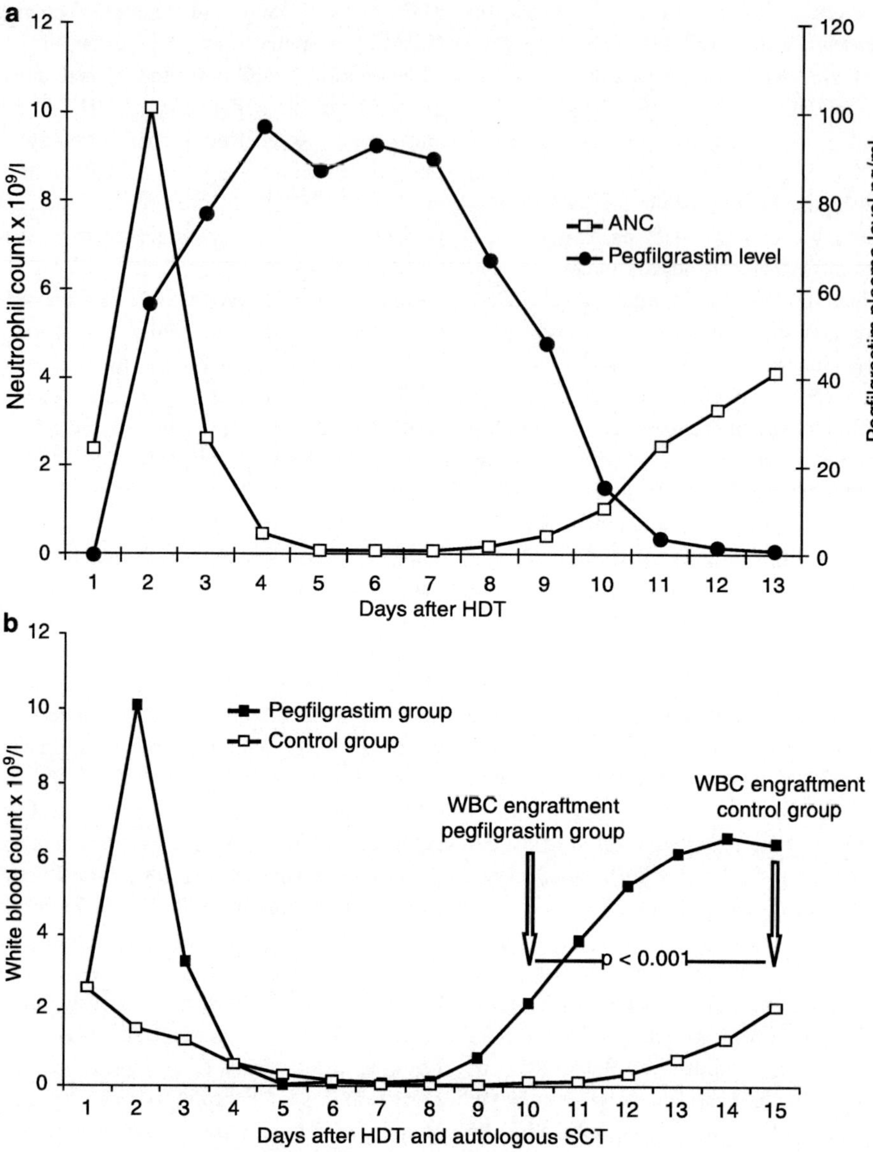

Fig. 10.5 (**a**) Neutrophil counts and pegfilgrastim levels of patients receiving 6 mg pegfilgrastim on day+1 after HDT and autoloogus SCT are shown. (**b**) Comparison of time to leucocyte recovery after HDT and autologous SCT of patients who received pegfilgrastim and a historical control group withour hematopoietic growth factor support

nine HDT trials (Koreth et al. 2007), which also included studies with older patients who had received double intermediate-dosed conditioning regimen, HDT was superior to conventional therapy as far as event-free was concerned but not with regard to survival. The duration of survival is influenced by the use of more or less effective salvage therapies, in particular since the introduction of novel agents (Kumar et al. 2008). Therefore, it is not surprising that HDT followed by autologous SCT remains the therapy of first choice for patients eligible for this treatment procedure.

10.3.6 Timing of High-Dose Chemotherapy

In principle, HDT with autologous PBSCT can be performed frontline as consolidation therapy following induction therapy or as salvage treatment at the time of relapse after a conventional first-line therapy. Two studies have addressed this question in a randomized fashion (Fermand et al. 2005; Barlogie et al. 2006a). Both studies did not observe a difference with regard to overall survival. In the study of Barlogie et al. (2006a), there was also no difference with regard to event-free survival. In contrast, Fermand et al. (2005) observed a significantly longer time of event-free survival in the "early" treatment group of patients with 39 versus 13 months in those receiving HDT following a previous relapse. More important, the time spent without therapy was longer in the "early" treatment group with 28 versus 22 months. In none of the studies, a comparison was made with respect to quality of life. It should be also considered that patients not receiving up-front HDT are usually on therapy for a longer period of time which is associated with a greater risk that organ complications acquired along the conventional therapy hamper a "late" HDT. In addition, there is a higher risk for developing a secondary myelodysplastic syndrome because of the long exposition to low-dose alkylating agents. Therefore, HDT as first-line therapy is recommended, while despite this general recommendation HDT is of therapeutic efficacy at any stage of the disease. In the light of this statement, peripheral blood stem cell collection should be performed following induction therapy, irrespective whether an "early" or "late" HDT is envisaged.

10.3.7 Tandem Autologous Transplantation

The experience with HDT and autologous SCT showed that patients achieving a complete or at least very good partial response had a longer overall survival than patients, who achieved only a partial remission (Lahuerta et al. 2008). In order to accomplish a CR in as many patients as possible dose intensification by means of sequential cycles of HDT and autologous PBSCT was proposed by several investigators. In particular, Barlogie and coworkers at the University of Arkansas (Barlogie et al. 1997) introduced double or tandem HDT as part of the "Total Therapy" program. The French IFM (Attal et al. 2003) was the first group to demonstrate feasibility and superiority of a tandem HDT in comparison to a single HDT in a randomized trial for patients up to the age of 60 years. Of all patients, 75% underwent a second transplantation and the treatment-related mortality was less than 5%. The 7-year event-free and overall survivals were 20% versus 10% and 42% versus 21% in favor for the tandem transplantation. However, the median difference in event-free and overall survival was – despite the statistical significance – only 2 and 10 months, respectively. Moreover, in a subgroup analysis the benefit of a second HDT was restricted to patients who did not achieve at least a very good partial response.

Five other randomized studies also investigated the efficacy of tandem versus single HDT and autologous PBSCT. In a recently published meta-analysis of all six trials (Kumar et al. 2009), taking into account 1,803 patients a significantly better response rate was obtained following tandem HDT that was associated with a significantly higher treatment-related mortality. As far as event-free and overall survivals were concerned there was no statistically significant difference whether one or two HDT were performed. Excluding one study from the meta-analysis in which single HDT in combination with thalidomide maintenance treatment was compared to tandem HDT without thalidomide resulted in a significant change in the hazard ratio favoring tandem transplantation with respect to EFS. Further, data in this meta-analysis did not permit a subgroup analysis according to the response following the first HDT. In conclusion, the therapeutic benefit of tandem HDT is not entirely clear. As with single HDT the role of tandem HDT has to be readdressed in the light of the availability of new therapeutic compounds.

10.3.8 The Role of Induction Treatment

The novel agents such as thalidomide (Glasmacher et al. 2006), bortezomib (Richardson et al. 2005) and lenalidomide (Dimopoulos et al. 2007; Weber et al. 2007) have shown high efficacy in patients with relapsed or refractory MM. Therefore, several investigators have moved these agents from the relapsed setting into front-line therapy. In the context of HDT and autologous PBSCT all three drugs have been used for induction therapy either in combination with dexamethasone or with conventional chemotherapy or with each other.

Studies using thalidomide in combination with dexamethasone and/or chemotherapy (Rajkumar et al. 2006; Cavo et al. 2005; Macro et al. 2006; Lokhorst et al. 2008) as induction therapy demonstrated higher response rates before HDT. Nevertheless, this early difference was neutralized by HDT, as response rates after HDT were not different anymore. Only a longer follow-up will show whether this minor benefit will translate into a longer time of event-free and overall survival. The incidence of deep-vein thrombosis is higher with thalidomide combinations necessitating the use of prophylactic anticoagulation.

Induction treatment with bortezomib results not only in a significant improvement of remission rates before transplant, difference that persists following HDT. The rate of at least very good partial responses with bortezomib and dexamethasone in the IFM trial in comparison to VAD is also significantly greater with 68% versus 47% (Harousseau et al. 2006). Preliminary data also show a benefit in terms of event-free survival. In addition, the high efficacy in patients with extramedullary disease favors this combination. The problem with an induction treatment including bortezomib is the high incidence of peripheral neuropathy, which develops in 46% of all patients including 7% with WHO grade 3 and 4.

Induction treatment with lenalidomide in combination with dexamethasone induces remissions in the majority of patients. A randomized comparison (Rajkumar et al. 2006) of lenalidomide with low-dose dexamethasone versus lenalidomide with high-dose dexamethasone resulted in a comparable therapeutic efficacy, but the toxicity was markedly reduced in patients receiving low-dose dexamethasone.

A longer follow-up is needed to estimate the therapeutic potential of the new drugs with regard to overall survival of patients. Until then, combinations with lower dosages of novel agents should be examined in order to reduce the toxicity of induction therapy without compromising the efficacy. Taken together, for patients outside of clinical trials, it is a reasonable approach to begin with conventional induction therapy and only change treatment to novel agents in case of unresponsiveness. This way, undue toxicity can be avoided. For high-risk patients with extramedullary disease or abnormal karyotype novel agents may also be considered as up-front therapy (Laura et al. 2006; Jagannath et al. 2007; Bahlis et al. 2006). In all studies with novel agents, peripheral blood stem cells could be collected for the majority of patients, while their number was reduced in comparison to patients receiving the conventional type of induction therapy. Therefore, a discontinuation of the novel agents is recommended before PBSC mobilization is initiated.

10.3.9 The Role of Consolidation or Maintenance Treatment

Besides induction therapy novel agents were also used after transplantation in order to further reduce residual tumor cells and prolong the duration of disease control. Maintenance therapy with interferon (INF) alpha or corticosteroids is associated with severe constitutional symptoms leading to a reduced quality of life. In addition, INF alpha has only a little effect on the course of the disease, if any effect at all (Myeloma Trialists' Collaborative Group 2001). Thus, with the availability of novel agents INF, alpha and corticosteroids are not used for maintenance therapy anymore.

Introduced by the Arkansas group (Barlogie et al. 2006b), thalidomide was continuously administered at different doses from the start of induction therapy, throughout tandem HDT and following HDT until disease progression. In a randomized comparison with patients not receiving thalidomide, treatment with thalidomide resulted in higher rates of complete remission with 62% versus 44%, while the 5-years survival rate was also superior with 56% versus 44%. Still, overall survival was not different in both treatment arms. After a follow-up time of 72 months, the group of patients with cytogenetic abnormalities showed had a better overall survival when they had received thalidomide (Barlogie et al. 2008).

The use of thalidomide only after HDT seems to be more effective. In a randomized study from the French IFM, 597 patients were randomized between three kind of maintenance therapies after tandem HDT and PBSCT (Attal et al. 2006). Patients received pamidronate, pamidronate plus thalidomide, or nothing. the Patients receiving thalidomide had the longest event-free survival at 3 years with a proportion of 52% versus 36% and an overall survival rate at 4 years of 87% versus 75%. Only patients with chromosome 13 deletion or with achievement of a complete or very good partial remission did not benefit from thalidomide treatment. Other studies (Abdelkefi et al. 2008; Spencer et al. 2006; Fenk et al. 2005b) have confirmed these results. Abdelkefi et al. (2008) showed that a maintenance therapy with thalidomide over a period of 6 months after a single HDT and autologous PBSCT is even superior to a tandem HDT without maintenance therapy.

The major side effect of thalidomide is a severe polyneuropathy forcing approximately 60% of the patients to discontinue the therapy (Barlogie et al. 2006b). This toxicity is very disadvantageous as patients, who are able to tolerate thalidomide for more than 10 months have a statistically significantly longer survival time than patients who had to abandon thalidomide due to adverse events (Lilienfeld-Toal et al. 2007). In addition, there is no consensus about the optimal treatment schedule and dose. Lenalidomide provides a useful alternative, as it is more potent in vitro and less toxic than thalidomide. It is also effective in high-risk patients with chromosome 13 deletions (Bahlis et al. 2006). Therefore, lenalidomide has the potential to improve remission rates, event-free, and overall survival following HDT without relevant toxicity. In principle, bortezomib may also be considered for maintenance, although a greater risk of developing polyneuropathies has to be envisaged in comparison to lenalidomide.

Another experimental alternative for maintenance therapy after HDT could be an isotype vaccination with dendritic cells (Abdalla et al. 2007; Curti et al. 2007; van Rhee 2007; Bogen et al. 2006). DC based vaccines for patients with malignant diseases generated under different culture conditions have been investigated for more than a decade. Despite these efforts, clinical results of DC vaccination studies showed therapeutic efficacy only in a limited number of patients so far (Nestle et al. 2005). In search of an alternative way for DC generation, we examined the molecular and functional characteristics of dendritic cells generated with interferon and GM-CSF (IFN-DC) and compared the results with dendritic cells generated with the classical protocol using IL-4 and TNF-alpha (IL-4/TNF-DC) (Korthals et al. 2007). We could show that both, IFN-DC and IL-4/TNF-DC, display typical DC characteristics, but also have distinct molecular and functional phenotypes. Our results from gene expression analysis show that IFN-DC have signs of a pronounced maturation state and an increased migratory capacity to the lymph nodes in comparison to IL-4/TNF-DC. Strikingly, IFN-DC showed a more plasmacytoid phenotype associated with NK cell characteristics on a molecular and protein level as well as a functional cytotoxic activity against tumor cells. We found a significant upregulation of 32 genes strongly related to NK cell functions in IFN-DC compared to IL-4/TNF-DC. These include NK cell receptors NKp80, NKp44, NKp46, and NKG2D that are synergizing the cytotoxic activity of NK cells (Bryceson et al. 2006; Moretta et al. 2001), as well as CD56 and cytotoxic effector molecules such as granzymes and TRAIL. Indeed, on protein level, we could detect intracellular pools of TRAIL and granzyme B in IFN-DC. Finally, as a further corroboration of the suggested cytotoxic capacity, IFN-DC, but not IL-4/TNF-DC, was able to kill K562 cells in vitro. These findings are of particular interest, as a new murine DC cell population has been recently described, termed interferon-producing killer dendritic cells (IKDC), that express molecular markers of plasmacytoid DC and NK cells (Chan et al. 2006; Taieb et al. 2006). IKDC exhibit specific cytolytic activity upon contact with tumor cells or activation with CpG oligonucleotides and subsequently upregulate costimulatory molecules, migrate to the lymph nodes and present antigen to T cells. Indeed, nine of the genes specifically expressed by IKDC, including granzymes, NKG2D, NKp46, and CD49b as determined by microarray analysis (Chan et al. 2006), were also differentially expressed by IFN-DC in comparison to IL-4/TNF-DC. Together with the pronounced migratory potential and the cytotoxic capacity of IFN-DC, the similarities between IFN-DC and mouse IKDC suggest that also in humans a molecular and functional relationship exists between DC and NK cells. In conclusion, IFN-DC, which can not only stimulate T cells but also can kill tumor cells by themselves, should be evaluated in clinical vaccination trials (Fig. 10.6).

10.3.10 Prognostic Factors

There are a number of prognostic factors, which can be used at the time of first diagnosis to estimate the risk of relapse. Among those are an advanced age, renal dysfunction, high ß2-microglobulin, low albumin, high CRP or LDH levels, thrombocytopenia, high plasma cell labeling index and most importantly chromosomal abnormalities with t(4;14) as the worst prognostic marker. The usefulness of gene expression studies defining high-risk profiles has to be evaluated prospectively. All these prognostic markers may

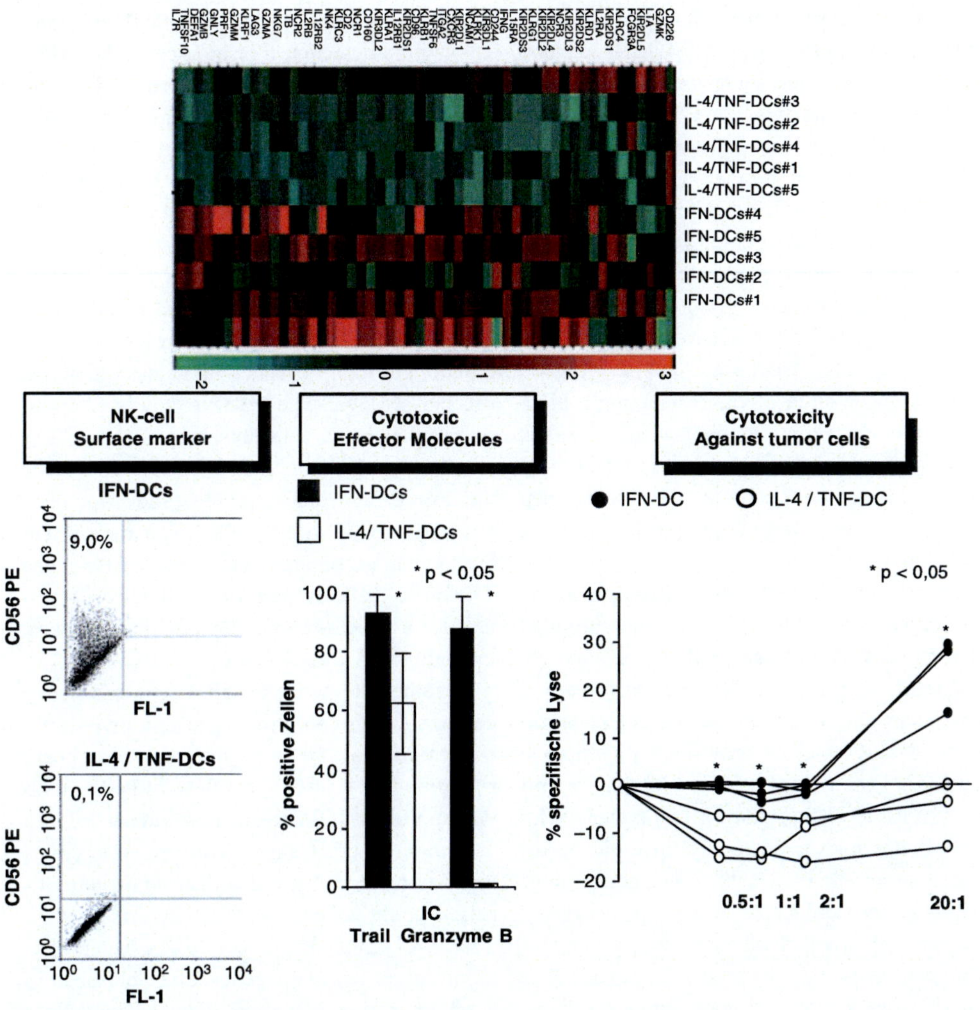

Fig. 10.6 IFN-DC have novel molecular, phenotypical and functional characteristics in comparison to IL-4/TNF-DC. (**a**) Hierarchical cluster analysis of 52 genes related to NK cell function for IFN-DC and IL-4/TNF-DC preparations with expression levels obtained by Affymetrix microarray analysis. (**b**) Expression of NK cell surface markers and (**c**) cytolytic effector molecules by DC as analysed by flow cytometray. CD56 and intracellular expression of TRAIL and granzyme B by IFN-DC and IL-4/TNF-DC. (**d**) Cytolytic activity of DC. Specific lysis of tumor cells by DC was measured by flow cytometric detection of propidium iodide uptake after coculture with K562 cells

be considered for clinical decision making in order to allocate patients to more or less intensive treatment regimen. Assessment of response by conventional diagnostic procedures is a dynamic parameter (Lahuerta et al. 2008). As mentioned above patients achieving at least a very good partial response after the first HDT have no further benefit from a second one (Attal et al. 2003). However, the prognostic implication of complete response is limited. Patients with a prior history of monoclonal gammopathy of undetermined significance (MGUS) or smoldering MM have the same treatment outcome after HDT as patients achieving a complete response even when they show a clear M-protein spike in the electrophoresis (Pineda-Roman et al. 2007). These patients had "returned"to their prior MGUS stage following eradication of the transformed MM tumor cell population as result of HDT. In this particular group of patients the achievement of CR or failure to reach this aim is not of prognostic relevance. Another group of patients with a disease type resembling a high-grade non-Hodgkins lymphoma may present with high levels of free light chains in the serum. Even if these patients achieve a complete remission, they have a very poor prognosis (van Rhee et al. 2007).

Another possibility to assess response during the course of therapy is the measurement of minimal residual disease (MRD) on a molecular level. This method is more sensitive and specific to detect tumor cells of clonal origin (Fenk et al. 2004a). It provides a quantitative estimate of the risk of relapse and may permit therapeutic decisions, as shown for patients with acute lymphoblastic or chronic myeloid leukemia (Szczepanski et al. 2001). The detection of MRD is of particular relevance, as novel agents are very effective in reducing the number of malignant cells and thus are leading to a higher rate of patients with very good partial and complete remissions. For patients with MM, a molecular remission as shown by qualitative immunoglobulin heavy chain (IgH)-PCR is associated with a better event-free survival after myeloablative allogeneic PBSCT (Corradini et al. 2003). Following HDT and autologous SCT bone marrow, samples of 87% of patients remain PCR-positive (Corradini et al. 1999). Therefore, a quantitative method is necessary. Using a limiting dilution assay for IgH-PCR, Bakkus et al. (2004) identified a threshold level of 0.015% clonotypic cells in bone marrow samples obtained 3 months after HDT and autologous SCT as prognostically relevant for the EFS. Another group used multiparameter flow cytometry with a detection threshold of 10^{-4} (0.01%) which is in the same range and reported similar results. Using real-time quantitative RCR as a third method, we defined a cut-off value of 0.03% clonotypic cells in the bone marrow determined before HDT and autologous PBSCT (Fenk et al. 2004b) as a prognostic marker for the probability of EFS. Patients falling below this threshold after induction and mobilization chemotherapy not only had longer EFS, but also a better OS than patients with values did above this cut-off level. The MRD level was found to be prognostically relevant independent of ISS stage, cytogenetics, and the kind of maintenance therapy. These results imply that induction therapy before HDT with SCT has to be improved at least for those patients with high MRD levels. Therefore, MRD monitoring provides a rationale for a patient-tailored therapy dependent on the individual response to a given treatment.

Another alternative to MRD monitoring may be gene expression profiling after a given drug is administered. Gene expression studies were performed 48 h after a test dose of bortezomib was applied to 142 untreated patients in order to determine whether any MM- or microenvironment-associated changes with prognostic implication could be observed (Shaughnessy et al. 2008). A high-risk score defined by the upregulation of proteasome genes after bortezomib application was associated with an extremely poor survival of less than 24 months and was an independent prognostic parameter in multivariate analysis. This kind of analysis will help us to get a better understanding of the pathophysiology of MM and mechanisms of drug resistance to novel drugs.

10.3.11 Targeted Versus High-Dose Chemotherapy

Novel therapies such as thalidomide, bortezomib, and lenalidomide necessitate redefining the role of HDT and autologous SCT. Further studies are needed to better understand how to use these agents in conjunction with HDT in patients with multiple myeloma. Some may ask whether in the era of novel agents HDT and autologous blood stem cell transplantation has any role. This opinion is supported by the results of a study comparing tandem HDT with low-dose melphalan and prednisone in combination with thalidomide in elderly patients (Facon et al. 2007). In this study, the combination of conventional chemotherapy with thalidomide was superior with regard to survival. Rather than comparing HDT with novel agents, the therapeutic efficacy of HDT in combination with novel agents should be investigated in order to improve remission rate and ultimately the duration of survival of the patients.

With the availability of a therapy based on a better understanding of the pathophysiology of the disease, we may undergo a transition from the general cytotoxic effect of HDT to an individualized specific effect of a small molecule, antibody, or other biological response modifier aiming at a particular structure within the malignant plasma cell or its precursor. This could be, for instance, the inhibition of pathophysiologically relevant pathways, which govern self-renewal, proliferation, and differentiation of the myeloma cell or protect it from apoptosis. Inhibition of particular pathways, which are known to play a role in MM cell growth, has not been successful so far (Ocio et al. 2008). This may be due to the evolutionary dynamic of human life, which is finding a new way, when one is blocked. More likely, the simultaneous inhibition of different pathways is probably required. One example may be the combined inhibition of the unfolded protein response, which is responsible for the detection and disposal of misfolded proteins. MM cells secrete large amounts of paraprotein, which are correctly folded by the chaperone system. If this process fails, two systems, the proteasome and the aggresome, eliminate the accumulating misfolded proteins. If this process also fails, cell death occurs because of accumulating toxic proteins. Inhibition of the chaperone system is possible with heat-shock protein inhibitors, whereas histone deacetylase inhibitors can inhibit the aggresome. Application of these novel drugs together with the proteasome inhibitor bortezomib has shown very promising results. Whether the inhibition of all three pathways will lead to a sustained clinical effect has to be awaited. As long as there is no effective targeted therapy available, high dose therapy with autologous peripheral blood stem cell transplantation is still the cornerstone of any therapy in combination with thalidomide, lenalidomide, and bortezomib.

References

Abdalla AO, Hansson L, Eriksson I, Nasman-Glaser B, Mellstedt H, Osterborg A (2007) Long-term effects of idiotype vaccination on the specific T-cell response in peripheral blood and bone marrow of multiple myeloma patients. Eur J Haematol 79:371–381

Abdelkefi A, Ladeb S, Torjman L, Othman TB, Lakhal A, Romdhane NB, Omri HE, Elloumi M, Belaaj H, Jeddi R, Aissaoui L, Ksouri H, Hassen AB, Msadek F, Saad A, Hsairi M, Boukef K, Amouri A, Louzir H, Dellagi K, Abdeladhim AB (2008) Single autologous stem-cell transplantation followed by maintenance therapy with thalidomide is superior to double autologous transplantation in multiple myeloma: results of a multicenter randomized clinical trial. Blood 111:1805–1810

Abonour R, Scott KM, Kunkel LA, Robertson MJ, Hromas R, Graves V, Lazaridis EN, Cripe L, Gharpure V, Traycoff CM, Mills B, Srour EF, Cornetta K (1998) Autologous transplantation of mobilized peripheral blood $CD34^+$ cells selected by immunomagnetic procedures in patients with multiple myeloma. Bone Marrow Transplant 22:957–963

Abraham R, Chen C, Tsang R, Simpson D, Murray C, Davidson M, Meharchand J, Sutton DM, Crump RM, Keating A, Stewart AK (1999) Intensification of the stem cell transplant induction regimen results in increased treatment-related mortality without improved outcome in multiple myeloma. Bone Marrow Transplant 24:1291–1297

10

Aiuti A, Webb IJ, Bleul C, Springer T, Gutierrez-Ramos JC (1997) The chemokine SDF-1 is a chemoattractant for human CD34+ hematopoietic progenitor cells and provides a new mechanism to explain the mobilization of CD34+ progenitors to peripheral blood. J Exp Med 185:111–120

Alexanian R, Haut A, Khan AU, Lane M, McKelvey EM, Migliore PJ, Stuckey WJ Jr, Wilson HE (1969) Treatment for multiple myeloma. Combination chemotherapy with different melphalan dose regimens. JAMA 208:1680–1685

Anagnostopoulos A, Aleman A, Ayers G, Donato M, Champlin R, Weber D, Alexanian R, Giralt S (2004) Comparison of high-dose melphalan with a more intensive regimen of thiotepa, busulfan, and cyclophosphamide for patients with multiple myeloma. Cancer 100:2607–2612

Attal M, Harousseau JL, Stoppa AM, Sotto JJ, Fuzibet JG, Rossi JF, Casassus P, Maisonneuve H, Facon T, Ifrah N, Payen C, Bataille R (1996) A prospective, randomized trial of autologous bone marrow transplantation and chemotherapy in multiple myeloma. Intergroupe Francais du Myelome. N Engl J Med 335:91–97

Attal M, Harousseau JL, Facon T, Guilhot F, Doyen C, Fuzibet JG, Monconduit M, Hulin C, Caillot D, Bouabdallah R, Voillat L, Sotto JJ, Grosbois B, Bataille R (2003) Single versus double autologous stem-cell transplantation for multiple myeloma. N Engl J Med 349:2495–2502

Attal M, Harousseau JL, Leyvraz S, Doyen C, Hulin C, Benboubker L, Agha IY, Bourhis JH, Garderet L, Pegourie B, Dumontet C, Renaud M, Voillat L, Berthou C, Marit G, Monconduit M, Caillot D, Grobois B, Avet-Loiseau H, Moreau P, Facon T (2006) Maintenance therapy with thalidomide improves survival in patients with multiple myeloma. Blood 108:3289–3294

Bahlis NJ, Mansoor A, Lategan JC, Valentine K, Thaell T, Blahey W, Savoie ML, Blaikie K, Kmet L, Roland B, Stewart DA (2006) Lenalidomide overcomes poor prognosis conferred by deletion of chromosome 13 and t(4;14) in multiple myeloma: MM016 trial. Blood 108(11):3557

Bakkus MH, Bouko Y, Samson D, Apperley JF, Thielemans K, Van Camp B, Benner A, Goldschmidt H, Moos M, Cremer FW (2004) Post-transplantation tumour load in bone marrow, as assessed by quantitative ASO-PCR, is a prognostic parameter in multiple myeloma. Br J Haematol 126:665–674

Barbui AM, Galli M, Dotti G, Belli N, Borleri G, Gritti G, Bellavita P, Viero P, Comotti B, Barbui T, Rambaldi A (2002) Negative selection of peripheral blood stem cells to support a tandem autologous transplantation programme in multiple myeloma. Br J Haematol 116:202–210

Barlogie B, Jagannath S, Vesole DH, Naucke S, Cheson B, Mattox S, Bracy D, Salmon S, Jacobson J, Crowley J, Tricot G (1997) Superiority of tandem autologous transplantation over standard therapy for previously untreated multiple myeloma. Blood 89:789–793

Barlogie B, Jagannath S, Desikan KR, Mattox S, Vesole D, Siegel D, Tricot G, Munshi N, Fassas A, Singhal S, Mehta J, Anaissie E, Dhodapkar D, Naucke S, Cromer J, Sawyer J, Epstein J, Spoon D, Ayers D, Cheson B, Crowley J (1999) Total therapy with tandem transplants for newly diagnosed multiple myeloma. Blood 93:55–65

Barlogie B, Kyle RA, Anderson KC, Greipp PR, Lazarus HM, Hurd DD, McCoy J, Moore DF Jr, Dakhil SR, Lanier KS, Chapman RA, Cromer JN, Salmon SE, Durie B, Crowley JC (2006a) Standard chemotherapy compared with high-dose chemoradiotherapy for multiple myeloma: final results of phase III US Intergroup Trial S9321. J Clin Oncol 24:929–936

Barlogie B, Tricot G, Anaissie E, Shaughnessy J, Rasmussen E, van Rhee F, Fassas A, Zangari M, Hollmig K, Pineda-Roman M, Lee C, Talamo G, Thertulien R, Kiwan E, Krishna S, Fox M, Crowley J (2006b) Thalidomide and hematopoietic-cell transplantation for multiple myeloma. N Engl J Med 354:1021–1030

Barlogie B, Pineda-Roman M, van Rhee F, Haessler J, Anaissie E, Hollmig K, Alsayed Y, Waheed S, Petty N, Epstein J, Shaughnessy JD Jr, Tricot G, Zangari M, Zeldis J, Barer S, Crowley J (2008) Thalidomide arm of Total Therapy 2 improves complete remission duration and survival in myeloma patients with metaphase cytogenetic abnormalities. Blood 112:3115–3121

Bellucci R, De Propris MS, Buccisano F, Lisci A, Leone G, Tabilio A, de Fabritiis P (1999) Modulation of VLA-4 and L-selectin expression on normal CD34+ cells during mobilization with G-CSF. Bone Marrow Transplant 23:1–8

Bensinger W (2008) Stem-cell transplantation for multiple myeloma in the era of novel drugs. J Clin Oncol 26:480–492

Bensinger WI, Longin K, Appelbaum F, Rowley S, Weaver C, Lilleby K, Gooley T, Lynch M,

Higano T, Klarnet J (1994) Peripheral blood stem cells (PBSCs) collected after recombinant granulocyte colony stimulating factor (rhG-CSF): an analysis of factors correlating with the tempo of engraftment after transplantation. Br J Haematol 87:825–831

Bensinger WI, Weaver CH, Appelbaum FR, Rowley S, Demirer T, Sanders J, Storb R, Buckner CD (1995) Transplantation of allogeneic peripheral blood stem cells mobilized by recombinant human granulocyte colony-stimulating factor. Blood 85:1655–1658

Bird JM, Bloxham D, Samson D, Marcus RE, Russell NH, Kelsey SM, Newland AC, Apperley JF (1994) Molecular detection of clonally rearranged cells in peripheral blood progenitor cell harvests from multiple myeloma patients. Br J Haematol 88:110–116

Bjorkstrand B (2001) European group for blood and marrow transplantation registry studies in multiple myeloma. Semin Hematol 38:219–225

Bjorkstrand B, Gahrton G (2007) High-dose treatment with autologous stem cell transplantation in multiple myeloma: past, present, and future. Semin Hematol 44:227–233

Blade J, Rosinol L, Sureda A, Ribera JM, Diaz-Mediavilla J, Garcia-Larana J, Mateos MV, Palomera L, Fernandez-Calvo J, Marti JM, Giraldo P, Carbonell F, Callis M, Trujillo J, Gardella S, Moro MJ, Barez A, Soler A, Font L, Fontanillas M, San MJ (2005) High-dose therapy intensification compared with continued standard chemotherapy in multiple myeloma patients responding to the initial chemotherapy: long-term results from a prospective randomized trial from the Spanish cooperative group PETHEMA. Blood 106:3755–3759

Bleul CC, Farzan M, Choe H, Parolin C, Clark-Lewis I, Sodroski J, Springer TA (1996) The lymphocyte chemoattractant SDF-1 is a ligand for LESTR/fusin and blocks HIV-1 entry. Nature 382:829–833

Blokhin N, Larionov L, Perevodchikova N, Chebotareva L, Merkulova N (1958) Clinical experiences with sarcolysin in neoplastic diseases. Ann NY Acad Sci 68:1128–1132

Bogen B, Ruffini PA, Corthay A, Fredriksen AB, Froyland M, Lundin K, Rosjo E, Thompson K, Massaia M (2006) Idiotype-specific immunotherapy in multiple myeloma: suggestions for future directions of research. Haematologica 91:941–948

Bourhis JH, Bouko Y, Koscielny S, Bakkus M, Greinix H, Derigs G, Salles G, Feremans W, Apperley J, Samson D, Bjorkstrand B, Niederwieser D, Gahrton G, Pico JL, Goldschmidt H (2007) Relapse risk after autologous transplantation in patients with newly diagnosed myeloma is not related with infused tumor cell load and the outcome is not improved by $CD34^+$ cell selection: long term follow-up of an EBMT phase III randomized study. Haematologica 92:1083–1090

Bruns I, Steidl U, Kronenwett R, Fenk R, Graef T, Rohr UP, Neumann F, Fischer J, Scheid C, Hubel K, Haas R, Kobbe G (2006) A single dose of 6 or 12 mg of pegfilgrastim for peripheral blood progenitor cell mobilization results in similar yields of $CD34^+$ progenitors in patients with multiple myeloma. Transfusion 46:180–185

Bruns I, Steidl U, Fischer JC, Czibere A, Kobbe G, Raschke S, Singh R, Fenk R, Rosskopf M, Pechtel S, von Haeseler A, Wernet P, Tenen DG, Haas R, Kronenwett R (2008) Pegylated granulocyte colony-stimulating factor mobilizes $CD34^+$ cells with different stem and progenitor subsets and distinct functional properties in comparison with unconjugated granulocyte colony-stimulating factor. Haematologica 93:347–355

Bryceson YT, March ME, Ljunggren HG, Long EO (2006) Synergy among receptors on resting NK cells for the activation of natural cytotoxicity and cytokine secretion 1. Blood 107:159–166

Cavo M, Zamagni E, Tosi P, Tacchetti P, Cellini C, Cangini D, De Vivo A, Testoni N, Nicci C, Terragna C, Grafone T, Perrone G, Ceccolini M, Tura S, Baccarani M (2005) Superiority of thalidomide and dexamethasone over vincristine-doxorubicindexamethasone (VAD) as primary therapy in preparation for autologous transplantation for multiple myeloma. Blood 106:35–39

Chan CW, Crafton E, Fan HN, Flook J, Yoshimura K, Skarica M, Brockstedt D, Dubensky TW, Stins MF, Lanier LL, Pardoll DM, Housseau F (2006) Interferon-producing killer dendritic cells provide a link between innate and adaptive immunity. Nat Med 12:207–213

Child JA, Morgan GJ, Davies FE, Owen RG, Bell SE, Hawkins K, Brown J, Drayson MT, Selby PJ (2003) High-dose chemotherapy with hematopoietic stem-cell rescue for multiple myeloma. N Engl J Med 348:1875–1883

Corradini P, Voena C, Astolfi M, Ladetto M, Tarella C, Boccadoro M, Pileri A (1995) High-dose

10

sequential chemoradiotherapy in multiple myeloma: residual tumor cells are detectable in bone marrow and peripheral blood cell harvests and after autografting. Blood 85:1596–1602

Corradini P, Voena C, Tarella C, Astolfi M, Ladetto M, Palumbo A, Van Lint MT, Bacigalupo A, Santoro A, Musso M, Majolino I, Boccadoro M, Pileri A (1999) Molecular and clinical remissions in multiple myeloma: role of autologous and allogeneic transplantation of hematopoietic cells. J Clin Oncol 17:208–215

Corradini P, Cavo M, Lokhorst H, Martinelli G, Terragna C, Majolino I, Valagussa P, Boccadoro M, Samson D, Bacigalupo A, Russell N, Montefusco V, Voena C, Gahrton G (2003) Molecular remission after myeloablative allogeneic stem cell transplantation predicts a better relapse-free survival in patients with multiple myeloma. Blood 102:1927–1929

Cremer FW, Kiel K, Sucker C, Wacker J, Atzberger A, Haas R, Goldschmidt H, Moos M (1997) A rationale for positive selection of peripheral blood stem cells in multiple myeloma: highly purified $CD34^+$ cell fractions of leukapheresis products do not contain malignant cells. Leukemia 11(Suppl 5): S41–S46

Cremer FW, Kiel K, Wallmeier M, Haas R, Goldschmidt H, Moos M (1998) Leukapheresis products in multiple myeloma: lower tumor load after mobilization with cyclophosphamide plus granulocyte colony-stimulating factor (G-CSF) compared with G-CSF alone. Exp Hematol 26:969–975

Cunningham D, Paz-Ares L, Gore ME, Malpas J, Hickish T, Nicolson M, Meldrum M, Viner C, Milan S, Selby PJ (1994) High-dose melphalan for multiple myeloma: long-term follow-up data. J Clin Oncol 12:764–768

Curti A, Tosi P, Comoli P, Terragna C, Ferri E, Cellini C, Massaia M, D'Addio A, Giudice V, Di BC, Cavo M, Conte R, Gugliotta G, Baccarani M, Lemoli RM (2007) Phase I/II clinical trial of sequential subcutaneous and intravenous delivery of dendritic cell vaccination for refractory multiple myeloma using patient-specific tumour idiotype protein or idiotype (VDJ)-derived class I-restricted peptides. Br J Haematol 139:415–424

Deichmann M, Kronenwett R, Haas R (1997) Expression of the human immunodeficiency virus type-1 coreceptors CXCR-4 (fusin, LESTR) and CKR-5 in $CD34^+$ hematopoietic progenitor cells. Blood 89:3522–3528

Dercksen MW, Rodenhuis S, Dirkson MK, Schaasberg WP, Baars JW, Van Der WE, Slaper-Cortenbach IC, Pinedo HM, von dem Borne AE, van der Schoot CE (1995) Subsets of $CD34^+$ cells and rapid hematopoietic recovery after peripheral-blood stem-cell transplantation. J Clin Oncol 13:1922–1932

Dimopoulos M, Spencer A, Attal M, Prince HM, Harousseau JL, Dmoszynska A, San MJ, Hellmann A, Facon T, Foa R, Corso A, Masliak Z, Olesnyckyj M, Yu Z, Patin J, Zeldis JB, Knight RD (2007) Lenalidomide plus dexamethasone for relapsed or refractory multiple myeloma. N Engl J Med 357:2123–2132

Dreger P, Haferlach T, Eckstein V, Jacobs S, Suttorp M, Loffler H, Muller-Ruchholtz W, Schmitz N (1994) G-CSF-mobilized peripheral blood progenitor cells for allogeneic transplantation: safety, kinetics of mobilization, and composition of the graft. Br J Haematol 87:609–613

Facon T, Mary JY, Hulin C, Benboubker L, Attal M, Pegourie B, Renaud M, Harousseau JL, Guillerm G, Chaleteix C, Dib M, Voillat L, Maisonneuve H, Troncy J, Dorvaux V, Monconduit M, Martin C, Casassus P, Jaubert J, Jardel H, Doyen C, Kolb B, Anglaret B, Grosbois B, Yakoub-Agha I, Mathiot C, Avet-Loiseau H (2007) Melphalan and prednisone plus thalidomide versus melphalan and prednisone alone or reduced-intensity autologous stem cell transplantation in elderly patients with multiple myeloma (IFM 99-06): a randomised trial. Lancet 370:1209–1218

Fenk R, Haas R, Kronenwett R (2004a) Molecular monitoring of minimal residual disease in patients with multiple myeloma. Hematology 9:17–33

Fenk R, Ak M, Kobbe G, Steidl U, Arnold C, Korthals M, Hunerliturkoglu A, Rohr UP, Kliszewski S, Bernhardt A, Haas R, Kronenwett R (2004b) Levels of minimal residual disease detected by quantitative molecular monitoring herald relapse in patients with multiple myeloma. Haematologica 89:557–566

Fenk R, Schneider P, Kropff M, Huenerlituerkoglu AN, Steidl U, Aul C, Hildebrandt B, Haas R, Heyll A, Kobbe G (2005a) High-dose idarubicin, cyclophosphamide and melphalan as conditioning for autologous stem cell transplantation increases treatment-related mortality in patients with multiple myeloma: results of a randomised study. Br J Haematol 130:588–594

Fenk R, Graef T, Bruns I, Ruf L, Fabian Z, Steidl U, Huenerlituerkoglu AN, Haas R, Kobbe G (2005b) Comparison of interferon versus thalidomide versus RIC allotransplant for maintenance/consolidation therapy after autologous stem cell transplantation in patients with multiple myeloma: a single center experience. Blood 106(11):1168

Fenk R, Hieronimus N, Steidl U, Bruns I, Graef T, Zohren F, Ruf L, Haas R, Kobbe G (2006) Sustained G-CSF plasma levels following administration of pegfilgrastim fasten neutrophil reconstitution after high-dose chemotherapy and autologous blood stem cell transplantation in patients with multiple myeloma. Exp Hematol 34:1296–1302

Fermand JP, Ravaud P, Chevret S, Divine M, Leblond V, Belanger C, Macro M, Pertuiset E, Dreyfus F, Mariette X, Boccacio C, Brouet JC (1998) High-dose therapy and autologous peripheral blood stem cell transplantation in multiple myeloma: up-front or rescue treatment? Results of a multicenter sequential randomized clinical trial. Blood 92:3131–3136

Fermand JP, Katsahian S, Divine M, Leblond V, Dreyfus F, Macro M, Arnulf B, Royer B, Mariette X, Pertuiset E, Belanger C, Janvier M, Chevret S, Brouet JC, Ravaud P (2005) High-dose therapy and autologous blood stem-cell transplantation compared with conventional treatment in myeloma patients aged 55 to 65 years: long-term results of a randomized control trial from the Group Myelome-Autogreffe. J Clin Oncol 23:9227–9233

Galimberti S, Morabito F, Guerrini F, Palumbo GA, Azzara A, Martino M, Benedetti E, Di Raimondo F, Petrini M (2003) Peripheral blood stem cell contamination evaluated by a highly sensitive molecular method fails to predict outcome of autotransplanted multiple myeloma patients. Br J Haematol 120:405–412

Glasmacher A, Hahn C, Hoffmann F, Naumann R, Goldschmidt H, Lilienfeld-Toal M, Orlopp K, Schmidt-Wolf I, Gorschluter M (2006) A systematic review of phase-II trials of thalidomide monotherapy in patients with relapsed or refractory multiple myeloma. Br J Haematol 132: 584–593

Goldschmidt H, Hegenbart U, Haas R, Hunstein W (1996) Mobilization of peripheral blood progenitor cells with high-dose cyclophosphamide (4 or 7 g/m^2) and granulocyte colony-stimulating factor in patients with multiple myeloma. Bone Marrow Transplant 17:691–697

Goldschmidt H, Hegenbart U, Wallmeier M, Hohaus S, Haas R (1997) Factors influencing collection of peripheral blood progenitor cells following high-dose cyclophosphamide and granulocyte colony-stimulating factor in patients with multiple myeloma. Br J Haematol 98:736–744

Goldschmidt H, Hegenbart U, Wallmeier M, Hohaus S, Engenhart R, Wannenmacher M, Haas R (1998) Peripheral blood progenitor cell transplantation in multiple myeloma following high-dose melphalan-based therapy. Recent Results Cancer Res 144:27–35

Haas R, Hohaus S, Egerer G, Ehrhardt R, Witt B, Hunstein W (1992) Recombinant human granulocyte-macrophage colony-stimulating factor (rhGM-CSF) subsequent to chemotherapy improves collection of blood stem cells for autografting in patients not eligible for bone marrow harvest. Bone Marrow Transplant 9:459–465

Haas R, Gericke G, Witt B, Cayeux S, Hunstein W (1993) Increased serum levels of granulocyte colony-stimulating factor after autologous bone marrow or blood stem cell transplantation. Exp Hematol 21:109–113

Haas R, Moos M, Karcher A, Mohle R, Witt B, Goldschmidt H, Fruhauf S, Flentje M, Wannenmacher M, Hunstein W (1994a) Sequential high-dose therapy with peripheral-blood progenitor-cell support in low-grade non-Hodgkin's lymphoma. J Clin Oncol 12:1685–1692

Haas R, Mohle R, Fruhauf S, Goldschmidt H, Witt B, Flentje M, Wannenmacher M, Hunstein W (1994b) Patient characteristics associated with successful mobilizing and autografting of peripheral blood progenitor cells in malignant lymphoma. Blood 83:3787–3794

Haas R, Mohle R, Pforsich M, Fruehauf S, Witt B, Goldschmidt H, Hunstein W (1995) Blood-derived autografts collected during granulocyte colony-stimulating factor-enhanced recovery are enriched with early Thy-1$^+$ hematopoietic progenitor cells. Blood 85:1936–1943

Haas R, Schmid H, Hahn U, Hohaus S, Goldschmidt H, Murea S, Kaufmann M, Wannenmacher M, Wallwiener D, Bastert G, Hunstein W (1997) Tandem high-dose therapy with ifosfamide, epirubicin, carboplatin and peripheral blood stem cell support is an effective adjuvant treatment for high-risk primary breast cancer. Eur J Cancer 33:372–378

Hamamura K, Matsuda H, Takeuchi Y, Habu S, Yagita H, Okumura K (1996) A critical role of VLA-4 in erythropoiesis in vivo. Blood 87:2513–2517

Harousseau JL, Attal M, Leleu X, Troncy J, Pegourie B, Stoppa AM, Hulin C, Benboubker L, Fuzibet JG, Renaud M, Moreau P, Avet-Loiseau H (2006) Bortezomib plus dexamethasone as induction treatment prior to autologous stem cell transplantation in patients with newly diagnosed multiple myeloma: results of an IFM phase II study. Haematologica 91:1498–1505

Heyll A, Sohngen D, Kobbe G, Schneider P, Bauser U, Thiele KP, Wehmeier A, Sudhoff T, Quenzel EM, Rieth C, Wernet P, Fischer J, Frick M, Aul C (1997) Idarubicin, melphalan and cyclophosphamide: an intensified high-dose regimen for the treatment of myeloma patients. Leukemia 11(Suppl 5): S32–S34

Hohaus S, Goldschmidt H, Ehrhardt R, Haas R (1993) Successful autografting following myeloablative conditioning therapy with blood stem cells mobilized by chemotherapy plus rhG-CSF. Exp Hematol 21:508–514

Hohaus S, Martin H, Wassmann B, Egerer G, Haus U, Farber L, Burger KJ, Goldschmidt H, Hoelzer D, Haas R (1998) Recombinant human granulocyte and granulocyte-macrophage colony-stimulating factor (G-CSF and GM-CSF) administered following cytotoxic chemotherapy have a similar ability to mobilize peripheral blood stem cells. Bone Marrow Transplant 22:625–630

Holmes FA, O'Shaughnessy JA, Vukelja S, Jones SE, Shogan J, Savin M, Glaspy J, Moore M, Meza L, Wiznitzer I, Neumann TA, Hill LR, Liang BC (2002) Blinded, randomized, multicenter study to evaluate single administration pegfilgrastim once per cycle versus daily filgrastim as an adjunct to chemotherapy in patients with high-risk stage II or stage III/IV breast cancer. J Clin Oncol 20:727–731

Hughes PE, Pfaff M (1998) Integrin affinity modulation. Trends Cell Biol 8:359–364

Jagannath S, Richardson PG, Sonneveld P, Schuster MW, Irwin D, Stadtmauer EA, Facon T, Harousseau JL, Cowan JM, Anderson KC (2007) Bortezomib appears to overcome the poor prognosis conferred by chromosome 13 deletion in phase 2 and 3 trials. Leukemia 21:151–157

Jagasia MH, Greer JP, Morgan DS, Mineishi S, Kassim AA, Ruffner KL, Chen H, Schuening FG (2005) Pegfilgrastim after high-dose chemotherapy and autologous peripheral blood stem cell transplant: phase II study. Bone Marrow Transplant 35:1165–1169

Johnson RJ, Owen RG, Smith GM, Child JA, Galvin M, Newton LJ, Rawstron A, Major K, Woodhead V, Robinson F, Jack A, Morgan GJ (1996) Peripheral blood stem cell transplantation in myeloma using CD34 selected cells. Bone Marrow Transplant 17:723–727

Johnston E, Crawford J, Blackwell S, Bjurstrom T, Lockbaum P, Roskos L, Yang BB, Gardner S, Miller-Messana MA, Shoemaker D, Garst J, Schwab G (2000) Randomized, dose-escalation study of SD/01 compared with daily filgrastim in patients receiving chemotherapy. J Clin Oncol 18:2522–2528

Ketterer N, Salles G, Raba M, Espinouse D, Sonet A, Tremisi P, Dumontet C, Moullet I, Eljaafari-Corbin A, Neidhardt-Berard EM, Bouafia F, Coiffier B (1998) High CD34(+) cell counts decrease hematologic toxicity of autologous peripheral blood progenitor cell transplantation. Blood 91:3148–3155

Khaldoyanidi S, Denzel A, Zoller M (1996) Requirement for CD44 in proliferation and homing of hematopoietic precursor cells. J Leukoc Biol 60:579–592

Khaldoyanidi S, Schnabel D, Fohr N, Zoller M (1997) Functional activity of CD44 isoforms in haemopoiesis of the rat. Br J Haematol 96:31–45

Kiel K, Cremer FW, Ehrbrecht E, Wallmeier M, Hegenbart U, Goldschmidt H, Moos M (1998) First and second apheresis in patients with multiple myeloma: no differences in tumor load and hematopoietic stem cell yield. Bone Marrow Transplant 21:1109–1115

Kinashi T, Springer TA (1994) Adhesion molecules in hematopoietic cells. Blood Cells 20:25–44

Kobbe G, Hieronimus N, Graef T, Bruns I, Cibere A, Zohren F, Steidl U, Germing U, Haas R, Fenk R (2006) Combined use of palifermin and pegfilgrastim significantly reduces toxicity of high-dose therapy and autologous blood stem cell transplantation in patients with multiple myeloma. Session type. Blood 108(11):5260

Korbling M, Przepiorka D, Huh YO, Engel H, van Besien K, Giralt S, Andersson B, Kleine HD,

Seong D, Deisseroth AB (1995) Allogeneic blood stem cell transplantation for refractory leukemia and lymphoma: potential advantage of blood over marrow allografts. Blood 85:1659–1665

Koreth J, Cutler CS, Djulbegovic B, Behl R, Schlossman RL, Munshi NC, Richardson PG, Anderson KC, Soiffer RJ, Alyea EP III (2007) High-dose therapy with single autologous transplantation versus chemotherapy for newly diagnosed multiple myeloma: a systematic review and meta-analysis of randomized controlled trials. Biol Blood Marrow Transplant 13:183–196

Korthals M, Safaian N, Kronenwett R, Maihofer D, Schott M, Papewalis C, Diaz BE, Winter M, Czibere A, Haas R, Kobbe G, Fenk R (2007) Monocyte derived dendritic cells generated by IFN-alpha acquire mature dendritic and natural killer cell properties as shown by gene expression analysis. J Transl Med 5:46

Kotto-Kome AC, Fox SE, Lu W, Yang BB, Christensen RD, Calhoun DA (2004) Evidence that the granulocyte colony-stimulating factor (G-CSF) receptor plays a role in the pharmacokinetics of G-CSF and PegG-CSF using a G-CSF-R KO model. Pharmacol Res 50:55–58

Kumar SK, Rajkumar SV, Dispenzieri A, Lacy MQ, Hayman SR, Buadi FK, Zeldenrust SR, Dingli D, Russell SJ, Lust JA, Greipp PR, Kyle RA, Gertz MA (2008) Improved survival in multiple myeloma and the impact of novel therapies. Blood 111:2516–2520

Kumar A, Kharfan-Dabaja MA, Glasmacher A, Djulbegovic B (2009) Tandem versus single autologous hematopoietic cell transplantation for the treatment of multiple myeloma: a systematic review and meta-analysis. J Natl Cancer Inst 101:100–106

Ladetto M, Omede P, Sametti S, Donovan JW, Astolfi M, Drandi D, Volpato F, Giaccone L, Giaretta F, Palumbo A, Bruno B, Pileri A, Gribben JG, Boccadoro M (2002) Real-time polymerase chain reaction in multiple myeloma: quantitative analysis of tumor contamination of stem cell harvests. Exp Hematol 30:529–536

Lahuerta JJ, Mateos MV, Martinez-Lopez J, Rosinol L, Sureda A, de la Rubia J, Garcia-Larana J, Martinez-Martinez R, Hernandez-Garcia MT, Carrera D, Besalduch J, de Arriba F, Ribera JM, Escoda L, Hernandez-Ruiz B, Garcia-Frade J, Rivas-Gonzalez C, Alegre A, Blade J, San Miguel JF (2008) Influence of pre- and post-transplantation responses on outcome of patients with multiple myeloma: sequential improvement of response and achievement of complete response are associated with longer survival. J Clin Oncol 26:5775–5782

Laura R, Cibeira MT, Uriburu C, Yantorno S, Salamero O, Blade J, Montserrat E (2006) Bortezomib: an effective agent in extramedullary disease in multiple myeloma. Eur J Haematol 76:405–408

Leavesley DI, Oliver JM, Swart BW, Berndt MC, Haylock DN, Simmons PJ (1994) Signals from platelet/endothelial cell adhesion molecule enhance the adhesive activity of the very late antigen-4 integrin of human $CD34^+$ hemopoietic progenitor cells. J Immunol 153:4673–4683

Lee KE, Mun YC, Nam SH, Kwon JM, Lee SM, Lee MA, Yoo ES, Ahn JY, Kim JH, Seong CM (2005) A prospective randomized study on the mobilization of $CD34^+$ cells comparing continuous intravenous vs subcutaneous administration of rhG-CSF in normal donors. Bone Marrow Transplant 36:1027–1031

Lemoli RM, Cavo M, Fortuna A (1996) Concomitant mobilization of plasma cells and hematopoietic progenitors into peripheral blood of patients with multiple myeloma. J Hematother 5:339–349

Lemoli RM, Martinelli G, Olivieri A, Motta MR, Rizzi S, Terragna C, Leopardi G, Benni M, Ronconi S, Cantori I, Rondelli D, Mangianti S, Leoni P, Montanari M, Cavo M, Tura S (1999) Selection and transplantation of autologous $CD34^+$ B-lineage negative cells in advanced-phase multiple myeloma patients: a pilot study. Br J Haematol 107:419–428

Lemoli RM, Martinelli G, Zamagni E, Motta MR, Rizzi S, Terragna C, Rondelli R, Ronconi S, Curti A, Bonifazi F, Tura S, Cavo M (2000) Engraftment, clinical, and molecular follow-up of patients with multiple myeloma who were reinfused with highly purified $CD34^+$ cells to support single or tandem high-dose chemotherapy. Blood 95:2234–2239

Lichterfeld M, Martin S, Burkly L, Haas R, Kronenwett R (2000) Mobilization of $CD34^+$ haematopoietic stem cells is associated with a functional inactivation of the integrin very late antigen 4. Br J Haematol 110:71–81

Liesveld JL, Winslow JM, Frediani KE, Ryan DH, Abboud CN (1993) Expression of integrins and examination of their adhesive function in

10

normal and leukemic hematopoietic cells. Blood 81:112–121
Lilienfeld-Toal M, Hahn-Ast C, Bertolini F, Bila J, Boulin M, Oakervee H, Cibeira T, Cook G, Fenk R, Waage A, Glasmacher A (2007) Longer duration of thalidomide monotherapy results in improved outcome in relapsed/refractory multiple myeloma. Blood [abstract] 110:2725
Lincz LF, Crooks RL, Way SL, Granter N, Spencer A (2001) Tumour kinetics in multiple myeloma before, during, and after treatment. Leuk Lymphoma 40:373–384
Lokhorst HM, Schmidt-Wolf I, Sonneveld P, Van Der HB, Martin H, Barge R, Bertsch U, Schlenzka J, Bos GM, Croockewit S, Zweegman S, Breitkreutz I, Joosten P, Scheid C, van Marwijk-Kooy M, Salwender HJ, van Oers MH, Schaafsma R, Naumann R, Sinnige H, Blau I, Delforge M, de Weerdt O, Wijermans P, Wittebol S, Duersen U, Vellenga E, Goldschmidt H (2008) Thalidomide in induction treatment increases the very good partial response rate before and after high-dose therapy in previously untreated multiple myeloma. Haematologica 93(1):124–127
Lopez-Perez R, Garcia-Sanz R, Gonzalez D, Balanzategui A, Chillon MC, Alaejos I, Mateos MV, Caballero MD, Mateo G, Nieto MJ, Gonzalez M, San Miguel JF (2000) The detection of contaminating clonal cells in apheresis products is related to response and outcome in multiple myeloma undergoing autologous peripheral blood stem cell transplantation. Leukemia 14:1493–1499
Lopez-Perez R, Garcia-Sanz R, Gonzalez D, Balanzategui A, Chillon MC, Alaejos I, Mateos MV, Caballero MD, Corral M, Orfao A, Gonzalez M, San Miguel JF (2001) Gene scanning of VDJH-amplified segments is a clinically relevant technique to detect contaminating tumor cells in the apheresis products of multiple myeloma patients undergoing autologous peripheral blood stem cell transplantation. Bone Marrow Transplant 28:665–672
Maas RE (2008) A comparison of the effect of prednisone and a placebo in the treatment of multiple myeloma. Cancer Chemother Rep 16:257–259
Macintyre W (1850) Case of mollities and fragilitas ossium accompanied with urine strongly charged with animal matter. Med Chir Trans Lond 33:211–232
Macro M, Divine M, Jaccard A, Bouscary D, Leblond V, Janvier M, Genet P, Castaigne S, Royer B, Allard C, Chevret S, Fermand J-P (2006) Dexamethasone + thalidomide compared to VAD as a pre-transplant treatment in newly diagnosed multiple myeloma: a randomized trial. Blood [abstract] 108:57
Martinelli G, Terragna C, Zamagni E, Ronconi S, Tosi P, Lemoli RM, Bandini G, Motta MR, Testoni N, Amabile M, Ottaviani E, Vianelli N, De Vivo A, Gozzetti A, Tura S, Cavo M (2000) Molecular remission after allogeneic or autologous transplantation of hematopoietic stem cells for multiple myeloma. J Clin Oncol 18:2273–2281
Martinelli G, Agazzi A, Laszlo D, Santoro P, Mancuso P, Pruneri GC, Greco P, Bertolini F (2003) Idarubicin containing regimen in multiple myeloma: preliminary results of a pilot study using a modified "TANDEM" transplant program. Leuk Lymphoma 44:299–302
Martin-Murea S, Voso MT, Hohaus S, Pforsich M, Fruehauf S, Goldschmidt H, Hegenbart U, Haas R (1998) The dose of granulocyte colony-stimulating factor administered following cytotoxic chemotherapy is not related to the rebound level of circulating $CD34^+$ haemopoietic progenitor cells during marrow recovery. Br J Haematol 101:582–585
McElwain T, Powles RL (1983) High-dose intravenous melphalan for plasma cell leukemia and myeloma. Lancet 2:822–824
Mitterer M, Lanthaler AJ, Schnabel B, Svaldi M, Oduncu F, Coser P, Emmerich B, Huemer H, Straka C (2001) Peripheral blood monoclonal B-cells predict the event free survival in multiple myeloma. Leuk Lymphoma 41:387–395
Miyake K, Medina KL, Hayashi S, Ono S, Hamaoka T, Kincade PW (1990) Monoclonal antibodies to Pgp-1/CD44 block lympho-hemopoiesis in long-term bone marrow cultures. J Exp Med 171:477–488
Miyake K, Weissman IL, Greenberger JS, Kincade PW (1991) Evidence for a role of the integrin VLA-4 in lympho-hemopoiesis. J Exp Med 173:599–607
Mohle R, Pforsich M, Fruehauf S, Witt B, Kramer A, Haas R (1994) Filgrastim post-chemotherapy mobilizes more $CD34^+$ cells with a different antigenic profile compared with use during steady-state hematopoiesis. Bone Marrow Transplant 14:827–832
Mohle R, Murea S, Kirsch M, Haas R (1995) Differential expression of L-selectin, VLA-4, and LFA-1 on $CD34^+$ progenitor cells from bone

marrow and peripheral blood during G-CSF-enhanced recovery. Exp Hematol 23:1535–1542

Mohle R, Moore MA, Nachman RL, Rafii S (1997) Transendothelial migration of CD34+ and mature hematopoietic cells: an in vitro study using a human bone marrow endothelial cell line. Blood 89:72–80

Mohle R, Bautz F, Rafii S, Moore MA, Brugger W, Kanz L (1998) The chemokine receptor CXCR-4 is expressed on CD34+ hematopoietic progenitors and leukemic cells and mediates transendothelial migration induced by stromal cell-derived factor-1. Blood 91:4523–4530

Moreau P, Facon T, Attal M, Hulin C, Michallet M, Maloisel F, Sotto JJ, Guilhot F, Marit G, Doyen C, Jaubert J, Fuzibet JG, Francois S, Benboubker L, Monconduit M, Voillat L, Macro M, Berthou C, Dorvaux V, Pignon B, Rio B, Matthes T, Casassus P, Caillot D, Najman N, Grosbois B, Bataille R, Harousseau JL (2002) Comparison of 200 mg/m(2) melphalan and 8 Gy total body irradiation plus 140 mg/m(2) melphalan as conditioning regimens for peripheral blood stem cell transplantation in patients with newly diagnosed multiple myeloma: final analysis of the Intergroupe Francophone du Myelome 9502 randomized trial. Blood 99:731–735

Moretta A, Bottino C, Vitale M, Pende D, Cantoni C, Mingari MC, Biassoni R, Moretta L (2001) Activating receptors and coreceptors involved in human natural killer cell-mediated cytolysis. Annu Rev Immunol 19:197–223

Myeloma Trialists' Collaborative Group (1998) Combination chemotherapy versus melphalan plus prednisone as treatment for multiple myeloma: an overview of 6,633 patients from 27 randomized trials. J Clin Oncol 16:3832–3842

Myeloma Trialists' Collaborative Group (2001) Interferon as therapy for multiple myeloma: an individual patient data overview of 24 randomized trials and 4012 patients. Br J Haematol 113:1020–1034

Nestle FO, Farkas A, Conrad C (2005) Dendritic-cell-based therapeutic vaccination against cancer. Curr Opin Immunol 17:163–169

Ocio EM, Mateos MV, Maiso P, Pandiella A, San-Miguel JF (2008) New drugs in multiple myeloma: mechanisms of action and phase I/II clinical findings. Lancet Oncol 9:1157–1165

Olivieri A, Scortechini I, Capelli D, Montanari M, Lucesole M, Gini G, Troiani M, Offidani M, Poloni A, Masia MC, Raggetti GM, Leoni P (2004) Combined administration of alpha-erythropoietin and filgrastim can improve the outcome and cost balance of autologous stem cell transplantation in patients with lymphoproliferative disorders. Bone Marrow Transplant 34:693–702

Oostendorp RA, Spitzer E, Brandl M, Eaves CJ, Dormer P (1998) Evidence for differences in the mechanisms by which antibodies against CD44 promote adhesion of erythroid and granulopoietic progenitors to marrow stromal cells. Br J Haematol 101:436–445

Palumbo A, Bringhen S, Petrucci MT, Musto P, Rossini F, Nunzi M, Lauta VM, Bergonzi C, Barbui A, Caravita T, Capaldi A, Pregno P, Guglielmelli T, Grasso M, Callea V, Bertola A, Cavallo F, Falco P, Rus C, Massaia M, Mandelli F, Carella AM, Pogliani E, Liberati AM, Dammacco F, Ciccone G, Boccadoro M (2004) Intermediate-dose melphalan improves survival of myeloma patients aged 50 to 70: results of a randomized controlled trial. Blood 104:3052–3057

Piccirillo N, Sica S, Laurenti L, Chiusolo P, La Barbera EO, Sora F, Leone G (1999) Optimal timing of G-CSF administration after CD34+ immunoselected peripheral blood progenitor cell transplantation. Bone Marrow Transplant 23:1245–1250

Pineda-Roman M, Bolejack V, Arzoumanian V, Anaissie E, van Rhee F, Zangari M, Walker R, Hollmig K, Shaughnessy JD Jr, Epstein J, Krishna S, Crowley J, Barlogie B (2007) Complete response in myeloma extends survival without, but not with history of prior monoclonal gammopathy of undetermined significance or smouldering disease. Br J Haematol 136:393–399

Prosper F, Stroncek D, McCarthy JB, Verfaillie CM (1998) Mobilization and homing of peripheral blood progenitors is related to reversible downregulation of alpha4 beta1 integrin expression and function. J Clin Invest 101:2456–2467

Rajkumar SV, Blood E, Vesole D, Fonseca R, Greipp PR (2006) Phase III clinical trial of thalidomide plus dexamethasone compared with dexamethasone alone in newly diagnosed multiple myeloma: a clinical trial coordinated by the Eastern Cooperative Oncology Group. J Clin Oncol 24:431–436

Reiffers J, Faberes C, Boiron JM, Marit G, Foures C, Ferrer AM, Cony-Makhoul P, Puntous M, Bernard P, Vezon G (1994) Peripheral blood progenitor cell transplantation in 118 patients with hematological malignancies: analysis of factors affecting the rate of engraftment. J Hematother 3:185–191

Richardson PG, Sonneveld P, Schuster MW, Irwin D, Stadtmauer EA, Facon T, Harousseau JL, Ben Yehuda D, Lonial S, Goldschmidt H, Reece D, San Miguel JF, Blade J, Boccadoro M, Cavenagh J, Dalton WS, Boral AL, Esseltine DL, Porter JB, Schenkein D, Anderson KC (2005) Bortezomib or high-dose dexamethasone for relapsed multiple myeloma. N Engl J Med 352: 2487–2498

Roberts AW, DeLuca E, Begley CG, Basser R, Grigg AP, Metcalf D (1995) Broad inter-individual variations in circulating progenitor cell numbers induced by granulocyte colony-stimulating factor therapy. Stem Cells 13:512–516

Rosel M, Khaldoyanidi S, Zawadzki V, Zoller M (1999) Involvement of CD44 variant isoform v10 in progenitor cell adhesion and maturation. Exp Hematol 27:698–711

Roussel M, Huynh A, Moreau P, Harousseau JL, Hulin C, Caillot D, Fruchart C, Marit G, Pegourie B, Attal M (2008) Bortezomib (BOR) and high dose melphalan (HDM) as conditioning regimen before autologous stem cell transplantation (ASCT) for de novo multiple myeloma (MM): final results of the IFM phase II study VEL/MEL. ASH Annual Meeting Abstracts 112:160

Schiller G, Vescio R, Freytes C, Spitzer G, Sahebi F, Lee M, Wu CH, Cao J, Lee JC, Hong CH (1995) Transplantation of $CD34^+$ peripheral blood progenitor cells after high-dose chemotherapy for patients with advanced multiple myeloma. Blood 86:390–397

Schmitz N, Dreger P, Suttorp M, Rohwedder EB, Haferlach T, Loffler H, Hunter A, Russell NH (1995) Primary transplantation of allogeneic peripheral blood progenitor cells mobilized by filgrastim (granulocyte colony-stimulating factor). Blood 85:1666–1672

Schofield R (1983) The stem cell system. Biomed Pharmacother 37(8):375–380

Shaughnessy JD Jr., Qu P, Edmondson R, Herman D, Zhou Y, Tian E, van Rhee F, Pineda-Roman M, Alsayed Y, Anaissie E, Qiang YW, Epstein J, Yaccoby S, Williams D, Zhan F, Stephens O, Hoering A, Crowley J, Barlogie B (2008) Changes in the expression of proteasome genes in tumor cells following short-term proteasome inhibitor therapy predicts survival in multiple myeloma treated with bortezomib-containing multi-agent chemotherapy. ASH Annual Meeting Abstracts 112:733

Simmons PJ, Masinovsky B, Longenecker BM, Berenson R, Torok-Storb B, Gallatin WM (1992) Vascular cell adhesion molecule-1 expressed by bone marrow stromal cells mediates the binding of hematopoietic progenitor cells. Blood 80:388–395

Socinski MA, Cannistra SA, Elias A, Antman KH, Schnipper L, Griffin JD (1988) Granulocyte-macrophage colony stimulating factor expands the circulating haemopoietic progenitor cell compartment in man. Lancet 1:1194–1198

Soligo D, Schiro R, Luksch R, Manara G, Quirici N, Parravicini C, Lambertenghi DG (1990) Expression of integrins in human bone marrow. Br J Haematol 76:323–332

Solly S (1844) Remarks on the pathology of mollities ossium with cases. Med Chir Trans Lond 27:435–461

Spencer A, Prince M, Roberts AW, Bradstok K, Prosser I (2006) First analysis of the Australian leukemia and lymphoma group trial of thalidomide and alternate day prednisolone following autologous stem cell transplantation for patients with multiple myeloma. Blood [abstract] 108:58

Staber PB, Holub R, Linkesch W, Schmidt H, Neumeister P (2005) Fixed-dose single administration of pegfilgrastim vs daily filgrastim in patients with haematological malignancies undergoing autologous peripheral blood stem cell transplantation. Bone Marrow Transplant 35:889–893

Steidl U, Fenk R, Bruns I, Neumann F, Kondakci M, Hoyer B, Graf T, Rohr UP, Bork S, Kronenwett R, Haas R, Kobbe G (2005) Successful transplantation of peripheral blood stem cells mobilized by chemotherapy and a single dose of pegylated G-CSF in patients with multiple myeloma. Bone Marrow Transplant 35:33–36

Stewart AK, Vescio R, Schiller G, Ballester O, Noga S, Rugo H, Freytes C, Stadtmauer E, Tarantolo S, Sahebi F, Stiff P, Meharchard J, Schlossman R, Brown R, Tully H, Benyunes M, Jacobs C, Berenson R, White M, DiPersio J, Anderson KC, Berenson J (2001) Purging of autologous peripheral-blood stem cells using CD34 selection does not improve overall or progression-free survival after high-dose chemotherapy for multiple myeloma: results of a multicenter randomized controlled trial. J Clin Oncol 19:3771–3779

Szczepanski T, Orfao A, van der Velden VH, San Miguel JF, van Dongen JJ (2001) Minimal residual disease in leukaemia patients. Lancet Oncol 2:409–417

Taieb J, Chaput N, Menard C, Apetoh L, Ullrich E, Bonmort M, Pequignot M, Casares N, Terme M, Flament C, Opolon P, Lecluse Y, Metivier D, Tomasello E, Vivier E, Ghiringhelli F, Martin F, Klatzmann D, Poynard T, Tursz T, Raposo G, Yagita H, Ryffel B, Kroemer G, Zitvogel L (2006) A novel dendritic cell subset involved in tumor immunosurveillance 1. Nat Med 12:214–219

Tarella C, Benedetti G, Caracciolo D, Castellino C, Cherasco C, Bondesan P, Omede P, Ruggieri D, Gianni AM, Pileri A (1995) Both early and committed haemopoietic progenitors are more frequent in peripheral blood than in bone marrow during mobilization induced by high-dose chemotherapy + G-CSF. Br J Haematol 91: 535–543

Teixido J, Hemler ME, Greenberger JS, Anklesaria P (1992) Role of beta 1 and beta 2 integrins in the adhesion of human CD34hi stem cells to bone marrow stroma. J Clin Invest 90:358–367

Thunberg U, Banghagen M, Bengtsson M, Christensen LD, Geisler CH, Gimsing P, Lenhoff S, Mortensen BT, Olofsson T, Simonsson B, Andersen NS, Sundstrom C, Swedin A, Sallstrom JF, Thuresson B, Westin J, Carlson K (1999) Linear reduction of clonal cells in stem cell enriched grafts in transplanted multiple myeloma. Br J Haematol 104:546–552

To LB, Haylock DN, Dowse T, Simmons PJ, Trimboli S, Ashman LK, Juttner CA (1994) A comparative study of the phenotype and proliferative capacity of peripheral blood (PB) $CD34^+$ cells mobilized by four different protocols and those of steady-phase PB and bone marrow $CD34^+$ cells. Blood 84:2930–2939

Tricot G, Gazitt Y, Leemhuis T, Jagannath S, Desikan KR, Siegel D, Fassas A, Tindle S, Nelson J, Juttner C, Tsukamoto A, Hallagan J, Atkinson K, Reading C, Hoffman R, Barlogie B (1998) Collection, tumor contamination, and engraftment kinetics of highly purified hematopoietic progenitor cells to support high dose therapy in multiple myeloma. Blood 91:4489–4495

Valteau-Couanet D, Faucher C, Auperin A, Michon J, Milpied N, Boiron JM, Bourhis JH, Gisselbrecht C, Vernant JP, Pinna A, Bendahmane B, Delabarre F, Benhamou E (2005) Cost effectiveness of day 5 G-CSF (Lenograstim) administration after PBSC transplantation: results of a SFGM-TC randomised trial. Bone Marrow Transplant 36:547–552

van Rhee F (2007) Idiotype vaccination strategies in myeloma: how to overcome a dysfunctional immune system. Clin Cancer Res 13:1353–1355

van Rhee F, Bolejack V, Hollmig K, Pineda-Roman M, Anaissie E, Epstein J, Shaughnessy JD Jr, Zangari M, Tricot G, Mohiuddin A, Alsayed Y, Woods G, Crowley J, Barlogie B (2007) High serum-free light chain levels and their rapid reduction in response to therapy define an aggressive multiple myeloma subtype with poor prognosis. Blood 110(3):827–832

Vanstraelen G, Frere P, Ngirabacu MC, Willems E, Fillet G, Beguin Y (2006) Pegfilgrastim compared with filgrastim after autologous hematopoietic peripheral blood stem cell transplantation. Exp Hematol 34:382–388

Verfaillie CM, McCarthy JB, McGlave PB (1991) Differentiation of primitive human multipotent hematopoietic progenitors into single lineage clonogenic progenitors is accompanied by alterations in their interaction with fibronectin. J Exp Med 174:693–703

Verfaillie C, Hurley R, Bhatia R, McCarthy JB (1994) Role of bone marrow matrix in normal and abnormal hematopoiesis. Crit Rev Oncol Hematol 16:201–224

Vescio RA, Han EJ, Schiller GJ, Lee JC, Wu CH, Cao J, Shin J, Kim A, Lichtenstein AK, Berenson JR (1996) Quantitative comparison of multiple myeloma tumor contamination in bone marrow harvest and leukapheresis autografts. Bone Marrow Transplant 18:103–110

Vescio R, Schiller G, Stewart AK, Ballester O, Noga S, Rugo H, Freytes C, Stadtmauer E, Tarantolo S, Sahebi F, Stiff P, Meharchard J, Schlossman R, Brown R, Tully H, Benyunes M, Jacobs C, Berenson R, DiPersio J, Anderson K, Berenson J (1999) Multicenter phase III trial to evaluate $CD34(^+)$ selected versus unselected autologous peripheral blood progenitor cell transplantation in multiple myeloma. Blood 93:1858–1868

Viardot A, Kronenwett R, Deichmann M, Haas R (1998) The human immunodeficiency virus (HIV)-type 1 coreceptor CXCR-4 (fusin) is preferentially expressed on the more immature $CD34^+$ hematopoietic stem cells. Ann Hematol 77:193–197

Voena C, Locatelli G, Castellino C, Omede P, Ladetto M, Zappone E, Milani R, Perfetti V, Boccadoro M, Pileri A, Lusso P, Villa C, Malnati M, Corradini P (2002) Qualitative and quantitative polymerase chain reaction detection of the residual myeloma cell contamination after positive selection of $CD34^+$ cells with small- and large-scale Miltenyi cell sorting system. Br J Haematol 117:642–645

Voermans C, Gerritsen WR, von dem Borne AE, van der Schoot CE (1999) Increased migration of cord blood-derived $CD34^+$ cells, as compared to bone marrow and mobilized peripheral blood $CD34^+$ cells across uncoated or fibronectin-coated filters. Exp Hematol 27:1806–1814

Weaver CH, Hazelton B, Birch R, Palmer P, Allen C, Schwartzberg L, West W (1995) An analysis of engraftment kinetics as a function of the CD34 content of peripheral blood progenitor cell collections in 692 patients after the administration of myeloablative chemotherapy. Blood 86:3961–3969

Weber DM, Chen C, Niesvizky R, Wang M, Belch A, Stadtmauer EA, Siegel D, Borrello I, Rajkumar SV, Chanan-Khan AA, Lonial S, Yu Z, Patin J, Olesnyckyj M, Zeldis JB, Knight RD (2007) Lenalidomide plus dexamethasone for relapsed multiple myeloma in North America. N Engl J Med 357:2133–2142

Whetton AD, Graham GJ (1999) Homing and mobilization in the stem cell niche. Trends Cell Biol 9:233–238

Winter JN, Lazarus HM, Rademakcr A, Villa M, Mangan C, Tallman M, Jahnke L, Gordon L, Newman S, Byrd K, Cooper BW, Horvath N, Crum E, Stadtmauer EA, Conklin E, Bauman A, Martin J, Goolsby C, Gerson SL, Bender J, O'Gorman M (1996) Phase I/II study of combined granulocyte colony-stimulating factor and granulocyte-macrophage colony-stimulating factor administration for the mobilization of hematopoietic progenitor cells. J Clin Oncol 14:277–286

Yamaguchi M, Ikebuchi K, Hirayama F, Sato N, Mogi Y, Ohkawara J, Yoshikawa Y, Sawada K, Koike T, Sekiguchi S (1998) Different adhesive characteristics and VLA-4 expression of CD34(+) progenitors in G0/G1 versus S + G2/M phases of the cell cycle. Blood 92:842–848

Yanai N, Sekine C, Yagita H, Obinata M (1994) Roles for integrin very late activation antigen-4 in stroma-dependent erythropoiesis. Blood 83:2844–2850

Zamboni WC (2003) Pharmacokinetics of pegfilgrastim. Pharmacotherapy 23:9S–14S

Zhou P, Zhang Y, Martinez C, Kalakonda N, Nimer SD, Comenzo RL (2003) Melphalan-mobilized blood stem cell components contain minimal clonotypic myeloma cell contamination. Blood 102:477–479

Therapy of Relapsed and Refractory Multiple Myeloma

11

Thomas Moehler and Hartmut Goldschmidt

Contents

Abstract Despite considerable improvements in first line treatment still the majority of patients experience relapse of multiple myeloma. Treatment decisions for relapse or refractory multiple myeloma should be based on a clinical decision path taking response and adverse events to previous therapy, myeloma specific complications and organ dysfunctions, overall clinical condition, age, cytogenetic information and prognostic factors into account. Bortezomib, thalidomide and lenalidomide have improved the therapeutic armentarium for patients with refractory or relapsed disease and are often used in combination with dexamethasone or chemotherapeutic agents. Combination therapies of novel agents in drug combination regimen are

T. Moehler (✉)
Department of Medicine V, University Hospital Heidelberg, Im Neuenheimer Feld 410, 69120 Heidelberg, Germany

Present Address:
i3 research, Wiesbaden, Germany
e-mail: thomas.moehler@i3global.com

T. Moehler and H. Goldschmidt (eds.), *Multiple Myeloma*,
Recent Results in Cancer Research 183, DOI: 10.1007/978-3-540-85772-3_11,

currently under investigation as well. For patients with a disease free survival of 12 month or longer after initial single or tandem high dose therapy and autologous stem cell transplantation (ASCT) repeat of high dose therapy with melphalan and ASCT should be considered in case of relapse. Radiotherapy and osteoplastic procedures can be used as adjunct to systemic therapy to treat local complications in particular vertebral pain caused by osteolytic bone disease. Cytogenetic tests, molecular techniques as gene expression profiling and other diagnostic will lead to a more individualized therapy. The integration of novel compounds into established regimen will be a major challenge for future clinical studies.

11.1 Introduction

Disease-free survival after first-line therapy of multiple myeloma has steadily increased in recent years. In addition, overall survival of myeloma patients has improved (Kumar et al. 2008).

After decades of stagnation, this development was possible by three different factors:

In addition to autologous blood stem cell transplantation which was introduced in myeloma treatment in the early 1990s, novel agents became available as bortezomib, thalidomide and lenalidomide. Novel agents not only improved the response rate and duration of elderly patients (above 65) but also improved treatment outcome of younger patients. These achievements are delineated in Chap. 11 on first-line therapy and maintenance. Along with the development of novel agents, the focus related to drug discovery for multiple myeloma has broadened from focusing on the myeloma cell to the relevance of the bone marrow microenvironment (Mitsiades et al. 2006).

More than 20 % have a chance of long-term remission over a period of 9 years after intensive first line treatment (Barlogie et al. 2008b).

Intensive treatment algorithms for first-line therapy that are associated with a significant percentage of patients in long-term remission use combination of hemo-therapeutic with novel agents for rapid remission induction followed by intensified therapy including autologous transplantation and subsequent post-remission or maintenance therapy.

Our review here intends to describe the approach to relapsed patients and tries to outline possible future avenues that might secure long-term remission for relapsed patients as well.

11.2 Diagnostic Workup of Patients at Relapse

Diagnostic procedures for myeloma patients are detailed in Chaps. 6 and 7. Diagnostic workup of patients with relapse principally does not differ from patients with first-line disease including radiological investigation, assessment of paraprotein in serum and urine. The relevance for serum-light chain test is described in Chap. 20. Due to advanced age, treatment, and disease-related complications, patients in relapse often present a reduced ECOG performance status and have more organ deficiencies such as compromised renal function. Relapse patients present more often with a lower ECOG status.

11.3 Conventional Treatment of Relapsed/Refractory Disease

A high-dose standard regimen for dexamethasone is 40 mg for 4 consecutive days on days 1, 9, 17 for a 28-day cycle achieves a response rate between 18% and 27%. Main problem with this regimen is the short 4–6 months duration of response (Richardson et al. 2005; Alexanian et al. 1986, 1992).

Due to short duration of response combined with a considerable set of adverse events as psychiatric disorders, diabetic metabolic events, and infections, dexamethasone single agent is not considered nowadays a standard treatment for relapsed disease. But dexamethasone is used in the short-term treatment of disease complications as cytopenias, renal complications.

Combination of high-dose dexamethasone regimen with chemotherapy has been found wide spread acceptance since the introduction of the VAD (vincristin, adriamycin, dexamethasone) regimen by Barlogie and colleagues in the early 1980s (Barlogie et al. 1984). A retrospective analysis indicated that the VAD regimen was more effective than high-dose dexamethasone alone in relapsed patients (65% vs. 21%) (Alexanian et al. 1986). The introduction of pegylated liposomal doxorubicin has added some advantage as it is administered via a peripheral vein, is less cardio toxic, and causes less alopecia (Hussein and Anderson 2004). Due to the neurotoxicity of vincristin these regimens are not first choice for treatment of relapsed multiple myeloma anymore.

A number of other chemotherapeutic combination regimens, the vast majority in combination with dexamethasone or prednisolone, have been used since then. In particular, the M2 regimen consisting of BCNU, melphalan, cyclophosmphamide, vincristine, and prednisone has been used since 1974 as regimen for relapsed myeloma (Lee et al. 1974).

The melphalan/prednisone (MP) regimen "Alexanian" has historically been used for those patient that achieved at least a 6-month remission with MP during first line. In recent years, bendamustine was found to have considerable activity in multiple myeloma. Poenisch et al. have even demonstrated in an open-label, randomized phase III study bendamustine to be superior to MP in the first-line setting with improved PFS, response rate in particular significantly higher CR rate of 35% compared to 13% with MP and time-to-treatment failure (TTF) (Ponisch et al. 2006). The activity of bendamustine was also shown for refractory/relapsed myeloma patients (Knop et al. 2005). The advantage of a bendamustine/prednisolone combination therapy is a short duration of treatment usually 2 days of intravenous infusion in combination with 5 days of oral corticosteroid treatment. Quality of life and ambulatory therapy is an important factor for relapsed and mostly frail patients.

The relevance of this historical development is largely based on the fact that nowadays previously established chemotherapeutic agents are now combined with novel agents to improve therapeutic efficacy (see below on combinations of novel agents with chemotherapeutic agents/corticosteroids) (Kropff et al. 2003). Use of chemotherapy without novel agents might be a treatment of choice for a minority of patients for third or subsequent lines, e.g., in case of resistance to novel agents or concomitant disease as severe neuropathy.

11.4 High-Dose Chemotherapy (HDCT) Supported by Autologous Stem Cell Transplantation

The rationale for high-dose chemotherapy (HDCT) followed by autologous stell cell transplantation (ASCT) in multiple myeloma was initially vague in particular because the proliferation rate of myeloma was known to be approximately 3% for the majority of patients. But the concept has finally evolved very strongly as described in Chap. 9. In vitro it could be shown that escalating doses of melphalan can overcome drug resistance in myeloma. Likely the effect of melphalan on tumor stroma and bone marrow has an important relevance for its therapeutic effect of melphalan and is probably a major reason for success of high-dose strategies for multiple myeloma (Podar et al. 2001; Basak et al. 2009).

High-dose therapy using melphalan and other conditioning regimen was initially developed in the setting of relapsed patients (Barlogie et al. 1987; Goldschmidt et al. 1997). Clinical studies have finally identified melphalan single agent conditioning regimen with 200 mg/m^2 as the regimen maximizing anti-myeloma effects with low transplant-related mortality (Goldschmidt et al. 2000) and Chap. 10 (Haas R. et al). Barlogie et al. could also demonstrate the efficacy of high-dose therapy in a complex chemotherapeutic regimen for the treatment of myeloma (Barlogie et al. 1999).

A number of clinical studies have addressed the question of timing of high-dose therapy in combination with autologous stem cell transplantation. Whereas Barlogie and colleagues did not identify significant differences comparing first-line high-dose therapy and high-dose therapy in relapse, Fermand et al. found a significant improvement for early high-dose therapy in their study (Barlogie et al. 2003; Fermand et al. 1998). Moreover, Fermand identified that time spent without therapy was longer in the "early" treatment group with 28 vs. 22 months. Longer time "on-therapy" results in an increased risk for organ complications and myelodysplastic syndrome. Myeloma cells acquire additional genetic alterations during disease duration and become increasingly drug resistance (De et al. 2006). As HDCT is currently considered an important element of a therapeutic strategy that might be able to cure a small but detectable number of patients, postponing HDCT would most likely endanger the "cure" concept (Barlogie et al. 2008a). These findings ultimately led to a firm integration of high-dose therapy in the first-line regimen for multiple myeloma. Despite considerable progress in the treatment of multiple myeloma using novel agents and combination regimen, it is still an accepted option to offer eligible patients HDCT at time of relapse if they have not received HDCT in first line. Whereas HDCT for first-line treatment is considered standard in the treatment of myeloma, only a few clinical studies have evaluated a second HDCT after relapse from first-line HDCT. Only retrospective nonrandomized studies are available addressing this important question. Olin et al. recently published a series of 41 patients that received a second HDCT in the relapse situation (Olin et al. 2009). They described an overall response rate in assessable patients of 55% and treatment-related mortality of 7%. Median progression-free survival (PFS) and overall survival (OS) were 8.5 months and 20.7 months, respectively. In a multivariate analysis of OS less than five, prior lines of therapy and a remission of more than 12 months after initial HDCT were predictive of OS after HDT. However, a third ABSCT for patients relapsing after tandem auto-transplantation did not contribute to long-term disease control (Lee et al. 2002).

In summary, second HDCT after failure of initial HDCT is feasible and can – if a selection of patients is performed – result in a clinically meaningful response rate and progression-free survival. As HDCT is not a strategy excluding novel therapies but rather part of a more complex approach including induction and possibly maintenance therapy, HDCT relapse treatment strategies containing novel agents and HDCT should be considered as an alternative to non-HDCT treatments for HDCT eligible patients. Unfortunately, there is no study group that has embarked on resolving the important question of second HDCT after initial HDCT; therefore, judgment will rely on retrospective studies.

11.5 Allogeneic Stem Cell Transplantation

Different strategies have been developed in the recent years to apply allogeneic blood stem cell transplantation for relapsed multiple myeloma (see also Chap. 10). The application of high-intensity conditioning regimen evaluated in clinical studies until late 1990 has more or less been stopped due to high transplant-related mortality between 25% and 50% (Bensinger 2009). Different regimens have been developed as alternative utilizing the (RIC) intensity conditioning approach developed by Storb et al. for multiple myeloma (Storb et al. 1999). Most clinical studies on allogeneic stem cell transplantation have so far been performed in relapsed multiple myeloma.

Similar to autologous stem cell transplantation in combination with HDCT, allogeneic stem cell transplantation (allo SCT) has initially been studied almost exclusively in relapsed/refractory patients.

Studies comparing conventional conditioning regimen with RIC have clearly shown that RIC have advantages for the majority of patients. Badros et al. have published on 31 patients that were treated with a RIC regimen and compared the results with 93 patients as historical controls receiving myeloablative conditioning in combination with allograft (Badros et al. 2001, 2002). Transplantation related mortality (TRM) for RIC was significantly superior to myeloablative regimen with 10 vs. 29%. This resulted in a significantly improved 1-year OS for the RIC with 71% vs. 45%.

To obtain a significant reduction in myeloma tumor burden immediately before allografting, several groups have developed auto/allo transplantation strategies that consist of HDCT with melphalan followed by nonmyeloablative conditioning for allografting approximately 6 weeks later. Long-term data on this approach for 102 patients with a median follow-up of 6.3 years were recently reported (Rotta et al. 2009). 5 years. Non-relapse mortality was 18%, 95% related to graft-vs-host-disease (GVHD) or infections. Among 95% with detectable disease, 59% achieved a complete remission. Median time to progression was 5 years, median PFS of 3 years and median OS not reached. The 5-year OS and PFS were 64% and 36%, respectively. Prognostic factors for reduced OS and PFS in multivariate analysis were $\beta_2$microglobulin of more than 3.5 mg/l at diagnosis and auto/allo HCT more than 10 months after treatment initiation. Forty-two percent of patients developed acute GVHD (aGVHD) and 74% extensive chronic GVHD (cGVHD). Lower TRM and adverse event rate during RIC regimens allows for transplantation of patients over the age of 55, and even myeloma patients 75 years of age have been successfully transplanted. It was also described that cGVHD is associated with an improved disease-free survival (Gerull et al. 2005).

A study combining data from several centers including approximately 120 patients described that relapse from prior autologous transplantation was the most significant risk factor for transplant mortality (hazard ratio 2.8; $p=0.02$), relapse (HR 4.14; $p < 0.001$), and death (HR 2.69; $p=0.05$). Planned tandem autologous, followed by reduced intensity allografting, has been reported in studies containing approximately 120 patients (Table 11.1). ASCT was performed approximately 2–6 months before planned allografting. The allograft regimens utilized melphalan 100–140 mg/m^2 plus fludarabine or 2 Gy TBI or cyclophosphamide plus fludarabine. These studies reported transplantation-related mortalities of 18–24%, cGVHD 7–60%, and survivals of 58–74% at 2 years, 86% at 3 years, and 69% at 5 years. CR rates ranged from 28% to 73%. cGVHD has been associated with a lower rate of disease recurrence, although this is still controversial as only occasional studies have shown benefit for cGVHD (Table 11.1).

Therefore, a number of clinical centers worldwide have developed strategies to combine autologous and RIC allogeneic transplantation for myeloma (Table 11.1 (Maloney et al. 2003; Kroger et al. 2002a, b; Vesole et al. 2009; Perez-Simon et al. 2003; Lee et al. 2002, 2003a)).

This and other studies clearly stated that long-term disease control and GVHD remain key issues for the further development of allografting in multiple myeloma. Up to now, this strategy should be performed within clinical studies or applied to selected patients that have

Table 11.1 Phase 2 trials of tandem autologous reduced intensity allogeneic transplantation from related and unrelated donors for the treatment of multiple myeloma

Reference	No.	Regimen	# Tandem auto	ProphGVHD	AGVHD %, 2–4	CGVHD %	TRM %	CR %	% Survival at (year)
Maloney et al. (2003)	54 (0)	TBI 2 Gy, Flu	54	CSA, Mmf	45	60	22	57	69 (5)
Lee et al. (2003)	45[a] (12)	HDM100 (TBI 2 Gy, Flu)	12	CSA	58	13	38, 10	64	36 (3), 86
Kroger et al. (2002b)	17 (8)	HDM100, Flu, ATG	17	CSA, Mtx	38	7	18	73	74 (2)
Kroger et al. (2002a)	21 (21)	HDM100–140, Flu, ATG	9	CSA, Mtx	38	12	24	40	74 (2)
Galimberti et al. (2005)	20 (0)	TBI 2 Gy, Flu (10) Cy, Flu (10)	20	CSA, Mmf	25	30	20	35	58 (2)
Perez-Simon et al. (2003)	29 (NR)	Mel, Flu	10	CSA, Mtx	41	51	21	28	60 (2)
Vesole et al. (2009)	23 (0)	Flu, Cy	23	CSA, steroid	17[b]	39	9	33	78 (2)

Source: Adapted from Bensinger (2009)

AGVHD acute graft-versus-host disease, *ATG* anti-thymocyte globulin, *CGVHD* chronic GVHD, *CR* complete response, *CSA* cyclosporine, *Cy* cyclophosphamide, *Flu* fludarabine, *Mmf* mycophenolic acid, *Mtx* methotrexate, *No.* total number of patients (number from matched unrelated donors), *NR* not reported, *ProphGVHD* graft-versus-host disease prophylaxis, *HDM* high-dose melphalan, # *Tandem auto* planned prior autologous transplant, *TBI* total body irradiation, *TRM* transplant-related mortality

[a]Fourteen patients given donor lymphocyte infusion, TRM or survival for tandem patients

[b]Only grade 3–4 GVHD reported

prognostic factors as low $\beta_2$microglobulin and less than 10 months between initial treatment and allografting or less than two prior lines of therapy. In a recent review of the EBMT of registry data containing 229 mostly pretreated patients, the TRM was 26% at 2 years and the 3-year OS and PFS were disappointing at 41% and 21% (Crawley et al. 2005). Younger patients (<65 years) with a first high-risk relapse such as occurring early (<2 years) after ASCT or with fulminant presentation are probably candidates for RIC allo-SCT in the context of clinical trials. Many of these trials are evaluating the role of posttransplantation strategies, which incorporate novel agents, to further improve outcome of RIC allo-SCT.

11.6 Thalidomide and Immunomodulatory Drugs

11.6.1 Thalidomide as Single Agent and Combined with Corticosteroids

Barlogie and coworkers were the first to discover the anti-myeloma effect of thalidomide (Singhal et al. 1999). Since the recognition that thalidomide has substantial anti-myeloma activity, several thalidomide analogues such as so-called IMiDs (immunomodulatory drugs) have been developed as lenalidomide. In the initial full publication of 84 patients, 32% responded (≥MR) to single agent thalidomide. An update confirmed the initial results and reported on a 2-year event-free survival and OS of 26% and 48%, respectively. An important milestone for the clinical investigation of thalidomide was the recently published, randomized, multicenter, open-label phase 3 OPTIMUM study that was designed to compare the efficacy of single-agent thalidomide with high-dose dexamethasone in patients with one to three prior lines of therapy (kropff et al. 2009). A total of 499 patients were randomized into four arms: thal 100, thal 200, thal 400, or dex as control arm. Median TTP with 9.9 months for thal 400 was significantly longer ($p=0.017$) compared to dex with 6.0 months. Median TTP for thal 100 and thal 200 were 6.7 and 7.3 months did not reach statistical difference to dex. Response rates (≥PR) validated by an independent review committee were similar for all groups with 24.6% for dex, 20.7% for thal 100, 18.0% for thal 200, 21.5% for thal 400. However, duration of response in months was found to be significantly superior for all thal treatment groups compared to dex (thal 100: 12.7; $p=0.046$; thal 200; 13.1, $p=0.005$; thal 400: 11.6, $p=0.016$; dex: 6.5). Thal 400 cause at least one grade 3 or grade 4 adverse events in 60.2% of patients compared to 39.5% in patients treated with dexamethasone. Thal caused more frequent nervous system events (16.4% versus 2.4%), blood and lymphatic system disorders (14.8% versus 4.8%), and general disorders (12.1% versus 8.1%). In contrast, infections ≥grade 3 were more frequently observed in the dexamethasone group (10.5% versus 8.6%). Venous thromboembolic events were similar in both groups (1.6% with dex with none with thal 400). Importantly, the median average daily dose was 99.5 for thal 100, 198.2 for thal 200, 255.5 mg for thal 400, and 40 mg for dex. The median treatment duration was shortest for dex with 144 days followed by 195, 179, and 185 days for thal 400, thal 200, and thal 100, respectively. In conclusion, this study confirmed that thalidomide is an important treatment option for patients with relapsed multiple myeloma but that the dosage of thalidomide with a maximum of 400 mg needs to be based on clinical considerations (Kropff et al. 2003).

The study has also provided novel insights that might be relevant for the future concepts of integrating thal in more complex multiagent treatment regimen. A increased thal 400 in combination with a stepwise dose reduction was superior in TTP and PFS indicating that an early progression can be prevented by a higher dose of thalidomide indicating that patients at start of treatment require higher doses whereas after response is achieved, a lower thal dosage as 100 or 200 mg might be sufficient. Indeed Attal et al. have shown that thal 100 as maintenance after ASCT can indeed prolong the PFS and OS compared to pamidronate as maintenance (Attal et al. 2004).

Recently, an update of the first thalidomide single-agent study was presented (van Rhee et al. 2008). From 169 patients., 17 patients remain alive and ten event-free with a median follow-up of 9.2 years. Multivariate analysis revealed cytogenetic abnormalities in 47% of patients and lambda-light chain isotype to significant affect overall and event-free survival adversely. Forty percent of 58 patients lacking these two unfavorable features, one-half of whom had no disease recurrence, survived at least 6 years. In contrast, fewer than 5% of patients with one or two risk factors ($p < 0.001$) survived for at least 6 years. This study confirmed initial observations that patients with thal doses in excess of 42 g enjoyed superior overall and event-free survival. The poor outcome in lambda-light chain type myeloma was attributed to an overrepresentation in molecularly defined high-risk disease.

11.6.2 Thalidomide in Combination with Chemotherapy/Corticosteroids

Although the OPTIMUM and other studies investigating thalidomide as single agent have enormous relevance for the development of thalidomide and other IMiDs, based on the rapid development in this area, single-agent thalidomide will be used only on rare occasions for myeloma patients. Instead thalidomide/dexamethasone or thal Chemotherapy combination will be used due to their greater efficacy. This consideration is supported by preclinical studies demonstrating a synergy between thalidomide and dexamethasone (Hideshima et al. 2000).

The combination of thalidomide/dexamethasone was superior to dexamethasone alone in relapsed patients after one or two lines of therapy. The combination therapy induced a statistically highly significant ($p < 0.0001$) increase in the response rate of 65% for PR/CR compared to 28% for single-agent dexamethasone treatment. A significant advantage was also found for 1-year progression-free survival with 46.5% for the combination and 31% for single-agent dexamethasone (p=0.009) (Fermand et al. 2006). The median time to response for the thal/dex combination is relatively short with 1–1.3 month which is particularly important for patients with imminent organ failure as renal insufficiency.

A systematic review has confirmed this results indicating superiority of thal/dex over Thal with and overall response rate of 51% for thal/dex with 29% for the single agent (von Lilienfeld-Toal et al. 2008).

Whereas the single-agent thalidomide did not significantly increase the DVT rate, the thal/dex combination was associated with up to 10% of DVT/PE events, and therefore, a prophylactic treatment for DVT/PE is recommended (Palumbo et al. 2008b). Major concern for thalidomide is neurotoxicity; moreover, sedation, somnolence, and constipation occur in more than 10% of patients (Table 11.3).

For first-line indication, a combination therapy of MPT was clearly shown to be superior to standard MP in a randomized study. Addition of thalidomide improved PR/CR response rate of 76% for MPT compared with 47.6% for MP, as well as the improved 2-year event-free survival (54% MPT vs. 27% MP) and 3-year overall survival (80% MPT vs. 64% MP) rates, event (Palumbo et al. 2006). Other studies in the first-line setting have confirmed this positive effect of thalidomide in combination with chemotherapy and have led to the approval of thalidomide for the combination with MP in first-line. Although a randomized study on thalidomide combination therapy has not been performed up to now, thal/dex has been further integrated into chemotherapy regimen. The first original publication on the combination therapy of thalidomide, cyclophosphamide, etoposide, and dexamethasone demonstrated a response rate (≥PR) of 68% (Moehler et al. 2001). Since then, a number of combination therapies have been investigated and found to be clinically applicable with response rates between 41% and 76% for relapsed/refractory myeloma patients (Lee et al. 2003b; Offidani et al. 2006; Garcia-Sanz et al. 2004; Dimopoulos and Anagnostopoulos 2003; Kyriakou et al. 2005) (overview presented in Table 11.2).

Table 11.2 Main adverse events profiles of novel agents

Thalidomide
• Peripheral polyneuropathy, somnolence, constipation, increased risk of VTE in combinations
• No dose adjustment in case of renal impairment
• Effective after bort-containing regimen, poor results after len-based therapy
• Thromboprophylaxis in thal-based combinations
Lenalidomide
• Myelosuppression, fatigue, increased risk of VTE in combinations
• Dose adjustment if creatinine clearance <50 ml/min*
• Effective after thal- or bort-containing regimens
• Thromboprohylaxis in len-based combinations
Bortezomib
• Peripheral polyneuropathy, thrombocytopenia, neutropenia, herpes zoster, gastrointestinal events
• No dose adjustment in case of renal impairment
• Effective after len- or thal-containing regimens
• VZV-prophylaxis

Adapted from van de Donk et al. (2010)

There is no randomized phase III study for relapsed/refractory myeloma patients that compared a regimen with the same regimen plus thalidomide. But comparison to historic control and the data of the first-line studies indicate that thalidomide combination therapy in the relapse is a powerful option particularly if the patient needs to achieve a rapid reduction in myeloma tumor burden.

An important consideration is the application of VTE prophylaxis for patients treated with thalidomide or lenalidomide. Palumbo et al. have summarized recommendations for VTE prophylaxis (Palumbo et al. 2008b). Various VTE prophylaxis strategies have been investigated in small, uncontrolled clinical studies. Individual risk factors for VTE are history of VTE, central venous catheter, comorbidities (infections, diabetes, and cardiac disease), immobilization, surgery, and inherited thrombophilia. Myeloma-related risk factors include cotreatment with dexamethasone or doxorubicin and hyperviscosity. VTE is very high in patients who receive dexamethasone, doxorubicin, or multiagent chemotherapy in combination with thalidomide or lenalidomide, but not with bortezomib. The panel recommended treatment with aspirin for patients with ≤1 risk factor. In fact, patients without risk factor and single-agent treatment VTE prophylaxis can be considered but is not mandatory according to currently available data.

Patients with two or more individual/myeloma-related risk factors require therapy with low-molecular-weight heparin (LMWH). LMWH is also recommended in case of combination treatment with high-dose dexamethasone or doxorubicin. Treatment with Vitamin K antagonists targeting an international normalized ratio (INR) of 2–3 can be considered as an alternative to LMWH although data in the literature are rare to support this strategy. A comparison of AE profile and characteristics of clinical efficacy is highlighted in Table 11.3.

Table 11.3 Thalidomide/dexamethasone + chemotherapy regimens for relapsed/refractory myeloma

	Study	*N*	ORR	Disease Status	TTP (mo)	OS
Thal/dex + PACE	Lee et al. (2003)	236	After two cycles 7% CR, 23% nCR, 70% PR	63% refractory to previous therapy	NR	NR
Thal/dex + cyclophosphamide (IV) + etoposide	Moehler et al. (2001)	50	4% CR, 64% PR	Primary refractory 9%, resistant relapse 59%	16 (PFS)	NR at 14 months
Thal/dex + pegylated liposomal doxorubicin	Offidani et al. (2006)	50	26% CR, 6% nCR, 6% VGPR, 38% PR	20% refractory	17 (EFS)	NR
Thal (200–800 mg/day), oral cyclophosphamide (50 mg/day) Dex (40 mg/day × 4 day) every 3 weeks	Garcia-Sanz et al. (2004)	71	10% CR, 45% (PR)	NA	2-year PFS = 57%	2-year OS – 66%
Thal (intermittent) + dex + cyclophosphamide orally	Dimopoulos et al. (2004)	53; *n* = 43 (81%) thalidomide-naive	60% ≥ PR, for Thalidomide-naive patients, 67% ≥ PR	27% primary refractory, 60% resistant relapse	12 (for responding patients)	17.5 months
Thal/dex + cyclophosphamide orally	Kyriakou et al. (2005)	52	17% (CR), 62% (PR)	42% primary refractory, 29% resistant relapse	34% (EFS) at 2 year	73% at 2 year

ORR overall response rate, *TTP* time to progression, *OS* overall survival, *Thal* thalidomide, *Dex* dexamethasone, *PACE* infusional cisplatin, doxorubicin, cyclophosphamide, and etoposide, *IV* intravenous, CR complete response, *nCR* near-complete response, *PR* partial response, *VGPR* very good partial response, *NA* not available, *NR* not reached, *PFS* progression-free survival, *EFS* event-free survival

11.6.3 Lenalidomide

Lenalidomide is an amino-substituted derivative of thalidomide which has more potent biologic activity in stimulating T cell proliferation; augmenting IL-2 and IFN-γ production; and inhibiting TNF-α, IL-6, and IL-1β production (Muller et al. 1999; Corral et al. 1999; List 2007).

In the initial phase of lenalidomide, the single-agent activity was evaluated and found to be significant with approximately 30% of patients with relapsed/refractory myeloma achieving at least a PR (Richardson et al. 2006b). The maximum tolerated dose (MTD) as single agent was determined with 25 mg. Most important for the development of lenalidomide was the observation that some of the typical adverse events observed for thalidomide were less pronounced or absent as somnolence, constipation, and neuropathy. Most commonly observed AEs with lenalidomide are fatigue, skin rash, thrombo-, and neutropenia. In contrast to thalidomide for which there is no direct evidence as of now for an accumulation or increased toxicity in patients with renal impairment, lenalidomide requires dose adaptation (Chen et al. 2007). Dose recommendations based on creatinine clearance are as follows: Cr Cl ≥50 ml/min: regular dose of 20 mg/day, Cr Cl 30–50 ml/min: 10 mg/d; CrCl <30 ml/min but not on dialysis: 15 mg every other day; patient on dialysis 15 mg thrice per week. With this dose adaptation, no increased toxicity is expected. There is no evidence that lenalidomide has any negative effects on renal or hepatic function.

11.6.4 Lenalidomide Combination Therapies

Dexamethasone was found to enhance the anti-myeloma effects of lenalidomide (Hideshima et al. 2000; Mitsiades et al. 2002). For this reason and the established role of dexamethasone in myeloma treatment this, combination was evaluated in several studies most notably in two randomized studies that led to the approval of lenalidomide for patients after first relapse. An overview of lenalidomide-based combination therapies is provided in Table 11.4.

In Europe, Lenalidomide achieved approval before thalidomide's approval for first line treatment. Lenalidomide approval for the relapsed refractory patients was based on two phase III studies MM-09 and MM-010, both comparing lenalidomide/Dex with high-dose dexamethasone/placebo for patients with one or two prior therapies. Both studies included more than 700 patients (Dimopoulos et al. 2006, 2009; Weber et al. 2007).

The response rate was significantly superior for len/dex as compared to dex/placebo with 59.1% vs. 23.9% for MM-0009 and 59.4% vs. 21.1% for MM-010. The median time to progression was more than double in the len/dex arm in both studies with 11.3 and 11.1 month in the Len/Dex arms and 4.7 months in both study for the dex/placebo arm ($p < 0.001$). In line with these results, the median overall survival was 29.6 months in MM-010 (not reached for MM-009) significantly prolonged as compared to 20.6 and 20.2 months for the control arm. Interestingly, len/dex achieved significantly ($p < 0.05$) higher response rates of 63% in thalidomide-sensitive patients compared to 43% in thalidomide-resistant patients. len/dex displayed also higher activity in patients at first relapse compared to patients in second or third relapse. Prior treatment with bortezomib did not affect the likelihood of response.

Regarding patient selection for len/dex combination therapy, a subanalysis of the open-label phase III study did not find t4:14 or del 13 as adverse prognostic parameters related to median time to progression and overall survival. In contrast, the 17p13 translocation was associated with a significant worse outcome with a median time to progression of 2.2 months ($p < 0.0019$)

Table 11.4 Lenalidomide-based regimens for relapsed/refractory myeloma

	Study	*N*	ORR/CR	No. of previous therapies (median/range)	TTP (months)	OS (months)
Lenalidomide	Richardson et al. (2006)	35 at Len 15 mg twice daily	29%	≥3 in 88%	3.9	27
		67 at Len 30 mg once daily	24%	>3 in 73%	7.7	27
Lenalidomide	Richardson et al. (2005)	222	25%	≥2	5.5	>15
Lenalidomide + dexamethasone	MM-009, Weber et al. (2007)	177	61%/14%	2 (1–3)	11.1	29.6
Lenalidomide + dexamethasone	MM-010, Dimopoulos et al. (2007)	176	60%/16%	2 (1–3)	11.3	NR
Lenalidomide + pegylated liposomal doxorubicin + vincristine + dexamethasone	Baz et al. (2006)	52	75%/29% (+nCR)	3 (1–7), 64% had refractory MM	12 (PFS)	NR
Lenalidomide + doxorubicin + dexamethasone	Knop et al. (2009)	41 at MTD	85%/24% nCR	2/NR	NR	NR
Lenalidomide + oral cyclophosphamide + dexamethasone	Morgan et al. (2007)	21	62%/5% (nCR)	4 (1–8)	5.6	5 of 21 patients died after a median follow-up of 8 mo
Cyclophosphamide + prednisone + lenalidomide	Reece et al. (2009)	31	94% ≥ PR/19%	Median: 2	Too early to evaluate	Too early to evaluate
Cyclophosphamide + lenalidomide + dexamethasone	Schey et al. (2010)	31	81% ≥PR/29%	Median: 3	Too early to evaluate	Too early to evaluate

ORR overall response rate, *TTP* time to progression, *OS* overall survival, *L* lenalidomide, *CR* complete response, *nCR* near-complete response, *PR* partial response, *NR* not reached, *PFS* progression-free survival, *EFS* event-free survival, *MTD* maximum tolerated dose, *MM* multiple myeloma and an overall survival of 4.6 months ($p < 0.001$) (Reece et al. 2009).

Both randomized len/dex studies described above established an increased risk for thromboembolic complications for patients treated with the len/dex combination. Lenalidomide as thalidomide increases rate of thrombosis in the combination with dexamethasone but also in combination therapy regimen. Several authors have therefore recommended combining the len/dex treatment with an antithrombotic approach as prophylactic treatment preferentially with low-molecular-weight heparin (Klein et al. 2009). Other more common observed AEs are skin rash and fatigue.

As a major advantage over thalidomide, Lenalidomide has a significant lower incidence of neuropathy, constipation, and somnolence.

To further investigate lenalidomide in combination therapy, several studies were performed in chemo/corticosteroid combinations (Table 11.4). Lenalidomide in conjunction with adriamycin and dexamethasone (RAD) in refractory and relapsed myeloma resulted in high response rate of 73% (≥PR). The RAD-combination led mainly to hematological and infectious adverse events (Knop et al. 2009). The combination of lenalidomide with cyclophosphamide (500 mg po) and corticosteroids was described using a completely oral regimen by (Morgan GJ et al. 2007). The response rate was 75% (≥MR) the median PFS was 6 months . Another similar regimen (REP) using oral combination of lenalidomide 10 mg, cyclophosphamide 100 mg, prednisolone was presented by van de Donk et al and led to an impressive 12 month PFS (van de Donk et al 2010b). In addition, lenalidomide has successfully been combined with pegylated liposomal doxorubicin (PLD), vincristine dexamethasone (≥PR: 75%), as well as with bendamustine and dexamethasone (≥PR: 67%) (Lentzsch 2009; Baz et al. 2006; Knop et al. 2009).

Another four-drug combination tested in refractory/relapsed lenalidomide-naive myeloma was lenalidomide, melphalan, prednisone, and thalidomide (RMPT). Initial results showed a high response rate with 75% of patients achieving at least a PR including 20% VGPR and 14% nCR/CR R38 (Cavallo et al. 2009; Palumbo et al. 2010). At the moment, there is no clear evidence that supports lenalidomide/thal combinations as long as other combinations with agents of other mechanism are available.

11.6.5 Pomalidomide

Pomalidomide (development name CC 4047) is another immunomodulatory analogue of thalidomide. The MTD of daily pomalidomide was identified as 2 mg in single-agent therapy (Schey et al. 2004). Fifty-four percent of patients enrolled in this study with a median of three prior regimens achieved a PR or better. The MTD for alternate day dosing was found to be 5 mg of pomalidomide (Streetly et al. 2008). Dose-limiting toxicity of pomalidomide was grade 4 neutropenia. Additional toxicity was thrombocytopenia (up to grade 3). Main (incidence >10%) of nonhematolological toxicity grade 1/2 was neuropathy (15%), constipation (approximately 15%); pomalidomide resulted in remarkable responses rates of 40%.

11.7 Bortezomib

11.7.1 Bortezomib Single Agent

The success story of this first-in-class reversible proteasome inhibitor started in 2003 when the approval was granted for third and subsequent relapse based on study data from CREST and SUMMIT studies (Richardson et al. 2003; Jagannath et al. 2004, 2008).

The APEX (Assessment of Proteasome Inhibition for Extending Remissions) trial led to the approval of the first-in-class proteasome inhibitor bortezomib for relapsed or refractory myeloma in 2005 (Richardson et al. 2005). The overall response rate for single-agent bortezomib is between 28% and 44% and CR rate between 2% and 9% for pretreated patients (Richardson et al. 2007a). The time to progression in patients. with two or more prior lines of therapy is between 6.2 and 9.5 months and was 13.7 months for patients with only one prior therapy. The median overall survival for patients in the bortezomib arm of the APEX trial was 29.8 months versus 23.7 months in the dexamethasone control arm although 62% of patients crossed over to the bortezomib arm.

Prolonged administration over 6 months or retreatment with bortezomib may be safe, and decision depends on the individual tolerability of bortezomib (Berenson et al. 2005). Major adverse events of bortezomib are fatigue, gastrointestinal event, peripheral neuropathy, and reversible thrombocytopenia. In the APEX study, increase in the number of herpes zoster infections was recorded as well. Because of the high rate of vermicelli zoster virus (VZV) reactivation, VZV prophylaxis is recommended during bortezomib treatment (Nucci and Anaissie 2009). Grade 3 peripheral neuropathy is the most common AE leading to treatment discontinuation (Lonial 2006). Thrombocytopenia and neutropenia are transient and cyclical (Richardson et al. 2005). Patients with low platelet counts ($<70 \times 10^9$/l) are at an increased risk for grade 3 or 4 thrombocytopenia (Lonial et al. 2005). As the bortezomib-induced thrombocytopenia is associated with a reversible interference with megakaryocyte function but not megakaryocyte ploidy or cellularity, bortezomib can be given to selected patients with myeloma-induced bone marrow suppression as long as a support with platelet transfusions is available to bypass until disease-related thrombocytopenia has resolved or at least substantially improved.

Bortezomib was more active when used for patients with one prior therapy as compared to two and three therapies. Major determinator for decision to treat with bortezomib is the status of peripheral neuropathy of the patient that can either be based on concomitant disease (e.g., diabetic polyneuropathy), be myeloma associated, or due to IMiDs and other neuropathic agents. In general, bortezomib as single agent of combination therapy is recommended for patients with peripheral neuropathy grade 0–1. Whereas fatigue, gastrointestinal events, and peripheral neuropathy (PNP) are the most common adverse events for bortezomib, grade 3 PNP is the most common reason for treatment discontinuation. Bortezomib-induced thrombocytopenia and neutropenia are cyclic, reversible, and in general, do not lead to treatment discontinuation. Bortezomib can safely be applied to patients with impaired renal function even in the situation of dialysis. Bortezomib single agent has been instrumental in rapid decrease of disease activity in combination therapies and thereby supported renal recovery.

11.7.2 Bortezomib Combination Therapy

A number of regimens have been developed that combine bortezomib with other anti-myeloma agents (s. Table 11.5; (Davies et al. 2007; Berenson et al. 2008; Orlowski et al. 2007; Kropff et al. 2007; Palumbo et al. 2008a; Reece et al. 2008)). For most of the reported combination regimen, no formal comparison between the regimens or with single-agent bortezomib has been performed.

Whereas the combination of bortezomib with vinca alkaloids is obsolete due to high risk of neuropathy, bortezomib has been investigated with alkylating agents and anthracyclines.

Table 11.5 Bortezomib-based regimens for relapsed/refractory myeloma

	Study	*N*	ORR/CR	Median no. of prior therapies (range)	TTP (months)	OS (months)
Bortezomib single agent	SUMMIT, Richardson et al. (2003)	193	28%/4%	6 (2–15)	7	17
Bortezomib single agent	CREST, Jagannath et al. (2004)	26	38%/4%	1	13.7	NR
Bortezomib single agent	APEX, Richardson et al. (2005)	27	30%/4%	2 (1–3)	9.5	26.7
Bortezomib single agent	MMY-3001, Orlowski et al. (2007)	333	43%/9%	≥2 in 66%	6.2	29.8
		322	44%/2%		6.5	75% at 14 mo
Bortezomib + pegylated liposomal doxorubicin	MMY-3001, Orlowski et al. (2007)	324	52%/4%	≥2 in 66%	9.3	82% at 14 mo
Bortezomib + melphalan	Berenson et al. (2008)	46	50%/4%	–	9 (PFS)	32
Bortezomib + IV melphalan + dexamethasone	Popat et al. (2009)	21	69%/19%	3 (1–5)	10 (PFS)	NR at 17 mo
Bortezomib + oral cyclophosphamide + dexamethasone	Kropff et al. (2009)	50	66%(≥PR)/16%	–	12 (EFS)	22
Bortezomib + oral cyclophosphamide + dexamethasone	Davies et al. (2007)	16	75%/31%	3 (1–5)	7 (PFS)	NR
Bortezomib + doxorubicin + dexamethasone	Palumbo et al. (2008a)	64	67% ≥ PR/9%	2	1-year EFS : 34%	1-year OS: 66%
Bortezomib + cyclophosphamide + prednisone	Reece et al. (2009)	37	68%≥ PR/ 32% CR/nCR	2	Median PFS: 15	Median OS: 24

ORR overall response rate, *CR* complete response, *nCR* near-complete response, *TTP* time to progression, *OS* overall survival, *PFS* progression-free survival, *EFS* event-free survival, *IV* intravenous, *SUMMIT* study of uncontrolled multiple myeloma managed with proteasome inhibition Therapy, *CREST* clinical response and efficacy study of bortezomib in the treatment of relapsing multiple myeloma *APEX* assessment of proteasome inhibition for extending remissions

All of these combinations (selection presented in Table 11.5) provided evidence for an at least additive therapeutic effect of bortezomib in the combination regimen (Kastritis et al. 2009).

Historical data and comparison of phase II data of course strongly suggest that bortezomib combination therapies have a substantial increased PFS rate and response rate compared to bortezomib single agent or bortezomib/dex combinations. In combination therapy with pegylated doxorubicin, improvements in time to progression (9.3 months vs. 6.5 months), overall response rate (52% vs. 44%), and survival advantage have been reported.

Bortezomib in combination with liposomal doxorubicin reached a CR+PR rate of 73% with CR/nCR of 36% (Orlowski et al. 2005) in a phase I study. The recommended dose for bortezomib was 1.3 mg/m^2 and liposomal doxorubicin 30 mg/m^2. A phase 3 study with 636 patients in relapse basically confirmed the phase I data and demonstrated a superior ORR of 52% (vs. 44% single agent bortezomib) and a CR/nCR rate of 17% vs. 13% single-agent bortezomib. The time to progression was significantly longer in the combination arm with 9.3 months compared to 6.5 months in the bortezomib arm (Orlowski et al. 2007). Sonneveld et al reported about the activity of the combination pegylated liposomal dosorubicin and bortezomib in patients treated with recurrent multiple myeloma who received (Sonneveld et al. 2009). However, there was an increase in neutropenia, thrombocytopenia, and gastrointestinal events in the combination group. Importantly, the response rate, TTP adverse event proile was independent of prior treatment with IMiDs. FDA has therefore approved the combination of liposomal doxorubicin with bortezomib for the treatment of relapsed and refractory multiple myeloma after failure of IMiD-containing regimen.

Bortezomib was also combined with oral and IV cyclophosphamide and melphalan and bendamustine, resulting in CR/PR rates between 65% and 95% (Fenk et al. 2007).

Nowadays, bortezomib is mostly used either in combination with dexamethasone as demonstrated in the APEX trial or in combination therapy regimen. The following features within the patient's medical history can be used as indicator for a beneficial effect of a combination therapy: short duration of previous therapy with the possibility of a drug-resistant myeloma variant, previous use of bortezomib with the possibility to induce a synergistic/additive effect with the combination therapy. Similarly, the choice and intensity of chemotherapy combination have to be balanced against expected therapeutic effects and concomitant diseases of the patients.

The decision on whether to use bortezomib as single agent, in combination with dexamethasone or in combination regimen either with IMiDs or with chemotherapy, has to be tailored to the individual situation of the patient and criteria set forward by the myeloma disease activity (Fig. 11.1). In general, a bortezomib/dexamethasone combination therapy appears to be the treatment of choice for bortezomib-naive patients that do not have a rapid progressing disease with imminent renal or other organ failure. At present there is no randomized data to indicate that more aggressive treatment strategies would be beneficial to the patients. As the primary treatment regimen becomes more aggressive and a certain percentage of patients obviously can enter into long-term complete remission, it will be of particular interest to start clinical trials that compare less and more aggressive second-line regimen with respect to the overall survival and long-term remission.

11.8 Novel Proteasome Inhibitors

Carfilzomib is an irreversible inhibitor or the proteasome and structural distinct from bortezomib (Chauhan et al. 2005b; Parlati et al. 2009). Preclinical data suggested that carfilzomib can be active even in bortezomib-resistant myeloma cells (Kuhn et al. 2007). Carfizomib (20 mg/m^2 d1, 2, 8, 9, 15, 16 of a 28-day cycle) induced a 45% response (≥PR) in 51 bortezomib-naïve patients and in 18% of 33 bortezomib-exposed patients (Siegel 2009). Peripheral neuropathy in carfilzomib-treated patients was uncommon indicating that polyneuropathy is not a class effect of proteasome inhibitors. (Siegel 2009)

NPI-0052 is another novel proteasome inhibitor, which inhibits all three catalytic activities of the 20S proteasome, whereas bortezomib and carfilzomib preferentially inhibit chymotrypsin-like activity. NPI-0052 has activity in bortezomib-resistant myeloma cells (Chauhan et al. 2005a). Initial results of two dose-finding trials of single agent NPI-0052 demonstrated clinical activity in relapsed/refractory myeloma (Spencer et al. 2009; Richardson et al. 2009b).

11.9 Combination of Novel Agents

The combination of bortezomib with IMiDs (thalidomide and lenalidomide) has received special attention (Table 11.6 (Pineda-Roman et al. 2008; Ciolli et al. 2008; Kim et al. 2010; Terpos et al. 2008; Palumbo et al. 2010)). In particular, the combination of bortezomib with lenalidomide and corticosteroids has several advantages as lenalidomide has a significant lower potential for polyneuropathy compared to thalidomide. In addition, preclinical data indicate that lenalidomide activates myeloma cell caspase 8 and thereby cooperates with bortezomib-induced dual activation of caspase 8 and 9, inducing a synergistic effect on myeloma cell apoptosis (Hideshima et al. 2000).

The lenalidomide/bortezomib/dexamethason (RVd) regimen was able to achieve an ORR of 79%, 33% with CR/nCR/VGPR in myeloma patients with relapse or refractory disease after one to three prior therapies. The overall survival with this regimen was approximately 22 months although most patients had previously received bortezomib- or thalidomide-containing regimen or single-agent therapy in previous treatment (Richardson 2006a; Richardson et al. 2007b; Richardson 2006; Richardson et al. 2010). Most important and in this respect clearly distinct form bortezomib/thalidomide combinations, RVd did not induce additional polyneuropathy even if treatment was extended to 3 years. The MTD level was found to be 15 mg/day lenalidomide for 14 days and for bortezomib 1.0 mg/m^2 on days 1, 4, 8, 11 of a 21-day cycle. The most common grade 3–4 treatment-related toxicities included reversible neutropenia, thrombocytopenia, and anemia. Another possibly synergistic effect in the RV(D)-combined treatment approach is that IMiDs including lenalidomide and bortezomib inhibit osteoclast function and thereby suppress myeloma bone disease (Terpos et al. 2007a, b; Breitkreutz et al. 2008).

Combination therapies of bortezomib and thalidomide as novel agent combination and in extended treatment regimens with chemotherapy and corticosteroids have been tested as well. Table 11.6 lists the treatment results and the neurological toxicity of this combination approach. In fact, in a phase II study investigating bortezomib/thalidomide/dexamethasone (VTD), 23% of patients had ≤ grade 2 polyneuropathy at trial onset and aggravation was infrequent (Pineda-Roman et al. 2008). The VTD regimen was then further intensified using PLD resulting in a 55% response rate in relapsed/refractory myeloma. Fatigue and polyneuropathy were the most common adverse events (Ciolli et al. 2006, 2008).

In general, more mature data have to be awaited related to polyneuropathy to generally recommend a bortezomib/thalidomide combination therapy. Unless there is a special reason to use VT combinations, the author's impression is that at present, RV combinations appear to be superior to VT combinations as the risk of polyneuropathy is lower and response rate and duration appear to be at least similar.

Table 11.6 Regimens with combinations of novel agents for relapsed/refractory myeloma

Regimen	Study	Type of study	Schedule	*N*	Response	No. of previous therapies	TTE	Key toxicities
Bortezomib + thalidomide + dexamethasone	Pineda-Roman et al. (2008)	Phase 1/2	Bort 1.3 mg/m on days 1, 4, 8, 11 of 21-day cycle Thal 150 mg day 1–21 of 21-day cycle Dex 20 mg on day 1, 2, 4, 5, 8, 9, 11, 12 of 21-day cycle in case of no PR after four cycles	85	All evaluable patients ≥PR: 63% nCR:16% CR: 6%	Median: ≥2 Thal: 74% Bort: 0% Len: NA	Median EFS: 6 months Median OS: 22 months	Dose-limiting toxicity: grade 4 thrombocytopenia and grade 4 neutropenia
Liposomal doxorubicin + bortezomib + thalidomide + dexamethasone	Ciolli et al. (2008)	Phase 2	Liposomal doxo 50 mg/m^2 (30 mg/m^2 for patients >75 years) on day 4 of a 28-day cycle Bort 1.0 mg/m^2 on days 1, 4, 8, 11 Dex 24 mg on days 1, 2, 4, 5, 8, 9, 11, 12 Thal 100 mg on days 1–28	42	≥PR: 74% nCR:29% CR: 24%	Median: 3 Thal: 64% Bort: 14% Len: NA	Median PFS: 15 months 2-year OS: 66%	% of patients Grade ≥ 3 neutropenia: 24% Grade ≥ 3 thrombocytopenia: 29% Grade ≥ 3 anemia: NA Grade ≥ 3 peripheral neuropathy: 2% Grade ≥ 3 venous thromboembolism: 0%

Bortezomib + cyclophosphamide + thalidomide + dexamethasone	Kim et al. (2010)	Phase 2	Bort 1.3 mg/m² on days 1, 4, 8, 11 of 21-day cycle Dex 20 mg/m² on days 1, 4, 8, 11 Cyclo: 150 mg/m² p.o. on days 1–4 Thal 50 mg day 1–21 of 21-day cycle	70	≥PR: 88% CR: 46%	Median: 2 Thal: ≥57% Bort: 0% Len: NA	Median TTP: 15 months Median OS: 32 months	% of cycles Grade ≥ 3 neutropenia: 4% Grade ≥ 3 thrombocytopenia: 12% Grade ≥ 3 anemia: 4% Grade ≥ 3 peripheral neuropathy: 3% Grade ≥ 3 venous thromboembolism: 1%
MTD: Lenalidomide + bortezomib + dexamethasone	Richardson et al. (2009)	Phase 1	MTD: Len 15 mg on days 1–14 of 21-day cycle Bort 1.0 mg/m² on days 1, 4, 8, 11 of 21-day cycle Dex 20 or 40 mg on days 1, 2, 4, 5, 8, 9, 11, 12 in case of progression after two cycles	38	All evaluable patients ≥MR: 61% CR/nCR: 8%	Median: 5 Thal: 87% Bort: 55% Len: 18%	Median TTP: 7.7 months Median OS: 37 months	% of patients Grade ≥ 3 neutropenia: 63% Grade ≥ 3 thrombocytopenia: 45% Grade ≥ 3 anemia: 18% Grade ≥ 3 peripheral neuropathy: 0% Grade ≥ 3 venous thromboembolism: 3%

(continued)

Table 11.6 (continued)

Regimen	Study	Type of study	Schedule	*N*	Response	No. of previous therapies	TTE	Key toxicities
MTD: Bortezomib + melphalan + prednisone + thalidomide	Palumbo et al. (2007)	Phase 1/2	MTD: Bort 1.3 mg/m^2 on day 1, 4, 15, 22 Mel 6 mg/m^2 p.o. on days 1-5 Pred 60 mg/m^2 on days 1–5 Thal 50 mg on days 1–35	30	All evaluable patients ≥PR: 67% VGPR: 27% CR: 17%	Median: 2 Thal: 30% Bort: NA Len: NA	1-year PFS: 61% 1-year OS: 84%	% of patients Grade ≥ 3 neutropenia: 43% Grade ≥ 3 thrombocytopenia: 33% Grade ≥ 3 anemia: 16% Grade ≥ 3 peripheral neuropathy: 6% Grade ≥ 3 venous thromboembolism: 0%
Bortezomib + melphalan + dexamethasone + thalidomide	Terpos et al. (2008)	Phase 2	Bort 1.0 mg/m^2 on day 1, 4, 8, 11 of a 28-day cycle Mel 0.15 mg/kg p.o. on days 1–4 Dex 12 mg/m^2 on days 1–4, 17–20 Thal 100 mg on days 1–4, 17–20	62	≥PR: 66% VGPR: 27% CR: 13%	Median: 2 Thal: 55% Bort: 10% Len: NA	Median TTP: 9.3 months 2-year OS: 63%	% of patients Grade ≥ 3 neutropenia: 10% Grade ≥ 3 thrombocytopenia: 23% Grade ≥ 3 anemia: 5% Grade ≥ 3 peripheral neuropathy: 10% Grade ≥ 3 venous thromboembolism: 0%

Lenalidomide + melphalan + prednisone + thalidomide	Palumbo et al. (2010)	Phase 1/2	Len 10 mg day 1–21 of a 28-day cycle Mel 0.18 mg/kg p.o. on days 1–4 Pred 2 mg/kg on days 1–4 Thal 50 mg or 100 mg on days 1–28 44	All evaluable patients ≥PR: 75% VGPR: 20% nCR/CR: 14%	Median: 1 Thal: 23% Bort: 20% Len: 0%	1-year PFS: 52% 1-year OS: 72%	% of patients Grade ≥ 3 neutropenia: 68% Grade ≥ 3 thrombocytopenia: 36% Grade ≥ 3 anemia: 32% Grade ≥ 3 neurotoxicity: 4.5% Grade ≥ 3 venous thromboembolism: 0%

CR complete response, *nCR* near-complete response, *VGPR*, very good partial response, *PR* partial response, *MR* minor response, *NA* not available, *TTE* time to events, *TTP* time to progression, *EFS* event-free survival, *OS* overall survival, *MTD* maximum tolerated dose

11

11.10 Emerging Therapies and Novel Pathways

Further therapeutic concepts to interfere with signaling cascades, apoptosis regulation, cell cycle, and myeloma cell interaction with microenvironment are currently in preclinical evaluation, and some have recently entered the clinical investigation. Those concepts that have entered clinical studies are discussed briefly in this paragraph but are also discussed in this book in the Chap. 8.

A number of preclinical data indicate that interference with the heat shock protein 90 (Hsp90) has anti-myeloma effects and more important exerts synergistic effects in combination with proteasome inhibitors. In relapse/refractory myeloma, this combination was well tolerated and associated with durable responses in both bortezomib-naïve and bortezomib-exposed patients (Badros 2009).

The degree of acetylation of histones influences their physical interaction with DNA and how DNA is packaged in the nucleus. This can have large-scale impact on gene expression. Inhibition of HDACs triggers accumulation of acetylated histones and induces differentiation and/or apoptosis of many types of malignant cells. Anti-myeloma effects were identified in in vitro experiments for vorinostat as well as other HDAC inhibitors such as LAQ824 and LBH589 (Catley et al. 2006; Bali et al. 2005).

In a phase I study in single-agent vorinostat in relapsed/refractory myeloma patients, 1 MR and 9 SDs were observed (Richardson et al. 2008). The study was closed prematurly before definitive identification of MTD based on the sponsor's decision. Maximum dose administered were 250 mg daily for 5 days/week of 4-week cycles and 200 mg twice daily for 14 days of 3-week cycles. Drug-related adverse events were fatigue (grade 3), other grade 2 or lower AEs: anorexia, dehydration, diarrhea, nausea. Subsequent phase I study combining vorinostat with bortezomib indicated a promising response rate with 8 of 16 patients achieving a CR or PR (Badros et al. 2009b).

The inhibition of the PI3-kinase/Akt pathway using perifosine and the mTOR pathway using temsirolismus/everolimus have shown promising activity in early-phase studies in relapsed/refractory patients (Gajate and Mollinedo 2007; Hideshima et al. 2006).

Elotuzumab an antibody directed against CS1, a cell surface glycoprotein, highly expressed in myeloma, generated encouraging results (Lonial 2009).

11.11 Prognostic Factors

Prognostic factors for multiple myeloma have been clearly identified in large cohorts of first-line myeloma patients. Many of these prognostic factors remain valid in the relapse situation including cytogenetic translocation t(4;14), t(14;16), deletion of chromosome 17 or 13, hypodiploidy, increased β_2-microglobulin, and decreased serum albumin.

Additional clinical challenges in the relapse situation include light chain and IgA isotype, renal failure, extramedullary disease, hyposecretory myeloma, and advanced bone disease.

11.12 Therapeutic Strategy for Relapsed/Refractory Myeloma Patients

The purpose of this chapter is to provide concluding remarks and summarize the data discussed in the sections above. References are only added as examples or if not already cited above.

The choice of relapse therapy is principally dependent on the age, performance status, previous therapeutic chain, and concomitant disease (van de Donk et al. 2010a). An overview of potential decision tree is given in Fig. 11.1. Particularly in the situation of first relapse, the careful evaluation of first-line therapeutic approach is very important to determine if an optimal combination approach was used.

HDCT should be considered for patients <70 years and/or in good general condition for those patients that did not receive HDCT as part of the first-line treatment. HDCT should also be considered if remission after first HDCT was equal to or more than 12 months.

In case of first-line HDCT with remission duration of less than 12 months, combination therapy of dexamethasone with one of the novel agents preferentially not used in first-line treatment should be used.

If there are no special clinical consideration as peripheral neuropathy or others that influence the treatment decision, therapy of first relapse will be using those novel agents in combination with dexamethasone that have not been part of the first-line treatment. A preference is to switch the class of novel compound e.g. IMiDs switch to proteasome inhibitors and vice versa.

Lenalidomide may be indicated when preexisting peripheral neuropathy exists, whereas a history of thromboembolism or presence of renal insufficiency may favor bortezomib-based therapy. Furthermore, in case of severe cytopenias, thalidomide with or without dexamethasone or single-agent dexamethasone can be useful and patients with poor tolerance of corticosteroids may benefit from a steroid-free regimen.

For treatment of first relapse as well as for later relapse, no clear guidance from clinical studies is available as to whether more intensified treatment, e.g., by using combination therapies of novel agents/chemotherapy/corticosteroid is preferable choice over novel agent/corticosteroid. Therefore, again the integration of clinical information is relevant to guide the treating physician. The urge to induce a rapid response, e.g., to prevent further deterioration of renal dysfunction or severe and rapid progressing osteolytic bone disease often argues for a more aggressive approach with combination of novel agents with chemotherapeutic agents if there are no significant comorbidities.

Radiotherapy or other local interventions as kyphoplasty need to be integrated in the treatment plan of patients with relapse disease, e.g., in case of extramedullary manifestation or painful osteolytic bone disease. In general, local intervention strategies should be performed after systemic treatment has controlled the overall disease activity.

For *elderly patients* who received MPT or len/dex for first line, second line bortezomib/dex or bortezomib/pegdox/dex should be considered. In case of contraindications to bortezomib, lenalidomide combination therapy can be used subsequent to failure of thalidomide-containing first-line regimen as it has been shown that lenalidomide can overcome resistance to thalidomide at least in a subset of patients. Conversely, in case of bortezomib/dex or bortezomib/chemotherapy/dex combinations in first-line lenalidomide or thalidomide in combination with dex and/or chemotherapy is recommended. The decision between lenalidomide and thalidomide could be based on comorbidity as neuropathy rate is clearly lower with lenalidomide compared to thalidomide.

In case of treatment with thalidomide or lenalidomide, a special consideration with regard to the risk of *venous thrombosis and embolism* (VTE) has to be given. In the first step, the individual and myeloma-related VTE risk for the patient have to be assessed. If there is no or one risk factor, treatment with aspirin is recommended. For patients receiving combination therapy with dexamethasone or doxorubicin or more than one risk factor, supportive treatment with LMWH or vitamin k antagonist is recommended.

A special challenge is patients with *renal failure* at the time point of relapse. As bortezomib clearance is independent of renal clearance,

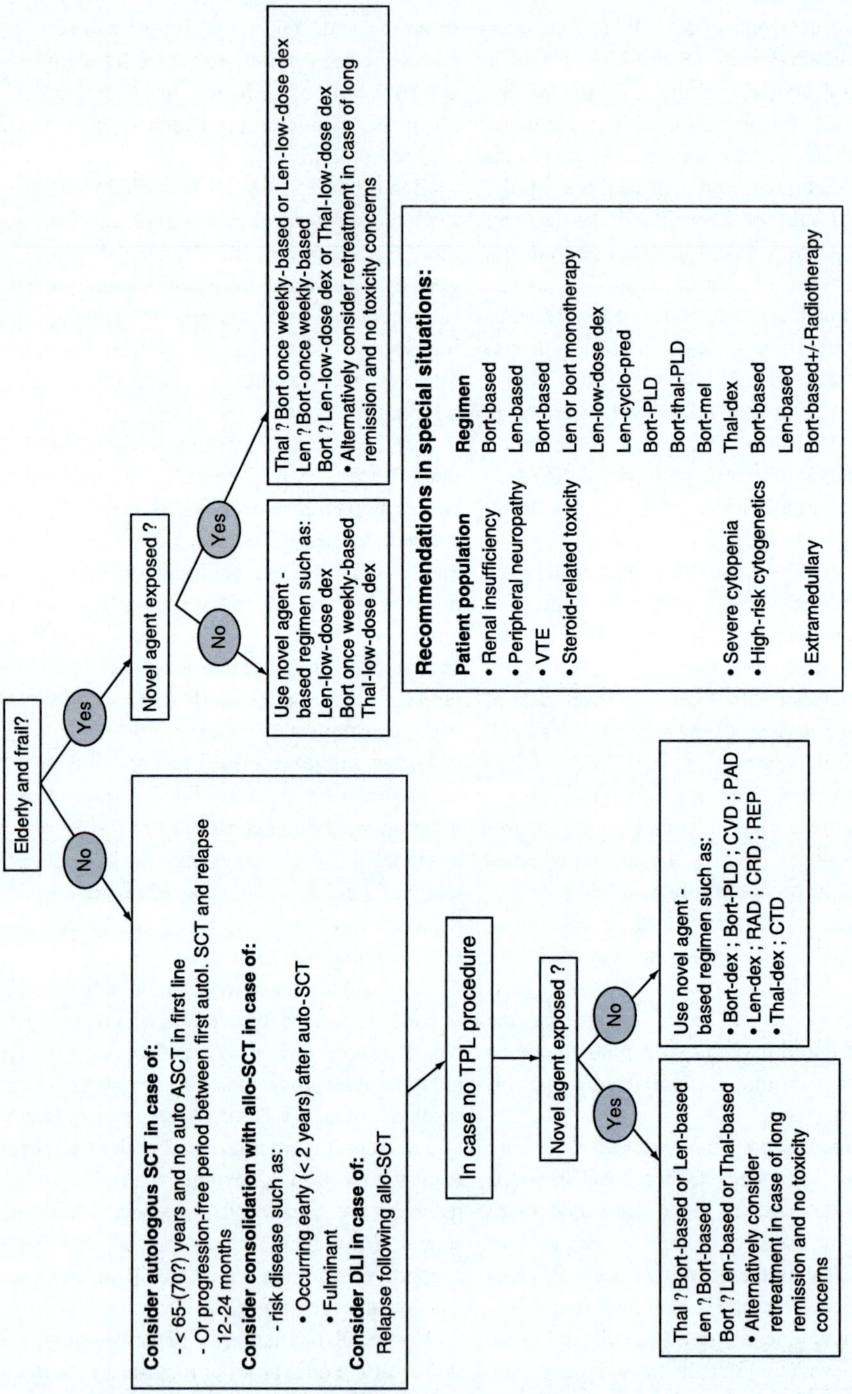

Fig. 11.1 Possible Treatment algorithm for patients with relapsed and refractory multiple myeloma. Modified according to van de Donk et al 2010a

bortezomib-containing regimen is a preferred strategy for these patients. Another option is thalidomide as thalidomide does not require dose reduction in case of renal impairment. Lenalidomide is a renally metabolized drug and requires dose reduction. A special consideration should be given to time to response of the regimen as regimen inducing a fast response is preferred–unless prohibited due to comorbidities–to prevent irreversible renal dysfunction.

The recommendation for *third-line therapy* or treatment of patients who were already treated with bortezomib, thalidomide, and lenalidomide would be inclusion of the following in clinical trial: a combination of novel agents with chemotherapeutics as low-dose oral cyclophosphamide or bendamustine or combinations of chemotherapeutic agents as EDAP (Barlogie et al. 1989). In addition, combination of novel agents in particular bortezomib/lenalidomide has been used successfully in this situation (Richardson et al. 2009a).

Altogether, at the moment, there is not enough evidence to recommend a specific treatment for relapsed myeloma patients with *high-risk cytogenetics*. More mature data from larger trials is needed. However, it seems that bortezomib may overcome the poor prognosis conferred by del(13q) and t(4;14), whereas conflicting results exist for lenalidomide regarding del(13q) and t(4;14).

A special challenge is the treatment of patients who relapse after *allogeneic stem cell transplantation* (see also Chap.10). In the early posttransplant period and still on immunosuppressive therapy, a rapid taper of immunosuppressive therapy in order to induce a graft-versus-myeloma (GvM) effect is recommended. As a next step donor lymphocyte infusion (DLI) can be considered. Novel agents have successfully been used in the treatment of allo-SCT and have been combined with immunological approaches to decrease tumor burden to allow immunological therapy to be effective. Response to IMiDs is frequently accompanied by a flare up of GVHD, suggesting immunostimulatory effects together with direct antimyeloma activity.

References

Alexanian R, Barlogie B, Dixon D (1986) High-dose glucocorticoid treatment of resistant myeloma. Ann Intern Med 105:8–11

Alexanian R, Dimopoulos MA, Delasalle K, Barlogie B (1992) Primary dexamethasone treatment of multiple myeloma. Blood 80:887–890

Attal M, Harousseau J-L, Leyvraz S, Doyen C, Hulin C, Benboubker L, Facon T, Bourhis J-H, Garderet L, Sotto JJ, Michallet M, Renaud M, Voillat L, Berthou C, Marrit G, Monconduit M, Coiffier B, Caillot D (2004) Maintenance treatment with thalidomide after autologous transplantation for myeloma: first analysis of a prospective randomized study of the Intergroupe Francophone du Myelome (IFM 99 02). Session type: oral session. Blood 104(11):155a

Badros A, Barlogie B, Morris C, Desikan R, Martin SR, Munshi N, Zangari M, Mehta J, Toor A, Cottler-Fox M, Fassas A, Anaissie E, Schichman S, Tricot G (2001) High response rate in refractory and poor-risk multiple myeloma after allotransplantation using a nonmyeloablative conditioning regimen and donor lymphocyte infusions. Blood 97: 2574–2579

Badros A, Barlogie B, Siegel E, Cottler-Fox M, Zangari M, Fassas A, Morris C, Anaissie E, Van RF, Tricot G (2002) Improved outcome of allogeneic transplantation in high-risk multiple myeloma patients after nonmyeloablative conditioning. J Clin Oncol 20(5):1295–1303

Badros A, Richardson PG, Albitar M, Jagannath S, Tarantollo S, Wolf JL, Messina M, Bermann D, Anderson KC (2009) Tanespimycin+Bortezomib in relapsed/refractory myeloma patients: results from the TIME-2 study. Am Soc Hematology 114:10

Badros A, Richardson PG, Albitar M, Jagannath S, Tarantollo S, Wolf JL, Messina M, Bermann D, Anderson KC (2009a) Tanespimycin + Bortezomib in relapsed/refractory myeloma patients: results from the TIME-2 study. Am Soc Hematology 114(1):10

Badros A, Burger AM, Philip S, Niesvizky R, Kolla SS, Goloubeva O, Harris C, Zwiebel J,

11

Wright JJ, Espinoza-Delgado I, Baer MR, Holleran JL, Egorin MJ, Grant S (2009b) Phase I study of vorinostat in combination with bortezomib for relapsed and refractory multiple myeloma. Clin Cancer Res 15:5250–5257

Bali P, Pranpat M, Bradner J, Balasis M, Fiskus W, Guo F, Rocha K, Kumaraswamy S, Boyapalle S, Atadja P, Seto E, Bhalla K (2005) Inhibition of histone deacetylase 6 acetylates and disrupts the chaperone function of heat shock protein 90: a novel basis for antileukemia activity of histone deacetylase inhibitors. J Biol Chem 280: 26729–26734

Barlogie B, Smith L, Alexanian R (1984) Effective treatment of advanced multiple myeloma refractory to alkylating agents. N Engl J Med 310: 1353–1356

Barlogie B, Alexanian R, Dicke KA, Zagars G, Spitzer G, Jagannath S, Horwitz L (1987) High-dose chemoradiotherapy and autologous bone marrow transplantation for resistant multiple myeloma. Blood 70:869–872

Barlogie B, Velasquez WS, Alexanian R, Cabanillas F (1989) Etoposide, dexamethasone, cytarabine, and cisplatin in vincristine, doxorubicin, and dexamethasone-refractory myeloma. J Clin Oncol 7: 1514–1517

Barlogie B, Jagannath S, Desikan KR, Mattox S, Vesole D, Siegel D, Tricot G, Munshi N, Fassas A, Singhal S, Mehta J, Anaissie E, Dhodapkar D, Naucke S, Cromer J, Sawyer J, Epstein J, Spoon D, Ayers D, Cheson B, Crowley J (1999) Total therapy with tandem transplants for newly diagnosed multiple myeloma. Blood 93:55–65

Barlogie B, Kyle R, Anderson K (2003) Comparable survival in multiple myeloma (MM) with high dose therapy (HDT) employing MEL 140 mg/m^2+TBI12Gy autotransplant versus standard dose therapy with VBMCP and no benefit from interferon (IFN) maintenance: result of Intergroup Trial S9321. Blood 102(11):42a

Barlogie B, Pineda-Roman M, van Rhee F, Haessler J, Anaissie E, Hollmig K, Alsayed Y, Waheed S, Petty N, Epstein J, Shaughnessy JD Jr, Tricot G, Zangari M, Zeldis J, Barer S, Crowley J (2008a) Thalidomide arm of total therapy 2 improves complete remission duration and survival in myeloma patients with metaphase cytogenetic abnormalities. Blood 112:3115–3121

Barlogie B, Shaughnessy JD Jr, Crowley J (2008b) Duration of survival in patients with myeloma treated with thalidomide. N Engl J Med 359: 210–212

Basak GW, Srivastava AS, Malhotra R, Carrier E (2009) Multiple myeloma bone marrow niche. Curr Pharm Biotechnol 10:345–346

Baz R, Walker E, Karam MA, Choueiri TK, Jawde RA, Bruening K, Reed J, Faiman B, Ellis Y, Brand C, Srkalovic G, Andresen S, Knight R, Zeldis J, Hussein MA (2006) Lenalidomide and pegylated liposomal doxorubicin-based chemotherapy for relapsed or refractory multiple myeloma: safety and efficacy. Ann Oncol 17:1766–1771

Bensinger WI (2009) Role of autologous and allogeneic stem cell transplantation in myeloma. Leukemia 23:442–448

Berenson JR, Jagannath S, Barlogie B, Siegel DT, Alexanian R, Richardson PG, Irwin D, Alsina M, Rajkumar SV, Srkalovic G, Singhal S, Limentani S, Niesvizky R, Esseltine DL, Trehu E, Schenkein DP, Anderson K (2005) Safety of prolonged therapy with bortezomib in relapsed or refractory multiple myeloma. Cancer 104:2141–2148

Berenson JR, Yang HH, Vescio RA, Nassir Y, Mapes R, Lee SP, Wilson J, Yellin O, Morrison B, Hilger J, Swift R (2008) Safety and efficacy of bortezomib and melphalan combination in patients with relapsed or refractory multiple myeloma: updated results of a phase 1/2 study after longer follow-up. Ann Hematol 87:623–631

Breitkreutz I, Raab MS, Vallet S, Hideshima T, Raje N, Mitsiades C, Chauhan D, Okawa Y, Munshi NC, Richardson PG, Anderson KC (2008) Lenalidomide inhibits osteoclastogenesis, survival factors and bone-remodeling markers in multiple myeloma. Leukemia 22:1925–1932

Catley L, Weisberg E, Kiziltepe T, Tai YT, Hideshima T, Neri P, Tassone P, Atadja P, Chauhan D, Munshi NC, Anderson KC (2006) Aggresome induction by proteasome inhibitor bortezomib and alpha-tubulin hyperacetylation by tubulin deacetylase (TDAC) inhibitor LBH589 are synergistic in myeloma cells. Blood 108:3441–3449

Cavallo F, Larocca A, Petrucci MT, Federico V, Falcone AP, Sanpaolo G, Canepa L, Crugnola M, Boccadoro M, Palumbo A (2009) A prospective randomized phase I/II study of lenalidomide, melphalan, prednisone and thalidomide (RMPT) for relapsed/refractory multiple myeloma patients. ASH Annual Meeting Abstracts (114):2864

Chauhan D, Catley L, Li G, Podar K, Hideshima T, Velankar M, Mitsiades C, Mitsiades N, Yasui H, Letai A, Ovaa H, Berkers C, Nicholson B, Chao TH, Neuteboom ST, Richardson P, Palladino MA, Anderson KC (2005a) A novel orally active proteasome inhibitor induces apoptosis in multiple myeloma cells with mechanisms distinct from bortezomib. Cancer Cell 8:407–419

Chauhan D, Li G, Podar K, Hideshima T, Neri P, He D, Mitsiades N, Richardson P, Chang Y, Schindler J, Carver B, Anderson KC (2005b) A novel carbohydrate-based therapeutic GCS-100 overcomes bortezomib resistance and enhances dexamethasone-induced apoptosis in multiple myeloma cells. Cancer Res 65:8350–8358

Chen N, Lau H, Kong L, Kumar G, Zeldis JB, Knight R, Laskin OL (2007) Pharmacokinetics of lenalidomide in subjects with various degrees of renal impairment and in subjects on hemodialysis. J Clin Pharmacol 47:1466–1475

Ciolli S, Leoni F, Gigli F, Rigacci L, Bosi A (2006) Low dose Velcade, thalidomide and dexamethasone (LD-VTD): an effective regimen for relapsed and refractory multiple myeloma patients. Leuk Lymphoma 47:171–173

Ciolli S, Leoni F, Casini C, Breschi C, Santini V, Bosi A (2008) The addition of liposomal doxorubicin to bortezomib, thalidomide and dexamethasone significantly improves clinical outcome of advanced multiple myeloma. Br J Haematol 141:814–819

Corral LG, Haslett PA, Muller GW, Chen R, Wong LM, Ocampo CJ, Patterson RT, Stirling DI, Kaplan G (1999) Differential cytokine modulation and T cell activation by two distinct classes of thalidomide analogues that are potent inhibitors of TNF-alpha. J Immunol 163:380–386

Crawley C, Lalancette M, Szydlo R, Gilleece M, Peggs K, Mackinnon S, Juliusson G, Ahlberg L, Nagler A, Shimoni A, Sureda A, Boiron JM, Einsele H, Chopra R, Carella A, Cavenagh J, Gratwohl A, Garban F, Zander A, Bjorkstrand B, Niederwieser D, Gahrton G, Apperley JF (2005) Outcomes for reduced-intensity allogeneic transplantation for multiple myeloma: an analysis of prognostic factors from the Chronic Leukaemia Working Party of the EBMT. Blood 105:4532–4539

Davies FE, Wu P, Jenner M, Srikanth M, Saso R, Morgan GJ (2007) The combination of cyclophosphamide, velcade and dexamethasone induces high response rates with comparable toxicity to velcade alone and velcade plus dexamethasone. Haematologica 92:1149–1150

De VJ, Hose D, Reme T, Tarte K, Moreaux J, Mahtouk K, Jourdan M, Goldschmidt H, Rossi JF, Cremer FW, Klein B (2006) Microarray-based understanding of normal and malignant plasma cells. Immunol Rev 210:86–104

Dimopoulos MA, Anagnostopoulos A (2003) Thalidomide in relapsed/refractory multiple myeloma: pivotal trials conducted outside the United States. Semin Hematol 40:8–16

Dimopoulos M, Spencer A, Attal M, Prince HM, Harousseau JL, Dmoszynska A, Yu Z, Olesnyckyj M, Zeldis JB, Knight RD (2006) Study of lenalidomide plus dexamethasone versus dex-amethasone alone in relapsed or refractory mul-tiple myeloma (MM): results of a phase 3 study (MM-010). Blood 106(11):6a

Dimopoulos M, Spencer A, Attal M, Prince HM, Harousseau JL, Dmoszynska A, San MJ, Hellmann A, Facon T, Foa R, Corso A, Masliak Z, Olesnyckyj M, Yu Z, Patin J, Zeldis JB, Knight RD (2007) Lenalidomide plus dexamethasone for relapsed or refractory multiple myeloma. N Engl J Med 357:2123–2132

Dimopoulos MA, Chen C, Spencer A, Niesvizky R, Attal M, Stadtmauer EA, Petrucci MT, Yu Z, Olesnyckyj M, Zeldis JB, Knight RD, Weber DM (2009) Long-term follow-up on overall survival from the MM-009 and MM-010 phase III trials of lenalidomide plus dexamethasone in patients with relapsed or refractory multiple myeloma. Leukemia 23:2147–2152

Fenk R, Michael M, Zohren F, Graef T, Czibere A, Bruns I, Neumann F, Fenk B, Haas R, Kobbe G (2007) Escalation therapy with bortezomib, dexamethasone and bendamustine for patients with relapsed or refractory multiple myeloma. Leuk Lymphoma 48:2345–2351

Fermand JP, Ravaud P, Chevret S, Divine M, Leblond V, Belanger C, Macro M, Pertuiset E, Dreyfus F, Mariette X, Boccacio C, Brouet JC (1998) High-dose therapy and autologous peripheral blood stem cell transplantation in multiple myeloma: up-front or rescue treatment? Results of a multicenter sequential randomized clinical trial. Blood 92:3131–3136

Fermand JP, Jaccard A, Macro M, Uzunhan Y, Allard C, Castaigne S (2006) A randomized comparison of dexamethasone thalidomide (Dex/Thal) vs Dex placebo (Dex/P) in patients (pts) with relapsing multiple myeloma (MM) [abstract ASH Annual Meeting]. Blood 108:3563

Gajate C, Mollinedo F (2007) Edelfosine and perifosine induce selective apoptosis in multiple myeloma by recruitment of death receptors and downstream signaling molecules into lipid rafts. Blood 109:711–719

Galimberti S, Benedetti E, Morabito F, Fazzi R, Pacini S, Andreazzoli F, Martino M, Iacopino P, Petrini M (2005) Chimerism does not influence graft-versus-myeloma and graft-versus-host disease in reduced intensity setting. Transpl Immunol 15:173–177

Garcia-Sanz R, Gonzalez-Porras JR, Hernandez JM, Polo-Zarzuela M, Sureda A, Barrenetxea C, Palomera L, Lopez R, Grande-Garcia C, Alegre A, Vargas-Pabon M, Gutierrez ON, Rodriguez JA, San Miguel JF (2004) The oral combination of thalidomide, cyclophosphamide and dexamethasone (ThaCyDex) is effective in relapsed/refractory multiple myeloma. Leukemia 18:856–863

Gerull S, Goerner M, Benner A, Hegenbart U, Klein U, Schaefer H, Goldschmidt H, Ho AD (2005) Long-term outcome of nonmyeloablative allogeneic transplantation in patients with high-risk multiple myeloma. Bone Marrow Transplant 36:963–969

Goldschmidt H, Hegenbart U, Wallmeier M, Hohaus S, Engenhart R, Wannenmacher M, Haas R (1997) High-dose therapy with peripheral blood progenitor cell transplantation in multiple myeloma. Ann Oncol 8:243–246

Goldschmidt H, Egerer G, Ho AD (2000) Autologous and allogeneic stem cell transplantation in multiple myeloma. Bone Marrow Transplant 25(suppl 2):S25–S26

Hideshima T, Chauhan D, Shima Y, Raje N, Davies FE, Tai YT, Treon SP, Lin B, Schlossman RL, Richardson P, Muller G, Stirling DI, Anderson KC (2000) Thalidomide and its analogs overcome drug resistance of human multiple myeloma cells to conventional therapy. Blood 96:2943–2950

Hideshima T, Catley L, Yasui H, Ishitsuka K, Raje N, Mitsiades C, Podar K, Munshi NC, Chauhan D, Richardson PG, Anderson KC (2006) Perifosine, an oral bioactive novel alkylphospholipid, inhibits Akt and induces in vitro and in vivo cytotoxicity in human multiple myeloma cells. Blood 107:4053–4062

Hussein MA, Anderson KC (2004) Role of liposomal anthracyclines in the treatment of multiple myeloma. Semin Oncol 31:147–160

Jagannath S, Barlogie B, Berenson J, Siegel D, Irwin D, Richardson PG, Niesvizky R, Alexanian R, Limentani SA, Alsina M, Adams J, Kauffman M, Esseltine DL, Schenkein DP, Anderson KC (2004) A phase 2 study of two doses of bortezomib in relapsed or refractory myeloma. Br J Haematol 127:165–172

Jagannath S, Barlogie B, Berenson JR, Siegel DS, Irwin D, Richardson PG, Niesvizky R, Alexanian R, Limentani SA, Alsina M, Esseltine DL, Anderson KC (2008) Updated survival analyses after prolonged follow-up of the phase 2, multicenter CREST study of bortezomib in relapsed or refractory multiple myeloma. Br J Haematol 143:537–540

Kastritis E, Palumbo A, Dimopoulos MA (2009) Treatment of relapsed/refractory multiple myeloma. Semin Hematol 46:143–157

Kim YK, Sohn SK, Lee JH, Yang DH, Moon JH, Ahn JS, Kim HJ, Lee JJ (2010) Clinical efficacy of a bortezomib, cyclophosphamide, thalidomide, and dexamethasone (Vel-CTD) regimen in patients with relapsed or refractory multiple myeloma: a phase II study. Ann Hematol 89:475–482

Klein U, Kosely F, Hillengass J, Hundemer M, Schmitt S, Neben K, Moehler T, Hegenbart U, Ho AD, Goldschmidt H (2009) Effective prophylaxis of thromboembolic complications with low molecular weight heparin in relapsed multiple myeloma patients treated with lenalidomide and dexamethasone. Ann Hematol 88:67–71

Knop S, Straka C, Haen M, Schwedes R, Hebart H, Einsele H (2005) The efficacy and toxicity of bendamustine in recurrent multiple myeloma after high-dose chemotherapy. Haematologica 90:1287–1288

Knop S, Gerecke C, Liebisch P, Topp MS, Platzbecker U, Sezer O, Vollmuth C, Falk K, Glasmacher A, Maeder U, Einsele H, Bargou RC (2009) Lenalidomide, adriamycin, and dexamethasone (RAD) in patients with relapsed and refractory multiple myeloma: a report from the German Myeloma Study Group DSMM (Deutsche Studiengruppe Multiples Myelom). Blood 113:4137–4143

Kroger N, Sayer HG, Schwerdtfeger R, Kiehl M, Nagler A, Renges H, Zabelina T, Fehse B, Ayuk F, Wittkowsky G, Schmitz N, Zander AR

(2002a) Unrelated stem cell transplantation in multiple myeloma after a reduced-intensity conditioning with pretransplantation antithymocyte globulin is highly effective with low transplantation-related mortality. Blood 100:3919–3924

Kroger N, Schwerdtfeger R, Kiehl M, Sayer HG, Renges H, Zabelina T, Fehse B, Togel F, Wittkowsky G, Kuse R, Zander AR (2002b) Autologous stem cell transplantation followed by a dose-reduced allograft induces high complete remission rate in multiple myeloma. Blood 100:755–760

Kropff MH, Lang N, Bisping G, Domine N, Innig G, Hentrich M, Mitterer M, Sudhoff T, Fenk R, Straka C, Heinecke A, Koch OM, Ostermann H, Berdel WE, Kienast J (2003) Hyperfractionated cyclophosphamide in combination with pulsed dexamethasone and thalidomide (HyperCDT) in primary refractory or relapsed multiple myeloma. Br J Haematol 122:607–616

Kropff M, Bisping G, Schuck E, Liebisch P, Lang N, Hentrich M, Dechow T, Kroger N, Salwender H, Metzner B, Sezer O, Engelhardt M, Wolf HH, Einsele H, Volpert S, Heinecke A, Berdel WE, Kienast J (2007) Bortezomib in combination with intermediate-dose dexamethasone and continuous low-dose oral cyclophosphamide for relapsed multiple myeloma. Br J Haematol 138:330–337

Kropff M, Baylon HG, Hillengass J, Robak T, Hajek R, Liebisch P, Goranov S, Hulin C, Blade J, Caravita T, Avet-Loiseau H, Moehler TM, Pattou C, Lucy L, Kuenburg E, Glasmacher A, Zerbib R, Facon T (2009) ASH Annual Meeting Abstracts 114:959

Kuhn DJ, Chen Q, Voorhees PM, Strader JS, Shenk KD, Sun CM, Demo SD, Bennett MK, van Leeuwen FW, Chanan-Khan AA, Orlowski RZ (2007) Potent activity of carfilzomib, a novel, irreversible inhibitor of the ubiquitin-proteasome pathway, against preclinical models of multiple myeloma. Blood 110:3281–3290

Kumar SK, Rajkumar SV, Dispenzieri A, Lacy MQ, Hayman SR, Buadi FK, Zeldenrust SR, Dingli D, Russell SJ, Lust JA, Greipp PR, Kyle RA, Gertz MA (2008) Improved survival in multiple myeloma and the impact of novel therapies. Blood 111:2516–2520

Kyriakou C, Thomson K, D'Sa S, Flory A, Hanslip J, Goldstone AH, Yong KL (2005) Low-dose thalidomide in combination with oral weekly cyclophosphamide and pulsed dexamethasone is a well tolerated and effective regimen in patients with relapsed and refractory multiple myeloma. Br J Haematol 129:763–770

Lee BJ, Sahakian G, Clarkson BD, Krakoff IH (1974) Proceedings: combination chemotherapy of multiple myeloma with alkeran, cytoxan, vincristine, prednisone, and BCNU. Cancer 33: 533–538

Lee CK, Barlogie B, Zangari M, Fassas A, Anaissie E, Morris C, Van RF, Cottler-Fox M, Thertulien R, Muwalla F, Mazher S, Badros A, Tricot G (2002) Transplantation as salvage therapy for high-risk patients with myeloma in relapse. Bone Marrow Transplant 30:873–878

Lee CK, Badros A, Barlogie B, Morris C, Zangari M, Fassas A, Van RF, Cottler-Fox M, Jacobson J, Thertulien R, Muwalla F, Mazher S, Anaissie E, Tricot G (2003a) Prognostic factors in allogeneic transplantation for patients with high-risk multiple myeloma after reduced intensity conditioning. Exp Hematol 31:73–80

Lee CK, Barlogie B, Munshi N, Zangari M, Fassas A, Jacobson J, van Rhee F, Cottler-Fox M, Muwalla F, Tricot G (2003b) DTPACE: an effective, novel combination chemotherapy with thalidomide for previously treated patients with myeloma. J Clin Oncol 21:2732–2739

Lentzsch S, O'Sullivan A, Lalo S (2009) A phase I study of Bendamustine combined with lenalidomide and dexamethasone in patients with refractory or relapsed multiple myelo114: 1856 ASH Annual Meeting Abstracts 114: 1856, 2009

List AF (2007) Lenalidomide – the phoenix rises. N Engl J Med 357:2183–2186

Lonial S (2006) Management of toxicities associated with bortezomib. Oncology (Williston Park) 20:1592–1593, 1597

Lonial S, Harousseau JL (2009) Phase 1/2 study of elotuzumab in combination with bortezomib in patients with multiple myeloma with one to three prior therapies: interim results. ASH Annual Meeting Abstracts 114:432

Lonial S, Waller EK, Richardson PG, Jagannath S, Orlowski RZ, Giver CR, Jaye DL, Francis D, Giusti S, Torre C, Barlogie B, Berenson JR, Singhal S, Schenkein DP, Esseltine DL, Anderson J, Xiao H, Heffner LT, Anderson KC (2005) Risk factors and kinetics of thrombocytopenia associated with bortezomib for relapsed, refractory multiple myeloma. Blood 106:3777–3784

Maloney DG, Molina AJ, Sahebi F, Stockerl-Goldstein KE, Sandmaier BM, Bensinger W, Storer B, Hegenbart U, Somlo G, Chauncey T, Bruno B, Appelbaum FR, Blume KG, Forman SJ, McSweeney P, Storb R (2003) Allografting with nonmyeloablative conditioning following cytoreductive autografts for the treatment of patients with multiple myeloma. Blood 102: 3447–3454

Mitsiades N, Mitsiades CS, Poulaki V, Chauhan D, Richardson PG, Hideshima T, Munshi NC, Treon SP, Anderson KC (2002) Apoptotic signaling induced by immunomodulatory thalidomide analogs in human multiple myeloma cells: therapeutic implications. Blood 99:4525–4530

Mitsiades CS, Mitsiades NS, Munshi NC, Richardson PG, Anderson KC (2006) The role of the bone microenvironment in the pathophysiology and therapeutic management of multiple myeloma: interplay of growth factors, their receptors and stromal interactions. Eur J Cancer 42: 1564–1573

Moehler TM, Neben K, Benner A, Egerer G, Krasniqi F, Ho AD, Goldschmidt H (2001) Salvage therapy for multiple myeloma with thalidomide and CED chemotherapy. Blood 98:3846–3848

Morgan GJ, Shey SA, Wu P, Srikanth M, Phekoo KJ, Jenner M, Davies FE (2007) Lenalidomide (Revlimide), in combination with cyclophosphamide and dexamethasone (RCD), is an effective and tolerated regimen for myeloma patients. Br J Hematol 137:268–269

Muller GW, Chen R, Huang SY, Corral LG, Wong LM, Patterson RT, Chen Y, Kaplan G, Stirling DI (1999) Amino-substituted thalidomide analogs: potent inhibitors of TNF-alpha production. Bioorg Med Chem Lett 9:1625–1630

Nucci M, Anaissie E (2009) Infections in patients with multiple myeloma in the era of high-dose therapy and novel agents. Clin Infect Dis 49:1211–1225

Offidani M, Corvatta L, Piersantelli MN, Visani G, Alesiani F, Brunori M, Galieni P, Catarini M, Burattini M, Centurioni R, Ferranti M, Rupoli S, Scortechini AR, Giuliodori L, Candela M, Capelli D, Montanari M, Olivieri A, Poloni A, Polloni C, Marconi M, Leoni P (2006) Thalidomide, dexamethasone, and pegylated liposomal doxorubicin (ThaDD) for patients older than 65 years with newly diagnosed multiple myeloma. Blood 108:2159–2164

Olin RL, Vogl DT, Porter DL, Luger SM, Schuster SJ, Tsai DE, Siegel DL, Cook RJ, Mangan PA, Cunningham K, Stadtmauer EA (2009) Second auto-SCT is safe and effective salvage therapy for relapsed multiple myeloma. Bone Marrow Transplant 43:417–422

Orlowski RZ, Voorhees PM, Garcia RA, Hall MD, Kudrik FJ, Allred T, Johri AR, Jones PE, Ivanova A, Van Deventer HW, Gabriel DA, Shea TC, Mitchell BS, Adams J, Esseltine DL, Trehu EG, Green M, Lehman MJ, Natoli S, Collins JM, Lindley CM, Dees EC (2005) Phase 1 trial of the proteasome inhibitor bortezomib and pegylated liposomal doxorubicin in patients with advanced hematologic malignancies. Blood 105: 3058–3065

Orlowski RZ, Nagler A, Sonneveld P, Blade J, Hajek R, Spencer A, San MJ, Robak T, Dmoszynska A, Horvath N, Spicka I, Sutherland HJ, Suvorov AN, Zhuang SH, Parekh T, Xiu L, Yuan Z, Rackoff W, Harousseau JL (2007) Randomized phase III study of pegylated liposomal doxorubicin plus bortezomib compared with bortezomib alone in relapsed or refractory multiple myeloma: combination therapy improves time to progression. J Clin Oncol 25: 3892–3901

Palumbo A, Bringhen S, Musto P, Caravita T, Capozzi R, Callea V, Cangialosi C, Montanaro M, Catalano L, Grasso M, Petti MC, Merla M, Falchi L, Omedè P, Ceccarelli M, Ambrosini MT, Avonto I, Gay F, Falco P, Boccadoro M (2006) Oral melphalan, prednisone and thalidomide for multiple myeloma. Blood 106(11):230

Palumbo A, Ambrosini MT, Benevolo G, Pregno P, Pescosta N, Callea V, Cangialosi C, Caravita T, Morabito F, Musto P, Bringhen S, Falco P, Avonto I, Cavallo F, Boccadoro M (2007) Bortezomib, melphalan, prednisone, and thalidomide for relapsed multiple myeloma. Blood 109:2767–2772

Palumbo A, Gay F, Bringhen S, Falcone A, Pescosta N, Callea V, Caravita T, Morabito F, Magarotto V, Ruggeri M, Avonto I, Musto P, Cascavilla N, Bruno B, Boccadoro M (2008a) Bortezomib, doxorubicin and dexamethasone in advanced multiple myeloma. Ann Oncol 19:1160–1165

Palumbo A, Rajkumar SV, Dimopoulos MA, Richardson PG, San MJ, Barlogie B, Harousseau J, Zonder JA, Cavo M, Zangari M,

Attal M, Belch A, Knop S, Joshua D, Sezer O, Ludwig H, Vesole D, Blade J, Kyle R, Westin J, Weber D, Bringhen S, Niesvizky R, Waage A, von Lilienfeld-Toal M, Lonial S, Morgan GJ, Orlowski RZ, Shimizu K, Anderson KC, Boccadoro M, Durie BG, Sonneveld P, Hussein MA (2008b) Prevention of thalidomide- and lenalidomide-associated thrombosis in myeloma. Leukemia 22:414–423

Palumbo A, Larocca A, Falco P, Sanpaolo G, Falcone AP, Federico V, Canepa L, Crugnola M, Genuardi M, Magarotto V, Petrucci MT, Boccadoro M (2010) Lenalidomide, melphalan, prednisone and thalidomide (RMPT) for relapsed/refractory multiple myeloma. Leukemia 24:1037–1042

Parlati F, Lee SJ, Aujay M, Suzuki E, Levitsky K, Lorens JB, Micklem DR, Ruurs P, Sylvain C, Lu Y, Shenk KD, Bennett MK (2009) Carfilzomib can induce tumor cell death through selective inhibition of the chymotrypsin-like activity of the proteasome. Blood 114:3439–3447

Perez-Simon JA, Martino R, Alegre A, Tomas JF, De LA, Caballero D, Sureda A, Sierra J, San Miguel JF (2003) Chronic but not acute graft-versus-host disease improves outcome in multiple myeloma patients after non-myeloablative allogeneic transplantation. Br J Haematol 121(1):104–108

Pineda-Roman M, Zangari M, Van RF, Anaissie E, Szymonifka J, Hoering A, Petty N, Crowley J, Shaughnessy J, Epstein J, Barlogie B (2008) VTD combination therapy with bortezomib-thalidomide-dexamethasone is highly effective in advanced and refractory multiple myeloma. Leukemia 22(7):1419–1427

Podar K, Tai YT, Davies FE, Lentzsch S, Sattler M, Hideshima T, Lin BK, Gupta D, Shima Y, Chauhan D, Mitsiades C, Raje N, Richardson P, Anderson KC (2001) Vascular endothelial growth factor triggers signaling cascades mediating multiple myeloma cell growth and migration. Blood 98:428–435

Ponisch W, Mitrou PS, Merkle K, Herold M, Assmann M, Wilhelm G, Dachselt K, Richter P, Schirmer V, Schulze A, Subert R, Harksel B, Grobe N, Stelzer E, Schulze M, Bittrich A, Freund M, Pasold R, Friedrich T, Helbig W, Niederwieser D (2006) Treatment of bendamustine and prednisone in patients with newly diagnosed multiple myeloma results in superior complete response rate, prolonged time to treatment failure and improved quality of life compared to treatment with melphalan and prednisone – a randomized phase III study of the East German Study Group of Hematology and Oncology (OSHO). J Cancer Res Clin Oncol 132:205–212

Popat R, Oakervee H, Williams C, Cook M, Craddock C, Basu S, Singer C, Harding S, Foot N, Hallam S, Odeh L, Joel S, Cavenagh J (2009) Bortezomib, low-dose intravenous melphalan, and dexamethasone for patients with relapsed multiple myeloma. Br J Haematol 144:887–894

Reece DE, Rodriguez GP, Chen C, Trudel S, Kukreti V, Mikhael J, Pantoja M, Xu W, Stewart AK (2008) Phase I-II trial of bortezomib plus oral cyclophosphamide and prednisone in relapsed and refractory multiple myeloma. J Clin Oncol 26:4777–4783

Reece D, Song KW, Fu T, Roland B, Chang H, Horsman DE, Mansoor A, Chen C, Masih-Khan E, Trieu Y, Bruyere H, Stewart DA, Bahlis NJ (2009) Influence of cytogenetics in patients with relapsed or refractory multiple myeloma treated with lenalidomide plus dexamethasone: adverse effect of deletion 17p13. Blood 114:522–525

Richardson PG, Barlogie B, Berenson J, Singhal S, Jagannath S, Irwin D, Rajkumar SV, Srkalovic G, Alsina M, Alexanian R, Siegel D, Orlowski RZ, Kuter D, Limentani SA, Lee S, Hideshima T, Esseltine DL, Kauffman M, Adams J, Schenkein DP, Anderson KC (2003) A phase 2 study of bortezomib in relapsed, refractory myeloma. N Engl J Med 348:2609–2617

Richardson PG, Sonneveld P, Schuster MW, Irwin D, Stadtmauer EA, Facon T, Harousseau JL, Ben-Yehuda D, Lonial S, Goldschmidt H, Reece D, San-Miguel JF, Blade J, Boccadoro M, Cavenagh J, Dalton WS, Boral AL, Esseltine DL, Porter JB, Schenkein D, Anderson KC (2005) Bortezomib or high-dose dexamethasone for relapsed multiple myeloma. N Engl J Med 352:2487–2498

Richardson P, Schlossmann R, Munshi N, Avigan D, Jagannath S, Alsina M, Doss D, McKenney M, Hande K, Farrell M, Gorelik S, Colson K, Warren D, Lunde L, Michelle R, Cole G, Mitsiades C, Hideshima T, Myers T, Knight R, Anderson K (2006a) A phase 1 trial of lenalidomide (REVLIMID) with bortezomib (VELCADE) in relapsed and refractory multiple myeloma. Blood 11:110a

Richardson PG, Blood E, Mitsiades CS, Jagannath S, Zeldenrust SR, Alsina M, Schlossman RL, Rajkumar SV, Desikan KR, Hideshima T, Munshi NC, Kelly-Colson K, Doss D, McKenney ML, Gorelik S, Warren D, Freeman A, Rich R, Wu A, Olesnyckyj M, Wride K, Dalton WS, Zeldis J, Knight R, Weller E, Anderson KC (2006b) A randomized phase 2 study of lenalidomide therapy for patients with relapsed or relapsed and refractory multiple myeloma. Blood 108: 3458–3464

Richardson P, Mitsiades C, Schlossman R, Ghobrial I, Hideshima T, Chauhan D, Munshi N, Anderson K (2007a) The treatment of relapsed and refractory multiple myeloma. Hematol Am Soc Hematol Educ Program 2007:317–323

Richardson PG, Jagannath S, Raje N, Jakubowiak A, Lonial S, Ghobrial I et al (2007b) Lenalidomide, bortezomib, and dexamethasone (Rev/Vel/Dex) in patients with relapsed or relapsed/refractory multiple myeloma (MM): preliminary results of a phase II study. Blood 110:2714

Richardson P, Mitsiades C, Colson K, Reilly E, McBride L, Chiao J, Sun L, Ricker J, Rizvi S, Oerth C, Atkins B, Fearen I, Anderson K, Siegel D (2008) Phase I trial of oral vorinostat (suberoylanilide hydroxamic acid, SAHA) in patients with advanced multiple myeloma. Leuk Lymphoma 49:502–507

Richardson PG, Weller E, Jagannath S, Avigan DE, Alsina M, Schlossman RL, Mazumder A, Munshi NC, Ghobrial IM, Doss D, Warren DL, Lunde LE, McKenney M, Delaney C, Mitsiades CS, Hideshima T, Dalton W, Knight R, Esseltine DL, Anderson KC (2009a) Multicenter, phase I, dose-escalation trial of lenalidomide plus bortezomib for relapsed and relapsed/refractory multiple myeloma. J Clin Oncol 27: 5713–5719

Richardson P, Hofmeister C, Jakubowiak A, Zimmerman TM, Spear MA, Palladino MA, Longenecker AM, Kelly SL, Neuteboom S, Cropp GF, Lloyd GK, Hannah AL, Anderson KC (2009b) Phase 1 clinical trial of the novel structure proteasome inhibitor NPI-0052 in patients with relapsed and relapsed/refractory multiple myeloma (MM). ASH Annual Meeting Abstracts (114):431

Richardson PG, Weller E, Lonial S, Jakubowiak AJ, Jagannath S, Raje NS, Avigan DE, Xie W, Ghobrial IM, Schlossman RL, Mazumder A, Munshi NC, Vesole DH, Joyce R, Kaufman JL, Doss D, Warren DL, Lunde LE, Kaster S, Delaney C, Hideshima T, Mitsiades CS, Knight R, Esseltine DL, Anderson KC (2010) Lenalidomide, bortezomib, and dexamethasone combination therapy in patients with newly diagnosed multiple myeloma. Blood 116:679–686

Rotta M, Storer BE, Sahebi F, Shizuru JA, Bruno B, Lange T, Agura ED, McSweeney PA, Pulsipher MA, Hari P, Maziarz RT, Chauncey TR, Appelbaum FR, Sorror ML, Bensinger W, Sandmaier BM, Storb RF, Maloney DG (2009) Long-term outcome of patients with multiple myeloma after autologous hematopoietic cell transplantation and nonmyeloablative allografting. Blood 113:3383–3391

Schey SA, Fields P, Bartlett JB, Clarke IA, Ashan G, Knight RD, Streetly M, Dalgleish AG (2004) Phase I study of an immunomodulatory thalidomide analog, CC-4047, in relapsed or refractory multiple myeloma. J Clin Oncol 22:3269–3276

Schey SA, Morgan GJ, Ramasamy K, Hazel B, Ladon D, Corderoy S, Jenner M, Phekoo K, Boyd K, Davies FE (2010) The addition of cyclophosphamide to lenalidomide and dexamethasone in multiply relapsed/refractory myeloma patients; a phase I/II study. Br J Haematol

Siegel D (2009) An ongoing open-label, phase II study of single-agent carfilzomib (CFZ) in patients with relapsed or refractory myeloma (MM): updated results from the bortezomib-treated cohort. ASH Annual Meeting Abstracts 114:303

Singhal S, Mehta J, Desikan R, Ayers D, Roberson P, Eddlemon P, Munshi N, Anaissie E, Wilson C, Dhodapkar M, Zeddis J, Barlogie B (1999) Antitumor activity of thalidomide in refractory multiple myeloma. N Engl J Med 341:1565–1571

Sonneveld P, Hajek R, Nagler A, Spencer A, Blade J, Robak T, Zhuang SH, Harousseau JL, Orlowski RZ (2008) Combined pegylated liposomal doxorubicin and bortezomib is highly effective in patients with recurrent or refractory multiple myeloma who received prior thalidomide/lenalidomide therapy. Cancer 112:1529–1537

Spencer A, Millward M, Mainwaring P, Harrison S, Catley L, Townsend A, Sukumaran S, Longenecker AM, Palladino MA, Lloyd GK, Neuteboom S, Padrik P, Spear MA, Price T (2009) Phase 1 clinical trial of the novel structure proteasome inhibitor NPI-0052. ASH Annual Meeting Abstracts (114):2693

Storb R, Yu C, Sandmaier B, McSweeney P, Georges G, Nash R, Woolfrey A (1999) Mixed hematopoietic chimerism after hematopoietic stem cell allografts. Transplant Proc 31:677–678

Streetly MJ, Gyertson K, Daniel Y, Zeldis JB, Kazmi M, Schey SA (2008) Alternate day pomalidomide retains anti-myeloma effect with reduced adverse events and evidence of in vivo immunomodulation. Br J Haematol 141:41–51

Terpos E, Dimopoulos MA, Sezer O (2007a) The effect of novel anti-myeloma agents on bone metabolism of patients with multiple myeloma. Leukemia 21:1875–1884

Terpos E, Sezer O, Croucher P, Dimopoulos MA (2007b) Myeloma bone disease and proteasome inhibition therapies. Blood 110:1098–1104

Terpos E, Kastritis E, Roussou M, Heath D, Christoulas D, Anagnostopoulos N, Eleftherakis-Papaiakovou E, Tsionos K, Croucher P, Dimopoulos MA (2008) The combination of bortezomib, melphalan, dexamethasone and intermittent thalidomide is an effective regimen for relapsed/refractory myeloma and is associated with improvement of abnormal bone metabolism and angiogenesis. Leukemia 22:2247–2256

van de Donk NW, Lokhorst HM, Dimopoulos M, Cavo M, Morgan G, Einsele H, Kropff M, Schey S, vet-Loiseau H, Ludwig H, Goldschmidt H, Sonneveld P, Johnsen HE, Blade J, San-Miguel JF, Palumbo A (2010a) Treatment of relapsed and refractory multiple myeloma in the era of novel agents. Cancer Treat Rev. Sep 20 [epub]

van de Donk NW, Wittebol S, Minnema MC, Lokhorst HM (2010b) Lenalidomide (RevlIMiD) combined with continuous oral cyclophosphamide (endoxan) and prednisone (REP) is effective in lenalidomide/dexamethasone-refractory myeloma. Br J Haematol 148:335–337

van Rhee F, Dhodapkar M, Shaughnessy JD Jr, Anaissie E, Siegel D, Hoering A, Zeldis J, Jenkins B, Singhal S, Mehta J, Crowley J, Jagannath S, Barlogie B (2008) First thalidomide clinical trial in multiple myeloma: a decade. Blood 112:1035–1038

Vesole DH, Zhang L, Flomenberg N, Greipp PR, Lazarus HM, Huff CA (2009) A Phase II trial of autologous stem cell transplantation followed by mini-allogeneic stem cell transplantation for the treatment of multiple myeloma: an analysis of Eastern Cooperative Oncology Group ECOG E4A98 and E1A97. Biol Blood Marrow Transplant 15:83–91

von Lilienfeld-Toal M, Hahn-Ast C, Furkert K, Hoffmann F, Naumann R, Bargou R, Cook G, Glasmacher A (2008) A systematic review of phase II trials of thalidomide/dexamethasone combination therapy in patients with relapsed or refractory multiple myeloma. Eur J Haematol 81:247–252

Weber DM, Chen C, Niesvizky R, Wang M, Belch A, Stadtmauer EA, Siegel D, Borrello I, Rajkumar SV, Chanan-Khan AA, Lonial S, Yu Z, Patin J, Olesnyckyj M, Zeldis JB, Knight RD (2007) Lenalidomide plus dexamethasone for relapsed multiple myeloma in North America. N Engl J Med 357:2133–2142

Allogeneic Transplantation in Multiple Myeloma

12

Gösta Gahrton

Contents

G. Gahrton
Department of Medicine, Karolinska Institutet and Karolinska University Hospital Huddinge, SE-141 86, Stockholm, Sweden
e-mail: gosta.gahrton@ki.se

Abstract Allogeneic hematopoietic stem cell transplantation in multiple myeloma has been performed since the 1980th, but is still a controversial treatment modality. The aim is to cure the disease and the rational is to eradicate myeloma cells by the dual effect of high dose myeloablative treatment, and the immune reaction against the myeloma cells by the graft (graft versus myeloma =GVM). At the same time the patient is saved from myeloablation by the normal allogeneic donor stem cells. Although outcome has improved with time the transplant related mortality using myeloablation is still high. Therefore reduced intensity non-myelablative conditioning (RIC) has increasingly substituted myeloablation and results have improved. Out of five published or ongoing prospective clinical trials using tandem autologous (ASCT) – RIC-allogeneic transplantation (RIC-allo) compared to tandem or single ASCT the tandem ASCT-RIC-Allo approach was superior. Attempts to improve outcome by adding new drugs (thalidomide, bortezomib or lenalidomide) or alternative cell therapies like donor T-cell infusions or NK cell treatment may improve results.

T. Moehler and H. Goldschmidt (eds.), *Multiple Myeloma*,
Recent Results in Cancer Research 183, DOI: 10.1007/978-3-540-85772-3_12,

12.1 Introduction

The idea of allogeneic transplantation for multiple myeloma is as in other malignant disorders fourfold. Firstly, high-dose cytotoxic drug or irradiation conditioning treatment before the transplant should eradicate as many malignant cells as possible. Secondly, the conditioning will suppress patient's immunocompetence to prevent graft failure. Thirdly, the graft should save the patient from the myeloablative effect of the conditioning by support with normal hematopoietic stem cells. Fourthly, immunocompetent cells in the graft will kill malignant cells by a graft-versus-myeloma (GVM) effect. The recently introduced so-called reduced-intensity non-myeloablative conditioning (RIC) accepts that the conditioning will eradicate less malignant cells than myeloablative treatment in order to diminish side effects. The RIC approach relies comparatively more on the GVM effect than myeloablative conditioning. Since none of the two approaches – myeloablative or RIC – seems to cure but perhaps a very small fraction of patients, additional treatments are frequently tried, such as posttransplant donor lymphocyte transfusion, posttransplant new drug treatments, etc. Recently, NK cell infusions have been tried both before and after transplantation.

12.2 Myeloablative High Dose Conditioning

The EBMT registry has now reports on more than 5,000 allogeneic myeloma transplants, of which somewhat less than 50% have been performed with myeloablative conditioning. Transplants using myeloablation have decreased somewhat since the introduction of RIC, and was about 150/year from 2002 to 2007. High-dose cyclophosphamide + total body irradiation (TBI) 10–12 Gy, fractionated or unfractionated with lung shielding, is the most commonly performed conditioning regimen, followed by melphalan + TBI (Gahrton et al. 2007). However, many other myeloablative protocols are used, such as busulfan + cyclophosphamide and combinations usually including parts of these regimens.

Myeloablative conditioning is hampered by high transplant-related mortality (TRM) reaching 30–40% (Gahrton et al. 1991). One reason is high incidence of severe graft-versus-host disease (GVHD). Another is significant relapse/progression rate (RL). Although RL was shown to be lower than with autologous transplantation already in 1996 in an EBMT retrospective case-matched analysis of 378 patients, the overall survival (OS) was at this time inferior due to the high transplant-related mortality (Bjorkstrand et al. 1996). However, in females, the treatment-related mortality was lower than in males, and therefore resulting in similar OS in females treated with autologous and allogeneic transplantation. Long-term survival appeared better in allogeneic transplants than in autologous ones in females, and was 30% at 9 years among the allotransplants. Later a large retrospective EBMT study (Gahrton et al. 2005) has confirmed the comparatively good results in females, in particular female to female transplants, while the worst results occurred in male patients irrespective of donor, apparently due to a lower RL but a higher TRM in sex-mismatched recipient/donor transplants, and the reverse in sex-matched male transplants. These differences seem to be due to the presence of female donor T cells that are specific for male minor histocompatibility antigens (H-Y) encoded by male Y chromosome genes. Attempts are presently being made to use or modulate minor histocompatibility antigens to improve GVM (Hambach et al. 2007).

Severe infections, often combined with severe GVHD, are the main causes of death following myeloablative allogeneic transplantation. New supportive treatment modalities, for example new antibiotics, better GVHD prevention methods, etc., seem to be reasons why myeloablative allogeneic transplant results improved dramatically with time, as shown in a comparison by EBMT of transplants performed before and after 1994 (Gahrton et al. 2001). TRM was reduced significantly, and the median OS for the later transplants was 50 months. However, the TRM was still high and myeloablative allogeneic transplantation is therefore now only rarely performed.

12.3 Molecular Remission

Molecular remissions are more frequent after myeloablative allogeneic transplantation than after autologous transplantation even when the intensity in the conditioning regimens is similar. Using clonal markers based on the rearrangement of immunoglobulin heavy-chain genes generated for each myeloma patient at diagnosis and used for polymerized chain reaction detection of residual myeloma cells after transplantation, in one study (Corradini et al. 1999), it has been shown that out of 29 patients who entered hematological remission after transplantation, 9 out of 14 entered molecular remission after allogeneic transplantation, and 2 out of 15 after autologous. In three of the allogeneic transplants, molecular remission occurred later than 3 years after transplant, while late molecular remissions were not seen in autologous transplants, indicating a GVM effect in allogeneic transplants. Further studies (Corradini et al. 2003) showed that in 48 patients who obtained a hematological remission following allogeneic transplantation, 16 (33%) obtained durable PCR-negativity after transplantation, while 13 (27%) remained persistently PCR-positive, and 19 (30%) showed a mixed pattern. The cumulative risk of relapse at 5 years was none for PCR-negative, 33% for PCR-mixed, and 100% for PCR-positive patients. Thus, molecular remission is more common in myeloablative allogeneic transplantation and molecular remission predicts for longer relapse-free survival. Attempts to induce molecular remission seem important, although it is not settled if myeloablation or GVM is the most important factor. Since myeloablation is associated with high TRM, attempts to obtain molecular remissions should focus on other means, such as new drugs, GVM, or specific antimyeloma cell therapy in combination with the RIC approach (below).

12.4 Source of Stem Cells

As in other malignant hematological malignancies treated with allogeneic stem cell transplantation, bone marrow (BM) was originally the stem cell source, but today most transplants are performed with peripheral blood stem cells (PBSC). In the EBMT registry, the great majority of reported allogeneic transplants are now performed with PBSC.

An EBMT analysis of 1,667 patients who had received a first allogeneic identical sibling donor transplant with BM or PBSC from 1994 to 2003 and reported to the EBMT data base was recently performed. Out of these patients 1,179 had received PBSC and 488 BM. The engraftment rate was more rapid with PBSC irrespective of the intensity in the conditioning regimen. Otherwise, there was no significant difference in TRM, RL, or response to treatment dependent on the source of stem cells. Overall, chronic GVHD (cGVHD) was more frequent with PBSC than with BM, while acute GVHD (aGVHD) was similar. In a multivariate analysis, the higher rate of chronic GVHD did not translate into any detectable difference in RL due to the cell source. Thus, even if there are minor differences in some parameters, the use

12

of PBSC or BM results in similar OS. For practical purposes, PBSC is today the most commonly used method.

12.5 Reduced Intensity conditioning (RIC)

12.5.1 Retrospective Studies

The Seattle Group developed an allogeneic transplant modality using considerably lower intensity in the conditioning regimen than had previously been used, i.e., 2 Gy total body irradiation followed posttransplant by GVHD prevention with mycophenolate moffetil and cyclosporin (Maloney et al. 2003). The rational was that the GVM effect may be more important than the intensity of the conditioning regimens.TRM was significantly reduced. Later, this regimen was used with added fludarabine (30 mg/m^2 x 3) in the conditioning in 24 refractory or relapsed patients that received an allogeneic transplant from an unrelated donor either preceded by an autologous transplant (13 patients) or proceeding directly to an allogeneic transplantation (11 patients) (Georges et al. 2007). At 3-year follow-up, OS was 61% for all patients and better in the tandem transplant group (77%).

Another RIC transplant modality is conditioning with melphalan 100–140 mg/m^2 + fludarabine 30 mg/m^2 × 5. Ayuk et al. (2008) used this conditioning in 57 patients. A fraction of patients received ATG (antithymocyte globulin) and other patients alemtuzumab. The treatment-related mortality was 11% at 100 days and 70% at 1 year in their first report, i.e., considerably lower than is seen with myeloablative conditioning. Fifty-five percent obtained complete remission and 27% partial remission, i.e., a response rate of 82%. Overall and disease-free survival were 68% and 42%, respectively, at 49 months.

RIC has recently been compared retrospectively to myeloablative conditioning by the EBMT (Crawley et al. 2007). Patients were generally in a relatively advanced stage of disease, and the median age was somewhat higher than in later prospective studies. A dose of melphalan less than 140 mg/m^2, a busulfan dose of 8 mg/kg or less, and a cyclophosphamide dose of less than 120 mg/kg were considered to be reduced intensity. If TBI was used, a dose of radiation less than 6 Gy or up to 6 Gy fractionated was accepted as RIC. With this definition, RIC was associated with lower TRM but higher RL than with myeloablative conditioning. The progression-free survival (PFS) was superior with myeloablative conditioning, but there was no significant difference in OS. Both ATG and alemtuzumab were associated with higher RL and alemtuzumab in addition with poorer PFS and OS.

12.5.2 Prospective Studies

There are currently five known ongoing or closed prospective studies comparing RIC allotransplants to autologous transplants. In these studies, the RIC allotransplant is performed after a first autologous transplant (Tables 12.1 and 12.2). They are based on so-called genetic randomization, i.e., patients with an HLA-identical sibling are offered a RIC allotransplant after the autologous transplant. Those patients that lack an HLA-identical sibling receive either one or two autologous transplants. Autologous stem cell transplantation is the standard method to treat patients with multiple myeloma up to 65–70 years of age. Autologous transplantation is usually performed after an induction period using combinations like VAD (vincristine, doxorubicine, dexamethasone) or recently combinations including thalidomide, bortezomib, or lenalidomide. The conditioning regimen is usually 200-mg melphalan/m^2.

Table 12.1 Patients and transplant characteristics in five prospective studies comparing RIC allotransplants with autotransplants

Group/author	Inclusion criteria	Conditioning for RIC allotransplantation	Study design
IFM/Garban et al. (2006), Moreau et al. (2008)	High-risk (high β_2 micro)	Fludarabine/busulfan/ATG	Auto/allo vs auto/auto
Italian Group/Bruno et al. (2007)	All patients	TBI 2 Gy	Auto/allo vs auto/auto
PETHEMA/Rosinol et al. (2008)	Patients < 70 years No CR/nCR after first Auto	Melphalan/fludarabine	Auto/allo vs auto/auto
HOVON/Lokhorst et al. (2008)	Patients < 66 years	TBI 2 Gy	Auto/allo vs auto/maintenance
EBMT/Björkstrand et al. (2008), Gahrton et al. (2009)	Patients < 70 years	TBI 2 Gy/fludarabine	Auto/allo vs auto or auto/auto

Table 12.2 Results of five studies comparing tandem autologous/RIC allotransplantation versus autologous transplantation

Group/author	No. of patients RICallo/auto	CR rate (%)	EFS months (median)	OS months (median)
IFM/Garban et al. (2006), Moreau et al. (2008)	Intention to treat 65/219 Received correct treatment 46/166	62 vs 51(CR + VGPR) (p=NS)	19 vs 22 (p=0.58)	34 vs 48 (p=0.07)
Italian Group/Bruno et al. (2007)	80 vs 82	55 vs 26 (p=0.004)	35 vs 29 (p=0.02)	80 vs 54 (p=0.01)
PETHEMA/Rosinol et al. (2008)	25 vs 85 failing nCR or CR after first auto	40 vs 11 (p=0.001)	PFS not reached vs 31 (p=0.08)	PFS not reached vs 58 (p=0.9)
HOVON/Lokhorst et al. (2008)	Intention to treat 126/141 Received correct treatment 101/115	45 vs 42	39% vs 34% at 4 years (p=NS)	56% vs 63% at 4 years (p=NS)
EBMT/Björkstrand et al. (2008), Gahrton et al. (2009)	Intention to treat 108/249 Received correct treatment 98 vs 250	51 vs 41	PFS 35% vs 18% at 60 months	65% vs 58% at 60 months

IFM (Intergroup Francais de Myelom) included 65 patients in the auto-allo group, and 219 patients in the auto-auto group in the first published prospective study. In the first report of this trial (Garban et al. 2006), there was no significant difference in event-free survival but a trend for better OS in the auto-auto group compared to the auto-allo group (median 48 vs 34 months; $p=0.07$) based on an intention to treat analysis. If only those patients who actually received the auto-allo transplant (46 patients) or tandem auto transplant (166 patients) were analyzed, there was still a trend for better OS in the auto-auto group (median OS 57 vs 41 months; $p = .08$). This study was recently updated after a median follow-up of 56 months (Moreau et al. 2008), and results were mainly the same, i.e., no significant difference between auto-auto and auto-allo transplantation neither with respect to OS ($p=0.07$) nor with respect to event-free survival, but a slight trend for superior OS in the auto-auto group both if analysis was made on an intention to treat basis and if comparing only those patients that actually received the correct transplant combination. No such trend was seen for event-free survival (EFS).

In this study, only patients under 65 years were included, and the serum beta-2 microglobulin had to be >3 mg/L and patients had to have deletion of chromosome 13. The reduced-intensity conditioning was busulfan + fludarabine and high-dose ATG. Thus the conditioning was very different from the original Seattle protocol, particularly concerning the high-dose ATG, which has been shown in retrospective EBMT studies to be an adverse prognostic factor (Crawley et al. 2007). Still, the result of the IFM study discouraged from performing allotransplants in multiple myeloma.

Later Bruno et al. (2007) showed a superior OS for patients who received auto-allo transplantation. Two hundred and forty-five patients were included at diagnosis. HLA typing was performed in 162: 80 of these had an HLA-identical sibling donor, and 82 patients had none and comprised the control group. Only 58 patients completed the auto-allo transplant and 46 the auto-auto transplant. Whether analyzed as an intention to treat, i.e., HLA typing had been performed, or based on the actual treatment, there was a significant advantage of having an identical sibling or performing an auto-allotransplantation, respectively. Patients were followed up to 84 months posttransplant. The survival advantage for the auto-allo regimen was seen after about 2-year follow-up. Thus, the major advantage was improved long-term survival in the auto-allo group.

The PETHEMA Group (Rosinol et al. 2008) has recently presented a third study. Only those patients who did not enter a complete remission or a near-complete remission at the first autologous transplantation were included in the comparison between auto-allo and auto-auto transplantation. One hundred and ten patients had a second transplant; 25 of them a RIC-allo transplant. Although, with this relatively small material, there was no significant difference between auto-RICallo transplants and auto–auto transplants in event-free survival or OS, the shapes of the curves were similar to those in the study by the Italian group (Bruno et al. 2007). The allo-RIC transplants deviated at around 2 years from transplant to form a horizontal curve, and the p value was 0.08.

The HOVON Group presented a fourth study at the ASH meeting in 2008 (Lokhorst et al. 2008). Following an autologous transplantation, patients were treated with either RIC-allo or maintenance with thalidomide or interferon, based on the availability of an identical sibling donor. The conditioning regimen was TBI 200 cGY, i.e., the original Seattly regiment and the same as in the Italian study. Out of 126 patients that had a donor, 101 received the RIC transplant, and out of 141 who had not 115 entered the study. After a median follow-up of 38 months, there was no significant difference between the two groups neither in OS nor in PFS. The 48 months OS was 56% and 63% and PFS 39% and 34% in the auto-allo and auto-maintenance group, respectively.

EBMT has an ongoing fifth study that started in 1999 (Björkstrand et al. 2008).

Previously untreated patients receive VAD or VAD-like induction treatment, and must have a response status of at least stable disease (CR, PR, or SD) at the time of inclusion at the first autologous transplantation. Patients with an HLA-identical sibling then proceed to RIC-allo, while those without a matched sibling receive no further treatment or a second autologous transplant. In the recently updated study (Gahrton et al. 2009), 357 patients are included, and median follow-up is 61 months. One hundred and eight patients were allocated to the RIC-allo group (91 actually received the allotransplant) and 249 to the Auto group. In an intention to treat analysis, OS at 60 months is 65% in the RIC-allo group and 58% in the auto group and PFS is 35% and 18%, respectively, at this time. The relapse/progression rate was lower with RIC allo and seen both in patients with and in those without the del13 chromosomal abnormality. Although the TRM at 24 months was expectedly higher (12%) in the RIC allo patients, the outcome overall was superior in this group.

The conditioning regimen before RIC-allo differs in the five studies. Only IFM used high-dose ATG. Fludarabine was as well used in the IFM study and also in the studies by PETHEMA and EBMT. The Italian and HOVON studies used only 2 Gy TBI without immunosuppression, i.e., the original Seattle regimen. Thus none of the studies showing a better outcome or a tendency for better outcome with RIC-allo as compared to autologous transplantation used ATG in the conditioning. The impact of ATG treatment on outcome has been debated (Gahrton and Bjorkstrand 2008). It may be possible that certain ATG types, like the Jurkart T-cell line–derived ATG, may have a GVHD preventive effect without significant prevention of GVM (Ayuk et al. 2008), while others have an adverse effect on outcome as shown in a retrospective EBMT study (Crawley et al. 2007).

12.6 How to Improve Results of Allogeneic Transplantation?

It is not obvious how to improve outcome with allogeneic transplantation. There are several different possibilities, among them including new drugs in the conditioning regimen or using them for induction pretransplant or for maintenance posttransplant. Other possibilities may be to optimize donor lymphocyte transfusions posttransplant, to use natural killer cells (NK) posttransplant either preemptive or at early signs of relapse or pretransplant. Also, using unrelated donors after high-resolution HLA typing may be as good, or even better than using sibling donors for long-term outcome.

12.6.1 Donor Lymphocyte Transfusions

Donor lymphocytes transfusions to treat relapse following allogeneic transplantations may induce about 30–40% responses in relapsed patients that may last for more than 2 years. Donor lymphocyte transfusions frequently cause GVHD, and the response is often associated with cGVHD. Escalating dosages of DLI were used in a multinational multicenter study (van de Donk et al. 2006) of 63 patients who were refractory or had relapsed after RIC allogeneic transplantation. Twenty-four patients responded – 12 of them with CR. The OS was 23.6 months from the time of DLI, and in responders, PFS was 27.8 months. Major toxicities were GVHD (38.1%) and chronic GVHD (42.9%), and seven patients (11.1%) died from treatment-related mortality.

This study illustrates that although responses of significant duration can be obtained with DLI, GVHD is rarely separated from GVM.

12.6.2 NK Cells Have Antimyeloma Effect and Moderate GVHD

There are experimental evidence that NK cells have an antimyeloma cell effect (Alici et al. 2007). Recent studies in a mouse myeloma model have shown improved survival following autologous NK cell treatment when used together with IL2. Also, in vitro studies have shown killing of human myeloma cells by expanded autologous human NK cells (Alici et al. 2008). In the allogeneic setting, NK cells have been related to increased efficacy and improved survival of patients with acute leukemia transplanted with haploidentical T-cell-depleted allogeneic stem cells and supported posttransplant by NK cells. NK cells were shown to be lytic against allogeneic targets that did not express their inhibitory KIR ligands. NK cells in this HLA-mismatched allogeneic setting improved engraftment, decreased the incidence of leukemia relapse, and did not cause GVHD (Ruggeri et al. 2002, 2005). Another approach attempted in multiple myeloma was to transfuse haploidentical T-cell-depleted KIR ligandmismatched NK cells after conditioning therapy with melphalan and fludarabine followed by delayed rescue with autologous stem cells (Shi et al. 2008). The NK cells killed the target myeloma cells in vitro. Engraftment was not hampered, and 50% of the patients entered CR despite only transient donor chimerism. Thus, pretransplant molecular high-resolution HLA typing of recipient and donor as well as KIR genotyping of the donor and direct assessment of the donor NK repertoire could identify donors with the potential for donor-versus-recipient NK cell alloreactivity. Expansion of NK cells may be crucial for potential application both in autologous and allogeneic transplantation either to prevent or to treat relapse/progression.

12.6.3 Role of Immunosuppressive Agents in the Conditioning Therapy

The role of including immunosuppressive drugs in the conditioning treatment is controversial.

In a retrospective EBMT study, Crawley et al. (2007) showed a significantly poorer outcome if alemtuzumab or ATG was included in the conditioning regimen. A higher relapse rate was seen with both agents. Alemtuzumab had the worst adverse effect. Other studies of other hematologic malignancies have also reported a higher relapse rate when ATG was included in the conditioning (Remberger et al. 2008).

However, in one study (Ayuk et al. 2008), ATG was claimed to be advantageous when used in the conditioning. Seventy-nine (57%) patients received ATG (Fresenius) and 59 (43%) did not. Other drugs in the conditioning regimen were melphalan 100–150 mg/m^2 administered intravenously in days -3 and -2, and fludarabine (median total dose 120 mg/m^2, range 90–180 mg/m^2) given days -7 to -3. The acute GVHD grade III-IV, as well as chronic GVHD was less in the ATG group. Also, the response rate was higher and there was a trend for improved EFS at 3 years. However, there was no significant improvement in OS.

The interpretation of these results must be taken cautiously. As suggested by Ayuk et al. (2008), these differences may be related to the source of ATG as well as to dosages. They used ATG-Fresenius in high dosages (up to 90 mg/kg) claiming that this might involve an antimyeloma effect, while other studies – including the one by Crawley et al. (2007) – frequently use Thymoglobuline in dosages of 8–12.5 mg/kg. ATG-Fresenius derives from the human Jurkart T-cell line, while Thymoglobuline is an antithymocyte globuline that derives from human thymocytes, which may also explain differences in action. However, it has to be pointed out that among the prospective studies described above, the best RIC-allo results were obtained by Bruno et al. (2007) and by EBMT (Björkstrand et al. 2008; Gahrton et al. 2009) that did not use ATG in the conditioning, while the poorest results were obtained by Garban et al. (2006) using high-dose ATG. Thus, further studies are needed for firm conclusion as to the value of ATG in the conditioning regimen.

12.6.4 Targeted Drugs Pretransplant or Posttransplant

Bortezomib is a proteosome inhibitor that blocks the activation of NF-κB, and is an important mediator of myeloma cell survival. It seems that bortezomib inhibits alloreactive mixed lymphocyte responses, still increasing T-cell-dependent killing of tumor cells (Sun et al. 2004). In a murine model, bortezomib, administrated together with an allogeneic stem cell transplant, prevented GVHD while preserving the graft-versus-tumor effect. However there are other conflicting reports claiming increased GVHD. Thus, although bortezomib is now one of the most effective drugs used in the treatment of multiple myeloma, its place in association with allogeneic stem cell transplantation is not clear (Mattei et al. 2005). Probably it can be used in progression and relapse following allotransplantation and also in the induction regimen, but it is unclear if it should be used in close association with transplantation or in association with DLI.

Lenalidomide is an immunomodulatory drug that has stimulatory effects on host antitumor T-cells and NK cells. In a recent study (Minnema et al. 2008), lenalidomide was given to 16 end-stage myeloma patients who relapsed after allogeneic transplantation resulting in 91% responses and CR in 3 out of 16 patients. Only three patients developed aGVHD and cGVHD was improved in two patients. Thus it is possible that lenalidomide is particularly valuable in relapses following allotransplantation. The NK stimulatory effect could be reason to try expanded NK cell treatment in association with lenalidomide in relapse following allogeneic transplantation

12.7 Conclusions

Allogeneic transplantation is a controversial treatment modality in multiple myeloma. Myeloablative transplantation is hampered by a high transplant-related mortality, and is presently not generally recommended except for clinical trials of selected patient groups. Reduced-intensity non-myeloablative conditioning (RIC) transplantation may be superior to autologous transplantation – single or tandem – but further studies have to be done for firm conclusion. Results seem to be dependant of the kind of RIC used – particularly the type of immune suppression. Alemtuzumab appears contraindicated as part of the conditioning regimen, but other immunosuppressive agents may be used, however, preferentially in clinical trials since the roles of ATG and fludarabine are unclear. New drugs, such as bortezomib, lenalidomide, and new cell therapies, such as NK cell treatment in association with RIC allogeneic transplantation, are potential candidates to improve results. Further studies are needed to find the right place for these possible approaches.

Acknowledgment This review was supported by the Swedish Cancer Fund and the Cancer Society of Stockholm.

References

Alici E, Konstantinidis KV, Sutlu T, Aints A, Gahrton G, Ljunggren HG, Dilber MS (2007) Anti-myeloma activity of endogenous and adoptively transferred activated natural killer cells in experimental multiple myeloma model. Exp Hematol 35:1839–1846

12

Alici E, Sutlu T, Bjorkstrand B, Gilljam M, Stellan B, Nahi H, Quezada HC, Gahrton G, Ljunggren HG, Dilber MS (2008) Autologous antitumor activity by NK cells expanded from myeloma patients using GMP-compliant components. Blood 111: 3155–3162

Ayuk F, Perez-Simon JA, Shimoni A, Sureda A, Zabelina T, Schwerdtfeger R, Martino R, Sayer HG, Alegre A, Lahuerta JJ, Atanackovic D, Wolschke C, Nagler A, Zander AR, San Miguel JF, Kroger N (2008) Clinical impact of human Jurkat T-cell-line-derived antithymocyte globulin in multiple myeloma patients undergoing allogeneic stem cell transplantation. Haematologica 93:1343–1350

Bjorkstrand BB, Ljungman P, Svensson H, Hermans J, Alegre A, Apperley J, Blade J, Carlson K, Cavo M, Ferrant A, Goldstone AH, de Laurenzi A, Majolino I, Marcus R, Prentice HG, Remes K, Samson D, Sureda A, Verdonck LF, Volin L, Gahrton G (1996) Allogeneic bone marrow transplantation versus autologous stem cell transplantation in multiple myeloma: a retrospective case-matched study from the European Group for Blood and Marrow Transplantation. Blood 88:4711–4718

Björkstrand B, Iacobelli S, Hegenbart U, Gruber A, Greinix H, Volin L, Narni F, Musto P, Beksac M, Bosi A, Milone P, Corradini P, Goldschmidt H, De Witte T, Morris C, Niederwieser D, Gahrton G (2008) Autologous stem cell transplantation (ASCT) versus ASCT followed by redued-intensity conditioning allogeneic SCT with identical sibling donor in previously untreated multiple myeloma: prelliminary analysis of a prospective controlled trial by the EBMT. Bone Marrow Transplant 41:S38

Bruno B, Rotta M, Patriarca F, Mordini N, Allione B, Carnevale-Schianca F, Giaccone L, Sorasio R, Omede P, Baldi I, Bringhen S, Massaia M, Aglietta M, Levis A, Gallamini A, Fanin R, Palumbo A, Storb R, Ciccone G, Boccadoro M (2007) A comparison of allografting with autografting for newly diagnosed myeloma. N Engl J Med 356:1110–1120

Corradini P, Voena C, Tarella C, Astolfi M, Ladetto M, Palumbo A, Van Lint MT, Bacigalupo A, Santoro A, Musso M, Majolino I, Boccadoro M, Pileri A (1999) Molecular and clinical remissions in multiple myeloma: role of autologous and allogeneic transplantation of hematopoietic cells. J Clin Oncol 17:208–215

Corradini P, Cavo M, Lokhorst H, Martinelli G, Terragna C, Majolino I, Valagussa P, Boccadoro M, Samson D, Bacigalupo A, Russell N, Montefusco V, Voena C, Gahrton G (2003) Molecular remission after myeloablative allogeneic stem cell transplantation predicts a better relapse-free survival in patients with multiple myeloma. Blood 102: 1927–1929

Crawley C, Iacobelli S, Bjorkstrand B, Apperley JF, Niederwieser D, Gahrton G (2007) Reduced-intensity conditioning for myeloma: lower nonrelapse mortality but higher relapse rates compared with myeloablative conditioning. Blood 109:3588–3594

Gahrton G, Bjorkstrand B (2008) Allogeneic transplantation in multiple myeloma. Haematologica 93:1295–1300

Gahrton G, Tura S, Ljungman P, Belanger C, Brandt L, Cavo M, Facon T, Granena A, Gore M, Gratwohl A et al (1991) Allogeneic bone marrow transplantation in multiple myeloma. European Group for Bone Marrow Transplantation. N Engl J Med 325:1267–1273

Gahrton G, Svensson H, Cavo M, Apperly J, Bacigalupo A, Bjorkstrand B, Blade J, Cornelissen J, de Laurenzi A, Facon T, Ljungman P, Michallet M, Niederwieser D, Powles R, Reiffers J, Russell NH, Samson D, Schaefer UW, Schattenberg A, Tura S, Verdonck LF, Vernant JP, Willemze R, Volin L (2001) Progress in allogenic bone marrow and peripheral blood stem cell transplantation for multiple myeloma: a comparison between transplants performed 1983–93 and 1994–98 at European Group for Blood and Marrow Transplantation centres. Br J Haematol 113:209–216

Gahrton G, Iacobelli S, Apperley J, Bandini G, Bjorkstrand B, Blade J, Boiron JM, Cavo M, Cornelissen J, Corradini P, Kroger N, Ljungman P, Michallet M, Russell NH, Samson D, Schattenberg A, Sirohi B, Verdonck LF, Volin L, Zander A, Niederwieser D (2005) The impact of donor gender on outcome of allogeneic hematopoietic stem cell transplantation for multiple myeloma: reduced relapse risk in female to male transplants. Bone Marrow Transplant 35:609–617

Gahrton G, Iacobelli S, Bandini G, Bjorkstrand B, Corradini P, Crawley C, Hegenbart U, Morgan G, Kroger N, Schattenberg A, Schonland SO, Verdonck LF, Volin L, de Witte T, Niederwieser

D (2007) Peripheral blood or bone marrow cells in reduced-intensity or myeloablative conditioning allogeneic HLA identical sibling donor transplantation for multiple myeloma. Haematologica 92:1513–1518

Gahrton G, Björkstrand B, Iacobelli S, Hegenbart U, Gruber A, Greinix H, Volin L, Narni F, Musto P, Beksac M, Bosi A, Milone G, Corradini P, Goldschmidt H, de Witte T, Morris C, Niederwieser D (2009) Tandem autologous(ASCT)/ allogeneic reduced intensity conditioning transplantation (RIC) with identical sibling donor versus ASCT in previously untreated multiple myeloma (MM): Long term follow up of a prospective controlled trial by the EBMT. Blood 114(abstr):52

Garban F, Attal M, Michallet M, Hulin C, Bourhis JH, Yakoub-Agha I, Lamy T, Marit G, Maloisel F, Berthou C, Dib M, Caillot D, Deprijck B, Ketterer N, Harousseau JL, Sotto JJ, Moreau P (2006) Prospective comparison of autologous stem cell transplantation followed by dose-reduced allograft (IFM99-03 trial) with tandem autologous stem cell transplantation (IFM99-04 trial) in high-risk de novo multiple myeloma. Blood 107:3474–3480

Georges GE, Maris MB, Maloney DG, Sandmaier BM, Sorror ML, Shizuru JA, Lange T, Agura ED, Bruno B, McSweeney PA, Pulsipher MA, Chauncey TR, Mielcarek M, Storer BE, Storb R (2007) Nonmyeloablative unrelated donor hematopoietic cell transplantation to treat patients with poor-risk, relapsed, or refractory multiple myeloma. Biol Blood Marrow Transplant 13:423–432

Hambach L, Spierings E, Goulmy E (2007) Risk assessment in haematopoietic stem cell transplantation: minor histocompatibility antigens. Best Pract Res Clin Haematol 20:171–187

Lokhorst H, Sonneveld P, van der Holt B, van Oers M, Raymakers R, Zweegman S, Minnema M, Zijlmans M (2008) Donor versus no donor analysis of newly diagnosed myeloma patients included in the HOVON 50/54 Study. Blood 112(abstr):461

Maloney DG, Molina AJ, Sahebi F, Stockerl-Goldstein KE, Sandmaier BM, Bensinger W, Storer B, Hegenbart U, Somlo G, Chauncey T, Bruno B, Appelbaum FR, Blume KG, Forman SJ, McSweeney P, Storb R (2003) Allografting with nonmyeloablative conditioning following cytoreductive autografts for the treatment of patients with multiple myeloma. Blood 102:3447–3454

Mattei D, Mordini N, Vigna Taglianti R, Bruno B, Rapezzi D, Gallamini A (2005) Bortezomib treatment followed by a second non-myeloablative allogeneic stem cell transplant in two previously autografted patients with multiple myeloma relapse. Haematologica 90:861–862

Minnema MC, van der Veer MS, Aarts T, Emmelot M, Mutis T, Lokhorst HM (2008) Lenalidomide alone or in combination with dexamethasone is highly effective in patients with relapsed multiple myeloma following allogeneic stem cell transplantation and increases the frequency of CD4(+) Foxp3(+) T cells. Leukemia. 2009; 23:605–607

Moreau P, Garban F, Attal M, Michallet M, Marit G, Hulin C, Benboubker L, Doyen C, Mohty M, Yakoub-Agha I, Leyvraz S, Casassus P, Avet-Loiseau H, Garderet L, Mathiot C, Harousseau JL (2008) Long-term follow-up results of IFM99-03 and IFM99-04 trials comparing non-myeloablative allotransplantation with autologous transplantation in high-risk de novo multiple myeloma. Blood 112:3914–3915

Remberger M, Mattsson J, Svahn B, Ringdén O (2008) Using reduced intensity conditioning and HLA-identcal sibling donors, antithymocyte globulin increases the risk of relapse, which can be overcome by a high stem cell dose Bone Marrow Transplant. 2008; 42:769–771

Rosinol L, Perez-Simon JA, Sureda A, de la Rubia J, de Arriba F, Lahuerta JJ, Gonzalez JD, Diaz-Mediavilla J, Hernandez B, Garcia-Frade J, Carrera D, Leon A, Hernandez M, Fernandez Abellan P, Bergua JM, San Miguel J, Blade J (2008) A prospective pethema study of tandem autologous transplantation versus autograft followed by reduced-intensity conditioning allogeneic transplantation in newly diagnosed multiple myeloma. Blood 112(9):3591–3593

Ruggeri L, Capanni M, Urbani E, Perruccio K, Shlomchik WD, Tosti A, Posati S, Rogaia D, Frassoni F, Aversa F, Martelli MF, Velardi A (2002) Effectiveness of donor natural killer cell alloreactivity in mismatched hematopoietic transplants. Science 295:2097–2100

Ruggeri L, Capanni M, Mancusi A, Martelli MF, Velardi A (2005) The impact of donor natural killer cell alloreactivity on allogeneic hematopoietic transplantation. Transpl Immunol 14: 203–206

Shi J, Tricot G, Szmania S, Rosen N, Garg TK, Malaviarachchi PA, Moreno A, Dupont B,

12

Hsu KC, Baxter-Lowe LA, Cottler-Fox M, Shaughnessy JD Jr, Barlogie B, van Rhee F (2008) Infusion of haplo-identical killer immunoglobulin-like receptor ligand mismatched NK cells for relapsed myeloma in the setting of autologous stem cell transplantation. Br J Haematol 143:641–653

Sun K, Welniak LA, Panoskaltsis-Mortari A, O'Shaughnessy MJ, Liu H, Barao I, Riordan W, Sitcheran R, Wysocki C, Serody JS, Blazar BR, Sayers TJ, Murphy WJ (2004) Inhibition of acute graft-versus-host disease with retention of graft-versus-tumor effects by the proteasome inhibitor bortezomib. Proc Natl Acad Sci USA 101:8120–8125

van de Donk NW, Kroger N, Hegenbart U, Corradini P, San Miguel JF, Goldschmidt H, Perez-Simon JA, Zijlmans M, Raymakers RA, Montefusco V, Ayuk FA, van Oers MH, Nagler A, Verdonck LF, Lokhorst HM (2006) Prognostic factors for donor lymphocyte infusions following nonmyeloablative allogeneic stem cell transplantation in multiple myeloma. Bone Marrow Transplant 37:1135–1141

Radiotherapy 13

Sonja Krause, Jürgen Debus, and Dirk Neuhof

Contents

S. Krause (✉)
Department of Radiation Oncology,
University of Heidelberg,
Im Neuenheimer Feld 400,
69120 Heidelberg, Germany
e-mail: sonja.krause@med.uni-heidelberg.de

Abstract Solitary plasmocytoma occurring in bone (solitary plasmocytoma of the bone, SBP) or in soft tissue (extramedullary plasmocytoma, EP) can be treated effectively and with little toxicity by local radiotherapy. Ten-year local control rates of up to 90% can be achieved.

Patients with multiple myeloma often suffer from symptoms such as pain or neurological impairments that are amenable to palliative radiotherapy. In a palliative setting, short treatment schedules and lower radiation doses are used to reduce toxicity and duration of hospitalization.

In future, low-dose total body irradiation (TBI) may play a role in a potentially curative regimen with nonmyeloablative conditioning followed by allogenic peripheral blood stem cell transplantation.

13.1 Solitary Plasmocytoma

Solitary plasmocytoma are rare neoplasms originating from plasma cells in bone (solitary plasmocytoma of the bone, SBP) or in soft tissue (extramedullary plasmocytoma, EP). SBP comprise about 10% of plasma cell neoplasms and are mainly found in the axial skeleton (Holland et al. 1992), while EP are even more

T. Moehler and H. Goldschmidt (eds.), *Multiple Myeloma*,
Recent Results in Cancer Research 183, DOI: 10.1007/978-3-540-85772-3_13,

rare (about 3%) with most manifestations in the head-and-neck region (Bachar et al. 2008). Patients typically present with symptoms caused by local tumor mass: pain and neurological deficits in the case of SBP; dysphagia, breathing problems, and epistaxis in the case of EP. Both SBP and EP can be treated effectively and with little toxicity by local radiotherapy (Kumar 2008; Michalaki et al. 2003).

13.1.1 Diagnostic Workup

Before starting local treatment of solitary plasmocytoma, thorough diagnostic workup is essential to rule out occult multiple myeloma, as patients having already progressed to multiple myeloma may require systemic treatment. Most authors define solitary plasmocytoma as one single, histologically confirmed lesion with normal bone marrow biopsy (<10% plasma cells), negative skeletal survey on plain film, normal blood count, normal serum calcium, and normal renal function (Tsang et al. 2001). The addition of whole-body MRI scans to diagnostic schedules may increase the sensitivity to detect multiple myeloma in up to 25% of patients initially considered to have solitary plasmocytoma (Wilder et al. 2002). In addition, MRI is helpful for definition of treatment volumes by clear delineation of soft tissue masses.

13.1.2 Radiotherapy of SBP

Concerning the definition of clinical target volumes of SBP, there is still ongoing debate whether the whole bone marrow of affected bones should be included. In the case of vertebral bodies, most authors recommend the inclusion of the affected bone and the two neighboring vertebral bodies (Tsang et al. 2001). If long bones are affected, some groups define clinical target volumes as radiographically visible mass surrounded by a 2–5 cm margin (Jyothirmayi et al. 1997; Ozsahin et al. 2006; Wilder et al. 2002) and achieve excellent local control rates. However, in a small retrospective series, Mayr et al. (1990) reported local relapse in three out of five patients with only partial bone irradiation compared to 100% local control in 12 patients with treatment of the whole bone. Unaffected regional lymph nodes were not included in the target volume. As to radiation doses, most authors recommend application of 40–50 Gy in 1.8–2.0 Gy fractions (Bolek et al. 1996; Holland et al. 1992; Kumar 2008) based on observations of Mendenhall et al. (1980) that doses >40 Gy resulted in local control rates of 94% compared to 69% after <40 Gy.

All studies reported excellent local control of SBP with 10-year local control rates of up to 90% (Liebross et al. 1998; Wilder et al. 2002). Tumor remission after radiotherapy was achieved after 3–5 months (Jyothirmayi et al. 1997). Interestingly, persistence of tumor mass after therapy had no influence on survival rates (Bolek et al. 1996). Local failure inside or outside the radiation field rarely occurred, and very few patients developed solitary lesions in other locations (Frassica et al. 1989). However, overall survival was diminished severely by a high rate of progression to multiple myeloma: About half the patients developed multiple myeloma after 1–3 years (Bolek et al. 1996; Holland et al. 1992) resulting in 5-year overall survival ranging from 32% (Bolek et al. 1996) to 74% (Frassica et al. 1989). Most studies observed a 10-year disease-free survival of about 25% (Frassica et al. 1989; Ozsahin et al. 2006). Given the high probability of systemic disease development, a small prospective study by Aviles et al. (1996) achieved much lower progression rates of 12% in patients treated with radiotherapy followed by administration of low-dose prednisone/melphalan over 3 years compared to 54% progression to myeloma in patients treated with radiotherapy alone. However, the question of adjuvant chemotherapy remains to be addressed by larger prospective studies.

13.1.3
Radiotherapy of EP

For radiation therapy of EP, especially in the head-and-neck region, most authors followed guidelines for squamous cell carcinoma in that location for definition of target volumes and radiation doses. Most groups applied doses of 40–60 Gy in 1.8–2.0 Gy fractions (Creach et al. 2009; Michalaki et al. 2003). Tournier-Rangeard et al. (2006) found a much better local control with doses to the target volume >45 Gy than with <45 Gy (100% vs. 50% 5-year local control rate) and even recommended a 10 Gy boost in case of bulky disease if toxicity is tolerable. For EP of nasal cavity or paranasal sinuses, three portal fields were used (one anterior and two lateral wedged fields), EP of nasopharynx, oropharynx, or hypopharynx were usually treated with two laterally opposing fields (Chao et al. 2005; Liebross et al. 1999). In recent years, more complex techniques have evolved that provide a better protection of uninvolved tissues with a high susceptibility to radiation such as the parotid or submandibular gland: Intensity-modulated radiotherapy (IMRT) with up to nine or more photon beams allows the formation of individually shaped treatment volumes.

Concerning the question whether unaffected cervical lymph nodes should be treated (elective neck irradiation, ENI), discussion is still ongoing. Some authors observed recurrences in cervical nodes in up to 30% of patients with untreated cervical lymph nodes and thus recommended ENI, at least for high-risk locations such as oral cavity, naso- and oropharynx and larynx and for bulky tumors (Chao et al. 2005; Liebross et al. 1999; Mayr et al. 1990; Tournier-Rangeard et al. 2006). Others finding recurrence rates in local lymph nodes of <4% advised against the application of ENI in order to reduce long-term toxicity (Chao et al. 2005; Jyothirmayi et al. 1997; Susnerwala et al. 1997).

EP can be controlled locally by radiotherapy in a similarly effective fashion as SBP: 5-year local control rates 72–100% were reported for EP (Liebross et al. 1999; Tournier-Rangeard et al. 2006). However, most studies observed a better overall survival for EP patients of 76% after 5 years (Bachar et al. 2008; Ozsahin et al. 2006) and 54–72% after 10 years (Chao et al. 2005; Ozsahin et al. 2006). Ten-year disease-free survival rates ranged from 55% to 75% (Chao et al. 2005; Ozsahin et al. 2006; Tournier-Rangeard et al. 2006). Concerning progression to multiple myeloma, EP patients seemed to have lower conversion rates of 10–32% after 10 years compared to SBP patients (Bachar et al. 2008; Bolek et al. 1996; Kumar 2008; Liebross et al. 1999).

13.1.4
Treatment Toxicity

Very little data can be found in literature addressing treatment toxicity, probably because of small patient numbers and a variety of different locations. Creach et al. (2009) described toxicity in 18 patients treated for EP in the head-and-neck region (10 patients received an additional irradiation of cervical lymph nodes): 10 of 18 patients reported xerostomia, 5 complained of nose bleedings. Other side effects were nasal obstruction, larynx edema, dysfunction of the lacrimal canal, hypothyreosis, problems related to the paranasal sinuses and Lhermitte's sign, each occuring in one patient. In this small group of patients, two developed a secondary malignoma: one patient suffered from a myxoid fibrous histiocytoma in the radiation field 6.5 years after radiotherapy, another developed a malignant brain tumor after 6.9 years. The reason for this unusually high rate of secondary malginoma remains unclear.

13.2
Palliative Treatment of Multiple Myeloma

In spite of considerable progress in the treatment of multiple myeloma, the disease still is not curable. Thus, effective palliation is an important issue in treatment concepts. Local radiotherapy is used in the palliative treatment of the most frequent symptoms of multiple myeloma: Reduction of pain due to osseous or soft tissue masses, prevention or additive treatment of bone fractures, and reduction of neurological symptoms due to spinal compression.

13.2.1 Pain Control

Local pain caused by irritation of spinal nerves or spinal cord is often the first and the most common symptom in patients with multiple myeloma, occurring in 55–90% of patients (Plasswilm and Belka 2004; Mose et al. 2000). Local radiotherapy has been an important part in the palliative treatment of painful spinal masses for a long time: A study published in 1975 (Mill 1975) reported the palliation of pain by local radiotherapy in 81% of 65 patients presenting with multiple myeloma. Over time, many groups achieved similar results (Rostom 1988; Yaneva et al. 2006). A complete elimination of pain could not be achieved in all patients, but most profited from radiotherapy by a reduction of their symptoms. Mose et al. (2000) reported complete elimination of pain in 34.4% of 71 treated volumes and partial analgesia in 50.7%.

The irradiated volume usually contained the whole affected bone, in the case of vertebral manifestations including the neighboring vertebral bodies, in order to prevent spreading via the dorsal venous vascular plexus connecting neighboring vertebral bodies (Wilkowski et al. 2002). However, Catell et al. (1998) have shown that in the case of long bones, effective pain reduction is possible by irradiation of only part of the respective bone. Planning should be based on CT scans for better evaluation of pasaosseous soft tissue masses (Wilkowski et al. 2002). Various techniques are applied for irradiation: In most cases, photon beams are used for treatment of bone lesions in a single-field or multi-field technique. Electron beams (with the maximum radiation dose occurring near the body surface) are used for treating superficial lesions (e.g., treatment of the rib cage or sternum).

Wilkowski et al. (2002) reported significant pain reduction by radiation doses as small as 10–15 Gy, but most groups applied higher doses of 25–30 Gy in 10–15 fractions (Bosch and Frias 1988; Leigh et al. 1993). However, hypofractionated irradiation (e.g., 1×8 Gy, 4×4 Gy, 4×5 Gy) was shown to relieve pain in a similarly effective manner (Falkmer et al. 2003).

Pain reduction was in some cases already perceived during radiation therapy but usually started 2–3 weeks after therapy (Plasswilm and Belka 2004). The analgetic effect was described as long-lasting, with relapse rates of 6% after a median of 16 months (Leigh et al. 1993).

A predictive factor for good clinical response was a high Karnofsky performance score of 80–90% (Mose et al. 2000). In addition, the simultaneous application of chemotherapy seemed to enhance the analgetic effect of radiotherapy. Mose et al. could induce pain reduction in 96.3% of patients receiving simultaneous chemotherapy and radiotherapy but only in 77.5% of patients treated with radiotherapy alone. Adamietz and Bottcher (1994) reported local response in 80% of patients under radiochemotherapy compared to 39.6% of patients under radiotherapy alone.

In summary, local radiotherapy has been shown to be an effective tool for pain control in multiple myeloma. However, it had no effect on survival rates (Mose et al. 2000; Yaneva et al. 2006).

13.2.2 Recalcification

Osseous instability, particularly of vertebral bodies, is another challenge in palliative treatment of multiple myeloma. The pathologically upregulated osteoclastic activity in multiple myeloma patients can be compensated for some time by increased osteoblast function, but in later disease stages, this compensation fails, and osteolytic lesions threaten spinal stability (Hjertner et al. 2006).

Local radiotherapy should be started as soon as possible after diagnosis of an unstable osteolytic lesion, as it has been shown that radiologically unstable lesions without actual fracturation of the bone responded much better to radiotherapy than already fractured bones (Liebross et al. 1998, 1999). Mose et al. could induce recalcification in 47.4% of irradiated bones. In a small series published by Lecouvet et al. (1997), fractures occurred in 5% of irradiated vertebrae compared to 20% of nonirradiated vertebrae. In addition, manifestation rates of new focal lesions could be reduced by spinal radiotherapy.

A comparatively small group of patients (about 10%) present with neurological impairments due to spinal compression. The most common causes for spinal compression are vertebral fractures, however, some patients suffer from weakness of limbs or inability to walk caused by extradural extension of plasmocytoma of an adjacent vertebra or extradural compression without bone disease. The therapeutic approach recommended by most authors is local radiotherapy, preferably after local decompression by laminectomy. Although life expectancy of patients with malignant spinal compression is limited and therefore short-course radiotherapeutic schedules (e.g., 1 × 8 Gy, 5 × 4 Gy) seem a sensible option, it has been shown that long-course schedules (e.g., 10 × 3 Gy) result in much better improvement of motor function. Rades et al. (2006) reported an improvement of motor function in 52% of patients with neurological impairments. Of 70 nonambulatory patients, 47% even regained the ability to walk.

13.3 Total Body Irradiation (TBI)

Autologous transplantation of peripheral blood stem cells after myeloablative conditioning has been shown to improve long-term survival but cannot achieve long-term cure. Until recently, the standard conditioning regimen comprised total body irradiation (TBI) with a radiation dose of 8 Gy followed by chemotherapy. This concept was changed by the publication of the Intergroupe Francophone du Myélome 9502 trial (Moreau et al. 2002): The authors observed equal event-free survival in patients conditioned with 8 Gy TBI plus melphalan 140 mg/m^2 compared to patients treated with melphalan 200 mg/m^2. However, toxicity was lower and 45-month survival slightly favorable in the latter group. Thus, TBI lost importance in a potentially curative setting.

In recent years, a new role for TBI in pretransplantation conditioning seems to emerge: Several studies described a potentially curative regimen with nonmyeloablative conditioning with 2 Gy TBI in one single fraction alone or combined with fludarabine followed by allogenic peripheral blood stem cell transplantation (PBST) and immunosuppressive treatment. In this concept, TBI causes a transient immunosuppression and helps to induce a graft-versus-myeloma effect with tolerable graft-versus-host disease (Gerull et al. 2005; Bruno et al. 2009; Georges et al. 2007).

The target volume for TBI are all tumor cells and all lymphatic tissues, so the whole body including the skin must be treated. This requires large radiation fields of up to 210 × 70 cm, compared to the radiation fields of 40 × 40 cm in 1 m distance from focus that conventional linear accelerators usually provide. Radiation Oncology departments developed different techniques for covering such large treatment volumes. One approach is to increase the distance between focus and patients by treating the patient sitting on a special chair and applying laterally opposing fields with a focus distance of 3.5 m.

References

Adamietz IA, Bottcher HD (1994) Estimation of radiotherapy effect in multiple myeloma. Int J Radiat Oncol Biol Phys 29:221

Aviles A, Huerta-Guzman J, Delgado S, Fernandez A, Diaz-Maqueo JC (1996) Improved outcome in solitary bone plasmocytomata with combined therapy. Hematol Oncol 14:111–117

Bachar G, Goldstein D, Brown D, Tsang R, Lockwood G, Perez-Ordonez B, Irish J (2008) Solitary extramedullary plasmocytoma of the head and neck–long-term outcome analysis of 68 cases. Head Neck 30:1012–1019

Bolek TW, Marcus RB, Mendenhall NP (1996) Solitary plasmocytoma of bone and soft tissue. Int J Radiat Oncol Biol Phys 36:329–333

Bosch A, Frias Z (1988) Radiotherapy in the treatment of multiple myeloma. Int J Radiat Oncol Biol Phys 15:1363–1369

Bruno B, Rotta M, Patriarca F, Mattei D, Allione B, Carnevale-Schianca F, Sorasio R, Rambaldi A, Casini M, Parma M, Bavaro P, Onida F, Busca A, Castagna L, Benedetti E, Iori AP, Giaccone L, Palumbo A, Corradini P, Fanin R, Maloney D, Storb R, Baldi I, Ricardi U, Boccadoro M (2009) Non-myeloablative allografting for newly diagnosed multiple myeloma: the experience of the Gruppo Italiano Trapianti di Midollo. Blood 113:3375–3382

Catell D, Kogen Z, Donahue B, Steinfeld A (1998) Multiple myeloma of an extremity: must the entire bone be treated? Int J Radiat Oncol Biol Phys 40:117–119

Chao MW, Gibbs P, Wirth A, Quong G, Guiney MJ, Liew KH (2005) Radiotherapy in the management of solitary extramedullary plasmocytoma. Intern Med J 35:211–215

Creach KM, Foote RL, Neben-Wittich MA, Kyle RA (2009) Radiotherapy for extramedullary plasmocytoma of the head and neck. Int J Radiat Oncol Biol Phys 73:789–794

Falkmer U, Jarhult J, Wersall P, Cavallin-Stahl E (2003) A systematic overview of radiation therapy effects in skeletal metastases. Acta Oncol 42:620–633

Frassica DA, Frassica FJ, Schray MF, Sim FH, Kyle RA (1989) Solitary plasmocytoma of bone: Mayo clinic experience. Int J Radiat Oncol Biol Phys 16:43–48

Georges GE, Maris MB, Maloney DG, Sandmaier BM, Sorror ML, Shizuru JA, Lange T, Agura ED, Bruno B, McSweeney PA, Pulsipher MA, Chauncey TR, Mielcarek M, Storer BE, Storb R (2007) Nonmyeloablative unrelated donor hematopoietic cell transplantation to treat patients with poor-risk, relapsed, or refractory multiple myeloma. Biol Blood Marrow Transplant 13: 423–432

Gerull S, Goerner M, Benner A, Hegenbart U, Klein U, Schaefer H, Goldschmidt H, Ho AD (2005) Long-term outcome of nonmyeloablative allogeneic transplantation in patients with high-risk multiple myeloma. Bone Marrow Transplant 36:963–969

Hjertner O, Standal T, Borset M, Sundan A, Waage A (2006) Bone disease in multiple myeloma. Med Oncol 23:431–441

Holland J, Trenkner DA, Wasserman TH, Fineberg B (1992) Plasmocytoma. Treatment results and conversion to myeloma. Cancer 69:1513–1517

Jyothirmayi R, Gangadharan VP, Nair MK, Rajan B (1997) Radiotherapy in the treatment of solitary plasmocytoma. Br J Radiol 70:511–516

Kumar S (2008) Solitary plasmocytoma: is radiation therapy sufficient? Am J Hematol 83:695–696

Lecouvet F, Richard F, Vande BB, Malghem J, Maldague B, Jamart J, Ferrant A, Michaux JL (1997) Long-term effects of localized spinal radiation therapy on vertebral fractures and focal lesions appearance in patients with multiple myeloma. Br J Haematol 96:743–745

Leigh BR, Kurtts TA, Mack CF, Matzner MB, Shimm DS (1993) Radiation therapy for the palliation of multiple myeloma. Int J Radiat Oncol Biol Phys 25:801–804

Liebross RH, Ha CS, Cox JD, Weber D, Delasalle K, Alexanian R (1998) Solitary bone plasmocytoma: outcome and prognostic factors following radiotherapy. Int J Radiat Oncol Biol Phys 41: 1063–1067

Liebross RH, Ha CS, Cox JD, Weber D, Delasalle K, Alexanian R (1999) Clinical course of solitary extramedullary plasmocytoma. Radiother Oncol 52:245–249

Mayr NA, Wen BC, Hussey DH, Burns CP, Staples JJ, Doornbos JF, Vigliotti AP (1990) The role of radiation therapy in the treatment of solitary plasmocytomas. Radiother Oncol 17:293–303

Mendenhall CM, Thar TL, Million RR (1980) Solitary plasmocytoma of bone and soft tissue. Int J Radiat Oncol Biol Phys 6:1497–1501

Michalaki VJ, Hall J, Henk JM, Nutting CM, Harrington KJ (2003) Definitive radiotherapy for extramedullary plasmocytomas of the head and neck. Br J Radiol 76:738–741

Mill WB (1975) Radiation therapy in multiple myeloma. Radiology 115:175–178

Moreau P, Facon T, Attal M, Hulin C, Michallet M, Maloisel F, Sotto JJ, Guilhot F, Marit G, Doyen C, Jaubert J, Fuzibet JG, Francois S, Benboubker L, Monconduit M, Voillat L, Macro M, Berthou C, Dorvaux V, Pignon B, Rio B, Matthes T, Casassus P, Caillot D, Najman N, Grosbois B, Bataille R, Harousseau JL (2002) Comparison of 200 mg/m^2 melphalan and 8 Gy total body irradiation plus 140 mg/m^2 melphalan as conditioning regimens for peripheral blood stem cell transplantation in patients with newly diagnosed multiple myeloma: final analysis of the Intergroupe Francophone du Myelome 9502 randomized trial. Blood 99:731–735

Mose S, Pfitzner D, Rahn A, Nierhoff C, Schiemann M, Bottcher HD (2000) Role of radiotherapy in the treatment of multiple myeloma. Strahlenther Onkol 176:506–512

Ozsahin M, Tsang RW, Poortmans P, Belkacemi Y, Bolla M, Dincbas FO, Landmann C, Castelain B, Buijsen J, Curschmann J, Kadish SP, Kowalczyk A, Anacak Y, Hammer J, Nguyen TD, Studer G, Cooper R, Sengoz M, Scandolaro L, Zouhair A (2006) Outcomes and patterns of failure in solitary plasmocytoma: a multicenter Rare Cancer Network study of 258 patients. Int J Radiat Oncol Biol Phys 64:210–217

Plasswilm L, Belka C (2004) Strahlentherapie beim Myelom. Der Onkologe 8:858–863

Rades D, Hoskin PJ, Stalpers LJ, Schulte R, Poortmans P, Veninga T, Dahm-Daphi J, Obralic N, Wildfang I, Bahrehmand R, Engenhart-Cabilic R, Schild SE (2006) Short-course radiotherapy is not optimal for spinal cord compression due to myeloma. Int J Radiat Oncol Biol Phys 64:1452–1457

Rostom AY (1988) A review of the place of radiotherapy in myeloma with emphasis on whole body irradiation. Hematol Oncol 6:193–198

Susnerwala SS, Shanks JH, Banerjee SS, Scarffe JH, Farrington WT, Slevin NJ (1997) Extramedullary plasmocytoma of the head and neck region: clinicopathological correlation in 25 cases. Br J Cancer 75:921–927

Tournier-Rangeard L, Lapeyre M, Graff-Caillaud P, Mege A, Dolivet G, Toussaint B, Charra-Brunaud C, Hoffstetter S, Marchal C, Peiffert D (2006) Radiotherapy for solitary extramedullary plasmocytoma in the head-and-neck region: a dose greater than 45 Gy to the target volume improves the local control. Int J Radiat Oncol Biol Phys 64:1013–1017

Tsang RW, Gospodarowicz MK, Pintilie M, Bezjak A, Wells W, Hodgson DC, Stewart AK (2001) Solitary plasmocytoma treated with radiotherapy: impact of tumor size on outcome. Int J Radiat Oncol Biol Phys 50:113–120

Wilder RB, Ha CS, Cox JD, Weber D, Delasalle K, Alexanian R (2002) Persistence of myeloma protein for more than one year after radiotherapy is an adverse prognostic factor in solitary plasmocytoma of bone. Cancer 94:1532–1537

Wilkowski R, Schymura B, Busch M, Zimmermann F (2002) Strahlentherapie. In: Bartl R (ed) Manual Multiples Myelom – Empfehlungen zur Diagnostik, Therapie und Nachsorge. Zuckschwerdt, München, pp S138–S142

Yaneva MP, Goranova-Marinova V, Goranov S (2006) Palliative radiotherapy in patients with multiple myeloma. J BUON 11:43–48

Osteoplastic Procedures for the Treatment of Vertebral Complications in Multiple Myeloma Patients

14

Christian Kasperk and Ingo Grafe

Contents

C. Kasperk (✉)
Department of Internal Medicine I
and Clinical Chemistry,
University of Heidelberg,
Im Neuenheimer Feld 410, 69120
Heidelberg, Germany
e-mail: christian.kasperk@med.uni-heidelberg.de

Abstract Pain induced by vertebral fracture in multiple myeloma can be treated by an osteoplastic procedure. The magnitude of the pain reduction by the procedure depends on the presence of additional causes for pain as spondylosis deformans, osteochondrosis, stenosis of the spinal canal, or intervertebral nerve compression. To identify additional reasons for pain apart from a verterbal fracture-induced pain, a detailed preoperative analysis of the patients complaints is crucial for the outcome after an osteoplastic procedure. In addition, the technical aspects for performing the procedure and potential complications have to be considered as well as the stability of the cortical bone of the respective verterbal body. A complete collapse of the vertebra (vertebra plana) is an unfavorable situation for any osteoplastic procedure. In case of inflammatory or infetctious vertebral lesions (e.g. spondylodiscitis) osteoplastic procedures are contraindicated. An interdisciplinary discussion of the individual case among oncologists, radiotherpists, trauma/spien surgeons, radiologists, and osteologists/endocrinologists is a prerequisite for the identification of patients who will truly benefit from an osteoplastic procedure and to avoid overtreatment of the patient and economical expoitation of healthcare providers.

T. Moehler and H. Goldschmidt (eds.), *Multiple Myeloma*,
Recent Results in Cancer Research 183, DOI: 10.1007/978-3-540-85772-3_14,

14.1 Introduction

Pain induced by vertebral fracture in multiple myeloma can be treated by an osteoplastic procedure. The magnitude of the pain reduction by the procedure depends on the presence of additional causes for pain as spondylosis deformans, osteochondrosis, stenosis of the spinal canal, or intervertebral nerve compression. To identify additional reasons for pain apart from a vertebral fracture–induced pain, a detailed preoperative analysis of the patient's complaints is crucial for the outcome after an osteoplastic procedure. In addition, the technical aspects for performing the procedure and potential complications have to be considered as well as the stability of the cortical bone of the respective vertebral body. A complete collapse of the vertebra (vertebra plana) is an unfavorable situation for any osteoplastic procedure. In case of inflammatory or infectious vertebral lesions (e.g., spondylodiscitis), osteoplastic procedures are contraindicated. An interdisciplinary discussion of the individual case among oncologists, radiotherapists, trauma/spine surgeons, radiologists, and osteologists/endocrinologists is a prerequisite for the identification of patients who will truly benefit from an osteoplastic procedure and to avoid overtreatment of the patient and economical exploitation of health-care providers.

14.2 Osteoplastic Procedures

Osteoplastic techniques such as balloon kyphoplasty and vertebroplasty use a quickly solidifying resin (polymer from polymethylmetacrylate PMMA) or calcium phosphate cement. In malignoma-associated osteolytic lesions, only PMMA should be used. An important aspect of osteoplastic procedures is the immediate stability for the treated fractured vertebra. Usually osteoplastic procedures are performed at thoracic vertebrae 4–12 and lumbar vertebrae 1–5; cervical vertebral fractures due to pathological lesions of the spine are not a standard situation for osteoplastic techniques. During osteoplastic procedures, the patient is positioned horizontally (face down with pillows under shoulders and iliac crests) in a hyperlordotic position. Patients with an instable thorax, painful rib fractures, or instable cervical vertebral fractures should not be treated by osteoplastic techniques.

14.3 Balloon Kyphoplasty

In 1998, balloon kyphoplasty has been introduced for the stabilization of vertebral fractures (Garfin et al. 2001). Today it is an established osteoplastic procedure for routine therapy of vertebral fractures or lesions due to primary or secondary osteoporosis.

Usually balloon kyphoplasty is performed in general anesthesia after intubation of the patient. The balloon catheter is inserted into the fractured vertebral body via a trans- or extrapedicular approach. The balloon is then inflated using a contrast fluid under fluoroscopic control until it extends to the endplates of the vertebral body. The balloon is deflated and removed from the vertebra so that within the fractured vertebral body an empty void remains. Goal of the balloon expansion procedure is to restore the initial height of the vertebra. As muscle relaxation during general anesthesia and the positioning of the patient prevent any compressive forces on the spine that might cause a collapse of the space created by the balloon, the cavum remains even after removal of the balloon. Hyperlordosis as a consequence of the positioning of the patient and general anesthesia in complete muscle relaxation support the reheightening process of partially collapsed or fractured vertebrae.

As the amount of contrast fluid is known that was used to inflate the balloon, the volume of the

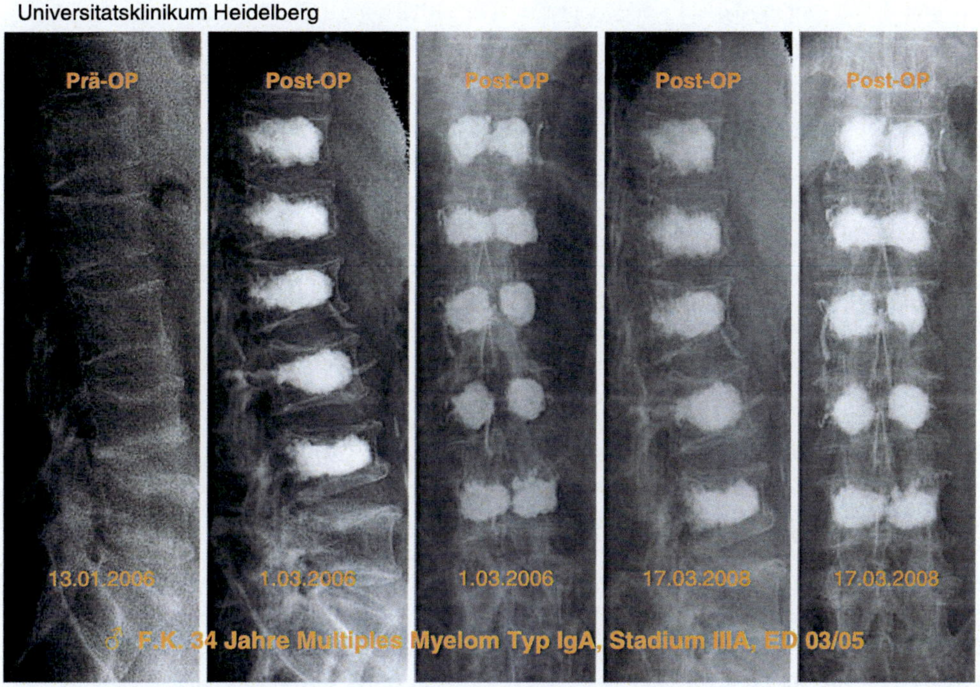

Fig. 14.1 Kyphoplasty in a 34-year-old patient was performed to improve severe lumbar back pain and to stop ongoing compression fracturing of all lumbar vertebrae due to myeloma. After 2 years, the X-rays demonstrate radio-morphologically a stable anatomical situation

balloon-created space is known and the same volume of PMMA plastic or other "cement" material is inserted into the void whereby only polymethylmetacrylate (PMMA) is used in malignoma-associated osteolytic lesions (Fig. 14.1). As PMMA and calcium phosphate cements solidify rapidly within the treated vertebral body, embolic events from PMMA or calcium phosphate cement are rare events.

14.4 Vertebroplasty

Vertebroplasty was established in 1984 for the internal stabilization of vertebral fractures and vertebral lesions (Galibert 1987; Gangi 1999). This technique is often applied by interventional radiologists in analgosedation under fluoroscopic or computer tomographic guidance.

Via a trans- or extrapedicular approach, a cannula is placed within the fractured vertebra and the PMMA plastic material is directly injected into the treated vertebra under fluoroscopic control.

In contrast to balloon kyphoplasty, vertebroplasty does not rely on the generation of a cavum of defined void within the treated vertebral body. Due to low viscosity of the PMMA plastic material and the overall technical procedure, a significant reheightening of the treated vertebra is not expected. The distribution of the PMMA plastic material within the treated vertebral body cannot be controlled; therefore, PMMA leakages are more frequent after vertebroplasty. A typical location for PMMA leakages after vertebroplasty is the venous plexus surrounding the vertebrae which – for most cases – does not have any clinical consequences.

14.5 Comparison of Kyphoplasty and Vertebroplasty

The major technical difference between these two osteoplastic techniques is the usage of a balloon catheter for balloon kyphoplasty as described above in more detail. The balloon creates a void of defined volume within the fractured vertebra that is subsequently filled with plastic (or "cement") material of high viscosity to internally stabilize the fractured vertebral body. Leakages of the used plastic or cement material are therefore significantly less likely after balloon kyphoplasty. Another advantage for balloon kyphoplasty is the compression of spongious bone material during the intravertebral expansion of the balloon which creates a condensed spongiosa layer surrounding the void which may close possible cortical perforations of the vertebral body and allows bone repair to occur on the surface of the implanted plastic or cement material. In case of malignant disease and pathological osteolytic lesions, the malignant tissue is compressed and relocated to subcortical areas supporting local control, e.g., by radiation or chemotherapy.

The extent and the direction of dissemination of the PMMA material are less controllable in vertebroplasty leading to leakages mainly in venous plexus surrounding the vertebrae or into the muscle tissue. The direction of the dissemination is determined by areas within the vertebral body providing the lowest resistance which may predispose to leakages. Vertebroplasty may be more beneficial for the patient at an early time point when the vertebral body containing a pathological lesion shows signs of collapse (e.g., MRI bone edema) but has not lost much of its initial height, yet.

14.6 Indications and Contraindications

Osteoplastic techniques such as the balloon kyphoplasty or vertebroplasty should be considered if a patient suffers from severe-to-moderate pain due to a vertebral fracture or due to an osteolytic lesion which cannot be sufficiently controlled by pain medication. In addition, it should be considered if these minimally invasive procedures could potentially prevent future neurological complications due to instable vertebral bodies compromising the function of the spinal cord or spinal nerves. This situation occurs most often in secondary osteoporosis caused by malignant diseases such as multiple myeloma which destroys the biomechanical stability of the vertebral bodies.

In order to perform osteoplastic procedures, the cortical bone of the analyzed vertebral body should be intact – particularly the ventral and dorsal wall of the respective vertebral body – to prevent leakages of plastic or cement material into the spinal canal. Pedicular structures have also to be intact to apply the osteoplastic insertion instruments safely under fluoroscopic control. There should be no major degenerative changes of the spine that would compromise the fluoroscopic visibility of crucial vertebral structures and orientation by the surgeon during surgery.

Osteoplastic procedures are contraindicated in case of local or systemic infections. In particular, spondylodiscitis has to be excluded preoperatively as cause of a vertebral destruction. For most traumatic vertebral fractures without primary or secondary osteoporosis, osteoplastic procedures are not recommended because bone fragments will be dislocated such that neurologic complications may occur or the morphological stability of the entire vertebral body may be jeopardized.

14.7 Randomized Controlled Studies of Osteoplastic Procedures for Vertebral Osteoporotic Fractures

No randomized, sham-controlled and blinded studies have so far been published on vertebral fractures and pain for malignancy-induced vertebral compression fractures. There is one randomized, controlled study in patients with multiple myeloma demonstrating a beneficial effect of kyphoplasty for at least 12 months as compared to non-standardized conservative management of painful vertebral fractures due to multiple myeloma (Berenson et al. 2009).

There are three randomized, controlled studies on osteoplastic procedures published for osteoporotic painful vertebral compression fractures.

The randomized FREE study (Wardlaw et al. 2009) investigated the balloon kyphoplasty in 300 patients with a mean age of 73 years. Ninety-five percent of the patients were diagnosed with primary and 5% with secondary osteoporosis. Patients had one to three vertebral fractures with a mean time interval between diagnosis of vertebral fracture and the kyphoplasty procedure of 5 weeks. All treated vertebrae had a minimum height reduction of 15% and a bone marrow edema in MRI. One hundred and thirty-eight patients treated with balloon kyphoplasty had postoperatively and also after 12 months a significant reduction in back pain and up to 6 months after kyphoplasty an improved mobility compared to the conservatively treated group. This study did not evaluate vertebral augmentation or a possible improvement of the kyphosis angle of the spine.

A double-blind randomized, sham-controlled study was published by Buchbinder et al. (2009) investigating vertebroplasty in 78 patients with a mean age of 76 years with painful osteoporotic vertebral fractures. Patients had one to two vertebral fractures not older than 12 months, and MRI confirmed bone marrow edema or fracture line. Thirty-five patients received vertebroplasty, and 36 patients underwent a sham procedure (local skin and periosteal anesthesia, synthetic material prepared to induce the PMMA smell in the operating room). In this study, no statistical difference of pain reduction between vertebroplasty and sham treatment group was noted postoperatively or 3 and 6 months after vertebroplasty.

Kallmes et al. (2009) investigated vertebroplasty in a randomized blinded, sham-controlled study in 131 patients at a mean age of 73 years with osteoporotic vertebral fractures. The patients were diagnosed with one to three vertebral fractures. The verum group ($n=68$) received mainly monopedicular vertebroplasty; for some vertebrae that did not contain "satisfactory amounts" of synthetic material, a bipedicular vertebroplasty was performed. A sham procedure was performed for control patients and a crossover of the patients was allowed after 1 month or at a later time point if pain reduction was not sufficient. Whereas the pain reduction was not significantly different between the two groups, more patients ($n=27$) in the sham-operated control group crossed over to verum. Only eight patients of the verum group crossed over to the alternative treatment.

In a competitive randomized study comparing balloon kyphoplasty to vertebroplasty (Liu et al. 2010), 50 patients per group at a mean age of 73 years were treated with vertebroplasty or balloon kyphoplasty. In the postoperative period as well as after 3 months, there was no significant difference in pain reduction between the two techniques. Vertebrae treated with balloon kyphoplasty were found to have a better vertebral augmentation and an improvement of the degree of the kyphosis.

In a non-randomized, controlled study (n=40), balloon kyphoplasty was compared to a standardized control treatment (n=20) for painful osteoporotic vertebral fractures. Balloon kyphoplasty was superior to conservative treatment regarding pain reduction over a period of at least 12 months and with regards to mobility in the first 6 months after kyphoplasty (Kasperk et al. 2005; Grafe et al. 2005). All vertebrae in the control group exhibited a progression of vertebral compression fracturing, whereas after balloon kyphoplasty a small but significant vertebral augmentation was recorded.

14.8 Studies Using Kyphoplasty and Vertebroplasty in Patients with Multiple Myeloma

Published reports on the outcome after minimal-invasive osteoplastic procedures (kyphoplasty and vertebroplasty) in patients with back pain due to multiple myeloma are based on prospective and retrospective, uncontrolled and unblinded cohort studies. In Tables 14.1–14.3, an overview on published trials utilizing kyphoplasty and vertebroplasty in patients with multiple myeloma is presented, including series with ≥10 patients with multiple myeloma.

In some of the published studies, the indication for an intervention is evaluated by an interdisciplinary team, and preoperative spine X-rays, MRI and CT scans are needed for this interdisciplinary assessment (Huber et al. 2009). Inclusion criteria for both kyphoplasty and vertebroplasty are localized painful vertebral fractures refractory to conservative treatment including opiate analgesia and/or physical therapy. In many cases, a desired more effective restoring of the height of a recently fractured vertebra leads to the selection of kyphopasty instead of vertebroplasty as the most appropriate procedure. Typical exclusion criteria for both interventions (kyphoplasty and vertebroplasty) include unstable fractures (i.e., with a destruction of the posterior wall of the vertebral body) or with retropulsed tumor tissue or bone fragments, epidural compression of neural elements, stenosis of the spinal canal, radicular pain, failure to localize symptomatic levels at the spine, intolerance to being positioned prone, significant medical contraindications (e.g., coagulopathy), or local or systemic infection. While kyphoplasty is typically performed in general anesthesia, vertebroplasty was usually conducted in local anesthesia in most patients. The treated levels by both kyphoplasty and vertebroplasty are mainly located in the thoracic and lumbar spines. There are few reports on vertebroplasty in cervical vertebral bodies (e.g., Pflugmacher et al. 2006b); however, cervical vertebral bodies are not treated routinely by osteoplastic procedures. The reported cement leakage rates are somewhat higher after vertebroplasty treatment (0–94%) compared to kyphoplasty (0–26%). In two retrospective studies, the included patients with multiple myeloma were treated either by kyphoplasty or by vertebroplasty (or both at different levels) (Fourney et al. 2003; Köse et al. 2006; Table 14.3). Köse et al. report a significantly better pain improvement after kyphoplasty compared to the vertebroplasty group after 6 and 12 months. However, due to the retrospective design and small group size as well as a possible selection bias by different indications for kyphoplasty and vertebroplasty, no direct comparison of efficacy and safety of both procedures is possible on the basis of these trials.

There is no randomized, blinded, sham-controlled clinical study to confirm the use of osteoplastic procedures in myeloma cases or other malignant entities causing osteolytic vertebral lesions. However, evidence from one randomized trial in myeloma patients (Berenson et al. 2009) and evidence provided from randomized trials in patients with primary osteoporosis are the current bases for the identification of myeloma patients most likely to benefit from osteoplastic procedures.

Table 14.1 Kyphoplasty in multiple myeloma patients

Author	Number of patients (mean age) Anesthesia	Number of levels treated	Follow-up	Outcome clinical[a]	Outcome radio-morphological	Complications
Prospective reports						
Pflugmacher et al. (2006a, b, 2007)	23 (63.5) GA	59	24 months	*64% pain reduction* VAS decreased from 8.6 to 2.4 (postoperatively) and to 3.1 (24 months) *57% improved disability* ODI improved from 78.1 to 37.3 (postoperatively) and to 33.6 (24 months)	Postoperative height improvement in 61% of vertebral bodies with height restoration of 3.5 mm (from 25 to 28.5 mm) After 2 years, slight height decrease by 1 mm Postoperative correction of kyphosis in 76.5% of patients by 8° After 2 years, slight loss of correction in 53.1% of patients by 3° Adjacent fractures in two patients	Cement leakage 10%
	20 (62.4) GA	48	12 months	*62% pain reduction* VAS decreased from 8.2 to 2.2 (3 days) and to 3.1 (12 months) *56% improved disability* ODI improved from 71.5 to 27.5 (3 days) and to 31.2 (12 months)	Postoperative height improvement in 64.5% of vertebral bodies with height restoration of 4.3 mm (47.3% of lost height) After 1 year, slight height decrease in 43.7% (21/48) of treated vertebral bodies by 1.1 mm Postoperative correction of kyphosis in 78.4% of patients by 6.3° After 1 year, slight loss of correction in 42% of patients by 1.8° One adjacent fracture after 2 weeks	Clinically asymptomatic cement leakage in 10.4%

(continued)

Table 14.1 (continued)

Author	Number of patients (mean age) Anesthesia	Number of levels treated	Follow-up	Outcome clinical[a]	Outcome radio-morphological	Complications
Lane et al. (2004)	19 (60.4) GA	46	3 months	*33% improved disability*ODI reduced from 48.9 to 32.6 Improvement in 84.2% (16/19 patients) No improvement with preoperative ODI <28	53.4% restoration of midvertebral height loss (in 42 of 46 levels) 37.8% restoration of anterior vertebral height loss (in 35 of 46 levels)	Cement leakage in 26.3%No clinical sequelae
Dudeney et al. (2002)	18 (63.5) No information on anesthesia	55	7.4 months (mean)	From SF36-questionnaire:Pain improved from 23.2 to 55.4 Physical function improved from 21.3 to 50.6	34% restoration of lost height	No major complications4% asymptomatic cement leakage
Retrospective reports						
Astolfi et al. (2009)	30 (63) GA [n=13]+LA [n=17]	45	4 years (median)	*56% pain reduction* VAS reduced from 8.7 to 2.8 (1 month), 2.1 (3 years), 3.8 (5 years) Complete pain relief in 59% Pain recurred in 10% between 3 and 12 months *58% improved disability* ODI improved from 87 to 45 (1 month), 21 (3 years), 37 (5 years) SF36 improved from 23 to 76.5 (1 month), 77.2 (3 years), 67.8 (5 years)	55% restoration of lost height, maintained to 5 years 6.8° correction of segmental kyphotic angle, decrease of 1.7° after 5 years Follow-up fractures in 14 patients (31.1%) after 18 months (mean)	Transiently increased back pain and pyrexia immediate postoperatively in two patients Two (4.4%) asymptomatic cement leakage No major complications

Table 14.2 Vertebroplasty in patients with multiple myeloma

Author	Number of patients (mean age)	Number of levels treated	Follow-up	Outcome clinical[a]	Outcome radio-morphological	Complications
Prospective reports						
Ramos et al. (2006)	12 (66) LA	19	3.2 years (median) [2–56 months]	*67% pain reduction* VAS reduced from 7.5 to 3.7 (1 day) and to 2.5 (3 years) 92% showed ≥75% pain reduction within 3 months *52% improved functional status* ECOG [0–4]reduced from 3.1 to 2.5 (1 day) and to 1.5 (3 years)	No further collapse of treated or neighboring vertebrae at last follow-up	Leakage in 94% (16/19) patients No clinical or neurological symptoms
Diamond et al. (2004)	7 (69) LA	14	6 weeks	*75% pain reduction*VAS [0–25] reduced from 19 to 4 After 1 day, six of seven patients (86%) had ≥50% decreased pain score *50–60% improved functional status* BI improved from 11.9 to 18.7 Of seven patients, three cease pain medication, three reduce analgesic >50% after 1 day	No information provided	No complications No paravertebral or foraminal leakages
Retrospective reports						
McDonald et al. (2008)	67 (66.2) LA + conscious sedation	114	12 months	Pain "at rest" improved from 3.9 to 2.7 (25%) (1 week) [69%] Pain "at activity" improved from 8.5 to 5.3 (48%) (1 week) [62%] RDQ improved from 19.5 to 11 (48%) (1 week) [56%] 70% of patients reported improvement in mobility after 1 week Clinical outcomes maintained for 1 year of follow-up Narcotics discontinued 16%, decreased 49%, increased 5%	No information provided	Twelve patients (17%) showed subsequent vertebral compression fractures, six within 12 months, Seven adjacent, five symptomatic treated with second VP 19% asymptomatic cement leakage

(continued)

14

Table 14.2 (continued)

Author	Number of patients (mean age)	Number of levels treated	Follow-up	Outcome clinical[a]	Outcome radio-morphological	Complications
Thang et al. (2008)	27 (65) LA: if 1 level treated GA: if >1 level treated	117	1 month (41 months)	1 month: *72% pain reduction* VAS reduced from 7.5 to 2.1 70–100% pain reduction in 70% 0–49% pain reduction in 16.7% *55% improved functional status* ECOG [1–5] reduced from 1.9 to 0.86 Opiate consumption interrupted in 59.3%, partially reduced in 22.2% 70.4% decrease in opiate dose	No evidence for progression at treated site after median follow-up of 41 months	No major complications One cement leakage L5 nerve root correlated with appearance of a transient sensory defect, which resolved within 3 weeks Eight clinically not relevant cement leakages (24%)
Shimony et al. (2004)	50 (62.7) Cancer patients 14 MM LA + conscious sedation	129	3 months (median)	Outcomes of myeloma subgroup not reported separately Pain reduction in 82% of patients Improved mobility in 52% of patients	No information provided	No major complications Increased pain in seven patients (with preoperative mild-to-moderate epidural involvement) (Immediately after VP in three patients, treated with epidural steroid injection of steroid infusion, after several weeks in four patients, treated by neuroforaminal epidural nerve root block)

Table 14.3 Reports including both kyphoplasty and vertebroplasty in patients with multiple myeloma

Author	Number of patients (mean age)Anesthesia	Number of levels treated	Follow-up	Outcome clinical[a]	Outcome radio-morphological	Complications
Retrospective reports						
Köse et al. (2006)[b]	34 KP: 18 (63.7) VP: 16 (62.2) LA + midazolam if needed	KP: 22 VP: 28	12 months	*KP: 73% pain reduction* KP: VAS [0–50] improved from 36 to 12.1 (6 weeks), 8.6 (6 months), 9.7 (12 months) *VP: 64% pain reduction* VP: VAS improved from 37.8 to 15.3 (6 weeks), 12.2 (6 M), 13.5 (12 months) → Significant better improvement after KP after 6 + 12 months compared to VP Decreased need of analgesics	Mean height restoration 54% No collapse of adjacent vertebrae	One superficial wound infection, resolved No neurologic or pulmonary complications No cement leakage
Fourney et al. (2003)[c]	56 (64) Cancer patients KP: 15 VP: 34 KP + VP: 7 (at separate levels) 21 MM: KP: 11 VP: 6 KP + VP: 4 KP: GA VP: GA or LA	97 KP: 32 VP: 65	4.5 months (median) [1 day–19.7 months]	Outcomes of myeloma subgroup not reported separately *Entire study group* VAS reduced from 7 to 2 Immediate pain improvement or complete relief after 84% of procedures (VP: 86%; KP: 80%) Maintained improvement through 1 year No significant functional improvement Decreased analgesic usage at 1 month	42% restoration of lost height and 4.1° improved kyphosis after kyphoplasty	9.2% (6/65) asymptomatic cement leakage after vertebroplasty No leakage after kyphoplasty No procedure-related clinical complications (2 patients subsequent spinal surgery not related to procedures)

(continued)

Table 14.3 (continued)

VAS Visual Analogue Score (Pain) [0–10]; differing ranges are indicated in brackets
ODI Oswestry Disability Index [0–100]
ECOG Eastern Cooperative Oncology Group scale [1–5] – functional status
BI Barthel Index, disability score [0 (worst disability) – 20 (no disability)]
RDQ Roland-Morris Disability Questionnaire [1–23]
SF36 Short Form 26 Health Survey [%]
MM Multiple myeloma
LA Local anesthesia
GA General anesthesia
KP Kyphoplasty
VP Vertebroplasty

[a]% Pain reduction and improved disability/functional status represents the percentage of change of the last reported follow-up compared to the preoperative value

[b]Indications for kyphoplasty: >50% loss of vertebral height vertebroplasty: <50% loss of vertebral height

[c]Indications for kyphoplasty: (1) kyphosis >20°, (2) disruption of posterior vertebral cortex, (3) significant vertebral collapse vertebroplasty: (1) severe vertebral collapse, when insertion of balloon device not possible, (2) GA or longer procedure time not tolerated

References

Astolfi S, Scaramuzzo L, Logroscino CA (2009) A minimally invasive surgical treatment possibility of osteolytic vertebral collapse in multiple myeloma. Eur Spine J 18(Suppl 1):115–121

Berenson JR, Pflugmacher R, Jarzem P, Zonder JA, Tillman JB, Ashraf T, Vrionis FD (2009) Final results of the first randomized trial comparing balloon kyphoplasty to non-surgical management among cancer patients with vertebral compression fractures: marked improvement in back function, quality of life and pain in the balloon kyphoplasty arm. Blood (ASH Annual Meeting Abstracts) 114: Abstract 2873

Buchbinder R, Osborne RH, Ebeling PR, Wark JD, Mitchell P, Wriedt C, Graves S, Staples MP, Murphy B (2009) A randomized trial of vertebroplasty for painful osteoporotic vertebral fractures. N Engl J Med 361:557–568

Diamond TH, Hartwell T, Clarke W, Manoharan A (2004) Percutaneous vertebroplasty for acute vertebral body fracture and deformity in multiple myeloma: a short report. Br J Haematol 124:485–487

Dudeney S, Lieberman IH, Reinhardt MK, Hussein M (2002) Kyphoplasty in the treatment of osteolytic vertebral compression fractures as a result of multiple myeloma. J Clin Oncol 20:2382–2387

Fourney DR, Schomer DF, Nader R, Chlan-Fourney J, Suki D, Ahrar K, Rhines LD, Gokaslan ZL (2003) Percutaneous vertebroplasty and kyphoplasty for painful vertebral body fractures in cancer patients. J Neurosurg 98(1 Suppl):21–30

Galibert P (1987) Note preliminaire sur le traitement des angiomes vertebraux par vertebroplastie acrylique percutanee. Neurochirurgie 33:166–167

Gangi A (1999) Computed tomography and fluoroscopy guided vertebroplasty: results and complications in 187 patients. Semin Intervent Radiol 16:137–142

Garfin SR, Yuan HA, Reiley MA (2001) New technologies in spine – kyphoplasty and vertebroplasty for the treatment of painful osteoporotic compression fractures. Spine 26:1511–1515

Grafe I, DaFonseca K, Hillmeier J, Meeder PJ, Libicher M, Nöldge G, Bardenheuer H, Pyerin W, Basler L, Weiss C, Taylor R, Nawroth P, Kasperk C (2005) Reduction of pain and fracture incidence after kyphoplasty: 1 year outcome of a prospective controlled trial of patients with primary osteoporosis. Osteoporos Int 16:2005–2012

Huber FX, McArthur N, Tanner M, Gritzbach B, Schoierer O, Rothfischer W, Krohmer G, Lessl E, Baier M, Meeder PJ, Kasperk C (2009) Kyphoplasty for patients with multiple myeloma is a safe surgical procedure: results from a large patient cohort. Clin Lymphoma Myeloma 9:375–380

Kallmes DF, Comstock BA, Haegerty PJ, Turner JA, Wilson DJ, Diamond TH, Edwards R, Gray LA, Stout L, Owen S, Hollingworth W, Ghdoke B, Annesley-Williams DJ, Ralston SH, Jarvik JG (2009) A randomized trial of vertebroplasty for osteoporotic spinal fractures. N Engl J Med 361:569–579

Kasperk C, Hillmeier J, Nöldge G, Grafe I, DaFonseca K, Raupp D, Bardenheuer H, Libicher M, Liegibel U, Sommer U, Hilscher U, Pyerin W, Vetter M, Meinzer H, Meeder PJ, Taylor R, Nawroth P (2005) Treatment of painful vertebral fractures by kyphoplasty in patients with primary osteoporosis: a prospective nonrandomized controlled study. J Bone Miner Res 20:604–612

Köse KC, Cebesoy O, Akan B, Altinel L, Dinçer D, Yazar T (2006) Functional results of vertebral augmentation techniques in pathological vertebral fractures of myelomatous patients. J Natl Med Assoc 98:1654–1658

Lane JM, Hong R, Koob J, Kiechle T, Niesvizky R, Pearse R, Siegel D, Poynton AR (2004) Kyphoplasty enhances function and structural alignment in multiple myeloma. Clin Orthop Relat Res 426:49–53

Liu JT, Liao WJ, Tan WC, Lee JK, Liu CH, Chen YH, Lin TB (2010) Balloon kyphoplasty versus vertebroplasty for treatment of osteoporotic vertebral compression fracture: a prospective, comparative, and randomized clinical study. Osteoporos Int 21:359–364

McDonald RJ, Trout AT, Gray LA, Dispenzieri A, Thielen KR, Kallmes DF (2008) Vertebroplasty in multiple myeloma: outcomes in a large patient series. AJNR Am J Neuroradiol 29:642–648

Pflugmacher R, Kandziora F, Schroeder RJ, Melcher I, Haas NP, Klostermann CK (2006a) Percutaneous balloon kyphoplasty in the treatment of pathological vertebral body fracture and deformity in multiple myeloma: a one-year follow-up. Acta Radiol 47:369–376

Pflugmacher R, Schleicher P, Schröder RJ, Melcher I, Klostermann CK (2006b) Maintained pain reduction in five patients with multiple myeloma

14

12 months after treatment of the involved cervical vertebrae with vertebroplasty. Acta Radiol 47:823–829

Pflugmacher R, Schulz A, Schroeder RJ, Schaser KD, Klostermann CK, Melcher I (2007) A prospective two-year follow-up of thoracic and lumbar osteolytic vertebral fractures caused by multiple myeloma treated with balloon kyphoplasty. Z Orthop Ihre Grenzgeb 145:39–47

Ramos L, de Las Heras JA, Sánchez S, González-Porras JR, González R, Mateos MV, San Miguel JF (2006) Medium-term results of percutaneous vertebroplasty in multiple myeloma. Eur J Haematol 77:7–13

Shimony JS, Gilula LA, Zeller AJ, Brown DB (2004) Percutaneous vertebroplasty for malignant compression fractures with epidural involvement. Radiology 232:846–853

Thang NNT, Abdo G, Martin JB, Seium-Neberay Y, Yilmaz H, Verbist MC, Rufenacht D, Sappino AP, Dietrich PY (2008) Percutaneous cementoplasty in multiple myeloma: a valuable adjunct for pain control and ambulation maintenance. Support Care Cancer 16:891–896

Wardlaw D, Cummings SR, Meirhaeghe J, Bastian L, Tillman JB, Ranstam J, Eastell R, Shabe P, Talmadge K, Boonen S (2009) Efficacy and safety of balloon kyphoplasty compared with non-surgical care for vertebral compression fracture (FREE): a randomized controlled trial. Lancet 373:1016–1024

Supportive Therapy in Multiple Myeloma

15

Heinz Ludwig and Niklas Zojer

Contents

Abstract In this chapter we want to give an overview on various supportive measures, which help to prevent or to fight complications of multiple myeloma, improve patient wellbeing and increase safety of administration of specific anti-myeloma therapy.

15.1 Introduction

Multiple myeloma is characterized by bone disease with osteolytic lesions, fractures and osteoporosis, renal impairment, anemia, and immunological impairment. These sequels of the disease and the toxicity of myeloma therapy

H. Ludwig (✉)
Department of Medicine I, Center of Oncology and Hematology, Wilhelminenspital, Montleartstr. 37, 1160 Vienna, Austria
e-mail: heinz.ludwig@wienkav.at

T. Moehler and H. Goldschmidt (eds.), *Multiple Myeloma*,
Recent Results in Cancer Research 183, DOI: 10.1007/978-3-540-85772-3_15,

often significantly reduce the physical, emotional, and psychosocial well-being of myeloma patients making supportive therapy an essential part of therapeutic management. Supportive care includes preventive measures such as vaccinations; prophylactic anti-infective measures; prophylaxis and treatment of myeloma bone disease and hypercalcemia; treatment of anemia, pain, infections, renal impairment; and psychological support. The concerted action of these interventions can significantly reduce morbidity and improve the patient's quality of life during the different phases of their disease.

15.2 Myeloma Bone Disease

Bone pain is a prominent symptom in myeloma. Typically, patients experience localized bone pain, but pain may be multifocal and/or migratory. At diagnosis, almost all patients have features of osteoporosis; 70% show osteolytic lesions on plain radiography and 30% have fractures (Kyle 1975). Initially, some patients show both increased bone degradation and elevated osteogenesis, but as the disease progresses, bone degradation by far outweighs bone formation (Taube et al. 1992). Thus, the typical radiologic appearance of bone lesions in myeloma are lytic foci without any accompanying sites of bone formation, known as "punched out" bone lesions (Terpos and Dimopoulos 2005).

15.2.1 Mechanisms of Bone Disease

In myeloma, several cytokines contribute to the increased formation, differentiation, and stimulation of osteoclasts and inhibition of osteoblasts. These cytokines are mainly secreted by bone marrow stromal cells and often induced by direct myeloma-stromal cell contact. Interleukin-1b (IL-1b), tumor necrosis factor (TNF)-α, TNF-β, interleukin-6 (IL-6), macrophage colony stimulating factor (M-CSF), vascular endothelial growth factor (VEGF), and other cellular growth hormones have all been implicated as major osteoclast activators (Bataille et al. 1997; Podar et al. 2001). Receptor activator of nuclear factor-kappaB ligand (RANKL) (Roux et al. 2002), which is produced by bone marrow stromal cells induces differentiation of osteoclast progenitors and activates mature osteoclasts by binding to its receptor (RANK) on the respective cell types. In normal bone tissue homeostasis, RANKL and its natural decoy receptor osteoprotegerin (OPG) are carefully balanced. In myeloma, an imbalance between OPG and RANKL is frequently observed, with impaired OPG production and sequestration of available OPG by binding to syndecan-1 (CD138) on myeloma cells. Macrophage inflammatory protein-1alpha (MIP-1alpha) is another inflammatory cytokine which recently has been shown to enhance RANKL- and IL-6-induced osteoclast formation (Han et al. 2001). Restoring the balance between RANKL and OPG not only stops myeloma-induced bone resorption (Croucher et al. 2001; Hofbauer et al. 2001), but also inhibits growth and survival of myeloma cells. The latter effect occurs only when the disease process is restricted to the bone marrow, whereas extramedullary myeloma cell clones seem to have a different growth pattern (Yaccoby et al. 2002). Recently, dickkopf protein1 (DKK1) (Tian et al. 2003) and frizzled related protein (sFRP)-2 (Oshima et al. 2005) have been identified as inhibitors of the Wnt signaling system that supports osteoblastogenesis. Both proteins are secreted in excess by myeloma cells and hence suppress bone formation.

15.2.2 Bone Fractures

Fractures of long bones occur most frequently as a result of bone rarefaction in the proximal parts of the upper arm and femora. They usually require stabilization by surgical fixation with connecting osteosynthesis. Radiotherapy may be used as sole treatment in selected cases but should be applied to all lesions prone to fracture. A single 8–10 Gy fraction is recommended (Terpos and Dimopoulos 2005).

15.2.3 Vertebral Lesions

Osteoporosis may prevail as the only bone sign of multiple myeloma. Frequently, one or more vertebral bodies are found to be affected by either osteolytic lesions and/or vertebral collapse. Painful sites should be irradiated (8–10 Gy within a single fraction). Vertebroplasty or kyphoplasty may be used for immediate pain control and for stabilization of the affected vertebral bodies in case osteolytic lesions are confined to one or few vertebra. Kyphoplasty will also result in complete or partial restoration of the collapsed vertebral body. Some patients may present or develop instability of their spine requiring complex orthopedic or neurosurgical interventions in order to reestablish stability.

15.2.4 Bisphosphonates

Bisphosphonates (BP) are derived from pyrophosphates by substitution of an oxygen atom with a carbon atom and modifying one or both lateral chains of the molecule. Their affinity for Ca^{2+} allows them to bind quickly and specifically to hydroxyapatite, the major calcium containing mineral in bone, especially in regions where resorption is occurring. When osteoclasts break down bone, bisphosphonates accumulate in the resorption space under these cells, exposing them to high bisphosphonate concentrations. Bisphosphonates inhibit the recruitment of osteoclasts from their precursor cells and suppress their subsequent cellular proliferation and differentiation (Siris 1997). They also inhibit the production of IL-6, the most important growth hormone for myeloma cells, and stimulate apoptosis of osteoclasts and myeloma cells (Abildgaard et al. 1998; Shipman et al. 1997, 1998; Takahashi et al. 2001). The efficacy of the bisphosphonates clodronate, pamidronate, and zoledronate in preventing bone lesions has been investigated in several randomized trials while for ibandronate few data from randomized trials are available.

Etidronate and clodronate have been studied as oral formulation. Because intestinal resorption for all oral bisphosphonates is poor (usually <3%), patients are required to fast for at least 1 h prior to and after ingesting the medication. Etidronate was found to be clinically ineffective (Belch et al. 1991; Daragon et al. 1993), although reduction of bone resorption was noted in one trial (Daragon et al. 1993). Treatment with 2.4 g clodronate per day resulted in a 50% reduction in the progression of osteolytic lesions, an increase in the proportion of patients with no pain, and greater decreases in serum and urinary calcium compared to the placebo-treated controls in a Finnish trial (Lahtinen et al. 1992). Interestingly, similar results were reported with a much lower dose of 1.6 g per day by the British MRC group (McCloskey et al. 1998). In this study, a 50% reduction in non-vertebral fractures and a decrease in hypercalcemic events as well as significantly fewer vertebral fractures were observed. Back pain and loss of body height was less in the clodronate group which also had better performance status after 24 months, but survival was not prolonged.

15

Table 15.1 Guidelines for use of bisphosphonates

Substance	Pamidronate	Zoledronate	Clodronate
Dose	90 mg	4 mg	1,600 mg
Application mode	3-h infusion	15-min infusion	2-h infusion or oral
Interval at onset of therapy	Monthly	Monthly	Monthly, or if oral daily
Treatment duration			
ASCO	2 years Monitor creatinine prior to each dose of pamidronate or zoledronate Monitor calcium, magnesium, phosphate, electrolytes, Hb/Hc		
IMWG	CR, VGPR, discontinue after 1 year, continue of <VGPR and/or ongoing active bone disease After 2 years: discontinue if no active bone disease, if active bone disease continue at your discretion		
Mayo	2 years After 2 years: discontinue if CR or stable plateau phase if active disease continue with prolonged treatment intervals (3 months)		
NCCN	No recommendation, chronic users should be monitored for renal function and ONJ Clodronate not mentioned		
ESMO	Long term, type of bisphosphonate not mentioned		

Pamidronate has only limited activity as oral formulation (Brincker et al. 1998) and hence, usually is administered as a 90 mg infusion (over 3–4h) in monthly intervals. Several trials confirmed its efficacy in reducing bone pain, episodes of hypercalcemia, and skeletal complications (Berenson et al. 1996, 1998). In patients starting pamidronate treatment during second-line or subsequent chemotherapy regimens, a prolongation of survival was also observed (Berenson et al. 1998). In a dose-escalation study evaluating tolerability and effectiveness of repeated pamidronate infusions, a close correlation was found between dose intensity and treatment effects. Dose intensities of 25–45 mg/week resulted in a significant palliative effect, whereas the best results were obtained with high doses of 60 or 90 mg pamidronate (Thürlimann et al. 1994) (Table 15.1). Disappointing results with pamidronate maintenance treatment have recently been reported in patients randomized to control, pamidronate, or pamidronate and thalidomide maintenance therapy after double autologous transplantation (Attal et al. 2006). The number of skeletal events was only marginally lower in patients on pamidronate maintenance therapy compared to controls (24% vs. 21%, ns) and slightly higher than in those on pamidronate plus thalidomide (18%). Likewise, overall survival was not affected by pamidronate maintenance therapy (4 year survival rate: control 77%, pamidronate 74%, pamidronate plus thalidomide 87%, $p<0.04$).

Among the newer more potent aminobisphosphonates, zoledronic acid (Berenson et al. 2001), ibandronate (Coleman et al. 1999), and incadronate (Shipman et al. 1998), zoledronic acid is the most widely used one that combines high activity with convenience of administration. A short infusion (5 min) of doses of 2 or 4 mg, is as effective as 2-h infusions of 90 mg pamidronate (Berenson et al. 2001). Because of its potential nephrotoxicity, the recommended infusion time is now 15 min using a dose of 4 mg, administered at monthly intervals. Zoledronic acid should be withheld in patients with renal impairment (creatinine level above normal, and in patients with >50% increase of their baseline creatinine) making testing of renal function prior to infusion mandatory. Nephrotoxic drugs such as NSAIDs, contrast media, and aminoglycoside antibiotics should be withheld on the day of zoledronate therapy. In contrast to an anecdotal prior report (Myers et al. 2002), we (Ludwig et al. 2009) and others (Rosen et al. 2001) did not observe any increase in episodes of renal impairment in patients treated with the combination of thalidomide and zoledronic acid. A comparison between zoledronate and pamidronate showed similar clinical efficacies between both drugs, only the bone resorption marker N-telopeptide of collagen type I (NTX) was more suppressed in the zoledronate cohort (Siris 1997; Abildgaard et al. 1998). A recent comparison in 1960 patients between intravenous zoledronate and oral clodronate revealed a moderate reduction of skeletal events (27% vs. 35%, ns) and significant prolongation of progression-free (19.5 vs. 17.5 months) and of overall survival (50 vs. 44.5 months) with monthly zoledronate therapy (Morgan et al. 2010).

Ibandronate, another highly effective aminobisphosphonate, offers the advantage of excellent renal tolerance (Jackson 2005), but so far has failed to render convincing results in the prevention and treatment of myeloma bone disease (Terpos et al. 2003; Menssen et al. 2002). Table 15.2 shows a synopsis of the main randomized, placebo-controlled trials on bisphosphonate treatment in myeloma patients (Belch et al. 1991; Daragon et al. 1993; Lahtinen et al. 1992; McCloskey et al. 1998; Brincker et al. 1998; Berenson et al. 1998, 2001; Attal et al. 2006; Rosen et al. 2001, 2003; Terpos et al. 2003; Menssen et al. 2002; Djulbegovic et al. 2001; McCloskey et al. 2001; Harvey and Lipton 1996).

15.2.4.1 Adverse Events of Bisphosphonates

Side effects of bisphosphonates depend on the type of drug and route of administration. Oral treatment can be associated with gastrointestinal adverse effects such as nausea, abdominal discomfort, slight anorexia, and diarrhea. A transient (up to 24 h) inflammatory reaction with flu-like symptoms, fever, and myalgia and arthralgia, particularly after the first infusion, can be seen with the use of aminobisphosphonates in about 30–40% of patients (Hewitt et al. 2005). Pamidronate has been associated with ocular inflammatory disease such as scleritis, uveitis, conjunctivitis, and also with blurred vision (Santaella and Fraunfelder 2007). Renal impairment is rare with clodronate, ibandronate, and pamidronate, but more frequently seen with zoledronate (Berenson 2005). However, in most patients bisphosphonate treatment is well tolerated.

Osteonecrosis of the Jaw (ONJ)

ONJ has emerged as the most important complication of therapy with bisphosphonates. Current evidence suggests that zoledronate confers a significant greater risk for this complication than other bisphosphonates and that the cumulative dose and duration of treatment play a role (Zervas et al. 2006). Dental procedures, impaired immune defense, local infections, treatment with corticosteroids, thalidomide, and cytotoxic drugs are likely contributors. Patients should have a dental exam and those with unresolved dental complications or with planned

Table 15.2 Prospective randomized trials with bisphosphonates in patients with myeloma or in patients with myeloma and breast cancer

Author	Number of patients	Bisphosphonate	Comparator	Comments
Belch (1991)	173	Etidronate 5 mg/kg, orally, daily	Placebo	No sig. difference in bone pain, fractures, episodes of hypercalcemia
Daragon (1993)	94	Etidronate 10 mg/kg, orally, daily for 4 months	Placebo	No sig. difference in clinical, biological and radiological parameters, but sig. ↓ bone resorption in etitronate-treated pts.
Lahtinen (1992)	350	Clodronate 2.4 g, orally, daily	Placebo	Sig. ↓ progression of bone lesions, ↓ progression of vertebral fractures, sig. ↑ painless, ↓ hypercalcemia
McCloskey (1998)	536	Clodronate 1,600 mg, orally, daily	Placebo	Sig. ↓ vertebral fractures, sig. ↓ height loss, sig. ↓ back pain, sig. ↓ poor PF, ↓ hypercalcemia
McCloskey (2001)	535	Clodronate 1,600 mg, orally, daily	Placebo	Previously reported
Harvey (1996)	377	Pamidronate 90 mg, i.v., every 4 weeks	Placebo	Sig. ↓ bone pain, sig. ↓ incidence and time to skeleton-related events
Berenson (1998)	392	Pamidronate 90 mg, 4-h infusion, every 4 weeks	Placebo	Sig. ↓ skeletal events, sig. ↑ survival on second-line therapy
Brincker (1998)	300	Pamidronate 300 mg, orally, daily	Placebo	Sig. ↓ severe pain, sig. ↓ reduction of body height
Menssen (2002)	198	Ibandronate 2 mg, i.v., monthly	Placebo	None, dose of ibandronate too low
Terpos (2003)	43	Ibandronate 4 mg, monthly infusion	Pamidronate 90 mg, monthly infusion	Pamidronate induced a greater reduction of bone resorption markers
Berenson (2001)	280	Zoledronate 0.4, 2.0, or 4.0 mg, 5-min infusion;	Pamidronate 90 mg, 2-h infusion	2.0 or 4.0 mg zoledronate or zoledronate 2.0 and 4.0 mg as effective as 90 mg pamidronate sig. ↓.need for radiation therapy to bone, ↓ skeletal-related events, ↓ hypercalcemia; 0.0 mg zoledronate not effective

Table 15.2 (continued)

Rosen (2001)	1.648 MM or breast cancer	Zoledronate 4.0 or 8.0 mg 15 min-infusion, q 4 weeks × 12	Pamidronate 90 MG, 2-h infusion	Similar efficacy and toxicity of both drugs (but 8.0 mg zoledronate associated with higher renal toxicity)
Rosen (2003)	194 MM 412 breast cancer	Zoledronate 4.0 mg, 4.0/8.0 mg, initially 5-min infusion, changed to 15-min infusion	Pamidronate 90 mg, 2-h infusion	Long term follow up of previous study. Zoledronate was similar effective than pamidronate in MM, and slightly more effective in breast cancer, 8 mg zoledronate was associated with higher renal toxicity
Attal (2006)	597	Pamidronate 90 mg, infusion time not specified	Pamidronate and thalidomide 90 mg, infusion time not specified, thal.: 50–400 mg/day and control	Skeletal events: pamidronate 21%, pamidronate-thalidomide 18%, control 24%, Survival@4 years: pam. 74%, pam.-thal.:84%, control: 77%
Morgan (2010)	1960	Zoledronate 4 mg, 15-min infusion, q 4 weeks vs Clodronate 1600 mg, per OS, daily		Skeletal events: zoledronate 27%, clodronate 35% Progression free survival: zoledronate 19.5, clodronate 17.5 Overall survival: zoledronate 50, clodronate 44.5 months
Djulbegovic (2001)	2,183 11 trials	Meta-analysis		Sig. prevention of pathological vertebral fractures, sig. amelioration of pain

invasive procedures should not be started on bisphosphonates. These and other preventive measures seem to reduce the incidence of osteonecrosis (Dimopoulos et al. 2009).

15.2.4.2 Guidelines for the Use of Bisphosphonates

Several international groups, such as American Society of Oncology (Kyle et al. 2007), National Comprehensive Cancer Network (NCCN) (Anderson and NCCN Multiple Myeloma Panel Members 2009), the Mayo Clinic (Lacy et al. 2006), the European Society for Medical Oncology (ESMO) (Harousseau and Dreyling 2008), and the International Myeloma Working Group (Durie 2007), issued guidelines regarding the use of bisphosphonates. According to the majority of these guidelines, all patients with active disease should be started on bisphosphonates. This therapy should be continued for 2 years. Due to the increasing risk of ONJ with increasing duration of therapy, bisphosphonates should be stopped in patients with CR or VGPR without active bone disease, but continued with 3 monthly treatment intervals (Lacy et al. 2006) in those with active bone disease and/or less than VGPR. None of the guidelines provides recommendations regarding the maximal treatment duration. Pamidronate is favored over zoledronic acid until more data are available on the risk of ONJ and other complications. Oral clodronate treatment may be preferred by some patients because of its ease of application and lower risk of ONJ, and may be offered as low cost alternative.

15.2.4.3 Prophylactic Measures for ONJ

Patients should receive a comprehensive dental examination and should be informed about the importance of optimal dental hygiene. Existing/high-risk dental conditions should be treated before initiating BP therapy. After therapy initiation, unnecessary invasive dental procedures should be avoided and dental status should be monitored on an annual basis. Dental problems should be managed conservatively. Temporary suspension of bisphosphonate treatment should be considered if invasive dental procedures are necessary. Initial therapy of ONJ should include discontinuation of bisphosphonates until healing occurs. The decision to restart bisphosphonate should be individualized, until prospective long-term studies are available, considering possible advantages and disadvantages of bisphosphonate therapy.

Presently, information on a possible benefit of bisphosphonates for the prevention of progression of patients with MGUS to multiple myeloma is not available. Further studies are also needed to evaluate their role in patients with smoldering myeloma.

15.3 Hypercalcemia

15.3.1 Diagnosis and Symptoms

Hypercalcemia, the most frequent metabolic complication of multiple myeloma, is predominantly caused by tumor-induced bone resorption. In myeloma patients with impaired kidney function, hypercalcemia can be aggravated by decreased renal calcium excretion.

Diagnosis of hypercalcemia solely based on increased serum calcium levels is unreliable, because binding of albumin to circulating calcium tends to lead to underestimations of biologically active calcium. For more accurate results, the concentration of ionized calcium should be determined. Alternatively, the calcium level should be corrected as follows (Payne et al. 1979):

$$\textit{Corrected serum} \\ \textit{calcium}(mmol/L) = \textit{measured serum calcium}\,(mmol/L) - [0.025 \times \textit{albumi}\,(g/L)] + 1$$

The frequency and intensity of the symptoms of hypercalcemia depend on its severity. Patients with slightly increased calcium levels (<3 mmol/L) are often asymptomatic, whereas more pronounced hypercalcemia (3–4 mmol/L) is associated with symptoms, such as dry mouth, nausea, vomiting, anorexia, constipation, polydipsia, polyuria, fatigue, depression, confusion, impairment of cognitive function or, rarely, even coma. Beyond levels of 4 mmol/L, the patient may develop a hypercalcemic crisis, which can be fatal, if not immediately treated.

15.3.2 Treatment of Hypercalcemia

15.3.2.1 Rehydration

Successful myeloma therapy is the best prophylaxis for myeloma-associated hypercalcemia. Treatment of symptomatic hypercalcemia should immediately be started with intravenous saline (3–6 L per day), for restoring extracellular volume depletion and for inducing calcium diuresis. Fluid repletion alone can reduce serum calcium levels by 0.3–0.5 mmol/L within 48 h.

Forced saline diuresis with the addition of high doses of loop diuretics (furosemide 80–100 mg/day) can be used to induce sodium-linked calcium diuresis, but requires careful monitoring of central venous pressure and frequent evaluations of serum electrolytes, with electrolyte replacements if appropriate. The load of intravenous fluid may be increased to 500–750 mL/h under intensive clinical observation. In patients who receive only moderate amounts of saline under routine monitoring conditions, diuretics may aggravate volume depletion and, therefore, are only recommended when fluid balance can be carefully monitored.

15.3.2.2 Bisphosphonates

Aside from adequate hydration, bisphosphonates, such as pamidronate, zoledronate or clodronate, have become the second mainstay of myeloma-associated hypercalcemia treatment (Body et al. 1998; Carano et al. 1990). Clodronate should be given either at a dose of 1,200 mg as a single infusion over 6 h or repeatedly at daily doses of 300–600 mg. Pamidronate may be given at a dose of 60–90 mg as a single 3-h infusion. Two to three days may elapse before decreases in calcium levels occur, and full treatment effect may take 10–14 days for clodronate and 20–30 days for pamidronate. Bisphosphonate treatment should be continued with oral clodronate (400 mg 3 times/day) or intermittent monthly clodronate (600–1,200 mg) or pamidronate (60–90 mg). Pamidronate treatment may induce transient pyrexia as adverse effect.

Ibandronate and zoledronic acid, third-generation bisphosphonates, are more potent than pamidronate in treatment of hypercalcemia. In addition, they allow shorter infusion periods. Ibandronate can even be applied as a slow intravenous injection and is highly active in hypercalcemia (Pecherstorfer et al. 2003). In patients with hypercalcemia, however, Ibandronate has been administered as a 2 h infusion (Pecherstorfer et al. 2003), at a dose of 2–6 mg and was found to reduce serum calcium levels sufficiently within 3–4 days and to maintain this reduction for up to 30 days (Body 2001). Zoledronic acid, given as a 15-min infusion at a dose of 4 mg, induced calcium normalization in a larger number of patients and prevented relapses for longer time periods than pamidronate, while still showing a good safety profile (Body 2001; Major and Coleman 2001).

15.3.2.3 Calcitonin and Corticosteroids

Additional treatment with calcitonin should be considered in patients who are at risk of developing a hypercalcemic crisis. Calcitonin effectively suppresses osteoclastic bone resorption, inhibits renal tubular calcium reabsorption, and reduces serum calcium levels within 2 h. The effect of calcitonin on bone resorption is short lived due to its down regulatory activity on osteoclast receptors, while its effect on renal calcium excretion is more persistent and important for long-term control of hypercalcemia (Ralston et al. 1985). Finally, corticosteroids, which are routinely included in several chemotherapy regimens for the treatment of myeloma, curb intestinal calcium absorption and can also inhibit bone resorption to some degree. Therefore, they are often included in combination therapies for hypercalcemia.

15.4 Anemia

15.4.1 Pathogenesis of Anemia

Anemia is a common complication of myeloma and its treatment (Birgegard et al. 2006). Twenty to 60% of patients already present with mild or moderate anemia at diagnosis, and almost all patients with uncontrolled long-standing disease become anemic. Myeloma-associated anemia is induced by one or several of a variety of factors, namely, erythropoietin deficiency (Musto 1998), which occurs in practically all patients with impaired kidney function and in about 25% of patients with normal creatinine levels (Beguin et al. 1992), decreased responsiveness of the erythron to proliferative signals of erythropoietin, insufficient numbers of erythroid precursor cells, a direct pro-apoptotic effect on erythroid precursor cells by FAS-ligand- and/or TRAIL-positive myeloma cells, a shortened lifespan of red blood cells, impaired iron utilization, and paraprotein-induced expansion of the plasma volume leading to dilutional anemia. In addition, myeloma therapy, chemo- as well as radiotherapy, may cause anemia or aggravate an already existing anemic state.

The blunted erythropoietin response to the anemic condition seen in the majority of anemic myeloma patients is mediated by inflammatory cytokines (IL-1, TNF-α, and interferon-γ) that suppress both erythropoietin synthesis (Faquin et al. 1992) and proliferation of erythroid precursor cells (Balkwill et al. 1987; Denz et al. 1990) and possibly by increased hepcidin levels that decrease intestinal iron resorption and inhibit the release of iron from storage pools, leading to functional iron deficiency. Another contributing factor to blunted erythropoietin response is increased plasma viscosity caused by high paraprotein levels (Singh et al. 1993). Activated macrophages also remove slightly damaged red blood cells from circulation, thus shortening their lifespan.

15.4.2 Clinical Symptoms of Anemia

Anemic myeloma patients may present with various symptoms. Almost all of them suffer from fatigue (Palumbo et al. 2005), which is often associated with depression, emotional disturbance, or impaired cognitive function. The peripheral hypoxia of moderate-to-severe anemia induces vasodilatation, which may lead to compensatory tachycardia, left ventricular hypertrophy, and, in cases with severe anemia, to congestive heart failure and pulmonary edema. As myeloma patients are typically elderly and often have other morbid conditions, the symptoms of anemia may be pronounced, even at moderately reduced hemoglobin levels.

15.4.3 Treatment of Anemia

15.4.3.1 Transfusions

Patients who are severely symptomatic due to anemia and in need for rapid improvement should receive red blood cell transfusions (RBC). One unit of red cells consists of roughly 1.7×10^{12} red cells in 270 mL, 0.1×10^{6} leukocytes, 0.2×10^{9} platelets, and 200–250 mg iron. Nowadays, special filters that reduce the contamination with white blood cells are applied to reduce the risk of alloimmunization and of transfusion reactions and also the risk of transferring CMV infections. The transfusion of 2 units of RBCs usually results in an immediate increment of 1–2 g in hemoglobin levels, but the improvement is only transient and unless the patient's condition is changing, repeated transfusions will be required in relatively short intervals (2–3 weeks). Transfusions are associated with several risks, such as immediate and late immunological reactions, transfer of infections, volume and iron overload, and in rare cases, even induction of graft versus host disease (Ludwig 2002). In addition, transfusions have been reported to increase the relapse rate in patients with colorectal cancer with the risk for recurrence increasing with the number of transfusions administered perioperatively (Amato and Pescatori 2006) and to reduce survival in general (Vamvakas and Taswell 1994).

In addition, transfusions that had been stored for more than 2 weeks were found to increase the mortality risk in patients undergoing cardiac surgery (Koch et al. 2008). Transfusions administered to critically ill patients increase morbidity and mortality (Marik and Corwin 2008).

Hence, data indicating serious safety concerns with transfusions are accumulating. Lastly, transfusions reduce the patient's autonomy and require substantial logistic support. Transfusions, however, are the only effective treatment in patients unresponsive to erythropoiesis-stimulating agents (ESAs).

15.4.3.2 Erythropoiesis-Stimulating Proteins (ESAs)

Treatment with ESAs is another treatment option for anemia, which, in contrast to the "old reasoning," is not interchangeable with red blood cell transfusions. ESAs have different indications (HB < 10 g/dL vs. Hb < 8 g/dL for RBCs), different response rates (60–70% vs. ~100% for RBCs), and different toxicities. The first documentation of their efficacy in myeloma had already been published as early as 1990 (Ludwig et al. 1990). Eighty-five percent of patients responded to erythropoietin alpha with an increase in hemoglobin of ≥2 g/dL. These initial findings have subsequently been confirmed by a series of prospective randomized phase 3 trials, most of them including patients with multiple myeloma together with patients with CLL and other non-Hodgkin's lymphomas. These trials (Table 15.3) compared either erythropoietin alpha, erythropoietin beta, or darbepoetin alpha with a placebo or untreated control group and documented a response rate (response being defined as increase in hemoglobin of ≥2 g/dL) of 60–75% (Dammacco et al. 1998, 2001; Garton et al. 1995; Osterborg et al. 1996, 2002; Cazzola et al. 1995, 2003; Silvestris et al. 1995; Hedenus et al. 2003). The response rates obtained in patients with multiple myeloma tended to be slightly higher compared to patients with other lymphomas (Osterborg et al. 1996; Cazzola et al. 1995), and importantly, responses were also noted in a fraction (0–21%) of the untreated controls, indicating that erythropoiesis can recover in patients responding to tumor

Table 15.3 Prospective randomized trials of erythropoietic proteins and response to therapy

First author, year of publication	*N*	Erythropoietin dose	Response criterion	Response rate	Other effects
Silvestris 1995	44	Epoetin alpha 150–300 U/kg, Sc. TIW	+ ≥2 g/dL hemoglobin	78%	Restoration of non-paraprotein immunoglobulin production in 5 pts on epoetin
Garton 1995	25	Epoetin alpha 150–300 U/kg Sc. TIW	+ ≥6% hematocrit	60% vs. 0%	Small randomized trial
Cazzola 1995	146, MM: 84	Epoetin beta 1,000–10,000 U Sc, daily	+ ≥2 g/dL hemoglobin	62% vs. 7%	Probability of response dose dependent, low serum Epo level correlated with response
Dammacco 2001	145	Epoetin alpha 150–300 U/kg Sc. TIW	Transfusion need, + ≥2 g/dL Hematopoietic response	75% vs. 21%	Significant reduction in transfusion need (28% vs. 47%, $P = 0.017$) significant improvement in more QOL measures ($p \leq 0.05$)
Osterborg 2002	349, MM: 117	Epoetin beta 150–300 U/kg Sc. TIW	+ ≥2 g/dL hemoglobin	76% vs. 29%	Significant reduction in transfusion need (risk reduction:66%, $p < 0.0001$)
Cazzola 2003	241, MM:~70%	Epoetin beta, 30,000 U vs. 10,000 Sc weekly vs. TIW	+ ≥2 g/dL hemoglobin	72% vs. 75%	Only patients with Epo level <100 mU/mL enrolled baseline Epo predictive of response ($p < 0.002$)
Hedenus 2003	344, MM: 173	Darbepoetin 2.25 µg/kg, Sc, weekly	+ ≥2 g/dL hemoglobin	60% vs. 18%	Significant reduction in transfusion need (31% vs. 48%, $p < 0.001$) significant improvement in FACT-fatigue subscore ($p < 0.032$)

treatment. Treatment of poor prognosis patients results in lower response rates as documented in one study reporting a ≥2 g/dL increase in Hb levels in 35% of patients only (Musto et al. 1997). This accords with the general experience that response to ESAs is poor in patients with rapidly progressive disease, acute infections or heavy inflammation, and shortly after autologous transplantation and after surgery.

15.4.3.3 Treatment Recommendations for ESAs

Treatment guidelines have been issued by ASCO/ASH (Rizzo et al. 2008), EORTC (Bokemeyer et al. 2007; Aapro and Link 2008), ESMO (Greil et al. 2008), and other organizations or groups. Due to increased mortality or recurrence rate reported in eight of more than 60 prospective randomized trials, the indication for ESA use has been restricted by the FDA and EMEA to patients undergoing concomitant chemotherapy. Treatment should be started in patients with Hb <10 g/dL or in those with significant symptoms at Hb levels <11 g/dL. Erythropoietin alpha or beta can be used at a dose of 10,000 U TIW, or 30,000 U or 40,000 U once weekly, and darbepoetin at 150 μg weekly or 500 μg every 3 weeks (Gabrilove et al. 2001). Hemoglobin values should be monitored weekly and the dosage of ESAs tapered, if necessary, to prevent overshooting of hemoglobin levels. In patients who fail to respond within 6 weeks, the initial dose may be doubled. Patients with absolute or relative deficiencies in endogenous erythropoietin (O/P, i.e., ratio of observed by expected hemoglobin level <0.9) (Cazzola et al. 1995, 2003) and with preserved marrow function as reflected by platelet counts >150,000/μL show the highest response rates to ESAs (Osterborg et al. 2005).

Additional benefits can be expected from iron supplementation during the phases of high iron demands from enhanced erythropoiesis. In patients with renal anemia, intravenous iron supplementation reduced the required weekly rhEPO dose by 30–70% (Sunder-Plassmann and Horl 1997). Parenteral iron should be administered in cancer patients with overt iron deficiency, as indicated by low transferrin saturation (<20%) and/or high numbers (>5%) of hypochromic red cells. It also enhances the response to ESAs in patients with functional iron deficiency and has been shown to overcome resistance to erythropoietin alpha in a small series of patients with multiple myeloma (Katodritou et al. 2004). At present, there is no generally accepted recommendation regarding the use of intravenous iron in general or regarding a specific iron preparation and its appropriate dose and schedule (Ludwig 2006). Oral iron treatment is only of very little benefit during erythropoietin therapy.

The most important benefit of ESA therapy pertains to the reduction of transfusion need and the improvement in quality of life (Demetri et al. 1998; Leitgeb et al. 1994) with a better sense of well-being, better exercise capacity, and less fatigue. The largest gain in quality of life from incremental increases of 1 g/dL hemoglobin occurs, when the hemoglobin increases from 11 to 12 g/dL (Crawford et al. 2002). Retrospective comparisons regarding the influence of ESA on survival are methodically flawed and yielded conflicting results. One study showed a positive impact of ESA therapy on survival (Baz et al. 2007), one was negative (Katodritou et al. 2008), and another one reported no survival difference (Richardson et al. 2008). For final clarification, a patient-level meta-analysis including all hitherto conducted studies and comparing ESA treated patients with controls would be required.

Thromboembolic complications are another important adverse effect of ESA therapy with a hazard ratio of 1.68 for patients with various cancers compared to controls (Bohlius et al. 2006). There is also a risk of thromboembolic complications associated with thalidomide or lenalidomide treatment (Knight et al. 2006), and in these patients, prophylactic anticoagulation with low molecular weight heparin or aspirin is recommended. Hypertension is rare, and other adverse effects are usually limited to slight pain or mild erythema at the injection site, which occurs in a minority of treated patients.

15.5 Infections

15.5.1 Causes of Infections

Infections, particularly those of bacterial origin, are frequent complications of multiple myeloma and are among the most common causes of death in myeloma patients (Peest et al. 1991). The susceptibility of myeloma patients to infections results mainly from suppression of production of polyclonal immunoglobulins and of T cell function as well as from granulocytopenia (Massaia et al. 1988; Jacobson and Zolla-Pazner 1986). Treatment-induced mucositis is an important risk factor for the intrusion of pathogenic microorganisms, and indwelling catheters, as used for the application of continuous therapy, pose patients at risk for catheter associated gram positive infections.

During active disease, the risk of infections is about four times higher than during remission (Hargreaves et al. 1995), and during the first 2 months of induction chemotherapy, bacterial infections occur twice as frequently as during later treatment episodes. Some of these early infections are serious and require hospitalization, some may even be fatal; often delay of chemotherapy is necessary (Oken et al. 1996). After reaching the plateau phase of their disease, patients at risk for serious infections are characterized by poor IgG responses to exogenous antigens, such as pneumococcal capsular polysaccharides or tetanus and diphtheria toxoids (Hargreaves et al. 1995). Mortality from infections is particularly high in immunosuppressed patients who have received allografts from unrelated donors (Mattsson et al. 1997). Patients on high-dose glucocorticoids are prone to newly acquired or reactivated viral and fungal infections, with the latter frequently manifesting as oral or oro-esophageal candidiasis.

The spectrum of microorganisms isolated during a febrile episode changes in the course of the disease. In early stage myeloma, the most common infections involve the respiratory tract, manifesting as bronchitis and pneumonia. These infections are predominantly caused by *Haemophilus influenzae* or *Streptococcus pneumoniae*. In patients with advanced myeloma and during the neutropenic phases of intensive chemotherapy, *Staphylococcus aureus* and gram-negative bacteria are more common. However, infections with gram-positive bacteria have recently become more frequent in neutropenic myeloma patients. They were the predominant cause of infections observed in 20–40% of patients after high-dose therapy and autologous stem cell transplantation (Salutari et al. 1998; Kolbe et al. 1997). Patients with advanced myeloma also tend to suffer from infections of the urinary tract and of septicemia. Table 15.4 lists microorganisms frequently involved in myeloma-associated infections.

Early diagnosis and treatment of infections is particularly important in myeloma patients. Diagnostic measures should include differential blood counts, urine tests, bacterial cultures, and viral isolates from blood, urine, and other specimens, chest X-rays and CT scan, serum electrophoresis, and quantitative assessment of immunoglobulins. If diarrhea is present, stool should be tested for clostridium difficile toxin, bacteria, viruses (CMV, rota-, adeno-, Norfolk-virus), and if indicated, for protozoa. Neutropenic patients may fail to show fever as a symptom of sepsis; suddenly emerging fatigue and weakness can be the only obvious symptoms of severe infections in these patients. In these cases,

Table 15.4 Microorganisms frequently involved in myeloma-associated infections

Class	Organism	Predominant Source
Gram-negative bacteria	*Escherichia coli, Klebsiella pneumonia, Pseudomonas aeruginosa*	Gastrointestinal tract
Gram-positive bacteria	*Staphylococcus aureus*	Oropharynx, skin, catheter locations
	Staphylococcus pneumonia, Haemophilus influenza	Respiratory tract
Fungi	*Candida* spp.	Skin mucosal surfaces
	Aspergillus spp.	Respiratory tract
Viruses	*Adenovirus*	Respiratory tract
	Herpes simplex varicella zoster cytomegalovirus	Latent infections

immediate treatment with adequate doses of broad-spectrum antibiotics is essential.

15.5.2 Prophylaxis of Infections

Risk of infections in myeloma patients can be reduced by the administration of immunoglobulin preparations. A randomized placebo-controlled study in plateau-phase patients using monthly immunoglobulin infusions (0.4 g/kg) for a period of 1 year showed significant reductions in frequency and severity of infections, with patients who responded poorly to pneumococcal immunization benefiting most from immunoglobulin infusions (Chapel et al. 1994). Another randomized trial in patients with lymphoproliferative syndromes or myeloma showed significant effects of nebulizations with IgA (every 12 h for 3 months) in preventing respiratory infections or at least delaying their onset (Bezares et al. 1997). Therefore, regular immunoglobulin substitution may be considered in myeloma patients who suffer from recurrent infections, but not in those without any history of infectious complications.

Effective infection prophylaxis in patients undergoing induction chemotherapy can be achieved by the administration of trimethoprim/sulfamethoxazole (co-trimoxazole, 160 mg/800 mg, twice daily, orally). In a randomized trial, the use of this regimen during the first 2 months of conventional induction chemotherapy resulted in significantly decreased frequencies and severities of bacterial infections (Oken et al. 1996). However, solid scientific data on prophylactic antimicrobial therapy in myeloma are scarce. Experience in several centers suggests that antibiotic prophylaxis should be based on the individual patient's risk profile. Important parameters are the patient's previous history of infections and, particularly, the type and dose of myeloma therapy. Patients on VAD, high-dose dexamethasone, or on a bortezomib-based regimen are at high risk of reactivation or new acquisition of herpetic infections. Those patients should receive antiviral prophylaxis with oral acyclovir, 800 mg, four times daily, or with one of the newer antiviral drugs, such as famciclovir or valacyclovir. Dose adaptation according to renal function is required.

Patients on high-dose dexamethasone are also at increased risk of acquiring fungal infections, in particular, candidiasis of the oral and upper gastrointestinal tract, warranting antifungal prophylaxis. For oro-esophageal candidiasis, oral amphotericin suspension, swallowed four times daily, or oral fluconazole, 50 mg daily, may be considered both for treatment and for antifungal prophylaxis.

15.5.3 Vaccination

Vaccinations against influenza, pneumococci, hemophilus, and meningococci may be considered, but the induction of protective antibodies is significantly lower than in healthy individuals. In one study, vaccination against influenza induced suboptimal titers in 81% and protective titers in 19% of patients only. Likewise, only 61% of patients produced protective antibodies against pneumococci while the response rate with a hemophilus vaccine (75%) was similar to results in the healthy population (Robertson et al. 2000). Studies documenting a possible clinical value of these vaccinations in myeloma are not available as yet.

15.5.4 Treatment of Infections

Empiric antibiotic treatment with a broad spectrum antibiotic must be started immediately (after blood cultures have been taken) without delay in patients with neutropenic fever. Some neutropenic patients may fail to show fever as a symptom of sepsis; suddenly emerging fatigue and weakness can be the only obvious symptoms of severe infections. Patients with low risk may be started on oral treatment either with a chinolone or macrolide antibiotic or with a second-generation cephalosporin, trimethoprim-sulfamethoxazole, or amoxicillin-clavulanic acid. Effectiveness of treatment must be monitored and in case of insufficient results changed to parenteral therapy. It should be kept in mind that these drugs usually do not provide coverage for coagulase-negative staphylococci, methicillin-resistant staphylococcus aureus, enterococci, some strains of penicillin-resistant streptococcus pneumonia, and viridans streptococci. In these cases, vancomycin is the treatment of choice, but its inherent nephrotoxicity may preclude its use. Linezolid or daptomycin may be used instead. In intermediate and high-risk patients, monotherapy with a fourth-generation cephalosporin such as ceftazidim, or alternatively, meropenem or imipenem, or duo treatment with an antipseudomonas beta-lactam and an aminoglycoside antibiotic is recommended.

Patients treated with high-dose dexamethasone, bortezomib, autologous or allogeneic transplantation are prone to viral infections. Herpetic infections should be treated with acyclovir, while ganciclovir, foscarnet, or cidofovir are the treatments of choice for cytomegalovirus infections; ribavirin is indicated for severe pulmonary infections by respiratory syncytial virus (RSV) and oseltamivir for infections caused by influenza viruses. Dosing of these antiviral drugs should be adjusted in patients with renal impairment.

Invasive aspergillosis and infections with other filamentous fungi, which may occur in neutropenic patients, particularly after allogeneic transplantation, have a high mortality rate (Lass-Florl et al. 1998; Pagano et al. 2001). Patients who develop cerebral abscesses and/or aspergillosis lesions in the vicinity of the pulmonary artery require emergency surgery, in addition to antifungal drugs (Bernard et al. 1997). For the treatment of invasive fungal infections, amphotericin B is still an established standard drug, and the degree of resistance of the invading aspergillus species to in vitro cultivation with amphotericin B is a reliable predictor of the clinical outcome of this antifungal treatment (Bernard et al. 1997). Caspofungin acetate, voriconazole, and posaconazole are relatively new antifungal agents, with even higher activity against aspergillosis and better tolerance than amphotericin.

Granulocyte colony-stimulating factor is routinely used to enhance the neutrophil recovery after autologous or allogeneic transplantation. A randomized trial in severely granulocytopenic myeloma patients after intensive chemotherapy showed that the addition of G-CSF (5 μg/kg/day) to broad-spectrum antibiotics improved the outcome of antibiotic treatment. In addition, it decreased the mortality rate, shortened the length of hospital stay, curbed superinfections, and prevented fungal infections (Aviles et al. 1996). However, in other cancer patients who were febrile and neutropenic, two placebo-controlled randomized trials failed to fully confirm these results (Maher et al. 1994; Anaissie et al. 1996). Patients who received antibiotic treatment in combination with G-CSF recovered earlier from neutropenia, but did not differ from controls with regard to days with fever and days in hospital (Maher et al. 1994). The addition of granulocyte–macrophage colony-stimulating factor (GM-CSF) to antibiotics significantly increased response rates, but failed to improve survival (Anaissie et al. 1996). Even though the growth factors G-CSF and GM-CSF have been reported to stimulate proliferation of myeloma cells in vitro (Klein et al. 1992), this effect has not been observed in vivo (Barlogie et al. 1990), and the use of G-CSF for prophylaxis and treatment of infections in neutropenic myeloma patients is considered safe.

15.6 Pain

15.6.1 Characteristics and Causes of Pain

Many myeloma patients suffer from moderate-to-severe pain in the skeleton, particularly in the lumbar spine. This type of pain is frequently the predominant symptom of myeloma at diagnosis, and also a common indicator of relapse or progressive disease. Microfractures and pathological fractures of vertebral bodies, ribs, pelvis, or long bones cause severe pain, which is characterized by its sudden onset. In addition, pain results from irritation of sensory nerves in the bone marrow by inflammatory cytokines and prostaglandins.

Other important causes of pain in myeloma are nerve root and spinal cord compression caused by extra-osseous extension of myeloma deposits or by compression fractures. These neurological impairments require rapid diagnosis and treatment in order to prevent possible mono- or paraplegia. Post-herpetic neuralgia, active herpetic virus infections, or mucosal ulcerations, possible complications of immunosuppression, and/or cytotoxic treatment, also cause considerable pain. A synopsis of the main causes of pain in myeloma patients is shown in Table 15.5.

Even though myeloma-associated pain usually subsides during effective chemotherapy and/or local irradiation, specific treatment for pain relief is required in most patients. It is noteworthy that the degree of pain, a subjective experience, is often differently estimated by patients, doctors, and nurses (Grossman et al. 1991), resulting in inadequate analgesia (Grossman 1993). Hence, the intensity of pain should be assessed by the patient with the use of pain scales to allow appropriate monitoring whether pain treatment is sufficient.

Table 15.5 Main causes of pain in multiple myeloma

Bone pain
Pathologic fractures
Microfractures
Osteolytic and/or osteoplastic bone lesions
Irritation of sensory nerves in the bone marrow
Neurological impairments
Nerve root and spinal cord compression
Therapy incluced neuroleptics
Lesions in skin and mucosal tissue
Post-herpetic neuralgia
Herpetic virus infections
Mucosal ulcerations

15

15.6.2 Medical Pain Treatment

In almost all myeloma patients, effective analgesia can be achieved by regular administration of oral medication. A three-step treatment plan, the so-called WHO pain treatment ladder (World Health Organization 1990) (Table 15.6) has been widely accepted for the treatment of tumor-related pain. Applying treatment with drugs of the first step, non-opioid drugs, may suffice even in patients suffering from severe pain. In case of persisting or increasing pain, treatment should readily be escalated to the second step, which covers weak opioid drugs. Strong opioids, drugs of the third step, are necessary if pain is still persisting or increasing. To all treatment steps, adjuvant analgesic drugs should be added as required.

Non-steroid anti-inflammatory drugs (NSAID) have analgesic as well as anti-inflammatory effects and may, in addition, retard prostaglandin-induced bone resorption. NSAIDs are useful in myeloma but should be used with caution in patients with renal impairment. However, common NSAIDs have partly been replaced or supplemented by some of the more recently developed cyclo-oxygenase-2 (COX-2) inhibitors, which have less gastrointestinal and possibly less renal toxicity (Michalowski 2002). Because the analgesic effects of the first-step drugs are limited and dose escalations beyond a certain level do not result in enhanced analgesia, insufficient pain control at the first step of the WHO pain treatment ladder requires the addition or sole application of weak opioids as soon as possible.

Typical opioids recommended by the WHO for the second step of pain treatment are codeine, dihydrocodeine, tramadol, and tilidine. These weak opioids exert their analgesic effect by binding to μ and to δ and κ receptors on brain cells. Both, affinity to these receptors and triggering of the intrinsic receptor activity, are important characteristics of opioids, but only the latter is responsible for the analgesic effect. Substances with a high potential for triggering intrinsic activity (morphine and pethidine) are agonists, whereas substances with high receptor affinity but lack of intrinsic activity (naloxone and naltrexone) are antagonists. Agonists/antagonists (buprenorphine and pentazocine) have both relatively high intrinsic activity and receptor affinity, thus potentially competing with agonists for the receptor binding site. Typical opioids for the third step of pain treatment are morphine, levomethadone, and buprenorphine, as well as transdermal fentanyl, which offers the advantages of long-term activity and better tolerance, particularly less gastrointestinal toxicity, but is more expensive. Buprenorphine is more potent than morphine, but when administered orally, it is subject to the first-pass effect of the liver. Its bioavailability is therefore low, unless it is administered transdermally, sublingually, or intravenously. Buprenorphine ampules, however, are available in few countries only because of the high addictive potency of the intravenous formulation of this drug. Transdermal opioids may be particularly helpful in patients who have difficulties swallowing medication.

A strict classification of opioids into second- and third-step drugs is not always possible.

Table 15.6 WHO pain ladder

Level 1	Level 2	Level 3
NSAIDs	Weak opioids	Strong opioids
Aspirin, ibuprofen, naproxen, COX-2 inhibitors	Codeine, dihydrocodeine, tramadol,tilidilate	Morphine, levomethadone, buprenorphine, fentanyl
Adjuvant medication (corticosteroid, antiemetics, neuroleptics, antidepressants, stool softener benzodiazepines) should be given as required		

Table 15.7 Recommended doses and treatment intervals of opioid analgesics

	Dose	Treatment interval (h)
Oral application		
Codeine	180–200 mg	3–4
Hydrocodone	30 mg	3–4
Morphine	10–30 mg	3–4
Buprenorphine	0.2 mg	6–8
Morphine, controlled release	90–120 mg	6–12
Levomethadone	2.5–5 mg	6–12
Transdermal application		
Fentanyl patch	25–100 μg/h	72
Buprenorphine patch	35–70 μg/h	72

Dosage plays an important role, and opioids vary widely in the duration of their analgesic effect and partly also in their adverse effects. In up to 70% of patients, a change from one to another opioid (opioid rotation) is needed to overcome diminishing analgesic activity and/or side effects. Table 15.7 lists recommended doses and treatment intervals for various opioids.

The adverse effects of opioids can frequently be well controlled by supportive measures (Cherny and Portenoy 1994), but in some patients, some difficulties may remain. At the start of treatment, nausea and emesis may prevail, requiring antiemetics; and dryness of mouth is a common complaint. Impairment of vigilance and temporary confusion may require transient dose reduction. Initial nausea and sedation often subsides or lessens during the course of treatment. Impairment of visceral motor function may manifest as inadequate colonic motility or bladder distension. As prophylaxis against constipation, a fiber-rich diet and adequate hydration should be recommended; treatment with laxatives may be necessary. In addition, patients should be aware of the fact that urinary retention, caused by opioid-induced increased detrusor muscle tension, is a possible complication of pain treatment with opioids. Respiratory depression, another possible adverse effect of opioids, however, occurs only rarely during pain treatment.

Sufficient dosing and adequate scheduling of pain treatment are essential in order to ascertain sufficient and continuous pain control. Combinations of opioids and NSAIDs may increase the efficacy of pain control and curb toxicities. Additional benefits may be achieved by adding glucocorticosteroids, antidepressants, or neuroleptics to pain treatment according to the WHO pain treatment ladder. In some patients, however, pain cannot be sufficiently controlled by these conventional forms of pain therapy. In those cases, sufficient pain control is often achieved by continuous intravenous infusion of morphines with portable pump systems or intrathecal application of morphines with or without potentiating drugs, such as calcium antagonists or ketamine.

15.7 Renal Failure

15.7.1 Prevalence and Causes of Renal Failure

Renal failure is a common feature of multiple myeloma, may provide a clue to diagnosis, cause major management problems, and may result in significant morbidity. Depending on the definition of renal failure, this complication occurs in 20–40% of newly diagnosed patients

15

with MM (Alexanian et al. 1990; Bladé et al. 1998; Kyle et al. 2003; Eleutherakis-Papaiakovou et al. 2007). Patients who present with acute severe renal failure have increased early mortality, reaching up to 30% within the first 2 months in some series (Bladé et al. 1998; Augustson et al. 2005). Renal impairment in patients with MM results from the toxic effects of monoclonal light chains, which can affect various segments of the nephron, glomeruli, tubules, interstitium, and blood vessels leading to different pathologic and clinical findings. Myeloma cast nephropathy (so-called myeloma kidney) is by far the most frequent form of renal damage. Other clinicopathological conditions include amyloidosis, light-chain deposition disease (LCDD) or, rarely, crystal-storing histiocytosis causing adult Fanconi syndrome. These entities may sometimes coexist in the same patient. Other contributing factors include dehydration, nephrotoxic drugs (antibiotics, NSAIDs), hypercalcemia, and perhaps use of contrast agents. Usually, these factors aggravate the toxic effects of light chains and are rarely the primary reason of renal failure (Dimopoulos et al. 2008). Although light-chain-induced nephropathy is highly likely in a patient with established diagnosis of multiple myeloma and significant urine light chain excretion, a renal biopsy is recommended to establish the specific type of light-chain-induced renal damage and to rule out or to establish additional pathologies.

15.7.2 Management of Myeloma-Induced Renal Failure

Supportive care measures in combination with anti-myeloma therapy should be initiated promptly. These include adequate hydration, avoidance of nephrotoxic drugs, and if required, treatment of hypercalcemia and/or hyperuricemia and of infections. The most important measure encompasses active myeloma therapy in order to eliminate or reduce the nephrotoxic paraproteins. Recovery of renal function has been reported in a significant proportion of patients treated with conventional chemotherapy, especially when high-dose dexamethasone is also used. Novel agents, such as thalidomide, bortezomib, and lenalidomide have significant activity in pretreated and untreated MM patients and should be used with high dose dexamethasone (Dimopoulos et al. 2008). Presently, it is impossible to favor a specific regimen but the ideal treatment should result in fast and complete response in order to prevent further damage to the kidney. As metabolism of thalidomide and of bortezomib is independent of renal function, both drugs can be administered without dose adaptations, while lenalidomide dosing has to be adapted to the glomerular filtration rate.

Mechanical methods such as removal of nephrotoxic light chains with plasma exchange can be combined with anti-myeloma therapy 2005; Pozzi et al. 1987; Zucchelli et al. 1988) but the largest randomized trial showed no improvement in renal function and myeloma outcome with plasma exchange (Clark et al. 2005). Removal of free light chains with dialysis is another alternative approach. A new hemodialysis membrane which recently has been developed to remove the circulating light chains more efficiently has been shown to lead to large reductions in the concentration of serum free light chains (Hutchison et al. 2007), but results from a randomized study comparing anti-myeloma therapy with and without the use of this dialysis membrane (Gambro 1100) approach are still pending.

Acknowledgments Supported by the Wilhelminen Cancer Research Institute of the Austrian Forum Against Cancer.

References

Aapro MS, Link H (2008) September 2007 update on EORTC guidelines and anemia management with erythropoiesis-stimulating agents. Oncologist 13(Suppl 3):33–36

Abildgaard N, Rungby J, Glerup H, Brixen K, Kassem M, Brincker H et al (1998) Long-term oral pamidronate treatment inhibits osteoclastic bone resorption and bone turnover without affecting osteoblastic function in multiple myeloma. Eur J Med 61:128–134

Alexanian R, Barlogie B, Dixon D (1990) Renal failure in multiple myeloma. Pathogenesis and prognostic implications. Arch Intern Med 150(8):1693–1695

Amato A, Pescatori M (2006) Perioperative blood transfusions for the recurrence of colorectal cancer. Cochrane Database Syst Rev (1):CD005033. Review

Anaissie EJ, Vartivarian S, Bodey GP, Legrand C, Kantarjian H, Abi-Said D et al (1996) Randomized comparison between antibiotics alone and antibiotics plus granulocyte–macrophage colony-stimulating factor (*Escherichia coli*-derived) in cancer patients with fever and neutropenia. Am J Med 100:17–23

Anderson KC and NCCN Multiple Myeloma Panel Members (2009) NCCN Clinical practice guidelines in oncology: multiple myeloma. Version 2 http://www.nccn.org/professionals/physician_gls/PDF/myeloma.pdf

Attal M, Harousseau JL, Leyvraz S, Doyen C, Hulin C, Benboubker L et al (2006) Inter-groupe Francophone du Myelome (IFM). Maintenance therapy with thalidomide improves survival in patients with multiple myeloma. Blood 108(10):3289–3294

Augustson BM, Begum G, Dunn JA et al (2005) Early mortality after diagnosis of multiple myeloma: analysis of patients entered onto the United Kingdom Medical Research Council trials between 1980 and 2002 – Medical Research Council Adult Leukaemia Working Party. J Clin Oncol 23(36):9219–9226

Aviles A, Guzman R, Garcia EL, Talavera A, Diaz-Maqueo JC (1996) Results of a randomized trial of granulocyte colony-stimulating factor in patients with infection and severe granulocytopenia. Anticancer Drugs 7:392–397

Balkwill F, Osborne R, Burke F, Naylor S, Talbot D, Durbin H et al (1987) Evidence for tumor necrosis factor/cachectin production in cancer. Lancet 330:ii1229–ii1232

Barlogie B, Jagannath S, Dixon DO, Cheson B, Smallwood L, Hendrickson A et al (1990) High-dose melphalan and granulocyte-macrophage colony-stimulating factor for refractory multiple myeloma. Blood 76:677–680

Bataille R, Manolagas SC, Berenson JR (1997) Pathogenesis and management of bone lesions in multiple myeloma. Hematol Oncol Clin North Am 11:349–361

Baz R, Walker E, Choueiri TK, Abou Jawde R, Brand C, McGowan B, et al (2007) Recombinant human erythropoietin is associated with increased overall survival in patients with multiple myeloma. Acta Haematol 117(3):162–167

Beguin Y, Yerna M, Loo M, Weber M, Fillet G (1992) Erythropoiesis in multiple myeloma: defective red cell production due to inappropriate erythropoietin production. Br J Haematol 82:648–653

Belch AR, Bergsagel DE, Wilson K, O'Reilly S, Wilson J, Sutton D, et al (1991) Effect of daily etidronate on the osteolysis of multiple myeloma. J Clin Oncol 9(8):1397–1402

Berenson JR (2005) Recommendations for zoledronic acid treatment of patients with bone metastases. Oncologist 10(1):52–62

Berenson JR, Lichtenstein A, Porter L, Dimopoulos MA, Bordoni R, George S et al (1996) Efficacy of pamidronate in reducing skeletal events in patients with advanced multiple myeloma. N Engl J Med 334:488–493

Berenson JR, Lichtenstein A, Porter L, Dimopoulos MA, Bordoni R, George S et al (1998) Long-term pamidronate treatment of advanced multiple myeloma patients reduces skeletal events. Myeloma Aredia Study Group. J Clin Oncol 16:593–602

Berenson JR, Rosen LS, Howell A, Porter L, Coleman RE, Morley W et al (2001) Zoledronic acid reduces skeletal-related events in patients with osteolytic metastases. Cancer 91:1191–1200

Bernard A, Caillot D, Couaillier JF, Casasnovas O, Guy H, Favre JP (1997) Surgical management of invasive pulmonary aspergillosis in neutropenic patients. Ann Thorac Surg 64:1441–1447

Bezares R, Murro H, Diaz A, Cavagnaro F, Caviglia D, Santome J (1997) Prevention of infections in patients with lymphoproliferative syndromes and myeloma by nebulization of an IgA concentrate [In Spanish]. Sangre 42:219–222

Birgegard G, Gascon P, Ludwig H (2006) Evaluation of anaemia in patients with multiple myeloma and lymphoma: findings of the European Cancer Anaemia Survey. Eur J Haematol 77(5):378–386

Bladé J, Rosiñol L (2005) Renal, hematologic and infectious complications in multiple myeloma. Best Pract Res Clin Haematol 18(4):635–652

15

Bladé J, Fernandez-Llama P, Bosch F et al (1998) Renal failure in multiple myeloma: presenting features and predictors of outcome in 94 patients from a single institution. Arch Intern Med 158(17):1889–1893

Body JJ (2001) Dosing regimens and main adverse events of bisphosphonates. Semin Oncol 28(Suppl 11):49–53

Body JJ, Bartl R, Burckhardt P, Delmas PD, Diel IJ, Fleisch H et al (1998) Current use of bisphosphonates in oncology. International Bone and Cancer Study Group. J Clin Oncol 16:3890–3899

Bohlius J, Wilson J, Seidenfeld J, Piper M, Schwarzer G, Sandercock J, et al (2006) Recombinant human erythropoietins and cancer patients: updated meta-analysis of 57 studies including 9353 patients. J Natl Cancer Inst 98(10): 708–714

Bokemeyer C, Aapro MS, Courdi A, Foubert J, Link H, Osterborg A, Repetto L, Soubeyran P, European Organisation for Research and Treatment of Cancer (EORTC) Taskforce for the Elderly (2007) EORTC guidelines for the use of erythropoietic proteins in anaemic patients with cancer: 2006 update. Eur J Cancer 43(2):258–270, Epub 2006 Dec 19. Review

Brincker H, Westin J, Abildgaard N, Gimsing P, Turesson I, Hedenus M et al (1998) Failure of oral pamidronate to reduce skeletal morbidity in multiple myeloma: a double-blind placebo-controlled trial. Danish-Swedish co-operative study group. Br J Haematol 101:280–286

Carano A, Teitelbaum SL, Konsek JD, Schlesinger PH, Blair HC (1990) Bisphosphonates directly inhibit the bone resorption activity of isolated avian osteoclasts in vitro. J Clin Invest 85:456–461

Cazzola M, Messinger D, Battistel V, Bron D, Cimino R, Enller-Ziegler L et al (1995) Recombinant human erythropoietin in the anemia associated with multiple myeloma or non-Hodgkin's lymphoma: dose finding and identification of predictors of response. Blood 86:4446–4453

Cazzola M, Beguin Y, Kloczko J, Spicka I, Coiffier B (2003) Once-weekly epoetin beta is highly effective in treating anaemic patients with lymphoproliferative malignancy and defective endogenous erythropoietin production. Br J Haematol 122(3): 386–393

Chapel HM, Lee M, Hargreaves R, Pamphilon DH, Prentice AG (1994) Randomised trial of intravenous immunoglobulin as prophylaxis against infection in plateau-phase multiple myeloma. The UK Group for Immunoglobulin Replacement Therapy in Multiple Myeloma. Lancet 343: 1059–1063

Cherny NI, Portenoy RK (1994) The management of cancer pain. CA Cancer J Clin 44:263–303

Clark WF, Stewart AK, Rock GA et al (2005) Plasma exchange when myeloma presents as acute renal failure: a randomized, controlled trial. Ann Intern Med 143(11):777–784

Coleman RE, Purohit OP, Black C, Vinholes JJ, Schlosser K, Huss H et al (1999) Double-blind, randomised, placebo-controlled, dose-finding study of oral ibandronate in patients with metastatic bone disease. Ann Oncol 10:311–316

Crawford J, Cella D, Cleeland CS, Cremieux PY, Demetri GD, Sarokhan BJ, et al (2002) Relationship between changes in hemoglobin level and quality of life during chemotherapy in anemic cancer patients receiving epoetin alfa therapy. Cancer 95(4):888–895

Croucher PI, Shipman CM, Lippitt J, Perry M, Asosingh K, Hijzen A et al (2001) Osteoprotegerin inhibits the development of osteolytic bone disease in multiple myeloma. Blood 98:3534–3540

Dammacco F, Silvestris F, Castoldi GL, Grassi B, Bernasconi C, Nadali G et al (1998) The effectiveness and tolerability of epoetin alfa in patients with multiple myeloma refractory to chemotherapy. Int J Clin Lab Res 28:127–134

Dammacco F, Castoldi G, Rodjer S (2001) Efficacy of epoetin alfa in the treatment of anaemia of multiple myeloma. Br J Haematol 113:172–179

Daragon A, Humez C, Michot C, Le Loet X, Grosbois B, Pouyol F, et al (1993) Treatment of multiple myeloma with etidronate: results of a multicenter double-blind study. Groupe d'Etudes et de Recherches sur le Myélome (GERM). Eur J Med 2(8):449–452

Demetri GD, Kris M, Wade J, Degos L, Cella D (1998) Quality-of-life benefit in chemotherapy patients treated with epoetin alfa is independent of disease response or tumor type: results from a prospective community oncology study. J Clin Oncol 16:3412–3425

Denz H, Fuchs D, Huber H, Nachbaur D, Reibnegger G, Thaler J et al (1990) Correlation between neopterin, interferon-gamma and haemoglobin in patients with haematological disorders. Eur J Haematol 44:186–189

Dimopoulos MA, Kastritis E, Rosinol L, Bladé J, Ludwig H (2008) Pathogenesis and treatment of renal failure in multiple myeloma. Leukemia 22:1485–1493

Dimopoulos MA, Kastritis E, Bamia C, Melakopoulos I, Gika D, Roussou M et al (2009) Reduction of osteonecrosis of the jaw (ONJ) after implementation of preventive measures in patients with multiple myeloma treated with zoledronic acid. Ann Oncol 20(1):117–120

Djulbegovic B, Wheatley K, Ross J, Clark O, Bos G, Goldschmidt H et al Bisphosphonates in multiple myeloma. Cochrane Database Syst Rev 2001: CD003188

Durie BG (2007) Use of bisphosphonates in multiple myeloma: IMWG response to Mayo Clinic consensus statement. Mayo Clin Proc 82(4):516–517, author reply 517–518

Eleutherakis-Papaiakovou V, Bamias A, Gika D et al (2007) Renal failure in multiple myeloma: incidence, correlations, and prognostic significance. Leuk Lymphoma 48(2):337–341

Faquin WC, Schneider TJ, Goldberg MA (1992) Effect of inflammatory cytokines on hypoxia-induced erythropoietin production. Blood 79: 1987–1994

Gabrilove JL, Cleeland CS, Livingston RB, Sarokhan B, Winer E, Einhorn LH (2001) Clinical evaluation of once-weekly dosing of epoetin alfa in chemotherapy patients: improvements in hemoglobin and quality of life are similar to three-times-weekly dosing. J Clin Oncol 19:2875–2882

Garton JP, Gertz MA, Witzig TE, Greipp PR, Lust JA, Schroeder G et al (1995) Epoetin alfa for the treatment of the anemia of multiple myeloma. A prospective, randomized, placebo-controlled, double-blind trial. Arch Intern Med 155:2069–2074

Greil R, Psenak O, Roila F, ESMO Guidelines Working Group (2008) Hematopoietic growth factors: ESMO recommendations for the applications. Ann Oncol 2(19 Suppl):ii116–ii118

Grossman SA (1993) Undertreatment of cancer pain: barriers and remedies. Support Care Cancer 1:74–78

Grossman SA, Sheidler VR, Swedeen K, Mucenski J, Piantadosi S (1991) Correlation of patient and caregiver ratings of cancer pain. J Pain Symptom Manage 6:53–57

Han JH, Choi SJ, Kurihara N, Koide M, Oba Y, Roodman GD (2001) Macrophage inflammatory protein-1alpha is an osteoclastogenic factor in myeloma that is independent of receptor activator of nuclear factor kappaB ligand. Blood 97:3349–3353

Hargreaves RM, Lea JR, Griffiths H, Faux JA, Holt JM, Reid C et al (1995) Immunological factors and risk of infection in plateau phase myeloma. J Clin Pathol 48:260–266

Harousseau JL, Dreyling M, On behalf of the ESMO Guidelines Working Group (2008) Multiple myeloma: ESMO clinical recommendations for diagnosis, treatment and follow-up. Ann Oncol 19(Supplement 2):ii55–ii57

Harvey HA, Lipton A (1996) The role of bisphosphonates in the treatment of bone metastases – the U.S. experience. Support Care Cancer 4: 213–217

Hedenus M, Adriansson M, San Miguel J, Kramer MH, Schipperus MR, Juvonen E, et al (2003) Efficacy and safety of darbepoetin alfa in anaemic patients with lymphoproliferative malignancies: a randomized, double-blind, placebo-controlled study. Br J Haematol 122(3):394–403

Hewitt RE, Lissina A, Green AE, Slay ES, Price DA, Sewell AK (2005) The bisphosphonate acute phase response: rapid and copious production of proinflammatory cytokines by peripheral blood gd T cells in response to aminobisphosphonates is inhibited by statins. Clin Exp Immunol 139(1):101–111

Hofbauer LC, Neubauer A, Heufelder AE (2001) Receptor activator of nuclear factor-kappaB ligand and osteoprotegerin: potential implications for the pathogenesis and treatment of malignant bone diseases. Cancer 92:460–470

Hutchison CA, Cockwell P, Reid S et al (2007) Efficient removal of immunoglobulin free light chains by hemodialysis for multiple myeloma: in vitro and in vivo studies. J Am Soc Nephrol 18(3):886–895

Jackson GH (2005) Renal safety of ibandronate. Oncologist 10(Suppl 1):14–18

Jacobson DR, Zolla-Pazner S (1986) Immunosuppression and infection in multiple myeloma. Semin Oncol 13:282–290

Katodritou E, Speletas M, Kapetanos D, Zervas K, Pavlitou A et al (2004) Evaluation of traditional and novel predictive markers of anemia response to recombinant human erythropoietin (rh-Epo) in patients with multiple myeloma and lymphoma: emerging role of functional iron deficiency. ASH Congress San Diego 2004. Blood 104(11):abstract 3690

15

Katodritou E, Verrou E, Hadjiaggelidou C, Gastari V, Laschos K, Kontovinis L, et al (2008) Erythropoiesis-stimulating agents are associated with reduced survival in patients with multiple myeloma. Am J Hematol 83(9):697–701

Klein JB, Scherzer JA, McLeish KR (1992) IFN-gamma enhances expression of formyl peptide receptors and guanine nucleotide-binding proteins by HL-60 granulocytes. J Immunol 148: 2483–2488

Knight R, DeLap RJ, Zeldis JB (2006) Lenalidomide and venous thrombosis in multiple myeloma. N Engl J Med 354(19):2079–2080

Koch CG, Li L, Sessler DI, Figueroa P, Hoeltge GA, Mihaljevic T, Blackstone EH (2008) Duration of red-cell storage and complications after cardiac surgery. N Engl J Med 358(12):1229–1239

Kolbe K, Domkin D, Derigs HG, Bhakdi S, Huber C, Aulitzky WE (1997) Infectious complications during neutropenia subsequent to peripheral blood stem cell transplantation. Bone Marrow Transplant 19:143–147

Kyle RA (1975) Multiple myeloma, review of 869 cases. Mayo Clin Proc 50:29–40

Kyle RA, Gertz MA, Witzig TE et al (2003) Review of 1027 patients with newly diagnosed multiple myeloma. Mayo Clin Proc 78(1):21–33

Kyle RA, Yee GC, Somerfield MR, Flynn PJ, Halabi S, Jagannath S, Orlowski RZ, Roodman DG, Twilde P, Anderson K (2007) American Society of Clinical Oncology clinical practice guideline update on the role of bisphosphonates in multiple myeloma. J Clin Oncol 25(17): 2464–2472

Lacy MQ, Dispenzieri A, Gertz MA, Greipp PR, Gollbach KL, Hayman SR et al (2006) Mayo clinic consensus statement for the use of bisphosphonates in multiple myeloma. Mayo Clin Proc 81(8):1047–1053

Lahtinen R, Laakso M, Palva I, Virkkunen P, Elomaa I (1992) Randomised, placebo-controlled multicentre trial of clodronate in multiple myeloma. Lancet 340:1049–1052

Lass-Florl C, Kofler G, Kropshofer G, Hermans J, Kreczy A, Dierich MP et al (1998) In-vitro testing of susceptibility to amphotericin B is a reliable predictor of clinical outcome in invasive aspergillosis. J Antimicrob Chemother 42: 497–502

Leitgeb C, Pecherstorfer M, Fritz E, Ludwig H (1994) Quality of life in chronic anemia of cancer during treatment with recombinant human erythropoietin. Cancer 73:2535–2542

Ludwig H (2002) Anemia of hematologic malignancies: what are the treatment options? Semin Oncol 29(3 Suppl 8):45–54

Ludwig H (2006) Iron metabolism and iron supplementation in anemia of cancer. Semin Hematol 43(4 Suppl 6):S13–S17

Ludwig H, Fritz E, Kotzmann H, Höcker P, Gisslinger H, Barnas U (1990) Erythropoietin treatment of anemia associated with multiple myeloma. N Engl J Med 322(24):1693–1699

Ludwig H, Hajek R, Tothova E, Drach J, Adam Z, Labar B, Egyed M, Spicka I, Gisslinger H, Greil R, Kuhn I, Zojer N, Hinke A (2009) Thalidomide-dexamethasone versus melphalan-prednisolone as first line treatment in elderly patients with multiple myeloma. Blood 113:3435–3442

Maher DW, Lieschke GJ, Green M, Bishop J, Stuart-Harris R, Wolf M et al (1994) Filgrastim in patients with chemotherapy-induced febrile neutropenia. A double-blind, placebo-controlled trial. Ann Intern Med 121:492–501

Major PP, Coleman RE (2001) Zoledronic acid in the treatment of hypercalcemia of malignancy: results of the international clinical development program. Semin Oncol 28(Suppl 3):17–24

Marik PE, Corwin HL (2008) Efficacy of red blood cell transfusion in the critically ill: a systematic review of the literature. Crit Care Med 36(9): 2667–2674

Massaia M, Dianzani U, Bianchi A, Camponi A, Boccadoro M, Pileri A (1988) Defective generation of alloreactive cytotoxic T lymphocytes (CTL) in human monoclonal gammopathies. Clin Exp Immunol 73:214–218

Mattsson J, Ringden O, Aschan J, Barkholt L, Dalianis T, Hagglund H et al (1997) A low incidence of grade II to IV acute GVHD, but high mortality from infection using HLA-A, -B, and -DR-identical unrelated donors and immunosuppression with ATG, cyclosporine, and methotrexate. Transplant Proc 29:735–736

McCloskey EV, Dunn JA, Kanis JA, MacLennan IC, Drayson MT (2001) Long-term follow-up of a prospective, double-blind, placebo-controlled randomized trial of clodronate in multiple myeloma. Br J Haematol 113:1035–1043

McCloskey EV, MacLennan IC, Drayson MT, Chapman C, Dunn J, Kanis JA (1998) A randomized trial of the effect of clodronate on skeletal morbidity in multiple myeloma. MRC Working Party on Leukaemia in Adults. Br J Haematol 100:317–325

Menssen HD, Sakalova A, Fontana A, Herrmann Z, Boewer C, Facon T et al (2002) Effects of long-term intravenous ibandronate therapy on skeletal-related events, survival, and bone resorption markers in patients with advanced multiple myeloma. J Clin Oncol 20(9):2353–2359

Michalowski J (2002) COX-2 inhibitors: cancer trials test new uses for pain drug. J Natl Cancer Inst 94:248–249

Morgan GJ, Davles FE, Gregory WM, Cocks K, Bell SE, Szubert AJ et al (2010) First-line treatment with zoledronic acid as compared with clodronic acid in multiple myeloma (MRC Myeloma IX): a randomised controlled trial. Lancet 376:1989–1999

Musto P (1998) The role of recombinant erythropoietin for the treatment of anemia in multiple myeloma. Leuk Lymphoma 29:283–291

Musto P, Falcone A, D'Arena G et al (1997) Clinical results of recombinant erythropoietin in transfusion-dependent patients with refractory multiple myeloma; role of cytokines and monitoring of erythropoiesis. Eur J Haematol 58:314–319

Myers B, Jones SG, McMillan AK et al (2002) Zoledronic acid, hypocalcaemia and renal dysfunction in thalidomide-treated myeloma patients. Blood 100:211a

Oken MM, Pomeroy C, Weisdorf D, Bennett JM (1996) Prophylactic antibiotics for the prevention of early infection in multiple myeloma. Am J Med 100:624–628

Oshima T, Abe M, Asano J, Hara T, Kitazoe K, Sekimoto E et al (2005) Myeloma cells suppress bone formation by secreting a soluble Wnt inhibitor, sFRP-2. Blood 106(9):3160–3165

Osterborg A, Boogaerts MA, Cimino R, Essers U, Holowiecki J, Juliusson G et al (1996) Recombinant human erythropoietin in transfusion-dependent anemic patients with multiple myeloma and non-Hodgkin's Lymphoma – a randomized multicenter study. The European Study Group of Erythropoietin (Epoetin Beta) treatment in multiple myeloma and non-Hodgkin's lymphoma. Blood 87:2675–2682

Osterborg A, Brandberg Y, Molostova V, Iosava G, Abdulkadyrov K, Hedenus M, Epoetin Beta Hematology Study Group et al (2002) Randomized, double-blind, placebo-controlled trial of recombinant human erythropoietin, epoetin Beta, in hematologic malignancies. J Clin Oncol 20:2486–2494

Osterborg A, Brandberg Y, Hedenus M (2005) Impact of epoetin-beta on survival of patients with lymphoproliferative malignancies: long-term follow up of a large randomized study. Br J Haematol 129(2):206–209

Pagano L, Girmenia C, Mele L, Ricci P, Tosti ME, Nosari A, GIMEMA Infection Program, Gruppo Italiano Malattie Ematologiche dell'Adulto et al (2001) Infections caused by filamentous fungi in patients with hematologic malignancies. A report of 391 cases by GIMEMA infection program. Haematologica 86:862–870

Palumbo A, Petrucci MT, Lauta VM, Musto P, Caravita T, Italian Multiple Myeloma Study Group et al (2005) Correlation between fatigue and hemoglobin level in multiple myeloma patients: results of a cross-sectional study. Haematologica 90(6):858–860

Payne RB, Carver ME, Morgan DB (1979) Interpretation of serum total calcium: effects of adjustment for albumin concentration on frequency of abnormal values and on detection of change in the individual. J Clin Pathol 32:56–60

Pecherstorfer M, Steinhauer EU, Rizzoli R, Wetterwald M, Bergstrom B (2003) Efficacy and safety of ibandronate in the treatment of hypercalcemia of malignancy: a randomized multicentric comparison to pamidronate. Support Care Cancer 11(8):539–547

Peest D, Coldewey R, Deicher H (1991) Overall vs. tumor-related survival in multiple myeloma. Eur J Cancer 27:672

Podar K, Tai YT, Davies FE, Lentzsch S, Sattler M, Hideshima T et al (2001) Vascular endothelial growth factor triggers signaling cascades mediating multiple myeloma cell growth and migration. Blood 98:428–435

Pozzi C, Pasquali S, Donini U et al (1987) Prognostic factors and effectiveness of treatment in acute renal failure due to multiple myeloma: a review of 50 cases. Report of the Italian Renal Immunopathology Group. Clin Nephrol 28(1):1–9

Ralston SH, Gardner MD, Dryburgh FJ, Jenkins AS, Cowan RA, Boyle IT (1985) Comparison of aminohydroxypropylidene diphosphonate, mithramycin and corticosteroids/calcitonin in treatment of cancer-associated hypercalcaemia. Lancet 2:ii: 907–ii: 910

15

Richardson P, Schlag R, Khuageva NK, Dimopoulos MA, Shpilberg O, Kropff MH et al (2008) Erythropoiesis-stimulating agents do not adversely affect long-term outcomes nor increase the risk of thromboembolic events in multiple myeloma patients treated in the phase III VISTA trial. Blood (ASH Annual Meeting Abstracts) 112:1741

Rizzo JD, Somerfield MR, Hagerty KL, Seidenfeld J, Bohlius J, Bennett CL, Cella DF, Djulbegovic B, Goode MJ, Jakubowski AA, Rarick MU, Regan DH, Lichtin AE, American Society of Clinical Oncology, American Society of Hematology (2008) Use of epoetin and darbepoetin in patients with cancer: 2007 American Society of Clinical Oncology/American Society of Hematology clinical practice guideline update. J Clin Oncol 26(1):132–149. Epub 2007 Oct 22. Erratum in: J Clin Oncol. 2008 Mar 1; 26(7):1192

Robertson JD, Nagesh K, Jowitt SN, Dougal M, Anderson H, Mutton K, Zambon M, Scarffe JH (2000) Immunogenicity of vaccination against influenza, **Streptococcus pneumoniae** and **Haemophilus influenzae** type B in patients with multiple myeloma. Br J Cancer 82(7):1261–1265

Rosen LS, Gordon D, Kaminski M, Howell A, Belch A, Mackey J et al (2001) Zoledronic acid versus pamidronate in the treatment of skeletal metastases in patients with breast cancer or osteolytic lesions of multiple myeloma: a phase III, double-blind, comparative trial. Cancer J 7(5): 377–387

Rosen LS, Gordon D, Kaminski M, Howell A, Belch A, Mackey J et al (2003) Long-term efficacy and safety of zoledronic acid compared with pamidronate disodium in the treatment of skeletal complications in patients with advanced multiple myeloma or breast carcinoma: a randomized, double-blind, multicenter, comparative trial. Cancer 98(8):1735–1744

Roux S, Meignin V, Quillard J, Meduri G, Guiochon-Mantel A, Fermand JP et al (2002) RANK (receptor activator of nuclear factor-kappaB) and RANKL expression in multiple myeloma. Br J Haematol 117:86–92

Salutari P, Sica S, Laurenti L, Leone F, Chiusolo P, Piccirillo N et al (1998) Incidence of sepsis after peripheral blood progenitor cells transplantation: analysis of 86 consecutive hemato oncological patients. Leuk Lymphoma 30:193–197

Santaella RM, Fraunfelder FW (2007) Ocular adverse effects associated with systemic medications: recognition and management. Drugs 67(1): 75–93

Shipman CM, Rogers MJ, Apperley JF, Russell RG, Croucher PI (1997) Bisphosphonates induce apoptosis in human myeloma cell lines: a novel anti-tumor activity. Br J Haematol 98:665–672

Shipman CM, Croucher PI, Russell RG, Helfrich MH, Rogers MJ (1998) The bisphosphonate incadronate (YM175) causes apoptosis of human myeloma cells in vitro by inhibiting the mevalonate pathway. Cancer Res 58:5294–5297

Silvestris F, Romito A, Fanelli P, Vacca A, Dammacco F (1995) Long-term therapy with recombinant human erythropoietin (rHu-EPO) in progressing multiple myeloma. Ann Hematol 70:313–318

Singh A, Eckardt KU, Zimmermann A, Gotz KH, Hamann M, Ratcliffe PJ et al (1993) Increased plasma viscosity as a reason for inappropriate erythropoietin formation. J Clin Invest 91:251–256

Siris ES (1997) Breast cancer and osteolytic metastases: can bisphosphonates help? Nat Med 3: 151–152

Sunder-Plassmann G, Horl WH (1997) Erythropoietin and iron. Clin Nephrol 47(3):141–157

Takahashi R, Shimazaki C, Inaba T, Okano A, Hatsuse M, Okamoto A et al (2001) A newly developed bisphosphonate, YM529, is a potent apoptosis inducer of human myeloma cells. Leuk Res 25:77–83

Taube T, Beneton MN, McCloskey EV, Rogers S, Greaves M, Kanis JA (1992) Abnormal bone remodelling in patients with myelomatosis and normal biochemical indices of bone resorption. Eur J Haematol 49:192–198

Terpos E, Dimopoulos MA (2005) Myeloma bone disease: pathophysiology and management. Ann Oncol 16(8):1223–1231

Terpos E, Viniou N, de la Fuente J, Meletis J, Voskaridou E, Karkantaris C et al (2003) Pamidronate is superior to ibandronate in decreasing bone resorption, interleukin-6 and beta 2-microglobulin in multiple myeloma. Eur J Haematol 70(1):34–42

Thürlimann B, Morant R, Jungi WF, Radziwill A (1994) Pamidronate for pain control in patients with malignant osteolytic bone disease: a prospective dose–effect study. Support Care Cancer 2:61–65

Tian E, Zhan F, Walker R, Rasmussen E, Ma Y, Barlogie B, Shaughnessy JD Jr (2003) The role of the Wnt-signaling antagonist DKK1 in the develop ment of osteolytic lesions in multiple myeloma. N Engl J Med 349(26):2483–2494

Vamvakas EC, Taswell HF (1994) Long-term survival after blood transfusion. Transfusion 34: 471–477

World Health Organization (1990) Cancer pain relief and palliative care: report of a WHO expert panel. WHO Technical Report 804. WHO, Geneva

Yaccoby S, Pearse RN, Johnson CL, Barlogie B, Choi Y, Epstein J (2002) Myeloma interacts with the bone marrow microenvironment to induce osteoclastogenesis and is dependent on osteoclast activity. Br J Haematol 116:278–290

Zervas K, Verrou E, Teleioudis Z, Vahtsevanos K, Banti A, Mihou D et al (2006) Incidence, risk factors and management of osteonecrosis of the jaw in patients with multiple myeloma: a single-centre experience in 303 patients. Br J Haematol 134(6):620–623, Epub 2006 Aug 1

Zucchelli P, Pasquali S, Cagnoli L et al (1988) Controlled plasma exchange trial in acute renal failure due to multiple myeloma. Kidney Int 33(6):1175–1180

Appendix: Staging and Prognosis Systems

Table A.1a Monoclonal gammopathy of undetermined significance (MGUS) or monoclonal gammopathy, unattributed/unassociated (MG[u])

M-protein in serum <30 g/l
Bone marrow clonal plasma cells <10% and low level of plasma cell infiltration in a trephine biopsy (if done)
No evidence of other B-cell proliferative disorders
*No related organ or tissue impairment (no end organ damage, including bone lesions)

Table A.1b Myeloma-related organ or tissue impairment (end organ damage) (ROTI) due to the plasma cell proliferative process

*Calcium levels increased: serum calcium > 0.25 mmol/l above the upper limit of normal or >2.75 mmol/l
*Renal insufficiency: creatinine >173 μmol/l
*Anaemia: haemoglobin 2 g/dl below the lower limit of normal or haemoglobin <10 g/dl
*Bone lesions: lytic lesions or osteoporosis with compression fractures (MRI or CT may clarify)
Other: symptomatic hyperviscosity, amyloidosis, recurrent bacterial infections (>2 episodes in 12 months)

*CRAB (calcium, renal insufficiency, anaemia or bone lesions)

Table A.1c Asymptomatic myeloma (smouldering myeloma)

M-protein in serum ≥ 30 g/l
and/or
Bone marrow clonal plasma cells ≥10%
No related organ or tissue impairment (no end organ damage, including bone lesions) or symptoms

T. Moehler
Department of Medicine V,
University Hospital Heidelberg,
Heidelberg, Germany
Present address:
i3 research, Wiesbaden, Germany
e-mail: thomas.moehler@med.uni-heidelberg.de

T. Moehler and H. Goldschmidt (eds.), *Multiple Myeloma*,
Recent Results in Cancer Research 183, DOI: 10.1007/978-3-540-85772-3,

Table A.1d Symptomatic multiple myeloma

M-protein in serum and/or urine
Bone marrow (clonal) plasma cells* or plasmacytoma
Related organ or tissue impairment (end organ damage, including bone lesions)

Source: International Myeloma Working Group (2003) Criteria for the classification of monoclonal gammopathies, multiple myeloma and related disorders: a report of the International Myeloma Working Group. Br J Haematol 121:749–757

*If flow cytometry is performed, most plasma cells (>90%) will show a 'neoplastic' phenotype

Some patients may have no symptoms but have related organ or tissue impairment

Table A.2 Historical myeloma staging system

Stage	Criteria	Measured myeloma cell mass (cells $\times 10^{12}/m^2$)*
I	*All* of the following: 1. Hemoglobin value > 10 g/100 ml 2. Serum calcium value normal 3. On roentgenogram, normal bone structure (scale 0) or solitary bone plasmacytoma only 4. Low M-component production rates a. IgG value < 5 g/100 ml b. IgA value < 3 g/100 ml c. Urine light chain M-component on electrophoresis < 4 g/24 hours	<0.6 (Low)
II	Fitting neither Stage I nor Stage III	0.6–1.20 (Intermediate)
III	*One or more* of the following: 1. Hemoglobin value < 8.5 g/100 ml 2. Serum calcium increased 3. Advanced lytic bone lesions (scale 3) 4. High M-component production rates a. IgG value > 7 g/100 ml b. IgA value > 5 g/100 ml c. Urine light chain M-component on electrophoresis > 12 g/24 hours	>1.20 (High)
Subclassification A = Relatively normal renal function (serum creatinine value < 2.0 mg/100 ml)** B = Abnormal renal function (serum creatinine value ≥ 2.0 mg/100 ml) Examples Stage IA = low cell mass with normal renal function Stage IIIB = high cell mass with abnormal renal function		

Source: Durie BG, Salmon SE (1975) A clinical staging system for multiple myeloma. Correlation of measured myeloma cell mass with presenting clinical features, response to treatment, and survival. Cancer 36:842–854

*10^{12} cells = approximately 1 kg or 2.2 Ibs; m^2 = square meter of body surface area

**If the serum creatinine value is not available, the blood urea nitrogen (BUN) value may be used as an indicator of renal function. (A BUN value of 30 mg/100 ml is roughly equal to a serum creatinine value of 2 mg/100 ml

Table A.3 International staging system

Stage	Criteria	Median Survival (months)
I	Serum β_2-microglobulin < 3.5 mg/L Serum albumin ≥ 3.5 g/dL	62
II	Not stage I or III*	44
III	Serum β_2-microglobulin ≥ 5.5 mg/L	29

Source: Greipp PR, San Miguel J, Durie BG, Crowley JJ, Barlogie B, Blade J, Boccadoro M, Child JA, Avet-Loiseau H, Kyle RA, Lahuerta JJ, Ludwig H, Morgan G, Powles R, Shimizu K, Shustik C, Sonneveld P, Tosi P, Turesson I, Westin J (2005) International staging system for multiple myeloma. J Clin Oncol 23:3412–3420

*There are two categories for stage II: serum β_2-microglobulin < 3.5 mg/L but serum albumin < 3.5 g/dL; or serum β_2-microglobulin 3.5 to < 5.5 mg/L irrespective of the serum albumin level

Table A.4 International myeloma working group uniform response criteria: CR and other response categories

Response subcategory	*Response criteria*[a]
sCR	CR as defined below plus Normal FLC ratio and absence of clonal cells in bone marrow[b] by immunohietochemistry or immunofluoreecence[c]
CR	Negative immunofixation on the serum and urine and Disappearance of any soft tissue plasmacytomas and ≤5% plasma oells in bone marrow[b]
VGPR	Serum and urine M-protein detectable by immunofixation but not on electrophoreaeais or 90% or greater reduction in serum M-protein plus urine M-protein level < 100 mg per 24 h
PR	≥50% reduction of serum M-protein and reduction in 24-hurinary M-protein by ≥90% or to <200 mg per 24h If the serum and urine M-protein are unmeasurable, a ≥50% decrease in the difference between involved and uninvolved Free light chain levels is required in place of the M-protein criteria if serum and urine M-protein are unmeasurable, and serum free light assay is also unmeasurable, ≥50% reduction in plasma cells is required in place of M-protein, provided baseline bone marrow plasma cell percentage was ≥30% In addition to the above listed criteria, if present at baseline, a ≥50% reduction in the size of soft tissue plasmacytomas is also required

(continued)

Table A.4 (continued)

Response subcategory	*Response criteria*[a]
SD (not recommended for use as an indicator of response; stability of disease is best described by providing the time to progession estimates)	Not meeting criteria for CR, VGPR, PR or progressive disease

Abbreviations: CR, complete response: FLC, free light chain; PR, pertial response; SD, stable disease; sCR, stringert complete response; VGPR, very good partial response

[a]All response categories require two consecutive assessments made at anytime before the institution of any new therapy; all categories also require no known evidence of progressive or new bone leaions if radiographic studies were performed. Radiographic studies are not required to satisfy these response requirements

[b]Confirmation with repeat bone manow biopsy not needed

[c]Presence/absence of clonal cells is base up on the k/λ ratio. An abnormal k/λ ratio by immunohistochemistry and/or immunofluorescence requires a minimum of 100 plasma cells for analysis. An abnomal ratio reflecting presence of an abnormal clone is k/λ of >4:1 or <1:2

Table A.5 International myeloma working group uniform response criteria: disease progression and relapse

Relapse subcategory	Relapse criteria
Progressive disease[a] To be used for calculation of time to progression and progression-free survival end points for all patients including those in CR (includes primary progressive disease and disease progression on or off therapy)	Progressive Disease: requires any one or more of the following: Increase of ≥ 25% from baseline in • Serum M-component and/or (the absolute increase must be ^{3} 0.5 g/dl)[b] • Urine M-component and/or (the absolute increase must be ^{3} 200 mg/24 h • Only in patients without measurable serum and urine M-protein levels: the difference between involved and uninvolved FLC levels. The absolute increase must be > 10 mg/dl. • Bone marrow plasma cell percentage: the absolute % must be ^{3} 10%[c] • Definite development of new bone lesions or soft tissue plasmacytomas or definite increase in the size of existing bone lesions or soft tissue plasmacytomas • Development of hypercalcemia (corrected serum calcium > 11.5 mg/dl or 2.65 mmol/l) that can be attributed solely to the plasma cell proliferative disorder

(continued)

Table A.5 (continued)

Relapse subcategory	Relapse criteria
Clinical relapse[a]	Clinical relapse requires one or more of: Direct indicators of increasing disease and/or end organ dysfunction (CRAB features)[b] It is not used in calculation of time to progression or progression-free survival but is listed here as as something that can be reported optionally or for use in clinical practice 1. Development of new soft tissue plasmacytomas or bone lesions 2. Definite increase in the size of existing plasmacytomas or bone lesions. A definite increase is defined as a 50% (and at least 1 cm) increase as measured serially by the sum of the products of the cross-diameters of the measurable lesion 3. Hypercalcemia (> 11.5 mg/dl) [2.65 mmol/l] 4. Decrease in hemoglobin of ³ 2 g/dl [1.25 mmol/l] (see Table 3 for further details) 5. Rise in serum creatinine by 2 mg/dl or more [177 μmol/l or more]
Relapse from CR[a] (To be used only if the end point studied is DFS)[d]	Any one or more of the following: • Reappearance of serum or urine M-protein by immunofixation or electrophoresis • Development of ³ 5% plasma cells in the bone marrowc • Appearance of any other sign of progression (i.e., new plasmacytoma, lytic bone lesion, or hypercalcemia see below)

Source: Durie BG, Harousseau JL, Miguel JS, Blade J, Barlogie B, Anderson K, Gertz M, Dimopoulos M, Westin J, Sonneveld P, Ludwig H, Gahrton G, Beksac M, Crowley J, Belch A, Boccadaro M, Turesson I, Joshua D, Vesole D, Kyle R, Alexanian R, Tricot G, Attal M, Merlini G, Powles R, Richardson P, Shimizu K, Tosi P, Morgan G, Rajkumar SV (2006) International uniform response criteria for multiple myeloma. Leukemia 20:1467–1473

Abbreviations: CR, complete response; DFS, disease-free survival

[a]All relapse categories require two consecutive assessments made at anytime before classification as relapse or disease progression and/or the institution of any new therapy

[b]For progressive disease, serum M-component increases of ≥ 1 gm/dl are sufficient to define relapse if starting M-component is ≥ 5 g/dl

[c]Relapse from CR has the 5% cutoff versus 10% for other categories of relapse

[d]For purposes of calculating time to progression and progression-free survival, CR patients should also be evaluated using criteria listed above for progressive disease